The Certified Occupational Therapy Assistant

Roles and Responsibilities

Edited by
Sally E. Ryan, COTA, ROH

SLACK Incorporated, 6900 Grove Road, Thorofare, New Jersey 08086

SLACK International Book Distributors

In Canada
McGraw-Hill Ryerson Limited
300 Water Street
Whitby, Ontario
L1N 9B6

In Australia and New Zealand
MacLennan & Petty Pty Limited
P.O. Box 425
Artarmon, N.S.W. 2064
Australia

In Japan
Igaku-Shoin, Ltd.
Tokyo International P.O. Box 5063
1-28-36 Hongo, Bunkyo-Ku
Tokyo 113
Japan

In Mexico
Manuel Moderno
Av. Sonaro 206
New Line Col. HIPODROMO
06100 Mexico DF

Foreign Translation Agent

John Scott & Company
International Publishers' Agency
417-A Pickering Road
Phoenixville, PA 19460
Fax: 215-988-0185

Executive Editor: Cheryl D. Willoughby
Publisher: Harry C. Benson

Printed in the United States of America

Library of Congress Catalog Card Number: 85-050367

ISBN: 1-55642-206-7

Published by: SLACK Incorporated
6900 Grove Road
Thorofare, NJ 08086-9447

Last digit is print number: 10 9 8 7 6 5 4

Dedicated to the Advancement
of the Profession of
Occupational Therapy

CONTRIBUTORS

PATTY L. BARNETT, COTA
Instructor
Occupational Therapy Department
University of Alabama in Birmingham
Regional Technical Institute
Birmingham, Alabama

B. JOAN BELLMAN, OTR
Chief Occupational Therapist
Department of Physical Medicine and Rehabilitation
District of Columbia General Hospital
Washington, District of Columbia

ROBERT K. BING, EdD, OTR, FAOTA
Professor and Chairman
Department of Occupational Therapy
Elizabethtown College
Elizabethtown, Pennsylvania

TERI BLACK, COTA
Instructor
Occupational Therapy Assistant Program
Madison Area Technical College
Madison, Wisconsin

TONÉ F. BLECHERT, COTA, ROH
Faculty Member
Occupational Therapy Assistant Program
St. Mary's Junior College
Minneapolis, Minnesota

BONNIE BROOKS, MEd, OTR
Assistant Director of Education
American Occupational Therapy Association
Rockville, Maryland

ILENNA BROWN, COTA, ROH
Senior Occupational Therapy Assistant
Clove Lakes Nursing Home and Health Related Facility
Staten Island, New York

MARIANNE F. CHRISTENSEN, OTR
Faculty Member
Occupational Therapy Assistant Program
St. Mary's Junior College
Minneapolis, Minnesota

SISTER MIRIAM JOSEPH CUMMINGS, CSJ, MA, OTR, FAOTA
Associate Professor and Chairperson
Department of Occupational Therapy
College of St. Catherine
St. Paul, Minnesota

SHERISE DARLAK, COTA
Staff Occupational Therapy Assistant
The Institute for Rehabilitation and Research
Texas Medical Center
Houston, Texas

MARGARET DRAKE, ABD, MA, OTR, ATR
Assistant Professor
Department of Occupational Therapy
University of Alabama in Birmingham
Regional Technical Institute
Birmingham, Alabama

MARY ELLEN LANGE DUNFORD, OTR/L
Pediatric Occupational Therapist
Mississippi Bend Area Education Agency 9
Clinton, Iowa

CYNTHIA F. EPSTEIN, MA, OTR, FAOTA
President and Director
Occupational Therapy Consultants, Inc.
Sommerville, New Jersey

M. LAURITA FIKE, MA, OTR
Director of Occupational Therapy
The Institute for Rehabilitation and Research
Texas Medical Center
Houston, Texas

LINDA FLOREY, MA, OTR, FAOTA
Associate Chief
Rehabilitation Services
Neuropsychiatric Institute
University of California, Los Angeles
Los Angeles, California

CAPTAIN FRANK E. GAINER, III, AMSC, MHS, OTR
Staff Occupational Therapist, Mental Health
Occupational Therapy Section
Walter Reed Army Medical Center
Washington, District of Columbia

ELNORA M. GILFOYLE, DSc (Honorary), OTR, FAOTA
Associate Professor and Head
Department of Occupational Therapy
Colorado State University
Fort Collins, Colorado

AZELA GOHL-GIESE, OTR
Associate Professor
Department of Occupational Therapy
College of St. Catherine
St. Paul, Minnesota

HARU HIRAMA, EdD, OTR/L
Professor and Coordinator
Occupational Therapy Assistant Program
Lehigh County Community College
Schnecksville, Pennsylvania

CAPTAIN BONNIE E. HOFFMAN, AMSC, MOT, OTR/L
Chief, Occupational Therapy Section
General Leonard Wood Army Community Hospital
Fort Leonard Wood, Missouri

ROBIN A. JONES, COTA/L
Senior Staff Therapist
Rehabilitation Institute of Chicago
Chicago, Illinois

SHERYL R. KANTOR, OTR/L
Director of Occupational Therapy
Bowman Therapeutic Associates, Ltd.
Morton Grove, Illinois

NANCY KARI, MPH, OTR
Assistant Professor
Department of Occupational Therapy
College of St. Catherine
St. Paul, Minnesota

BARBARA A. LARSON, COTA, ROH
Occupational Therapy Student
University of Minnesota
Minneapolis, Minnesota

M. JEANNE MADIGAN, EdD, OTR, FAOTA
Professor and Chairperson
Department of Occupational Therapy
Virginia Commonwealth University
Richmond, Virginia

WILLIAM MATTHEW MARCIL, COTA
Assistant Therapist
Hospice Buffalo, Inc.
Buffalo, New York

SUSAN M. McFADDEN, MEd, OTR, FAOTA
Private Practitioner and Consultant
Memphis, Tennessee

KATHRYN MELIN-EBERHARDT, COTA/L
Occupational Therapy Assistant
Occupational Therapy Department
Rehabilitation Unit
Mercy Hospital and Medical Center
Chicago, Illinois

JOYCE L. PACKER, MA, OTR
Instructor
Occupational Therapy Assistant Program
Wayne County Community College
Detroit, Michigan

KATHLYN L. REED, PhD, OTR/L, FAOTA
Formerly Professor and Chairperson
Department of Occupational Therapy
College of Allied Health
Health Sciences Center
University of Oklahoma
Oklahoma City, Oklahoma

MAJOR DENISE A. ROTERT, AMSC, MA, OTR
Head, Occupational Therapy Division
Tri-Service Alcohol Recovery Department
Naval Hospital Bethesda, NMC-NCR
Bethesda, Maryland

BRIAN J. RYAN, BSEE
Senior Rehability Engineer
Honeywell Corporation
Hopkins, Minnesota

SALLY E. RYAN, COTA, ROH
Faculty Assistant
Department of Occupational Therapy
College of St. Catherine
St. Paul, Minnesota

PHILLIP D. SHANNON, MA, MPA, OTR, FAOTA
Chair and Associate Professor
Department of Occupational Therapy
University at Buffalo
State University of New York
Buffalo, New York

KENT NELSON TIGGES, MS, OTR, FAOTA
Associate Professor, Associate Chair
University at Buffalo
State University of New York
Buffalo, New York
Director of Occupational Therapy
Hospice Buffalo, Inc.
Buffalo, New York

JAVAN E. WALKER JR., MA, OTR/L
Director, Occupational Therapy Assistant Program
Illinois Central College
East Peoria, Illinois

TONI WALSKI, MS, OTR
Director, Occupational Therapy Assistant Program
Madison Area Technical College
Madison, Wisconsin

PATRICIA M. WATSON, OTR
Home Care Therapist
Sister Kenny Institute
Minneapolis, Minnesota

MELANIE WIENER, OTR
Senior Staff Therapist
The Institute for Rehabilitation and Research
Houston, Texas

DORIS Y. WITHERSPOON, MA, OTR
Director, Occupational Therapy Assistant Program
Wayne County Community College
Detroit, Michigan

CONTENTS

Section I. Historical Perspectives

Section II. Core Knowledge

Section III. Intervention Strategies

Section IV. Models of Practice

Section V. Concepts of Practice

Section VI. Contemporary Issues and Trends

EXPANDED CONTENTS

Section I. Historical Perspectives

Section II. Core Knowledge

Section III. Intervention Strategies

Section IV. Models of Practice

Section V. Concepts of Practice

Section VI. Contemporary Issues and Trends

Appendices

OCCUPATIONAL THERAPY—A PROFILE*

Occupational therapy is the art and science of directing a person's participation in selected tasks to restore, reinforce, and enhance performance; to facilitate learning of skills and functions essential for adaptation and productivity; to diminish or correct pathology; and to promote and maintain health. Its fundamental purpose is the development and maintenance of a person's capacity, throughout life, to perform with satisfaction to self and others those tasks and roles essential to productive living and the mastery of self and the environment.

Since the primary focus of occupational therapy is on the development of adaptive skills and performance capacity, its concern is with factors that serve as barriers or impediments to the individual's ability to function, as well as those factors that promote, influence, or enhance performance.

Occupational therapy provides service to those individuals whose abilities to cope with tasks of living are threatened or impaired by developmental deficits, aging, poverty, cultural differences, physical injury or illness, or psychosocial and social disability.

The title "occupation" refers to a person's goal-directed use of time, energy, interest, and attention.

The practice of occupational therapy is based upon concepts that acknowledge the following principles:

1. Activities are primary agents for learning and development and an essential source of satisfaction.
2. When engaging in activities, the individual explores the nature of his or her interests, needs, capacities, and limitations; develops motor, perceptual, and cognitive skills; and learns a range of interpersonal and social attitudes and behaviors sufficient for coping with life tasks and mastering elements of the environment.
3. Task occupation is an integral part of human development; it represents or reflects life-work situations and is a vehicle for acquiring or redeveloping those skills essential to the fulfillment of life roles.
4. Activities matching or relating to the developmental needs and interests of the individual not only afford the necessary learning for development or restoration, but provide an intrinsic gratification that promotes and sustains health and evokes a strong investment in the restorative process.
5. The end product inherent in a task or an activity provides concrete evidence of the ability to be productive and to have an influence on one's environment.
6. Activities are "doing," and such a focus upon productivity and participation teaches a sense of self as a contributing participant rather than as a recipient.

These principles are applied in practice through programs reflecting the profession's commitment to comprehensive health care.

*Adapted with permission from "Occupational Therapy—Its Definition and Functions," *Reference Manual of Official Documents of the American Occupational Therapy Association.* © 1980 (revised 1983), American Occupational Therapy Association, Inc.

PREFACE

Work on this text began in the spring of 1984. That year was particularly significant because it marked the 25th anniversary of certified occupational therapy assistants (COTAs) working in the profession.

The project was given impetus from the fact that there was no comprehensive book written expressly for occupational therapy assistants. Discussions with technical level faculty, occupational therapists (OTRs) serving as clinical supervisors, and assistants emphasized the need for a text which would focus on the basic principles of the profession; a book which would provide both an extensive and a realistic view of the roles and functions of certified occupational therapy assistants in entry-level practice and beyond; a book which would provide examples of how to successfully build intraprofessional relationships; and, finally, a book which could be used in the clinic as well as the classroom. These objectives were adopted as a foundation for developing, organizing, and sequencing content areas.

Four documents published by the American Occupational Therapy Association (AOTA) also served as primary guides for content development: the *Entry-Level OTR and COTA Role Delineation*, the *Essentials of an Approved Educational Program for the Occupational Therapy Assistant*, *Uniform Terminology for Reporting Occupational Therapy Services*, and the *1982 Member Data Survey*. All but the latter are included as appendices.

The book is divided into six major sections. The first section (Historical Perspectives) introduces the themes and perspectives of the book. Section II focuses on the core knowledge of occupational therapy, which includes philosophical and theoretical material as well as principles of human development and basic influences contributing to health. The daily living skills of self-care, work, and play/leisure are also addressed as the primary foundations of the profession, along with descriptions of some of the skills necessary for effective therapeutic intervention. Emphasis is placed on the teaching/learning process, interpersonal communication, group dynamics, and the occupational therapy process.

In Section III (Intervention Strategies), case studies demonstrate the roles of occupational therapy assistants and occupational therapists working with selected patients to illustrate specific ways in which the profession's role delineation can be used to provide efficient and effective health care delivery.

Section IV (Models of Practice) provides numerous examples of the team approach in working with patients of varying ages in a variety of traditional and nontraditional treatment settings. The roles of the OTR/COTA team in a hospice setting are delineated, and the roles of the COTA in work and productive occupation programs and as an activities director are addressed.

Concepts of Practice are reviewed in Section V, which includes discussions of contemporary media techniques as well as management and supervision principles and issues.

The final section (Contemporary Issues) discusses ways of enhancing intraprofessional relationships through the effective use of supervision, mentoring, and conflict management fundamentals, and reviews the maturation process of the assistant and related professional socialization elements. Principles of occupational therapy ethics are presented, and future trends for the profession are outlined.

In addition to the main chapter designations, all important chapter sub-headings appear in the Table of Contents. Their titles reflect the major objectives of the writer(s) and editor. *The Certified Occupational Therapy Assistant: Roles and Re-*

sponsibilities Workbook, also published by SLACK, Inc., provides the student with study and discussion questions and exercises, as well as additional learning resources.

Every effort has been made to use gender inclusive language throughout the book. In some instances, it was necessary to use "him or her," recognizing that this may be awkward for the reader.

No preface would be complete without some discussion of the highly skilled contributing authors. Their work, individually and collectively, is the great strength of this text. Individual therapists and assistants, as well as eleven OTR/COTA authoring teams, have provided their extensive knowledge and expertise in preparing manuscripts. They come from diverse practice, education, and research backgrounds; four of the OTR contributors were former COTAs. Many of the 40 authors have been actively involved in leadership roles in their state associations, as well as in the American Occupational Therapy Association. The contributions of an electrical engineer have enhanced a chapter on computers. It has been a great privilege to work with these outstanding writers, and I convey my most sincere thanks to each of them.

I would also like to offer my thanks to the reviewers who provided critiques of the manuscript. Their objectivity and critical analyses of the content were most helpful.

My deepest appreciation is extended to Ellie Gilfoyle. She "planted the seed" and gave me sage advice, nurturing, and support during many phases of this project. Her belief in my abilities spurred me on.

Anne Just, editor at SLACK, Inc., provided me with numerous resources, advice, critiques, and over-all editorial assistance. Her generosity of time and talent as well as her expert problem solving skills helped me immeasurably in this enormous task. Publication of this text would not have been possible without her expert assistance and the generous help of the SLACK Book Division.

I would like to acknowledge and express my personal gratitude to Sister Miriam Joseph Cummings, Chairperson, and all of the members of the faculty of the Department of Occupational Therapy at the College of St. Catherine for their support and encouragement during the many phases of this task. Their willingness to share resources and offer critiques was of great help.

To the many therapists, assistants, friends, and family members who provided ideas, listened to my concerns, and responded to my endless questions, I offer my most sincere appreciation. I regret that space does not allow me to list each of them individually.

Thanking my husband Brian is most difficult. He filled many supportive roles which included consultant, reviewer, typist, errand runner, telephone monitor, and household manager. Suffice it to say that this project would never have been accomplished without his sense of humor, inspiration, insight, patience, and remarkable ability to adapt. I am ever grateful.

In conclusion, it is my belief that this book will serve as a model and a guidepost for occupational therapy teamwork in the delivery of patient services. It will serve as an incentive for technically and professionally educated practitioners to discover the many ways in which their skills and roles complement each other. It will also serve as a catalyst for developing new skills and roles in response to the ever changing needs of our society.

The former President of the American Occupational Therapy Association, Carolyn Manville Baum, summed it up best in her 1980 Eleanor Clarke Slagle Address when she stated,

> *As a profession and as professionals, let us put our resources, intelligence, and emotional commitment together and work diligently toward the ascent of our profession. The health care system, the clients (patients) we serve, and each of us individually will benefit from our commitment.*

Sally E. Ryan, COTA, ROH
Editor

SECTION I

Historical Perspectives

History may be defined as a recorded narrative of events which have occurred in the past. It is a collection of information drawn from many sources which include speeches, letters, minutes of meetings, photographs, diaries, articles, and interviews.

This first section details important aspects of the history of occupational therapy, and also provides a chronology of the significant events in the development, education and utilization of occupational therapy assistants. This section provides the reader with an appreciation for, and an understanding of, the important roots of the profession. It gives insight to the rich legacy of events and experiences drawn from history which provide a foundation for present and future practice. According to Bing, "Too often we are disposed to think that those lessons another generation learned do not apply to the present generation." He goes on to remind us that we learn in two ways—through our own first-hand experiences and from others "who made discoveries" in both the recent and distant past. He concludes that "The experience of others is a magnificent heritage, and the more we learn from them, the less time we waste in the present, proving what has already been proved."

CHAPTER 1

Occupational Therapy Revisited: A Paraphrastic Journey*

Robert K. Bing, OTR

Introduction

Occupational therapy's roots are in the sub-soil of the moral movement developed in Europe during the Age of Enlightenment. Philippe Pinel, a French philosopher-physician, and William Tuke, an English merchant-philanthropist, developed and applied the principles to the institutionalized insane. Moral treatment came to the United States as part of the Quakers' religious and intellectual luggage. It expanded rapidly in private, as well as public, institutions for the insane. During the last quarter of the 19th century moral treatment disappeared. It re-emerged in the early decades of the 20th century as occupational therapy.

A diverse group of women and men developed principles and definitions and founded an organization to support the practice of the retitled moral treatment and management. Susan Tracy, a nurse; George Barton, an architect; William Rush Dunton, Jr., a physician; Eleanor Clarke Slagle, a partially trained social worker who was also trained in invalid occupations; and Adolf Meyer, another physician, figure prominently in the development of this century's occupational therapy.

A second generation of occupational therapists elaborated, codified, and applied the founders' principles. Their efforts and successes are exemplified through one individual: Beatrice D. Wade, OTR, FAOTA.

Patterns and Themes

Let us start this paraphrastic journey. There are some significant landmarks to notice along the way. These are recurring patterns and themes of the past 200 years which give us today's relevance.

1. There is an inextricable union of the mind and the body; the employment of activity or occupation must be based on this precept, which is unique to occupational therapy.

2. Activity inherently contains modes the patient may employ to gain understanding of and

*Adapted from Bing, RK: Occupational therapy revisited: A paraphrastic journey, *The American Journal of Occupational Therapy*, 35:499–518, © 1981. Used with permission of the publisher.

ascendancy over one's feelings, actions, and thoughts; these modes include the habits of attention and interest; the perceived usefulness of occupation; creative expression; the processes of learning; the acquisition of skills; and seeing evidence of accomplishment.

3. Activity provides a balance between the practical and intellectual components of experience; therefore, a wide variety of activities must be accessible to meet human objectives for work, leisure, and rest.

4. One's approach to the patient is as significant to treatment and rehabilitation as are the selection and utilization of an activity.

5. Essential elements of occupational therapy practice are continuous observation, experimentation, empiricism, and analysis.

6. An appreciation of the pain which accompanies any illness or disability, a strong desire to reduce or remove it, a gentle firmness, and a knowledge of the patient's needs are fundamental characteristics of the provider of therapeutic occupations.

7. Therapeutic processes and modes of treatment are synonymous with the processes of learning and methods of education.

8. The patient is the product of his or her own efforts, not the article made or the activity accomplished.

A Theory of Experience

We could go back to the Garden of Eden to begin this story, if time permitted, since occupational therapy could well have started in that idyllic spot. Dr. Dunton, one of the founders of the 20th century movement, insisted that those fig leaves had to have been crocheted by Eve, who was trying to get over her troubles. They had something to do with her being beholden to Adam and his rib. We will unfortunately pass over all of that and begin the modern epoch with a brief description of what was taking place in Europe approximately 200 years ago.

The Age of Enlightenment

It was the Age of Enlightenment, or as some prefer, the Age of Reason. The roots of 20th century occupational therapy are visible in the empiricism of John Locke, an English philosopher and physician, who fostered confidence in human reason and human freedom; in Etienne de Condillac, a French philosopher, who advanced the dualism of body and mind; and in Pierre Cabanis, a French physician and theorist, who offered an explanation of the importance of the moral and social sciences in perfecting the art of medicine. These three, along with others, popularized the new ideas. Indeed, it was the best of times, a clear demarcation in the emergence of the modern world.

John Locke

If one were to combine the thoughts of these three, one would arrive at a theory of experience. John Locke, in his famous *Essay Concerning Human Understanding*, published in 1890,[1] examines the nature of the human mind and the processes by which it learns and comes to know about the world. When born, the human is a blank tablet (*tabula rasa*). Because of innate ability to receive sensations from the outside world, the human can assimilate and organize impressions. As contact with the environment stimulates the senses and causes impressions, the mind receives and organizes these into ideas and concepts. Since the human mind does not already contain innate ideas, all must come from without.[2]

There is a second source for the accumulation of experience, according to Locke. It is the mind itself, "the perception of the operations of our own mind, . . . (such as) thinking, doubting, believing, reasoning, knowing, . . . this source of ideas every man has wholly within himself." [3] Locke strongly holds that the body and mind exist as real entities and that they interact. He speaks of the aim of education as the process of knowing and learning through experience and of striving toward happiness. Ideally, he contends, one should work toward a sound mind in a healthful body. To achieve this ideal, Locke advocates physical exercise as a hardening process, and an exposure to a wide variety of sensations from the physical and social worlds.

Etienne de Condillac

Condillac was Locke's apologist. He tried to simplify Locke's fundamental theory by arguing that all conscious experiences are the result of passive sensations. They are the raw materials from which one forms complex and interrelated ideas. Learning consists of noting incomplete ideas, considering each separately, combining them into relationships, and ordering them. This process results in retaining the strongest degrees of association. Condillac asserts, "Then we shall grasp (ideas) easily and clearly and shall understand their origins entirely."[3]

Elsewhere in his writings, Condillac presents his thoughts on analysis. One cannot have the proper conception of a thing until one is in a position to analyze it. "To analyze," claims Condillac, "is nothing more than to observe in successive order the qualities of an object, . . . the simultaneous order in which they exist."[4]

Pierre Cabanis

The third philosopher, Pierre Cabanis, tends to apply medicine to philosophy and philosophy to medicine. Cabanis considers illness and its impact upon the formulation of values and ideas. Through the social sciences, which emerged in the Age of Enlightenment, he explains *morals* as psychological phenomena on a physiological base.

He concludes that moral impressions can have both physiological and pathological results. At last, there is a rational explanation for the psychological production of disease in which the so-called moral (emotional) passions play a significant part.[5] Cabanis contributed a socially based theoretical explanation of human experience which became the cornerstone for the moral management of the insane.

The Age of Enlightenment and Moral Treatment

Moral treatment of the insane was one result of the Age of Enlightenment. It sprang from the fundamental attitudes of the day: a set of principles which govern humanity and society, faith in the ability of the human to reason, and the supreme belief in the individual. The rapid changes due to this new philosophy advanced the disappearance of the notion that the insane were possessed of the devil. Mental diseases became legitimate concerns of humanitarians and physicians. The discontinuance of the idea that crime, sin, and vice were at the core of insanity brought forth humane treatment. Up to this time the insane had been housed and handled no differently from criminals or paupers, often in chains.

Two men living in the 18th century, working in different countries and unknown to each other, initiated the moral treatment movement. "No two men could possibly have been chosen out of all Europe at that time of whom it could be said more truly that they were cradled, and nursed, and educated among widely differing social, political, religious influences."[6] Philippe Pinel was a child of the French Revolution, a physician, scholar, and philosopher. He is described as "far exceeding the bounds of pure humanitarianism . . . to encompass the goals of a naturalist, . . . a reformer, a clinician, . . . and, above all, a philosopher."[7] William Tuke was a devout member of the Society of Friends (Quakers) and, because of his wealth and influence, conducted numerous philanthropic endeavors.

Philippe Pinel: Physician-Reformer

Whenever Philippe Pinel's name comes up in a conversation among health professionals, he is immediately mentioned as the striker of the chains at two French hospitals. His efforts and contributions go way beyond that reformational act. As a physician, he began his most serious work in 1792, as superintendent of Bicetre, the asylum for incurable males in Paris.

As a natural scientist, Pinel achieved exceptional skill in the observation of human behavior and the bringing of "some order into the chaos of . . . treatment methods by means of critical and objective investigations."[5] Pinel said, "Desirous of better information, I resolved for myself the facts that were presented to my attention; and forgetting the empty honours of my titular distinction as a physician, I viewed the scene that was opened to me with the eye of common sense and unprejudiced observation."[8] From his own experience, he urged that observations "be the basis upon which (one) should decide what opinions to believe."[9] Throughout his work, he constantly held before himself his own motto of independent thought: to seek to avoid all illusion, all prejudice, all opinion taken on authority.[10]

Pinel's descriptions of the mentally deranged provide insight into his compassionate nature. For him, the loss of reason was the most calamitous of human afflictions. The ability to reason principally separates the human from other living forms. Because of mental illness, the human's character "is always perverted, sometimes annihilated. His thoughts and actions are diverted . . . (and) his personal liberty is at length taken from him."[8]

What Pinel calls the *revolution morale* (moral revolution) is the ultimate insight of the insane into the delusional and absurd nature of their experiences.[7] This, to him, is the basis for treatment. Some historians believe that he is stating that moral treatment is synonymous with the human approach. His own writings do not bear this out. Each patient must be critically observed and analyzed; then treatment may be commenced. "To apply the principles of moral treatment, with undiscriminating uniformity, would be . . . ridiculous and unadvisable."[8] The moral method is well reasoned and carefully planned for the individual patient.

Moral Management

According to Pinel, moral management is a maintained continuity of approach, a predictable routine infused with vigor by personnel who inspire confidence. Moreover, moral treatment calls for a constant observed study of patients' behavior and performance. It includes a gentle approach, but one with firmness. Each patient is given as much liberty within the institution as he can tolerate. The approach is designed to give the patient a feeling of security with a respect for authority. Pinel asserted that "the atmosphere should be the same as in a family where the parents are quite strict. To establish this relationship, the doctor must convince the patient that he wishes to help him and that recovery is a real possibility."[9]

Occupations

Occupations figure prominently in Pinel's conception of moral treatment. Activities are employed to take the patients' thoughts away from their emotional problems and to develop their abilities. He considered literature and music equally effective in altering patients' emotions. Physical exercise and work should be part of every institution's fundamental program and be employed in accord with individual tastes. He concludes that "(this) method is primarily designed and intended to reach man at his best which . . . means human understanding, intelligence, and insight."[8]

The concept of moral treatment belongs solely to Philippe Pinel. His fundamental belief is that its purpose is to restore the patient to himself, "to use the patient's own emotions to balance his emotional excesses."[9] Truly, Pinel and his efforts, rooted in the Age of Enlightenment, mark the beginning of the modern epoch in the care of the mentally ill.

William Tuke: Philanthropist-Humanitarian

Across the channel in England, things were astir at the same time. King George III, who was giving the American colonies fits, was himself in similar trouble. In 1788 it became public knowledge that the King was seized with mania. Questions arose about his fitness to continue ruling. Nevertheless, public sentiment was on the side of the King. For the first time, insanity and its treatment formed a topic of public discussion. "The subject had been brought out of concealment in a way which defeated the conspiracy of silence."[11] This being the Age of Enlightenment, the public openly sympathized with the sufferer; there was no condemnation. No one suggested that the King was being visited by the Devil, or that he was being punished for his sins.

William Tuke, a devout Quaker, wealthy merchant, and renowned philanthropist, was made aware of the deplorable conditions in the insane asylum in York, England. There were tales of extreme neglect and possible cruelty. He was an unusual man, not given to listening to sensational reports and acting in a rash manner.[14] At a Friend's Quarterly Meeting in the spring of 1792, Tuke presented his concern that an institution for the insane, under the direction of the Society, be established in York. At first he was met with considerable resistance by those who believed that there were too few mentally ill Quakers and that it was not proper to concentrate them in such a lovely, quiet locale.[15]

The York Retreat

Initially, Tuke was disheartened, yet he pressed on, and within six months The Retreat for Persons Afflicted with Disorders of the Mind, or simply The Retreat, came into being. Until now the term "retreat" had never been applied to an asylum. Tuke's daughter-in-law suggested the term to convey the Quaker belief that such an institution might be "a place in which the unhappy might obtain refuge; a quiet haven in which (one) . . . might find a means of reparation or of safety."[16] The cornerstone stated simply the purpose of the institution: "The charity or love of friends executed this work in the cause of humanity."[15]

William Tuke became the superintendent. Thomas Fowler, an unusually open-minded man, was appointed visiting physician. After a trial and error period, they came to believe that moral treatment methods were preferable to those involving restraint and use of harsh drugs. The new approach was a product of Tuke's humanitarianism and Fowler's empiricism.

Kindness and Consideration

Several fundamental principles became evident within a short time. The approach was primarily one of kindness and consideration. The patients were not thought to be devoid of reason, feeling, and honor. The social environment was to be as nearly like that of a family as possible, with an atmosphere of religious sentiment and moral feeling.[16]

Occupation and the Habit of Attention

Tuke and Fowler strongly believed that most insane people retain a considerable amount of self-command. Upon admission, the patient was informed that treatment depended largely upon his own conduct. Employment in various occupations was expected as a way for the patient to maintain control over his disorder. As Tuke reported, "regular employment is perhaps the most efficacious; and those kinds of employment . . . to be preferred . . . are accompanied by considerable bodily action."[16] The staff endeavored to gain the patient's confidence and esteem, to arrest the attention and fix it upon objects opposite to any illusion one might have. The fundamental purpose of employment and recreation was to facilitate the regaining of the habit of attention, as Tuke calls it. Various learning exercises were used, such as mathematical problems, to help the patient gain ascendancy over faulty habits of attention.

Indolence

Tuke and Fowler determined that "indolence has a natural tendency to weaken the mind, and to induce ennui and discontent"[16] A wide range of occupations and amusements were available. Those not engaged in useful occupations were allowed to read, draw, or play various games. Tea parties, walks, and visitations away from the institution were regularly used in preparation for the patient returning home. All activities were closely analyzed through observation so that individualization of patients' needs could be accomplished.

The pioneer work of William Tuke and his son, Samuel, who wrote the definitive treatise on The Retreat, opened a new chapter in the history of the care of the insane in England. Mild management methods infused with kindness and the building of self-esteem through the judicious use of occupations resulted in the excitation and elicitation of superior, human motives. Patients recovered, left The Retreat, and rarely needed to return for further care. The entire regimen was carefully patterned "to accord (patients) the dignity and status of sick human beings."[17]

Moral Treatment Expansion

No sooner had Pinel's major work on moral treatment (1801) and Samuel Tuke's description of The Retreat been published (1813), than there was a rush toward implementing many reforms in other hospitals, particularly in England and the United States. In both countries occupations were introduced as an integral part of moral treatment.[18] Some unusual experiments were undertaken by Sir William Charles Ellis, a physician, who became the superintendent of a pauper lunatic asylum. The mainstay of his asylum management was useful occupations. He moved well ahead of mere amusements and "introduced a gainful employment of patients on a large scale and even had them taught a trade."[19] In conjunction with his wife, other reforms were undertaken. She organized the women patients into supervised groups to make useful and fancy articles.

Another innovation by Ellis was the development of what would eventually be called halfway houses. Keenly aware of environmental and social influences of insanity, Ellis suggested "after-care houses and night hospitals as a stepping stone from the asylum to the world by which . . . the length of patients' stay would be reduced and in many cases the cure completed."[17] He insisted that convalescing patients should go out and mix with the world before discharge. His proposals were made in the 1830s!

In the United States, very few public and private asylums existed in the post-Revolutionary era; however, institutional reforms did need to be undertaken. Any recounting of this period must include two very important individuals and their work: Benjamin Rush and Dorothea Lynde Dix. Their efforts did not overlap; they did not know one another, nor was one influenced by the other. As in the case of Pinel and Tuke, no two individuals on this side of the Atlantic could have been more unlike one another in background, education, or experience. Nevertheless, each recognized the hapless plight of the institutionalized insane, and they set for themselves the alleviation of dire conditions and the inauguration of moral treatment, including occupations and exercise.

Benjamin Rush: Father of American Psychiatry

Benjamin Rush, often referred to as the father of American psychiatry, was a Philadelphia physician in the latter half of the 1700s. Through his training in Europe and several visitations there, he adopted many of Pinel's practices; however, Rush did not adopt moral principles until later. As a member of the staff of Pennsylvania Hospital, he was placed in charge of a separate section set aside for the insane, the first such section in America. He was appalled by the conditions and appealed to the staff and the public for change. Change did come and humane treatment was instituted. Rush saw to it that "certain employments be devised for such of the deranged people as are capable of working."[20] This was based upon his philosophical stance that man, by his very nature, is meant to be active. Even in paradise, he was employed in the healthful and pleasant exercises of cultivating a garden. "Happiness, consisting in folded arms, and in pensive contemplation . . . by the side of brooks, never had any existence, except in the brains of mad poets, and love-sick girls and boys."[21]

In another place in his major writing, *Medical Inquiries and Observations Upon the Diseases of the Mind*, Rush clearly differentiates between goal-directed activity and aimless exercise. "Labour has several advantages over exercise, in being not only more stimulating, but more endurable in its effects; . . . it is calculated to arrest wrong habits of action, and to restore such as regular and natural."[21]

Dorothea Lynde Dix: Humanitarian-Reformer

Dorothea Lynde Dix, a reform-minded humanitarian of the middle 1800s, vehemently pressed for improved conditions for the insane who were incarcerated in jails and almshouses. She presented a number of *Memorials* to state legislatures, believing that the public had an obligation to care for such individuals. By 1848 numerous states had responded to her efforts, and she decided to tackle a more formidable object, the federal government. Dix envisioned the sale of public lands to finance the building of a federal system of hospitals for the indigent blind, deaf, and mute, as well as the insane. For six years she wheedled and cajoled members of Congress. Finally, in 1854, the bill was ready for President Franklin Pierce's signature. He was a close friend of Miss Dix and she felt highly confident of the outcome. However, the President vetoed the bill, claiming unconstitutionality. "Every human weakness or sorrow would take advantage of this bill if it became law. . . . It endangers states' rights."[22] Through her contacts with physicians in several states, she embraced moral treatment as the most humane method. She strongly advocated "decent care, quiet, affection, and normal activity (as) the only medicine for the insane."[22]

The United States: Individual Treatment, Occupations, and Education

The Quakers brought moral treatment to the United States as part of their intellectual and religious heritage. Through published accounts of The Retreat in York, some private asylums were established in which moral principles were practiced. A number of public institutions altered their programs to include individualized treatment, occupations, and education. Those patients who had remained for years as unimproving and listless, even on the verge of apathy were "seen in encouraging instances, when transferred to attendants who have more disposition to attend to them . . . to waken from their torpor, to become animated, active, and even industrious."[23]

Moral management also was taking on a new facet, the influence of a sane mind upon an insane mind. Those who daily attended the sick were to impress upon the insane the influences of their own character, designed to specifically improve the patients' behavior. Personnel must possess observational skills to see the "actual condition of the patient's mind . . . and a faculty of clear insight."[23] Other required traits included "seeing that which is passing in the minds of (patients) . . . a firm will, the faculty of self-control, a sympathizing distress at moral pain, (and) a strong desire to remove it."[23]

Arguments appeared in the literature relative to the moral use of firmness and gentleness. Strong cases were made for both extremes; however, it took two alienists (the precursors to psychiatrists), John Bucknill and D. Hack Tuke, grandson of Samuel Tuke, to settle the dispute in 1858. "The truth, as usual, lies between; and the (individual) who aims at success in the moral treatment of the insane must be ready to be all things to all men, if by any means he might save some."[23] They elaborate on their thesis by stating that self-reliance "requires widely different manifestations, to repress excitement, to stimulate inertia, to check the vicious, to comfort the depressed, to direct the erring, to support the weak, to supplant every variety of erroneous opinion, to resist every kind of perverted feeling, and to check every form of pernicious conduct."[23]

Bucknill and Tuke also wrote that moral treatment included the gaining of the patient's confidence, fixing his attention on interesting and wholesome objects of thought, diverting his mind from introspection, and loosening his hold on concentrated emotion. "For (these) purposes useful occupation is far superior to any form of amusement. The higher the purpose, and the more appellant the nature of the occupation . . . the more likely it is to draw him from the contemplation of self-wretchedness, and effect the triumph of moral influences."[23]

The next step in the rise of institutional occupations was the growth of emphasis on education. It was determined that those occupations which require a process of learning and thought are far preferable, from a curative point of view, to those which require none. "Moral treatment is as wide as that of education; . . . it is education applied to the field of mental phenomena."[23] Therefore, it was not unusual to find specific mental activities included with occupations. The purpose was to educate the individual in order to provide him with "the power of controlling his feelings, and his thoughts, and his actions."[24]

With continued experience, a number of alienists decided that occupations and amusements also could serve as a prophylaxes against insanity. One interesting prescription for the return and maintenance of sanity was "rest in bed, occupation, exercise, and amusements."[25] D. Hack Tuke declared, "If idleness is a curse to the sane, it is the parent of mischief and ennui to the insane, especially to the pubescent and adolescent."[26] He urged that the same approach be taken with the sane and the insane. "Employment, Nature's universal law of health, alike for body and mind, is specially beneficial . . . seeing that it displaces ideas by new and healthy thoughts, revives familiar habits of daily activity, (and) restores self-respect while it promotes the general bodily health."[26]

The Decline of Moral Treatment

Moral management and treatment by occupations reached its zenith in the United States just prior to the outbreak of the Civil War. Corporate and private asylums continued to expand their efforts, but state and public institutions withdrew their programs, so that by the last quarter of the 19th century virtually no moral treatment was taking place.

Several reasons for this decline and eventual disappearance can be identified. The nation warring on itself is one. Bockhoven cites others: 1) the founders of the U.S. movement retired and died, leaving no disciples or successors; 2) the rapidly increasing influx of foreign-born and poor patients greatly overtaxed existing facilities and required more institutions to be built with diminished tax support; 3) racial and religious prejudices on the part of the alienists, now beginning to be called psychiatrists, reduced interest in treatment; and 4) state legislatures became increasingly more interested in less costly custodial care.[27]

Essentially, there was no place in the public institutions for moral treatment. "The inferior physical plants and facilities, poorly trained and insufficient staff, . . . and, worst of all, overcrowding, prohibited any attempts to practice moral management."[28] A belief emerged that many of the insane were incurable. One eminent psychiatrist stated, "I have come to the conclusion that when a man becomes insane, he is about used up for this world."[29] Such pessimism was predominant in this country for almost a century. Custodial care had come to stay for a long time.

As we shall see, moral principles and practices emerged in the early years of the 20th century through the efforts of individuals and then by a group who founded an organization dedicated to those principles. They, in collaboration with others, established the definition and fundamental principles which have carried over through several generations of specifically educated practitioners of occupational therapy.

Once again, as with Pinel and Tuke and Rush and Dix, the individuals who founded and pioneered the 20th century occupational therapy movement could not have been more diverse in terms of background, experience, and education. They included a nurse, two architects, a physician, a social worker, and a teacher.

Susan Tracy: Occupational Nurse

Susan Tracy was this century's first proponent of occupations for invalids. A trained nurse herself, she initiated instruction in activities to student nurses as early as 1905, as part of their expanding responsibilities. She also developed the term "occupational nurses" to signify specialization.[30] By 1912 she decided to devote her full-time energies to patient activities, and she distinquished herself by applying moral treatment principles to acute conditions. As Tracy states, "the application of this most rational remedy to ordinary, everyday sick people, as found in the general hospital, is almost unknown."[31] She strongly claims that remedial treatments "are classified according to their physiological effects as stimulants, sedatives, anesthetics, . . . etc. Certain occupations possess like properties."[31] The physician may select stimulating occupations, such as water coloring and paper folding, or sedative ones, such as knitting, weaving, or basketry.

Throughout Tracy's many years of work she employed experimentation and observation to enhance her practice. Her carefully worded writings provide ample evidence of her intense desire to bring scientific principles to the application of invalid occupations. In 1918 she published a remarkable research paper on 25 mental tests derived from occupations. An example includes the following: by instructing the patient in using a piece of leather and a pencil, "require him to make a line of dots at equal distances around the margin and at uniform distant from the edge. This constitutes a Test of Judgement in estimating distances."[32] Continuing with the same piece of leather, the patient is instructed to punch a hole at each dot. "In order to do this he must consider the two sides of leather, the two parts of his tool, and bring these together, thus making a simple Coordination Test."[32] Other tests in the fabrication of the leather purse include Aesthetic Coordination and Rhythm, Differentiation of Form and Size, and Purposeful Relation. In all 25 tests, she stresses a completed, useful and "not unbeautiful" object.

Tracy's other writings state the value and usefulness of discarded materials to successful ward work.[33] She also emphasizes high quality of workmanship. "It is now believed that what is worth doing at all is worth doing well, and that practical, well-made articles have a greater therapeutic value than a useless, poorly made article."[34] A premium is placed upon originality and the "adoption of the occupation to the condition and natural tastes of the patient."[35] Further, she believes that "the patient is the product, not the article that he makes."[33]

Tracy's major work, *Studies in Invalid Occupation*,[36] published in 1918, is a revealing compendium of her observations and experiences with different kinds of patients, including the child of poverty, the child of wealth, the impatient boy, the grandmother, and the businessman.

By 1921 Susan Tracy had adopted the term "occupation therapy," originally coined by William Rush Dunton, Jr., defined it, and differentiated it from vocational training. She felt that this was necessary because of the rising confusion between the two concepts following World War I. "What is occupation? The treatment of disease by occupation . . . The aim of occupation is to get the man well; that of vocational training is to provide him with a job. Any well man will look for a job, but the sick man is looking for health."[37]

Throughout her writings she states that nothing is "too small to be pressed into the service of (a) resourceful mind and trained hands toward . . . the establishment of a healthy mind in a healthy body."[33]

George Barton: Re-education of Convalescents

George Edward Barton, by profession an architect, contracted tuberculosis in his adult life, which plagued him for the remainder of his years. His consistent struggle led him into a life of service to the physically handicapped. Out of his own personal concerns came the establishment of Consolation House, an early prototype of a rehabilitation center. He was an effective speaker and writer, often given to hyperbole; nevertheless, he gained his point with the listening or reading public.

Barton's central themes were hospitals and their responsibility to the discharged patient; the conditions the discharged patient faces; the need to return to employment; and occupations and re-education for convalescents. These were intense concerns to him because of his own health problems.

His first published article, derived from a speech given to a group of nurses, points out a weakness he perceives in hospitals: "We discharge from them not efficients, but inefficients. An individual leaves almost any of our institutions only to become a burden upon his family, his friends, the associated charities, or upon another institution. . . . I say to discharge a patient from the hospital, with his fracture healed, to be sure, but to a devastated home, to an empty desk and to no obvious sustaining employment, is to send him out to a world cold and bleak. . . . Occupation would shorten convalescence and improve the condition of many patients. . . . It is time for humanity to cease regarding the hospital as a door closing upon a life which is past and to regard it henceforth as a door opening upon a life which is to come."[38]

Barton established Consolation House in Clifton Springs, New York. Those referred to his institution underwent a thorough review, including a social and medical history and a consideration of education, training, experience, successes, and failures. "By considering these in relation to the condition (the patient) must presumably or inevitably be in for the remainder of his life, we can find some form of occupation for which he will be fitted."[39] He claimed that Consolation House was "getting down to our social difficulties."[39]

By 1915 Barton had adopted Dunton's term, occupation therapy, but preferred the adjectival form: occupational therapy. He declared, "If there is an occupational disease, why not an occupational therapy? . . . The first thing to be done . . . is for occupational therapy to provide an occupation which will produce a similar therapeutic effect to that of every drug in materia medica. An exercise for each separate organ, joint, and muscle of the human body. An exercise? An occupation. An occupation? A useful occupation! Then (occupational therapy) can fill the doctor's prescriptions . . . written in the terms of materia medica."[40] He even advocated a laxative by occupation, which is open to interpretation and speculation.

Re-education entered Barton's terminology with the aftermath of World War I. He viewed hospitals taking on a different mission than previously adopted. A hospital should become "a re-educational institution through which to put the waste products of society back and into the right place. . . . By a catalystic concatenation of contiguous circumstances we were forced to realize that when all is said and done, what the sick man really needed and wanted most was the restoration of his ability to work, to live independently and to make money."[11]

Barton's major contribution to the re-emergence of moral treatment is the awakening of physical reconstruction and re-education through the employment of occupations. Convalescence, to him, is a critical time for the inclusion of something to do. Activity "clarifies and strengthens the mind by increasing and maintaining interest in wholesome thought to the exclusion of morbid thought . . . and a proper occupation . . . during convalescence may be made the basis of the corollary of a new life upon recovery. . . . I mean a job, a better job, or a job done better than it was before."[42] With Susan Tracy, Barton held that the major consideration of occupations "should be devoted to the therapeutic and education effects, not to the value of the possible product."[43]

William Rush Dunton, Jr.: Judicious Regimen of Activity

Of the founders of the 20th century movement, William Rush Dunton, Jr., was the most prolific and influential. He published in excess of 120 books and articles related to occupational therapy and rehabilitation; served as President of the National Society for the Promotion of Occupational Therapy; and, for 21 years, was editor of the official journal. As a physician, he spent his professional career treating psychiatric patients in an institutional setting. The key to his treatment methods was occupational therapy, a term he coined to differentiate aimless amusements from those occupations definitely prescribed for their therapeutic benefits. Before embarking on what he called a judicious regimen of activity, he read the works of Tuke and Pinel, as well as the efforts of significant alienists of the 19th century.

From his readings and from observations of patients in Sheppard Asylum, a Quaker institution in Towson, Maryland, Dunton concluded that the acutely ill are generally not amenable to occupations or recreation. There is a weakened power of attention. Occupations at this time would be fatiguing and harmful. The prevailing prescription is "to let the patient alone, meanwhile improve (his) condition, restore and revivify exhausted mental and physical forces."[44] Later, activities should be selected which use energies not needed for physical restoration. Stimulating attention and directing the thoughts of the patient in regular and healthful paths would ensure an early release from the hospital. A wide variety of activities was developed by Dunton, from knitting and crocheting to printing and the repair of dynamos, in order to gain the attention and interest and meet the needs of all patients.

Dunton's proclivities for history and research led him to extensive readings and experimentation, all of which related to the human need for work, leisure, rest, and sleep; the causal factors of mental aberrations; and various cures of mental illness. Each excursion brought him back to a judicious regimen of activity as the treatment of choice, regardless of whether one was mentally or physically ill. He became more and more convinced that attention and interest in one's work and play are as efficacious, if not more so, than the many and varied medications available. "It has been found that a patient makes more rapid progress if his attention is concentrated upon what he is making and he derives stimulating pleasure in its performance."[45]

At the second annual meeting of the National Society for the Promotion of Occupational Therapy (later the AOTA) in 1918, Dunton unveiled his nine cardinal rules to guide the emerging practice of occupational therapy, and to ensure that the new discipline would gain acceptance as a medical entity. Any activity in which the patient engages should have as its objective a cure. It should be interesting; have a useful purpose other than merely to gain the patient's attention and interest; preferably lead to an increase in knowledge on the patient's part; and preferably be carried on with others, such as in a group. The occupational therapist should make a careful study of the patient in order to know his needs and attempt to meet as many as possible through activity. The therapist should stop the patient in his work before he reaches a point of fatigue, and encouragement should be genuinely given whenever indicated. Finally, work is much to be preferred over idleness, even when the end product of the patient's labor is of a poor quality or is useless.[46]

The major purposes of occupation in the case of the mentally ill were outlined in Dunton's first book.[47] The primary objective is to divert the attention either from unpleasant subjects, as is true with the depressed patient, or from day-dreaming or mental ruminations, as in the case of the patient suffering from *dementia praecox* (schizophrenia), to divert the attention to one main subject.

Another purpose of occupation is to re-educate, to train the patient in developing mental processes through "educating the hands, eyes, muscles, just as is done in the developing child."[47] Fostering an interest in hobbies is a third purpose. Hobbies serve as both present and future safety valves and render a recurrence of mental illness less likely. A final purpose may be to instruct the patient in a craft until he has enough proficiency to take pride in his work. "While this is proper, I fear . . . specialism is apt to cause a narrowing of one's mental outlook. . . . The individual with a knowledge of many things has more interest in the world in general."[47]

Dunton continued to write and publish his observations, each one elaborating on a previous one. His texts became required reading for students preparing for practice. Even in his nineties, well beyond his retirement from practice, he maintained his interest in the profession and continued to offer his counsel.

Eleanor Clarke Slagle: Founder and Pioneer

Eleanor Clarke Slagle qualifies both as a founder and pioneer. She was at the birth of the American Occupational Therapy Association in 1917. Prior to that time she had received part of her education in social work and had completed one of the early "Special Courses in Curative Occupations and Recreation" at the Chicago School of Civics and Philanthropy. Following this, she taught two courses for attendants of the insane, directed the Occupations Program at the Henry Phipps Clinic of Johns Hopkins Hospital under Dr. Adolf Meyer, and returned to Chicago to become the Superintendent of Occupational Therapy at Hull House. Later, Mrs. Slagle moved to New York where she pioneered in developing occupational therapy in the State Department of Mental Hygiene. In addition, she served with high distinction in every elective office of the American Occupational Therapy Association, including President (1919-1920), and as a paid Executive Secretary for fourteen years.[48,49,50,51]

She finds occupational therapy to be "an awkward term" but feels "it has been well defined as a form of remedial treatment consisting of various types of activities . . . which either contribute to or hasten recovery from disease or injury . . . carried on under medical supervision and . . . consciously motivated." Further, she emphasizes that occupational therapy must be "a consciously planned, progressive program of rest, play, occupation and exercise."[52] In addition, she explains that it is "an effort toward normalizing the lives of countless thousands who are mentally ill . . . (using) the normal mechanism of a fairly well balanced day."[53] She enjoyed quoting C. Charles Burlingame, a prominent psychiatrist of her day: "What is an occupational therapist? She is that newer medical specialist who takes the joy out of invalidism. She is the medical specialist who carries us over the dangerous period between acute illness and return to the world of men and women as a useful member of society."[52]

Slagle places considerable emphasis upon the personality factor of the therapist: "the proper balance of qualities, proper physical expression, a kindly voice, gentleness, patience, ability and seeming vision, adaptability . . . to meet the particular needs of the individual patient in all things. . . . Personality plus character also covers an ability to be honest and firm, with infinite kindness."[54]

The issue of the use of handicrafts as a therapeutic measure in the machine age would constantly arise. Her response is a classic. "Handicrafts are so generally used, not only because they are so diverse, covering a field from the most elementary to the highest grade of ability; but also, and greatly to the point, because their development is based on primitive impulses. They offer the means of contact with the patient that no other medium does or can offer. Encouragement of creative impulses also may lead to the development of large interests outside oneself and certainly leads to social contact, an important consideration with any sick or convalescent patient."[52]

Habit Training

Habit training was first attempted at Rochester (New York) State Hospital in 1901, and Slagle adopted the basic principles, developing a greater perspective and use among mental patients who had been hospitalized from five to twenty years and who had steadily regressed. The fundamental plan is "to arrange a twenty-four hour schedule . . . in which physicians, nurses, attendants and occupational therapists play a part."[54] It is a re-education program designed to overcome some disorganized habits, to modify others, and to construct new ones, with the goal that habit reaction will lead toward the restoration and maintenance of health. "In habit training, we show clearly an academic philosophy factor . . . that is, the necessity of requiring attention, of building on the abit of attention—attention thus becomes application, voluntary and, in time, agreeable."[54]

The purposes of habit training are two-fold: the reclamation and rehabilitation of the patient with the eventual goal of discharge or parole; and, if this is not reasonable, assisting the patient in becoming less of an institutional problem (i.e., less destructive and untidy).

A typical habit training schedule calls for the patients to arise in the morning at 6:00, wash, use the toilet, brush teeth, and air beds; breakfast; return to ward and make beds; sweep; and then classwork for 2 hours, consisting of a variety of simple crafts and marching exercises. After lunch there is a rest period and then continued class work and outdoor exercises, folk dancing, and lawn games. Following supper, there is music and dancing on the ward, followed by toileting, washing, brushing teeth, and preparing for bed.[55]

Once the patient has received maximum benefit from habit training, he is ready to progress through three phases of occupational therapy. The first is what Slagle called the kindergarten group. "We must show the ways and means of stimulating the special sense. The employment of color, music, simple exercises, games and story-telling along with occupations, the gentle ways and means . . . (used) in educating the child are equally important in reeducating the adult."[54] Occupations are graded from the simple to the complex.

The next phase is ward classes in occupational therapy "graded to the limit of accomplishment of individual patients."[58] When this is tolerated, the patient joins in group activities.

The third and final phase is the occupational center. "This promotes opportunities for the more advanced projects; . . . (a) complete change in environment; . . . comparative freedom; . . . actual responsibilities placed upon patients; the stimulation of seeing work produced; . . . all these carry forward the readjustment of patients."[56]

This founder, pioneer, and distinguished member of the profession provides a summary of her own accomplishments and philosophy. "Of the highest value to patients is the psychological fact that the patient is working for himself. . . . Occupational Therapy recognizes the significance of the mental attitude which the sick person takes toward his illness and attempts to make that attitude more wholesome by providing activities adapted to the capacity of the individual patient and calculated to divert his attention from his own problems."[54] Further, "It is directed activity, and differs from all other forms of treatment in that it is given in increasing doses as the patient improves."[57]

Adolf Meyer: The Philosophy of Occupational Therapy

Dr. Adolf Meyer is cited in this account of the evolution of occupational therapy because of his unusual support, and because his approach to clinical psychiatry was entirely consistent with the emerging occupational therapy movement. Adolf Meyer, a Swiss physician, immigrated to the United States in 1892 and initially accepted a position as pathologist at the Eastern Illinois Hospital for the Insane in Kankakee. Over the next 14 years he held various positions in the United States, and became professor of psychiatry at Johns Hopkins University in 1910. Throughout this period he developed the fundamentals of what was to become the psychobiological approach to psychiatry, a term he coined to indicate that the human is an indivisible unit of study, rather than a composite of symptoms. "Psychobiology starts not from a mind and a body or from elements, but from the fact that we deal with biologically organized units and groups and their functioning . . . the 'he's' and 'she's' of our experience, the bodies we find in action."[58] Meyer takes strong issue with those in medicine "who wish to reduce everything to physics and chemistry, or to anatomy, or to physiology, and within that to neurology."[58] His enlightened point of view is that one can only be studied as a total being in action and that this "whole person represents an integrate of hierarchically arranged functions."[59]

His commonsense approach to the problems of psychiatry is his keynote. "The main thing is that your point of reference should always be life itself. . . . I put my emphasis upon specificity. . . . As long as there is life there are positive assets action, choice, hope, not in the imagination but in a clear understanding of the situation, goals, and possibilities. . . . To see life as it is, to tend toward objectivity is one of the fundamentals of my philosophy, my attitude, my preference. It is something that I would recommend if it can be kept free of making itself a pest to self and to others."[60]

From the very beginning of his work in Illinois, he concerned himself with meaningful activity. In time, it becomes the fundamental issue in treatment. "I thought primarily of occupation therapy," he states, "of getting the patient to do things and getting things going which did not work but which could work with proper straightening out."[60] In a report to the Governor of the State of Illinois in 1895, Meyer wrote: "Occupation is, with good right, the most essential side of hygienic treatment of most insane patients."[60]

By 1921, Meyer had become Professor of Psychiatry at Johns Hopkins University, and he had had extensive experiences with other leaders in the occupational therapy movement such as William Rush Dunton, Jr., Eleanor Clarke Slagle, and Henrietta Price. At the Fifth Annual Meeting of the National Society for the Promotion of Occupational Therapy in October 1921, Meyer brought together his fundamental concepts of psychobiology to produce his paper, *The Philosophy of Occupation Therapy*. Through time, this has become a classic in occupational therapy literature.

Psychobiology is clearly visible in his statement that "the newer conceptions of mental problems (are) problems of living, and not merely diseases of a structural and toxic nature. . . . Our Conception of man is that of an organism that maintains and balances itself in the world of reality and actuality by being in active life and active use."[61]

Because of the nature of his paper, Meyer emphasizes occupation, time, and the productive use of energy. Interwoven are the elements of psychobiology. "The whole of human organisation has its shape in . . . rhythm. . . . There are many . . . rhythms which we must be attuned to: the larger rhythms of night and day, of sleep and waking hours . . . and finally the big four, work and play and rest and sleep, which our organism must be able to balance even under difficulty. The only way to attain balance in all this is actual doing, actual practice; a program of wholesome living is the basis of wholesome feeling and thinking and fancy and interests."[61]

A fundamental issue in the treatment of the mentally ill is "the proper use of time in some helpful and gratifying activity. . . . There is in all this a development of the valuation of time and work which is not accidental. It is part of the great espousal of the values of reality and actuality rather than of mere thinking and reasoning . . . (and) in giving opportunities rather than prescriptions. There must be opportunities to work, opportunities to do and to plan and create, and to learn to use material. . . . It is not a question of specific prescriptions, but of opportunities . . . to adapt opportunities."[61] He concludes his philosophic essay by returning once again to time and occupations. "The great feature of man is his new sense of time, with foresight built on a sound view of the past and present. Man learns to organize time and he does it in terms of doing things, and one of the many things he does between eating, drinking and . . . the flights of fancy and aspiration, we call work and occupation."[61]

Near the end of his working life, Meyer did a summing up. He wrote of dealing with individuals and groups from the viewpoints of good sense; of science, "with the smallest number of assumptions for search and research;" and of philosophy and religion as "a way of trust and dependabilities in life."[62]

Occupational Therapy: Definitions and Principles

As the founders and pioneers were experimenting with and writing their concepts, a definition of occupational therapy was emerging. It is remarkable that a definition could be developed so early in the formation of the movement and stand for several decades and several generations of occupational therapists.

H. A. Pattison, M.D., Medical Officer of the National Tuberculous Association, advanced his definition at the annual conference of the National Society for the Promotion of Occupational Therapy in September 1919. It was also adopted by the Federal Board of Vocational Education: "Occupational Therapy may be defined as any activity, mental or physical, definitely prescribed and guided for the distinct purpose of contributing to and hastening recovery from disease or injury."[63] In 1931 John S. Coulter, M.D., and Henrietta McNary,

OTR, added one phrase: "and assisting the social and institutional adjustment of individuals requiring long and indefinite periods of hospitalization."[64] This was inserted in order to recognize occupational therapy's involvement in chronicity.

By 1925 a committee made up of four physicians, including William Rush Dunton, compiled an outline for lectures to medical students and physicians.[65] Though their document never received the official imprimatur of the AOTA, it nevertheless stood for several years as a guide for practice.[68] Fifteen principles were described. "Occupational therapy is a method of training the sick or injured by means of instruction and employment in productive occupation . . . to arouse interest, courage, confidence; to exercise mind and body in . . . activity; to overcome disability; and to re-establish capacity for industrial and social usefulness."[65] Application calls for as much system and precision as other forms of treatment; activity is to be prescribed, administered and supervised under constant medical advice. Individual patient needs are paramount.

"Employment in groups is . . . advisable because it provides exercise in social adaptation and stimulating influence of example and comment."[65] In selecting an activity, the patient's interests and capabilities are to be considered, and as strength and capability increase, so should the occupation be altered, regulated, and graded accordingly. "The only reliable measure of the treatment is the effect on the patient."[65] Inferior workmanship may be tolerated, depending upon the patient's condition, but there should be consideration of "standards worthy of entirely normal persons . . . for proper mental stimulation."[65]

Articles made are to be useful and attractive, and meaningful tasks requiring healthful exercise of mind and body provide the greatest satisfaction. "Novelty, variety, individuality, and utility of the products enhance the value of an occupation as a treatment measure."[65] While quality, quantity, and the salability of articles made may be of benefit, these should not take precedence over the treatment objectives. As adjuncts to occupations, physical exercise, games, and music are of considerable benefit and fall into two main categories: gymnastics and calisthenics, and recreation and play.

One last principle speaks of the qualities of the occupational therapist: "good craftsmanship, and ability to instruct are essential qualifications; . . . understanding, sincere interest in the patient, and an optimistic, cheerful outlook and manner are equally essential."[65]

Occupational Therapy's Second Generation

The die was cast. Practice rapidly expanded in a phenomenal number of settings following the establishment of the founders' principles and definition. A second generation of therapists emerged during the late 1920s and the 1930s. They were the practitioners and educators who elaborated, codified, and applied the initial theory upon which present-day practice is based. A chronicle of their efforts would offer a highly valuable and valued study in itself. The names of Louis Haas, Mary Alice Coombs, Winifred Kahmann, Henrietta McNary, Harriet Robeson, Marjorie Taylor, and Helen Willard would prominently figure in such an account.

For the purpose of this history, a composite of these and others is drawn into one individual who exemplifies the spirit and deeds of the second generation of occupational therapists, those whose efforts are lasting and ensure present and future education and practice.

This idealized therapist would devote a professional career to either teaching, practicing, or administering. Quite possibly he or she would combine two or more of these and would acquire an expertise in one area of practice, such as the mentally ill.

A belief in the treatment of the total patient would guide the therapist's thoughts and actions because "since its founding occupational therapy has concerned itself with the basic tenet—the treatment of the total patient. This approach is unique to occupational therapy among the . . . health disciplines. . . . There has always existed a strong component concerned with the behavior of the physically ill or disabled, as well as the mentally sick; with the entirety of man and his functioning as a patient. This occupational therapy concept prevented (as has occurred in medical practice) an undesired separation of the psychiatric therapist from those who develop knowledge and skills centered in the treatment of the physically disabled."[86] Stated another way, "The major emphasis in occupational therapy is not the body as such but the individual as such. The therapist's background is strongly weighted in an understanding of personality adjustment and reactions to social situations . . . and in the patients' attitudes toward an adjustment to acute and chronic disabilities."[67]

At some point in her work, she would be asked to serve as consultant to one or more medical facilities, possibly a state hospital system. In time, she would produce a report. "The goal of all treatment in a modern mental hospital is the physical, social, and economic rehabilitation of the patient. . . . The accepted function (of occupational therapy) . . . is the scientific utilization of mental and physical activities for the purpose of raising the patient to the highest level of integration; to assist him in making his initial adjustment to the hospital; to sustain him while his body responds to physical treatment and his mind to psychotherapy; or to assist him in making a satisfactory adjustment to chronic illness."[68]

In the report she also would call for as normal an atmosphere as possible, where a patient can be encouraged to respond as normally as possible to a balanced program of work and play, with flexibility to meet individual needs. There must be organized a succession of steps through which the patient will be gradually led to his "highest level of integration. . . . At each level . . . the patient experiences a feeling of success and self-respect. One cannot overemphasize the importance of careful planning . . . in order that there be a systematic progression up this ladder of integration."[68]

In another context, supportive care, as a vital concern to the therapist, would also be described, particularly in the care of the physically disabled. To name only a few of its treatment objectives, occupational therapy may function as "a diagnostic evaluative instrument; as corrective treatment . . . or a design for effecting prevocational evaluation. Incorporated in each . . . is a treatment phase referred to as supportive care. This is a most fundamental and yet less definitive and indeed the least spectacular element of the total rehabilatory program. In supportive care, the occupational therapist (is concerned) with the behavioral factors which have and will affect the patient's response to the rehabilitation program. . . . It can be said with conviction that successful rehabilitation can be effected only when the patient has attained a true state of rehabilitation readiness."[69]

The true therapist might well become active with a group of former patients and assist in organizing an association of and for individuals who have been hospitalized, for instance, the mentally ill. Through such an experience she would conclude: "One difficulty which presented itself again and again was the need to instill in these (former) patients a philosophy toward their own rehabilitation . . . an organized effort beyond the hospital which would offer special training, guidance, and professional evaluation of their potentials."[70]

This would lead her to even greater endeavors on behalf of a whole category of patients. As an example, she would find that the 1920 Federal Vocational Rehabilitation Act excludes former psychiatric patients. In the manner of Dorothea Lynde Dix, whom she probably emulates, she would wage a relentless battle to right such a wrong. By enlisting the assistance of physicians' associations and veterans' groups, she would see the legislation change. As part of her campaign she would write, "The former mental patient, in his struggle for economic rehabilitation, incurs the burden imposed on the physically handicapped *plus* the stigmatization based on the popular misconception of mental disease. He must cast aside self-pity or the idea that the world owes him a living. The world does owe him understanding and guidance."[71] Finally, she would see amendments to Public Law 118 passed and signed by President Franklin Roosevelt, allowing psychiatric patients to qualify for the benefits of the Vocational Rehabilitation Act.

With such efforts the therapist's personal beliefs about emotional illness would become even more strongly felt. "The majority of mentally ill are (sick) through no fault of their own . . . any more than one who has contracted a physical illness. Persons suffering from mental disease are generally ill as a result of an accumulation of unsuccessful efforts . . . to adjust to (their) environment."[71]

Two continuing concerns of occupational therapists include the qualifications of the therapist and the utilization of media. One is as signficant as the other. "The personality of the therapist," she would say, "must command respect, admiration, hope and confidence, . . . for no therapy is better than the therapist who directs it."[71] Therapeutic media have a number of inherent qualities, such as providing a vehicle for recording patient performance objectively and affording the patient opportunities for "creative expression and evidence of accomplishment. The therapist should have a wide variety of activities (available) in accordance with the interests, aptitudes, and mental state of the patient."[17] A mind oriented to one modality of craft has no place in preparing such a program.

The accumulation of experiences as a clinician, an educator, or an administrator, or possibly as a combination of these, would lead this therapist of the second generation to arrive at a new definition of occupational therapy. It would precede by several years an altered definition by the national organization. It would incorporate the social and behavioral sciences with a diminished emphasis upon medicine. Human development would appear for the first time as a focus for the treatment of physical and psychosocial dysfunction. She would declare, "Occupational therapy's function is to provide skilled assistance in influencing human objectives; its approach is inextricably conjoined with the behavioral factors involved. It is interested in how the process of growth and development is modified by hospitalization, chronic illness or a permanent handicap."[72]

This refocus of occupational therapy would stress the totality of the human organism. The therapist would say, "It was inevitable, therefore, that there (would) evolve an ever increasing emphasis in occupational therapy . . . a greater understanding of the part that the developmental process plays in the preventive and therapeutic factors of this form of treatment."[73]

This description is based on one individual, Miss Beatrice D. Wade, OTR, FAOTA.

The story is far from finished. Without a doubt, someone will chronicle the lives and works of those who are still making contributions, from that era to the present generation. Among them are Marjorie Fish, Virginia Kilburn, Mary Reilly, Ruth Robinson, Clare Spackman, Ruth Brunyate Weimer, Carlotta Welles, and Wilma West, each of whom continues to serve in clarifying and defining reasonable and reasoned alternatives. As counselors they confirm old values and clearly point out new directions, as well as our faithfulness or infidelity to those timeless principles established by our professional ancestors.

Lessons from Our History

The history of occupational therapy is often neglected. However, it is reassuring to note that records and accounts still exist which are extremely relevant to today's endeavors. Lessons can and must be learned.

Mind and Body Inextricably Conjoined

We must refuse to accept any alternative to the belief in the wholeness of the human, that the mind and body are inextricably conjoined. Illness, treatment, and the return to a healthful state simultaneously affect the physiological and emotional processes. Indeed, should these processes ever become separated, occupational therapy would be of no value.

The Natural Science of the Human

The inextricable unity of the human leads to another lesson. The science fundamental to practice is the natural science of the human. No amount of neurophysiology, psychology, sociology, or child development alone can determine the differential diagnosis, treatment, or prognosis of the patient undergoing occupational therapy. The current trend toward specialization, with its varying emphases upon one or another science to the neglect of other sciences, and indeed to the neglect of other nonscientific aspects of occupational therapy, borders on superstition and mythology. It is the continuous acquisition and scientific synthesis of the ingredients of the human organism and its surroundings that guarantee authentic occupational therapy.

The Human Organism's Involvement in Tasks

Occupational therapy is the only major health profession that focuses upon the total human organism's involvement in tasks in making or doing. In spite of the many grafts effected, its roots remain in the sub-soil of the art, the craft: a paradigm of the total activity of the human. Like those who have come before us, we think of ourselves and others fundamentally as makers, as users, as doers, as tools. We look at "craft as a way in which man may create and cross a bridge within himself and center himself in his own essential unity."[74] The procedures one goes through in rearranging and reassembling the basic elements in art or craft operate upon and within; "his material modifies him as he modifies it, in proportion to his openness, his awareness of the exchange that is taking place."[74]

The Differentiation of Occupational Therapy

Any definition, description, or differentiation between ourselves and other health providers must have occupation and leisure as its major theme. Otherwise, we become a blurred copy of a host of others: physical therapists, social workers, psychologists, nurses, physicians, and psychiatrists.

Without the dynamics of human motion inherent in purposeful activity, we become quasi-physical therapists. Without the interaction between human objects and the objects of work and leisure, we become quasi-social workers, psychologists, or nurses. Without the demonstrated and proven interrelationships between healthful, normal growth and development, activity, and the pathology of illness and handicapping conditions, we become quasi-physicians and psychiatrists.

The Legacy of Experience

Too often there is the disposition to think that those lessons another generation learned do not apply to the present. We should be mindful that there are two ways to learn: by our own experience and from those who have made discoveries, regardless of how long ago they were made. The experience of others is a magnificent heritage, and the more we learn from them, the less time we waste in the present proving what has already been proved.

It is, however, of great importance to realize that we are influenced by those who came before us more than we can truly know. Who they were and what they did have immeasurable bearing upon what we are and what we do. No generation is capable of isolating itself from its past. The past, what we are, and what we do greatly assist in fashioning our future.

The archives, the portraits and photographs, the published accounts, and the personal memorabilia and scrapbooks are records of considerable moment. In the least, they are a profound reminder of the possibility that someday, someone may be looking back and may be wondering who we were and what we did.

Conclusion

I will conclude with the observations of two former Presidents of the AOTA, Mr. Thomas B. Kidner and Mrs. Eleanor Clarke Slagle. In 1930 Mr. Kidner offered a personal impression of the state of occupational therapy at the annual meeting of the Connecticut Occupational Therapy Society. He urged us to "look on occupational therapy with increased faith as the years go by as a natural means of aiding in the restoration of the sick and disabled to health and working capacity (which means happiness) because it appeals to all our human attributes."[57]

Mrs. Slagle, one year after she retired in 1937, observed that "the story of the profession of occupational therapy will never be fully told, nor will that of the patients who have so abundantly appreciated the opportunities of the service. There has been no fanciful crusading 'for the cause;' it has meant that a few have perhaps borne many burdens, but in the slow process that makes permanent things of great value, it can be said that there is a fine body of professional workers, experienced and well trained, coming forward and being welcomed to a really great human service, that of helping to show the way to the person with large disabilities to make the best of his incomplete self."[75] "The integrity of your profession is in your hands. I bid you all Godspeed in your work."[76]

References

1. Locke, J: *An Essay Concerning Human Understanding: Two Volumes*, New York: Dover Press, 1894.

2. Frost, SE: *Basic Teachings of the Great Philosophers*, New York: Barnes and Noble, 1942.

3. Riese, W: *The Legacy of Philippe Pinel: An Inquiry into Thought on Mental Alienation*, New York: Springer Publishing Co., 1969.

4. de Condillac, EB: *Oeuvres Philosophiques de Condillac*, Paris: Presse Universataires de France, 1947.

5. Ackerknecht, EH: *A Short History of Psychiatry*, New York: Hafner, 1968.

6. Tuke, DH: *A Dictionary of Psychological Medicine: Volume One*, Philadelphia: P. Blakiston, 1892.

7. Pinel, P: *Traite Medico-Philosophique sur l'Alienation Mentale*, Paris: Richard, Caille & Rover, 1801.

8. Pinel, P: *A Treatise on Insanity in Which Are Contained the Principles of a New and More Practical Nosology of Maniacal Disorders*, Translated by DD Davis, London: Cadell & Davis, 1806. Facsimile published by Hafner Publishing Co., New York, 1962.

9. Mackler, B: *Philippe Pinel: Unchainer of the Insane*, New York: Franklin Watts, 1968.

10. Folsom, CF: *Diseases of the Mind: Notes on the Early Management, European and American Progress*, Boston: A. Williams & Co., 1877.

11. Jones, K: *Lunacy, Law, and Conscience; 1744 - 1845: The Social History of Care of the Insane*, London: Routledge & Kegan Paul, 1955.

12. Dillenberger, J and Welch, C: *Protestant Christianity: Interpreted Through Its Development*, New York: Charles Scribner's Sons, 1954.

13. *Philadelphia Yearly Meeting of the Religious Society of Friends: Faith and Practice, Philadelphia: Philadelphia Yearly Meeting, 1972.*

14. Tuke, DH: *Reform in the Treatment of the Insane. Early History of the Retreat, York; Its Objects and Influence*, London: J & A Churchill, 1872.

15. Tuke, DH: *Reform in the Treatment of the Insane: An Early History of the Retreat, York: Its Objects and Influence*, London: J & A Churchill, 1892.

16. Tuke S: *Description of The Retreat, An Institution Near York for Insane Persons of the Society of Friends: Containing an Account of Its Origins and Progress, The Modes of Treatment, and a Statement of Cases*, York, England: Alexander, 1813.

17. Hunter, R and Macalpine, I: *Three Hundred Years of Psychiatry, 1535 - 1860: A History Presented in Selected English Texts*, London: Oxford University Press, 1963.

18. Conolly, J: *The Treatment of the Insane Without Mechanical Restraints*, London: Smith, Elder & Co., 1856. Facsimile published, Pall Mall, England: Dawson's, 1973.

19. Ellis, WC: *A Treatise on the Nature, Symptoms, Causes, and Treatment of Insanity*, London: Holdsworth, 1888.

20. Goodman, N: *Benjamin Rush: Physician and Citizen, 1746-1813*, Philadelphia: University of Pennsylvania Press, 1934.

21. Rush, B: *Medical Inquiries and Observations Upon the Diseases of the Mind,* 4th ed., Philadelphia: J Grigg, 1830.

22. Buckmaster, H: *Women Who Shaped History*, New York: Macmillan, 1966.

23. Bucknill, JC and Tuke, DH: *A Manual of Psychological Medicine*, New York: Hafner, 1968. Facsimile of 1858 Edition.

24. Barlow, J: *Man's Power Over Himself to Prevent or Control Insanity*, London: William Pickering, 1843.

25. Skultans, V: *Madness and Morals: Ideas on Insanity in the Nineteenth Century*, London: Routledge & Kegan Paul, 1975.

26. Tuke, DH: *A Dictionary of Psychological Medicine: Volume Two*, Philadelphia: P. Blakiston Son & Co., 1892.

27. Bockhoven, JS: *Moral Treatment in American Psychiatry*, New York: Springer, 1963.

28. Dain, N: *Concepts of Insanity in the United States, 1789-1865*, New Brunswick, NJ: Rutgers University Press, 1964.

29. Deutsch, A: *The Mentally Ill in America: A History of Their Care and Treatment from Colonial Times*, 2nd ed. New York: Columbia University Press, 1949.

30. Tracy, SE: The development of occupational therapy in the Grace Hospital, Detroit, Michigan, *Trained Nurse and Hosp Review*, 66:5, May 1921.

31. Tracy, SE: The place of invalid occupations in the general hospital, *The Modern Hospital*, 2:5, June 1914.

32. Tracy, SE: Twenty-five suggested mental tests derived from invalid occupations, *Maryland Psychiatric Quarterly*, 8, 1918.

33. Barrows, M: Susan E. Tracy, RN. *Maryland Psychiatric Quarterly*, 6, 1916-1917.

34. Tracy, SE: Treatment of disease by employment at St. Elizabeths Hospital, *The Modern Hospital*, 20:2, February 1923.

35. Parsons, SE: Miss Tracy's work in general hospitals, *Maryland Psychiatric Quarterly*, 6, 1916-1917.

36. Tracy, SE: *Studies in Invalid Occupation*, Boston: Whitcomb and Barrows, 1918.

37. Tracy, SE: Power versus money in occupation therapy, *Trained Nurse and Hosp Review*, 66:2, February 1921.

38. Barton, GE: A view of invalid occupation, *Trained Nurse and Hosp Review*, 52:8, June 1914.

39. Barton, GE: Occupational nursing, *Trained Nurse and Hosp Review*, 54:6, June 1915.

40. Barton, GE: Occupational therapy, *Trained Nurse and Hosp Review*, 54:3, March 1915.

41. Barton, GE: The existing hospital system and reconstruction, *Trained Nurse and Hosp Review*, 69:4, October 1922.

42. Barton, GE: What occupational therapy may mean to nursing, *Trained Nurse and Hosp Review*, 64:4, April 1920.

43. Barton, GE: *Re-education: An Analysis of the Institutional System of the United States*, Boston: Houghton Mifflin, 1917.

44. Sheppard Asylum: *Third Annual Report of the Sheppard Asylum*, Towson, MD: unpub., 1895.

45. Dunton, WR: The relationship of occupational therapy and physical therapy, *Arch Phys Ther*, 16, January 1935.

46. Dunton, WR: The principles of occupational therapy, *Proceedings of the National Society for the Promotion of Occupational Therapy: Second Annual Meeting*, Catonsville, MD: Spring Grove State Hospital, 1918.

47. Dunton, WR: *Occupation Therapy: A Manual for Nurses*, Philadelphia: WB Saunders, 1915.

48. Komora, PO: Eleanor Clarke Slagle, Mental Hygiene, 27:1, January 1943.

49. Pollock, HM: In Memoriam: Eleanor Clarke Slagle, 1876-1942, *Amer J Psych*, 99:3, November 1941.

50. *Then and Now, 1917-1967*, New York: American Occupational Therapy Association, 1967.

51. Loomis, B and Wade, BD: *Chicago . . . Occupational Therapy Beginnings: Hull House, The Henry B. Favill School of Occupations and Eleanor Clarke Slagle*, unpub.

52. Slagle, EC: Occupational therapy: Recent methods and advances in the United States, *Occup Ther & Rehab*, 13:5, October 1934.

53. Slagle, EC: History of the development of occupation for the insane, *Maryland Psychiatric Quarterly*, 4, May 1914.

54. Slagle, EC: Training aides for mental patients, *Arch Occup Ther*, 1:1, February 1922.

55. Slagle, EC and Robeson, HA: *Syllabus for Training of Nurses in Occupational Therapy*, Utica, NY: State Hospital Press, no date.

56. Slagle, EC: A year's development of occupational therapy in New York state hospitals, *Modern Hospital*, 22:1, January 1924.

57. Kidner, TB: Occupational therapy, its development, scope and possibilities, *Occup Ther & Rehab*, 10:1, February 1931.

58. Meyer, A: The psychological point of view. In Brady, JP (ed): *Classics in American Psychiatry*, St. Louis: Warren H Green, 1975.

59. Arieti, S: *American Handbook of Psychiatry: Volume Two*, New York: Basic Books, 1959.

60. Lief, A: *The Commonsense Psychiatry of Dr. Adolf Meyer: Fifty-two Selected Papers*, New York: McGraw-Hill, 1948.

61. Meyer, A: The philosophy of occupation therapy, *Arch Occup Ther*, 1:1, February 1922. Reprinted in *Amer J Occup Ther*, 31:10, November - December 1977.

62. Meyer, A: The rise to the person and the concept of wholes or integrates, *Amer J Psych*, 100, April 1944.

63. Pattison, HA: The trend of occupational therapy for the tuberculous, *Arch Occup Ther*, 1:1, February 1922.

64. Coulter, JS and McNary, H: Necessity of medical supervision in occupational therapy, *Occup Ther & Rehab*, 10:1, February 1931.

65. An outline of lectures on occupational therapy to medical students and physicians, *Occup Ther & Rehab*, 4:4, August 1925.

66. Wade, BD: Occupational therapy: A history of its practice in the psychiatric field, paper presented at 51st Annual Conference, American Occupational Therapy Association, Boston, October 19, 1967.

67. Advisory Committee in Occupational Therapy: The basic philosophy and function of occupational therapy, *University of Illinois Faculty-Alumni Newsletter of the Chicago Professional Colleges*, 6:4, January 1951.

68. Wade, BD: A survey of occupational and industrial therapy in the Illinois state hospitals, *Illinois Psych J*, 2:1, March 1942.

69. Wade, BD: Supportive care, *Bulletin of the Rehabilitation Institute of Chicago*.

70. Wade, BD: Hospital industries and the rehabilitation of the mentally ill, paper presented to the Department of Public Welfare, State of Minnesota, June 26, 1958.

71. Willard, HS, and Spackman, CS: *Principles of Occupational Therapy*, First Edition, Philadelphia: JB Lippincott, 1947.

72. Wage, BD: The development of clinically oriented education in occupational therapy: The Illinois plan, paper presented at the 49th Annual Conference, American Occupational Therapy Association, Miami, November 2, 1965.

73. Wade, BD: *The Preparation of Occupational Therapy Students for Functioning with Aging Persons and in Comprehensive Health Care Programs: A Manual for Educators*, Chicago: University of Illinois Medical Center, 1969.

74. Dooling, EM: *Way of Working*, Garden City, NY: Anchor Press/Doubleday, 1979.

75. Slagle, EC: Occupational Therapy, *Trained Nurse & Hosp Review*, 100:4, April 1938.

76. Slagle, EC: Editorial: From the heart, *Occup Ther & Rehab*, 16:5, October 1937.

Acknowledgments

A study of this nature and scope is not possible without the valuable and valued assistance of numerous individuals and sources. I wish to recognize the incomparable services provided by the staffs of the Moody Medical Library, The University of Texas Medical Branch at Galveston; the Quine Library, University of Illinois at the Medical Center, Chicago; the McGoogan Library of Medicine, University of Nebraska Medical Center, Omaha; and the Archives, Shapiro Developmental Center (Eastern Illinois State Hospital), Kankakee.

I am also grateful to all the following people: Lillian Hoyle Parent, OTR, Kathryn Reed, OTR, William C. Levin, MD, John G. Bruhn, PhD, Chester R. Burns, MD, PhD, James L. Cantwell, PhD, Charles H. Christiansen, EdD, Suzanne Hooker, DipOT, Lillian Hoyle Parent, MW, Eleanor Porter, Shirley H. Carr, OTR, Barbara Loomis, OTR, Margaret Mirenda, OTR, Beatrice D. Wade, OTR, Kay B. Hudgens, OTR, James Garibaldi, Mardy Hick, Betty Cox, Randall Rogers, W. Gregory Hunicurt, Judy Hargett, Daniel L. Creson, MD, PhD, Lucille M. Burnworth, Adele Jaco, Laura Reed, Judy Grace, and Frances Sawyer.

CHAPTER 2

The COTA: A Chronological Review

Haru Hirama, OTR/L

Editor's Note

The history of the certified occupational therapy assistant is presented as a chronology of the significant events in the development, education, and utilization of assistants in the delivery of occupational therapy services from 1949 to 1985.

The initial need for assistants grew out of manpower shortages in psychiatric occupational therapy, and developed over the years to the point where assistants were finding employment opportunities in all areas of practice. As the number of certified occupational therapy assistants increased, and the tasks delegated to them expanded, role and relationship problems and conflicts were identified. While many of the issues have been successfully resolved, others are in the process of resolution. Figure 2-1 at the conclusion of this chapter provides a summary of some of the most significant milestones in the history of the COTA.

The Beginning - A Plan to Extend Occupational Therapy Service

At the March 1949 meeting of the Board of Management of the American Occupational Therapy Association (AOTA) a proposal was made to establish a one year educational program for occupational therapy assistants in psychiatric hospitals. The plan was referred to the Committee on Psychiatry, Sub-Committee on Research for study.[1] The history of the certified occupational therapy assistant (COTA) began with that proposal.

On October 1, 1956, the AOTA Board of Management approved a plan to recognize aide-level occupational therapy personnel. The committee to implement the plan, chaired by Marion Crampton, was named the Committee on the Recognition of Occupational Therapy Aides (CROTA).

The committee was to develop a plan to recognize and train aides in occupational therapy.[2]

Crampton reported on the committee's progress to Colonel Ruth A. Robinson, President of the AOTA and the AOTA Board of Management, on October 20, 1957, in Cleveland, Ohio. The Board voted that "Certified Occupational Therapy Assistant" appear on an insignia to be worn to identify the COTA. The document, *Requirements of an Acceptance Program and the Curriculum Guide*, was accepted. Committee recommendations covered curriculum, workshops for instructors, and providing personnel, time, and space at the AOTA office to implement the plan. It was voted to authorize the expenditure of funds for whatever cost was to be involved in the implementation of the plan. The 5,233 registered occupational therapists (OTRs) in the U.S. were insufficient to meet the demand for services, so it was essential to add assistants to the work force as soon as possible. The committee chairman and the executive director were charged with the responsibility of implementation.[3,4] The plan was officially implemented in October 1958 when letters were sent to "state commissioners of mental health and other appropriate agencies and individuals"[5] recognizing the occupational therapy assistant.

Progress was reported in *The American Journal of Occupational Therapy*. The COTA insignia was available from AOTA to graduates of approved occupational therapy assistant programs, and to those who had worked two years in a disability area prior to the establishment of national standards. Satisfactory recommendations from three qualified individuals, one being the current registered occupational therapist supervisor, were required. It was agreed that qualification by work experience (grandfather clause) would terminate three years after the establishment of AOTA training standards. COTAs were not to have a vote in AOTA affairs, or representation in the House of Delegates or on the Board of Management[5].

The training programs for COTAs were established in the type of facility requiring the services of a COTA. One instructor was required for every 15 students. Admission to the program required that the individual be a high school graduate or equivalent, employed as an occupational therapy aide, in good physical and emotional health, 18 to 55 years of age, intelligent, mature, emotionally stable, flexible, cooperative, have the ability to establish and maintain effective interpersonal relationships, and be recommended for the program by a qualified person. The curriculum required 12 weeks for 460 hours, which included a minimum of 140 clock hours of didactic content, specialty skills, and supervised practical experience. The curriculum prepared the individual to work in psychiatric hospitals.[5]

The Executive Director's report in the 1958 AOTA annual report confirmed the completion of plans for the proposed COTA training program. Aides could apply to become COTAs under the grandfather clause. The CROTA acted as a review board to determine the qualifications of applicants.[6]

The 1960s - Early Education

The Board of Management reported that 336 COTAs joined AOTA under the grandfather clause by April 1, 1960. Approval was given for a plan to recognize and certify occupational therapy assistants in general practice. The curriculum for COTAs in general practice was scheduled to be implemented by October 1960. An annual recertification fee for COTAs was established.[7]

Many nursing homes in Maryland were interested in hiring occupational therapy assistants to conduct activity programs for their residents. A grant was obtained in Montgomery County, Maryland, to train COTAs in a nursing home setting. The 3 month course, scheduled from February 27 to June 2, 1961, enrolled 14 students, ranging in age from 21 to 55, whose backgrounds included business school and college. The program required 400 classroom hours plus supervised clinical practice.[8]

At the 1963 Board of Management meeting held in St. Louis, concern over the growing number of COTAs was voiced. The desirability of a "purely professional" association was discussed. The possibilty of assisting COTAs to achieve independence as a group was even considered. Others pointed out the increased need for COTAs to provide direct service, as more OTRs acquired graduate degrees and did not provide direct service. The need for defining the roles of the assistant and the therapist was raised. It was suggested that more meaningful COTA participation in the profession could be encouraged by membership workshops planned especially for COTAs, and by allowing some type of voting privilege. The Board of Management established three membership categories: 1) OTRs; 2) students enrolled in an approved occupational therapy school; and 3) COTAs. Voting privileges and the right to hold office were to be limited to OTRs. The COTA membership did not receive the privilege of receiving the association journal.[9]

There were 768 COTAs by August 20, 1963 (656 in psychiatry and 112 in general practice). Certified occupational therapy assistant programs were operated by a variety of organizations such as the Senior Centers of Metropolitan Chicago, which was endorsed for training COTAs in general practice. The Committee on Occupational Therapy Assistants requested Board action for authority to:

1 establish combined psychiatry and general practice programs;
2 establish OTA programs based on area of needs in educational institutions;
3 establish programs in junior colleges or community colleges and extend the programs beyond eighteen weeks;
4 re-interpret the AOTA policy that COTA programs will not be in institutions where professional occupational therapy curricula are conducted; and
5 seek guidance in replying to inquires requesting approval to establish programs.[9]

At the annual conference in St. Louis, the AOTA Council on Education began discussions on how to channel COTAs to the OTR level.[10] At the mid-year meeting in Indianapolis, the Council focused on educating OTRs to supervise COTAs.[11]

In August 1964, 863 COTAs were listed by AOTA. The total included 527 grandfathered COTAs (454 in psychiatry and 73 in general practice) and 336 from endorsed programs (219 in psychiatry and 117 in general practice). Mount Aloysius Junior College in Pennsylvania and St. Mary's Junior College in Minnesota began occupational therapy assistant programs in 1964 and 1965 respectively.[12]

The first advertisement for employment of a COTA appeared in the *American Journal of Occupational Therapy* in 1965.[13] The same issue published the first article by a certified occupational therapy assistant, entitled "Tool Holder," by Alene A. Johnson.[14]

In 1966 Adamson and Anderson publish a survey of 75 psychiatric and 76 physical disabilities facilities to determine utilization of COTAs and aides. One hundred respondents reported a total of 64 COTAs, 128 uncertified assistants, and 125 aides whose duties and responsibilities were undifferentiated. Functional programs were planned and conducted by aides and assistants in both psychiatric and physical disabilities services. The COTAs functioned with guidance and consultation from OTRs. In physical disabilities facilities, the aides prepared projects and transported patients. Ninety percent responded that trained assistants could alleviate the shortage of OTRs, 5 percent responded that assistants could not, and 5 percent had no comment. The authors emphasized the need for AOTA to define the role of the COTA, the OTR's role in guidance and supervision, and the supervisory structure, and to state a philosophy.[15]

The final endorsement of occupational therapy assistant training programs was designated to be a function of the Accreditation Committee. In 1964 Mount Aloysius Junior College graduated its second class of COTAs, and St. Mary's Junior College graduated its first class. Colonel Ruth A. Robinson was appointed project director of a workshop on the role and function of the COTA in relation to the OTR.[16]

The 1965 Delegate Assembly passed a resolution to charge the COTA one fee instead of the two previously required of those certified in both psychiatry and general practice. There were three "grandfathered" COTAs certified in both areas. A pilot program combined the study of psychiatry and general practice. Graduation from the pilot program entitled COTAs to a dual certification. A resolution giving COTAs a proportional vote in AOTA affairs, representation on governing bodies, and a section within AOTA for expressing their interests and concerns was defeated.[17] The first dual trained class of assistants worked in a general hospital providing diversional activities for 15 to 20 patients per day, ordering equipment and supplies, and making adapted equipment designed by the OTR.[18]

In 1966 there were 12 occupational therapy assistant educational programs in operation, two of which granted associate degrees. All future COTA educational programs were to prepare graduates to work in psychiatry and general medicine.[19]

In 1967 the Social Security Administration certified 3,500 nursing homes as extended care facilities to render acute post-hospital care to Medicare patients. Carr[20] advocated the use of COTAs with OTR consultants to fill the anticipated 15,000 occupational therapy positions in nursing homes.

In a review of the first 50 years of AOTA, President Brunyate[21] described the OTR/COTA relationship as abrasive. She saw the relationship as the OTR's attempt to protect the OTR role and the COTA's definsive reaction. Brunyate reminded the membership that OTRs and COTAs are part of the same profession, with each group having a distinct role.

A Guide for the Supervision of the Certified Occupational Therapy Assistant, established by AOTA in 1967, stated that the COTA was to be supervised by an OTR, an experienced COTA, or an OTR designate. Mildred Schwagmeyer, Director of Technical Education Services, reported that there were 1,102 COTAs, of which 313 were AOTA members and 789 nonmembers. The first COTA meeting was held at the annual conference in 1967. Forty-seven people representing nine states attended.[22] Fifty OTRs met at Hot Springs, Arkansas, to discuss trends in occupational therapy and to find solutions to the shortage of OTRs. The group considered having OTRs supervise COTAs, who would then carry out assigned duties.[23]

Ten years after the implementation of training programs for occupational therapy assistants, there were 20 training programs and over 1,200 COTAs. AOTA President Cromwell asked for a role identification of the OTR and COTA, as well as the integration of the COTA into association and work activities. She recognized the COTAs' reticence to seek avenues for their own recognition and appealed to the membership to work toward this goal.[24] By 1968, 1,213 COTAs were members of AOTA, and eight were serving on AOTA committees.[25]

Schwagmeyer acknowledged the 10th birthday of the COTA by reviewing the history of the occupational therapy assistant. Results of a 1968 COTA survey revealed that half of the 819 COTAs employed were employed under job titles other than occupational therapy assistant. The titles included: occupational therapy instructor, activity therapist, and director of occupational therapy; 361 had job descriptions, 247 did not. Of 223 job descriptions received by the author, many were not descriptive of a COTA position. Seventy-three percent of the COTAs stated that they had no OTR supervision. Of 727 COTAs employed full-time, most received the minimum wage or less.[26]

Cantwell suggested a change in the title of the COTA from "assistant" to "associate." Three COTA levels were suggested:

1 an occupational therapy aide requiring a 5 month education program;
2 a COTA to carry out patient care requiring a 1 year program;
3 a COTA to carry out treatment programs and administrative tasks, and to assist in research requiring a 2 year associate degree.

He suggested that the role of the COTA and the academic program be reviewed because of the growing health care needs in the United States.[27]

The annual report of the forty-ninth AOTA conference showed the 1968-69 period to have the greatest increase in the number of occupational therapy assistant programs in any one year period. There were 26 approved programs, of which seven were associate degree programs and nine were one year academic programs. An estimated eight new programs were to begin enrollment in Fall 1970. There were 1,349 COTAs and 9,463 OTRs in 1969. Eleven COTAs with associate degrees were enrolled in programs leading toward baccalaureate degrees in occupational therapy.[28]

Bolton reported that 29 COTAs attended the 1969 annual AOTA conference, and that 13 served on national committees. The possibility that COTAs were not taking advantage of privileges existing in the AOTA bylaws was raised. However, it was noted that COTAs did not receive the bylaws and thus were not aware of their privileges. The Executive Board approved enclosure of a copy of the bylaws in the 1970 mailing of the *Member Directory*.[29]

The 1970s - COTA Education and Qualifications Defined

At the 1970 Annual Conference, a number of resolutions that related to COTAs were acted on. A resolution was adopted to evaluate methods of measuring the skills and qualifications for becoming a COTA. A resolution to change the name of COTA to "certified occupational therapy technician" failed. A resolution to establish a membership category for COTAs wishing to receive the *American Journal of Occupational Therapy* was withdrawn. A resolution to make military occupational therapy technicians eligible for certification as occupational therapy assistants was adopted as amended. The individual was required to be in military service, to have been employed in occupational therapy for at least 12 months within the previous 2-year period, and to have a recommendation from an OTR. The resolution enabled military-trained occupational therapy technicians to apply for AOTA certification in January 1971. As a result, 17 Army, 14 Air Force, and 11 Navy occupational therapy technicians became COTAs. A resolution was adopted that the Council on Standards study and suggest alternative eligibility qualifications for becoming a COTA. A resolution to phase out specialty COTA programs by January 1975 failed. Approval of specialty programs for COTAs was to be discontinued by 1972 or at the time of the program's re-approval.[30]

Ritvo, Lyons, and Howe[31] emphasized the need to anticipate the future role of the COTA and plan accordingly. They suggested that the roles of the COTA and OTR be flexible and responsive to human needs as well as to local situations and requirements. They stressed the need for the OTR to have supervisory skills in order to work with the COTA. The authors recommended that training prepare COTAs for possible problems they would encounter on the job. Problems identified included the OTR and COTA relationship, conflict between OTR and COTA goals, and lack of definite program role expectations.

In 1971 a proposal was made to require a national examination for the initial certification of occupational therapy assistants. The AOTA membership billing form gave COTAs the choice of receiving the association journal, previously denied them. A resolution was proposed to develop eligibility criteria and procedures whereby COTAs would be allowed to take the registration exam to become OTRs.[32]

April 1971 COTA statistics showed that 11 percent of the 738 reporting were male. For the first time, the 1971 AOTA Registry and Directory combined the listing of OTRs and COTAs in one volume.[32] Wiemer recommended a clear delineation of the COTA role. She stated that the individual differences and potential skills of the COTA needed to be recognized and maximized.[33]

The University of Maryland was the site of an AOTA-funded workshop on OTR/COTA relationships in July 1972. Sally Ryan, COTA, served as the liaison between COTAs and the Council on Development. The focus was to help COTAs identify with AOTA and take a greater part in formulating association policies.[34]

The abrasive relationship identified earlier by Brunyate was publicly noted. Keith, an OTR, wrote that she drove 60 miles to a district occupational therapy meeting and was in a "state of shock" from the meeting. She questioned why there was a push for COTA programs when schools and employment were crowded with OTRs. She stated that she hated to be replaced by someone who was able to receive a license to practice occupational therapy in only one or two years.[35] Spelbring responded that other OTRs voiced similar apprehensions; however, many COTAs performed at a level equal to that of some OTRs. Administrators had a responsibility to hire the least costly personnel capable of filling the position.[36]

Hunter, an OTR, stated that she became "riled" after reading the newsletter item about the OTR/COTA workshop. She saw no need for COTAs to take on a role in the management and development of the profession, and considered the primary reason for the existence of the COTA to be the provision of direct service to patients. The resolution that COTAs be given full rights and privileges in AOTA seemed equivalent to the child telling the parent what to do.[37] Oliver, a COTA, responded to Hunter's letter by pointing out that large numbers of COTAs provide services previously provided by OTRs.[38] Jeanne Poggen, COTA, stated that some COTAs have grown beyond the basic standards set for COTAs because they have increased their knowledge, demonstrated their abilities, and been given the freedom to function at increasingly higher levels. She questioned why

OTRs were not doing the same. She felt that the profession needed both the COTA and the OTR.[39]

The first book review by a COTA appeared in the *American Journal of Occupational Therapy* in 1972, when Ruth L. Knapp, R.N., B.S., COTA, reviewed *Activity Programs for Senior Citizens* by Fish.[40] Bette Ackerman, COTA, wrote that OTRs need not feel threatened by the COTA's consideration of a title change. COTAs cannot function in the same capacity as OTRs, but in most instances are not assistants to OTRs. Norma Mahoney, COTA, wrote to encourage COTAs to take an active role in AOTA and voice their thoughts not as children to parents, but in an adult to adult dialogue.[41]

All specialty occupational therapy assistant educational programs were to terminate by December 31, 1972. The Wisconsin Division of Mental Hygiene, where classes had been conducted since 1959, graduated its sixteenth and last class in November 1972.[42] The Council on Standards voiced concern over the existing certification system requiring only graduation from an approved educational curriculum and recommendation from the program director to become a COTA.[42] It was felt that a more stringent method was needed.

Sally Ryan, COTA, expressed her concern for the quality and competence of COTAs and the certification plans. She noted that the 9 month, 11 month, and 2 year college degree programs all produced COTAs.[43]

Resolution 311-71 allowed COTAs who meet established criteria to sit for the AOTA registration examination. The criteria were approved by the Council on Standards in April 1972.[42] On February 12, 1973, the Executive Board endorsed the statement on career mobility, which allowed those COTAs with relevant work experience to sit for the AOTA registration examination.[44]

The Delegate Assembly met in Warrenton, Virginia, in April, 1973. The *Essentials for an Occupational Therapy Assistant Educational Program* were being written, and roles and functions of occupational therapy personnel were being delineated to serve as a basis for developing proficiency examinations. Six levels of occupational therapy personnel were identified: 1) aide; 2) entry-level COTA; 3) experienced COTA;4) entry-level therapist; 5) experienced therapist; and 6) specialized practitioner, program administrator, researcher, or clinical and/or academic instructor. Resolution 356-73 amended the bylaws, making COTAs eligible for election as Members-at-Large to the Executive Board of AOTA. The American Occupational Therapy Association listed 10,464 OTRs and 1,928 COTAs in December 1972.[45]

AOTA membership in December 1973 was 12,080 OTRs and 2,578 COTAs. Dolores Cook, COTA, served on the Council on Development. Toné Blechert, COTA, served on the Government Affairs Committee. A motion that the bylaws be amended to require COTAs to receive *The American Journal of Occupational Therapy* failed.[46]

Under the career mobility plan, 24 COTAs applied to take the January 1974 OTR examination. Of the nine COTAs who became OTRs through the plan, six completed additional field work in order to meet criteria for admission. Their work experience as COTAs ranged from five to nine years.[46] Three COTAs wrote an article in the *American Journal of Occupational Therapy* describing a self-learning method for teaching craft and activity techniques.[47]

The 1975 Delegate Assembly acted on five resolutions concerning COTAs. A resolution to change the bylaws to enable COTAs to be eligible for positions of Delegate and Alternate Delegate failed, as did a resolution to make COTAs eligible for the AOTA Roster of Fellows. A resolution to establish a COTA Award of Excellence was adopted. Another successful resolution stated new criteria for COTA entry to the professional-level certification examination. Beginning in January 1976, the requirements to sit for the examination included current certification with AOTA, field work experience, and four years of work experience as a COTA.[48]

In 1975 COTAs became eligible to be nominated for the Award of Merit (the highest honor of the AOTA) and the Eleanor Clarke Slagle Lectureship (the academic honor of the AOTA).[49] The *Essentials of an Approved Educational Program for the Occupational Therapy Assistant* (the *Essentials*) were established and adopted by AOTA in April 1975. COTA educational programs assumed responsibility for ensuring that the *Essentials* were met and maintained.[50]

A special session of the Delegate Assembly was held in Milwaukee on October 15-18, 1975. Among the resolutions adopted were that COTAs receive *AJOT* as a regular membership benefit, that membership fees for retired COTAs be waived, and that a certification examination for COTAs be developed.[51]

At the twelfth annual meeting of the Delegate Assembly in Atlanta, the legislative and policy-making body of AOTA was changed from Delegate Assembly to Representative Assembly. A motion to make COTAs eligible for election to the Representative Assembly was defeated. The Representative Assembly adopted a resolution to require all occupational therapy assistant candidates completing approved programs after October 31, 1976, to pass a written certification examination. The first COTA certification examination was scheduled for June 1977.[52]

The final meeting of the Delegate Assembly was held in San Francisco in October 1976, with President Jerry A. Johnson presiding. Another attempt to change the COTA title failed. Adopted resolutions stated policy for admission to the certification examination for COTAs, policy for recertification of COTAs whose certification had lapsed, and changes in fieldwork requirements for COTAs applying to take the professional-level occupational therapy certification examination.[53] Sally Ryan, COTA, was elected Executive Board Member-at-Large.[54]

A resolution for a name change was again defeated by the 1978 Representative Assembly.[55] A decision was made at the annual business meeting to award a designated COTA with the Roster of Honor.[56]

The 1979 Representative Assembly adopted a policy that "the initials 'COTA' shall be restricted for use by COTAs currently certified by AOTA. Assistants licensed by the state and not holding AOTA certification shall use other designations and initials required by the state."[57]

The 1980s - COTA Concerns and Role Defined

At the 1980 annual conference in Denver, the Executive Board was charged to develop a plan to enable COTAs to enhance their professional commitment and participation. It was noted that COTAs had no formal means of communicating their needs to the Association, and that their input had been limited. A two year COTA advocacy position was funded.[58]

In 1981 the COTA Task Force, chaired by Toné Blechert, COTA, developed a chart of COTA concerns. Nine educational needs were identified:

1 accepted role delineation;
2 relevant and affordable continuing education;
3 COTA role models to assist in the education of technical and professional-level students in college systems to demonstrate the working relationships between the two levels;
4 a clear AOTA position on "non-traditional" laddering;
5 increased preparation for entry-level COTAs concerning program administration, working in systems, and assertiveness;
6 official field work performance reports for COTA students;
7 increased theoretical entry-level knowledge;
8 refresher courses for COTAs re-entering the field; and
9 non-traditional class schedules within college systems to facilitate career mobility, (i.e.,.evening or weekend occupational therapy programs).[59]

Eight practice concerns were listed:

1 opportunities for career advancement as a COTA;
2 a recertification process that promotes personal/professional growth;
3 appropriate state/federal classification for COTAs;
4 a clear policy on supervision of the COTA;
5 a title change (due to dissatisfaction with the term "assistant");
6 clear guidelines for COTA pay scales;
7 COTA representation on licensure boards; and
8 AOTA support when states restrict COTA responsibilities.[59]

Professional involvement concerns included the following:

1 COTA orientation to the structure, function, and communication channels of AOTA;
2 more involvement of COTAs in the state affiliate organizations;
3 COTA advocacy at the national level;

4 COTA advocacy at the state and regional levels;
5 having professional publications include more material relevant to the clinical practice of COTAs;
6 having COTAs contribute written work to the *American Journal of Occupational Therapy* and the *Occupational Therapy Newspaper* and speak at workshops and conferences;
7 fuller representation in the Representative Assembly and on national committees; and
8 public relations material to increase the visability of COTAs.[59]

Three resolutions were developed from the list of concerns:

1 that three seats filled by COTAs be added to the Representative Assembly;
2 that a COTA advocacy position be established at the National Office to address COTA issues from membership; and
3 that a national COTA committee be established to assist state affiliate committees with their goals and objectives.

Three motions were to:

1 recommend that continuing education workshops be developed by AOTA for COTAs;
2 inform members of salary levels through the *Occupational Therapy Newspaper*; and
3 continue the COTA Task Force as an ad hoc committee of the Executive Board for the purpose of monitoring proposed actions, providing information to the Representative Assembly at conferences, serving as a clearing house for COTA concerns, providing information, and promoting COTA involvement.[60]

Data were collected in 1976 to study the COTA in practice in an effort to delineate the roles of the COTA and OTR. The role delineation was to serve as the basis for a criterion-referenced entry exam for COTAs. Entry-level was defined as "the role assumed by personnel during the first 12 months of practice following initial AOTA certification." Direct service was defined as including all tasks performed for the care of clients. Data were collected from: 1) the worker log, 2) the observation interview, 3) the structured checklist inventory (SCI), and 4) the supervisor-structured checklist inventory (SSCI). The 223 COTAs certified in 1974, 1975, and 1976 were requested to complete a worker log. The five-consecutive day log listed each task performed, including why, how, to whom, and the amount of time spent. Thirty-five COTAs completed logs, and 33 COTAs certified in 1976 were interviewed. Of the 429 COTAs certified in 1976 who were mailed the SCI, 108 returned a form. Of 100 supervisors of entry-level COTAs, 64 returned an SSCI. Findings were that 48.1 percent of COTAs worked in physical rehabilitation, half of the COTAs were the only occupational therapy personnel at the facility, and 13.9 percent were supervised by the administrator of the facility.[61]

The 1981 Representative Assembly adopted the *Entry-Level OTR and COTA Role Delineation* developed from the preceding information. AOTA membership fees were waived for permanently disabled, unemployed COTAs, and fees were reduced for COTAs over 65 years of age.[62] The *Occupational Therapy Newspaper* invited COTAs to submit articles for publication. A column for COTAs was made available for a six month trial period.[63]

AOTA President Hightower-Vandamm identified flaws in the career mobility program, which permitted COTAs to become OTRs without formal education. Some states which had occupational therapy licensure laws did not recognize the OTR designation awarded by the career mobility program.[64] The 1982 Representative Assembly voted to terminate the career mobility program. A resolution to have COTA Members-at-Large on the Representative Assembly was also defeated.[65]

Bissell and Mailloux surveyed OTRs on the role of crafts in occupational therapy for physical dysfunctions. The majority of OTR respondents who used crafts in treatment carried out treatment and documented patient performance themselves, even though half of the therapists worked with assistants. The authors questioned whether COTAs could take on more responsibility in these programs.[66]

Curley, COTA, expressed a feeling of professional alienation after reading an article in which the OTR author included COTAs with "other disciplines." She suggested that the paucity of COTA involvement in the profession may be the result

FIGURE 2-1 SIGNIFICANT MILESTONES IN THE HISTORY OF THE COTA

1949 Proposal made to establish a one year program for training psychiatric assistants.

1956 Board of management approved plan to recognize aide-level occupational therapy personnel.

1958 Education and certification plan for occupational therapy assistants implemented; grandfather clause established.

1959 134 assistants certified by AOTA to practice in psychiatry.

1960 336 assistants certified by AOTA under grandfather clause.

1961 Program implemented in Maryland to train OTAs in a nursing home setting.

1963 Board of management established an AOTA membership category for COTAs.

1964 COTAs certified in general practice.

1965 First article written by a COTA appeared in AJOT.

1966 All future educational programs to train assistants in both psychiatry and general practice.

1967 Guide for supervision of the COTA established by AOTA; first COTA meeting held at the annual conference.

1968 Eight COTAs serving on AOTA committees.

1969 Tenth anniversary of COTAs acknowledged by Schwagmeyer history.

1970 Change in title from "assistant" to "associate" suggested; resolution to change "assistant" to "technician" failed.

1971 Military occupational therapy technicians became eligible for AOTA certification.

1972 National OTR/COTA relationships workshop held; first book review written by a COTA published in AJOT.

1973 Career mobility plan endorsed by the executive board; COTAs became eligible for election as a member-at-large of the executive board.

1974 First COTAs take certification examination as a part of the career mobility plan to become a registered occupational therapist.

1975 Second article written by COTAs published in AJOT; COTA Award of Excellence established; COTAs became eligible to receive the Award of Merit and the Eleanor Clark Slagle Lectureship; COTAs began receiving AJOT as a membership benefit.

1976 First COTA elected member-at-large of the executive board.

1977 First national certification examination given to occupational therapy assistants.

1978 Roster of honor award established.

1979 Policy adopted stating the initials "COTA" can be used only by assistants currently certified by AOTA.

1980 Two year COTA advocacy position funded.

1981 COTA Task Force established; eight COTAs served as members of the faculty of professional level O.T. educational programs; entry-level OTR and COTA role delineation adopted.

1982 Career mobility plan terminated; COTA Share column introduced in *Occupational Therapy Newspaper.*

1983 Representative assembly agreed that a COTA member-at-large elected to the assembly would have both voice and vote.

1985 First COTA representative and alternate representative of the representative assembly elected; AOTA estimates indicate that there will be 7500 COTAs in the United States by the end of the year.

Compiled by Sally E. Ryan, COTA, Editor

of COTAs' common feeling of alienation from OTRs.[67]

The COTA "concerns column" (started in the *Occupational Therapy Newspaper* established by the Executive Board in 1981) continued beyond the six month trial period as COTAs enthusiastically wrote of their achievements and goals.[68,69,70,71,72,73,74] The column was renamed "COTA Share." In 1981, eight COTAs were faculty members of professional-level occupational therapy education programs.[75]

In 1983 the southeastern region held its fourth annual COTA conference with 50 in attendance.[76] The 1983 Representative Assembly adopted the Occupational Therapy Assistant Fieldwork Evaluation Form, and the COTA Task Force received budget support for another year. It was agreed that the COTA Member-at-Large elected to the Representative Assembly would have voice and vote.[77] Jones and Hawkins received the COTA service award.[78] There were 11 COTAs who presented formal sessions at the AOTA annual conference in Portland, Oregon.[79] School systems were the third most common employment setting for COTAs, following nursing homes and general hospitals.[80]

Bloss-Brown and Schoening stated that all graduates of their COTA education program found employment.[81] The 1983 AOTA annual report showed 6,628 COTA and 27,719 OTR members.[82] Even with these numbers, the shortage of occupational therapy personnel is as prevalent today as it was when COTAs were created to alleviate the shortage.[83]

In 1985, Robin Jones and Ilenna Brown were elected to serve in the Representative Assembly as the COTA Representative and Alternate, respectively.[84] Jones also became the chairperson of the COTA Task Force.

Summary

The shortage of occupational therapists following World War II prompted therapists to propose an assistant level. Occupational therapy aides were the first to receive formal education and training to become certified occupational therapy assistants. The shortage of therapists continued as greater numbers of people requested occupational therapy. The late 1960s showed a rapid increase in educational programs and in the number of COTAs.

In the 1970s, the responsibilities delegated to COTAs increased. Education standards were upgraded, qualifications were identified, and formal testing was required before certification. Many states began licensure laws to cover occupational therapy. Some COTAs and new assistants chose to practice only with a state license rather than become certified by AOTA. The term COTA, which had become a familiar acronym, changed for those who selected the designation "licensed occupational therapy assistant" (LOTA) or "occupational therapy assistant, licensed" (OTA/L).

Whatever initials were chosen, assistants began to strongly voice their concerns about the assistant's place in relationship to a therapist and in professional organizations. These concerns were heard and continue to be heard and resolved. Figure 2-1 provides a listing of important events in the development of the COTA.

The 1980s have shown increased requests for occupational therapy assistants to fill positions. The number of COTAs should continue to increase as more educational programs develop to meet these service needs.

References

1. Committee Reports: Education Committee, *Am J Occup Ther*, 4:221, 1949.
2. Board of Management Minutes, *Am J Occup Ther*, 11:41, 1957.
3. Abstracts of Annual Reports, *Am J Occup Ther*, 12:38, 1958.
4. West W: From the treasurer, *Am J Occup Ther*, 12:31, 1958.
5. Crampton MW: The recognition of occupational therapy assistants, *Am J Occup Ther*, 12:269-275, 1958.
6. Executive Director's Report: *Am J Occup Ther* 13:36, 1959.
7. Board of Management: Midyear meeting reports, *Am J Occup Ther*, 14:232, 1960.
8. Caskey VL: A training program for OTA, *Am J Occup Ther*, 15:157-159, 1961.
9. Board of Management Meeting: *Am J Occup Ther*, 18:34-35, 45, 1964.
10. Annual Business Meeting Report: *Am J Occup Ther*, 18:80, 1964.
11. Midyear Meeting Report: *Am J Occup Ther*, 18:268, 1964.
12. Board of Management Report: *Am J Occup Ther*, 19:100, 1965.
13. Classified Advertising: *Am J Occup Ther*, 19:185, 1965.
14. Johnson AA: Tool Holder, *Am J Occup Ther*, 19:214, 1965.
15. Adamson MJ and Anderson MA: A study of the utilization of occupational therapy assistants and aides, *Am J Occup Ther*, 20:75-79, 1966.

16. Minutes of the Annual Business Meeting: *Am J Occup Ther*, 20:109, 1966.

17. Delegate Assembly Minutes: *Am J Occup Ther*, 20:49-53, 1966.

18. Kirschman MM and Howard B: The role of the certified assistant in a general hospital, *Am J Occup Ther*, 20:293-297, 1966.

19. Annual Business Meeting: *Am J Occup Ther*, 21:95, 1967.

20. Carr SH: A modification of role for nursing home service, *Am J Occup Ther*, 21:126-127, 1967.

21. Brunyate RW: After fifty years, what status do we hold? *Am J Occup Ther*, 21:262-267, 1967.

22. Annual Business Meeting, *Am J Occup Ther*, 22:99-118, 1968.

23. Ainsley J, Barnes SS, Grove ES, et al: On change,*Am J Occup Ther*, 22:186-189, 1968.

24. Crowell FS: The newest of our member category: The COTA, *Am J Occup Ther*, 22:377-379, 1968.

25. Annual Business Meeting: *Am J Occup Ther*, 23:168-169,194, 1969.

26. Schwagmeyer M: The COTA today, *Am J Occup Ther*, 23:69-74, 1969.

27. Cantwell JL: The community-junior college: Challenges to occupational therapy education, *Am J Occup Ther*, 24:576-579, 1970.

28. Annual Report, *Am J Occup Ther*, 24:59-62, 1970.

29. 50th Annual Conference: Minutes of the 1970 annual business meeting, *Am J Occup Ther*, 25:128, 1971.

30. Delegate Assembly Minutes, *Am J Occup Ther*, 24:438-443, 1970.

31. Ritvo MM, Lyons M, Howe MC: Planned or haphazard change, *Am J Occup Ther*, 24:404-412, 1970.

32. Delegate Assembly Minutes, *Am J Occup Ther*, 25:371-382, 1971.

33. Weimer RB: Some concepts of prevention as an aspect of community health, *Am J Occup Ther*, 26:1-9, 1972.

34. 51st Annual Conference Minutes of Annual Business Meeting, *Am J Occup Ther*, 26:95-113, 1972.

35. Keith NA: To the editor (Letters to the editor), *Am J Occup Ther*, 26:50, 1972.

36. Spelbring LM: To the editor (Letters to the editor), *Am J Occup Ther*, 26:160, 1972.

37. Hunter MH: To the editor (Letters to the editor), *Am J Occup Ther*, 26:18, 1972.

38. Oliver R: To the editor (Letters to the editor), *Am J Occup Ther*, 26:218, 1972.

39. Paggen J: To the editor (Letters to the editor), *Am J Occup Ther*, 26:219, 1972.

40. Knapp RL: Activity programs for senior citizens (Book reviews), *Am J Occup Ther*, 26:224, 1972.

41. Ackerman B, Mahoney N: To the editor (Letters to the editor), *Am J Occup Ther*, 26:381-382, 1972.

42. 52nd Annual Conference: Minutes of the annual business meeting, *Am J Occup Ther*, 27:85-106, 1973.

43. Ryan S: To the editor (Letters to the editor), *Am J Occup Ther*, 27:53, 1973.

44. The American Occupational Therapy Association, Inc.: Statement on career mobility, *Am J Occup Ther*, 27:157-158, 1973.

45. Delegate Assembly, *Am J Occup Ther*, 27:412-426, 1973.

46. Delegate Assembly, *Am J Occup Ther*, 28:549-566, 1974.

47. Blechert T, Torgrimson S, Schoeneberger SR: Autotutorial method for teaching manual skills, *Am J Occup Ther*, 29:219-221, 1975.

48. Delegate Assembly, *Am J Occup Ther*, 29:552-564, 1975.

49. Association: Guidelines for AOTA recognition, *Am J Occup Ther*, 29:632-633, 1975.

50. AOTA: Essentials of an approved educational program for the occupational therapy assistant, *Am J Occup Ther*, 30:245-263, 1976.

51. Delegate Assembly, *Am J Occup Ther*, 30:168-180, 1976.

52. Delegate Assembly, *Am J Occup Ther*, 30:576-590, 1976.

53. Delegate Assembly, *Am J Occup Ther*, 31:177-194, 1977.

54. Annual Business Meeting, *Am J Occup Ther*, 31:196-203, 1977.

55. The Association: 1978 Representative Assembly 58th Annual Conference, *Am J Occup Ther*, 32:648-669, 1978.

56. Annual Business Meeting, *Am J Occup Ther*, 32:671-677, 1978.

57. The Association: 1979 Representative Assembly, 59th Annual Conference, *Am J Occup Ther*, 33:780-813, 1979.

58. The Association: 1980 Representative Assembly 60th Annual Conference, *Am J Occup Ther*, 34:844-870, 1980.

59. COTA Task Force: Chart of COTA concerns, *Occup Ther Newspaper*, 35(April): 8, 1981.

60. Barnett P: COTA Task Force Report, *Occup Ther Newspaper*, 35 (August): 8, 1981.

61. Shapiro D and Brown D: The delineation of the role of entry-level occupational therapy personnel, *Am J Occup Ther*, 35:306-311, 1981.

62. The Association: 1981 Representative Assembly 61st Annual Conference, *Am J Occup Ther*, 35:792-808, 1981.

63. Division of Professional Development: I'm glad you asked, *Occup Ther Newspaper*, 35 (March): 1981.

64. Hightower-Vandamm M: Soaring into the '80s New directions, *Am J Occup Ther*, 35:767-774, 1981.

65. The Association: 1982 Representative Assembly 62nd Annual Conference, *Am J Occup Ther*, 36:808-826, 1982.

66. Bissell JC and Mailloux Z: The use of crafts in occupational therapy for the physically disabled, *Am J Occup Ther*, 35:369-374, 1981.

67. Curley JS: Reacts to statement (Letters to the editor), *Am J Occup Ther*, 36:48, 1982.

68. Schwope CJ: COTA concerns, *Occup Ther Newspaper*, 36(March): 3, 1982.

69. Linroth R: (COTA share), *Occup Ther Newspaper*, 36(April): 3, 1982.

70. Guthman C: (COTA share), *Occup Ther Newspaper*, 36(May): 3, 1982.

71. Davy J: (COTA share), *Occup Ther Newspaper*, 36(June): 3, 1982.

72. Kurpick EJ: (COTA share), *Occup Ther Newspaper*, 36(July): 3, 1982.

73. White B: The homemaking rehabilitation program for the. mentally retarded (COTA share), *Occup Ther Newspaper*, 36(August): 3, 1982.

74. Brown L: (COTA share), *Occup Ther Newspaper*, 36(September): 3, 1982.

75. Research Information Division: Dataline, *Occup Ther Newspaper*, 36(March): 3, 1982.

76. Adams SR: Southeastern COTA's meetings on target with mutual concerns, *Occup Ther Newspaper*, 36(April): 1983.

77. The Association: 1983 Representative Assembly 63rd Annual Conference, *Am J Occup Ther*, 37:831-840, 1983.

78. The Association: 1983 Awards, *Am J Occup Ther*, 37:592, 1983.

79. 1983 Annual Conference Program: Insert in *Am J Occup Ther*, 37, 1983.

80. AOTA Ad Hoc Manpower Commission: Report to the AOTA. Representative Assembly, 3/31/83, AOTA 1983 Annual Conference.
81. Bloss-Brown SL, Schoening MR: Application of humanistic learning theory in an associate degree program for occupational therapy assistants, *Am J Occup Ther*, 37:392-398, 1983.
82. The American Occupational Therapy Association, Inc.: *1983 Annual Report*, Rockville, MD: AOTA, 1984.
83. Dataline: OT among fastest growing occupations, *Occup Ther Newspaper*, 38(June): 1, 1984.
84. Newly elected officers for 1985-86, *Occup Ther News*, 39 (May): 1, 1985.

Acknowledgments

The author and editor wish to thank Kathlyn L. Reed, PhD, OTR/L, FAOTA, for her content and editorial suggestions.

SECTION II

Core Knowledge

Section II focuses on the generic aspects of learning, which are the foundation for occupational therapy practice. This body of knowledge is introduced through the discussion of philosophical considerations—the values and beliefs about the nature of human existence and the nature of the profession which serve as a guide for action. These actions are further discussed in terms of theoretical frameworks and approaches frequently used as a basis for the delivery of occupational therapy services. The core elements of human development as they relate to motor, cognitive and psychosocial areas are also addressed as another important aspect of core knowledge.

The individualization of occupational therapy is stressed with an emphasis on the many ways environment, society, change, and prevention serve as health determinants. Consideration of the unique needs of the whole person is a prevailing theme throughout this segment. It is particularly prominent in relation to daily living skills, an important cornerstone of occupational therapy practice, which is presented as another one of the essential foundations. Self-care, and play/leisure and work activities, according to Witherspoon, "assist individuals in adapting to society, in assuming their occupational roles, in receiving gratification, and in reaching their full potential."

Other concentrations in this section focus on the teaching/learning process, interpersonal communication skills, group dynamics, and principles of therapeutic intervention. These important people-to-people skills and processes help prepare the occupational therapy assistant for entry-level practice.

CHAPTER 3

Philosophical Considerations for the Practice of Occupational Therapy

Phillip D. Shannon, OTR

Introduction

A vital aspect of the educational preparation of the occupational therapy assistant is an appreciation of the philosophy on which the practice of occupational therapy is based. Why is this so vital? There are at least four reasons.

First, the philosophy of any profession represents the profession's views on the nature of existence, including the reasons for its own existence in responding to the needs of the population served by that profession's practitioners. For example, a somewhat complex question addressed in philosophy is: "What is man?" Is man a physical being, a psychological being, a social being, or is man all of these? If man is perceived by a profession as a physical being only, then in responding to the needs of "man the patient" the action is quite clear: the practitioner deals only with the body, not with the mind. As inconceivable as this particular belief might appear, the practices of some professions reflect a narrow perspective of man. Sometimes, as will be discussed later, a profession does not practice what it believes.

Guided by its philosophical beliefs, a grand design evolves to specify the purposes or goals of the profession. Lacking an understanding of the philosophical basis for this grand design, the practitioner cannot be sure that the goals he or she is pursuing are worth pursuing, or that the services provided are worth providing.

A second reason for understanding the philosophy of the profession is that philosophy guides action. Indeed, it is only within the context of a profession's philosophy that actions have meaning. Attending to the leisure needs of the patient, for instance, is one of the major concerns of occupational therapy. Why? The answer is not simple; essentially, however, occupational therapists believe that man seeks a sense of quality in his life. One aspect of a quality life is a satisfying leisure life. Consequently, using the arts and crafts to promote the leisure interests and skills of the patient and, therefore, the quality of life of the patient, is an action that makes sense because the action has philosophical meaning.

One of the primary reasons for studying philosophy, according to Thomas, is to clarify beliefs so that the action "which stems from those beliefs is sound and consistent."[1] Clarifying the beliefs of the profession should be regarded as a critical component of the occupational therapy assistant's education to ensure that his or her actions are indeed sound and consistent. In other words, the occupational therapy assistant's entry-level behaviors should be based on, and consistent with, a set of guiding philosophical beliefs.

A third rationale for understanding the philosophy of occupational therapy is that there is a direct relationship between the growth of the profession and the ability of its practitioners to explain their "reasons for existence." In the present era of accountability, when the justification for programs and the competition for resources to support these programs is greater than in previous years, one cannot assume that those external to the profession, such as physicians, will perceive occupational therapy as an "intrinsically good" or essential service. Claims of "goodness" must be substantiated with evidence. That evidence must be supported philosophically, or it may lack a context for interpretation. For example, documented evidence that a patient's range of motion in the left elbow was increased by five degrees as a result of occupational therapy's intervention is important. However, what strengthens this evidence are the reasons for intervening in the first place. These reasons are linked to the philosophical beliefs of the profession.

Finally, it is not enough that the occupational therapy assistant should be skilled in applying the techniques of the profession. On the contrary, the occupational therapy assistant must have some appreciation, philosophical and theoretical, of the reasons why these techniques are applied. Lacking this appreciation, the techniques will be applied without the ability to communicate their value to the patient, thereby failing to motivate the patient's active involvement in his or her own treatment.

Certainly from the initial stage of patient referral to the last stage of discontinuing the patient's treatment, the philosophical beliefs of the profession must remain in the foreground. For the occupational therapy assistant who has major responsibilities along the entire continuum of health care, these beliefs and the actions which stem from them must be understood and practiced. Indeed, this is the first duty of the occupational therapy assistant.

What Is Philosophy?

To appreciate fully the philosophy of occupational therapy, one must first have an appreciation and understanding of philosophy in general and the types of questions and concerns that philosophy addresses. Basically, philosophy is concerned with the "meaning of life, and the significance of the world in which man finds himself."[2] Man is by nature a philosophical creature. Questions such as "who am I?; what is my destiny?; what do I want from life?" concern all human beings. Each individual, in responding to questions such as these, develops a personalized view of the world, commonly referred to as a "philosophy of life." This philosophy of life represents a fundamental set of values, beliefs, truths, and principles that guide the person's behavior from day to day, from year to year.

The philosophy of a profession also represents a set of values, beliefs, truths, and principles that guides the actions of the profession's practitioners. Typically, as with individuals, these evolve over time, and they sometimes change as a profession matures. Each profession, in shaping and reshaping its philosophy, has choices to make in three philosophical dimensions: the three major branches of philosophy. These include metaphysics, epistemology, and axiology.

Metaphysics

Metaphysics is concerned with questions about the ultimate nature of things, including the nature of man. With regard to the nature of man in particular, of special interest to the philosopher is the mind/body relationship. Are mind and body two separate entities, one superior to the other, or are mind and body a single entity representative of the "whole," the whole person? The first position, that of mind/body separation, is the dualistic position. The second position, that of mind/body as one entity, is the position of holism.

While most (if not all) professions claim to be holistic, the truth in this claim is seen to the extent to which the actions of the profession are consistent with its principles. Assume, for example, that the actions of "profession x" are directed toward exercise as the means for promoting a healthy body (i.e., a healthy "physical" body). Assume also that profession x claims to be holistic, asserting a concern for the whole person. In actuality it is dualistic, because the body is viewed as superior to the mind; the end goal of exercise, in this case, is a healthy body and not a healthy body *and* a healthy mind. There is a contradiction, therefore, in what profession x believes and what it does. Its actions do not follow from its beliefs, and the claim of holism is illegitimate. When exercise is seen as promoting the health of the "whole," a more holistic approach is demonstrated.

Epistemology

The second dimension pertinent to shaping and reshaping the philosophy of a profession is the dimension of epistemology, which is concerned with questions of truth. What is truth? How do we come to know things? How do we know that we know? One way of knowing is by experience. One knows, for example, that the flame of a fire brings pleasure in terms of the warmth it provides, but also that it produces pain if it is touched by the bare hand. Usually, one only needs to experience this pain once to "know that he or she knows." Is experience, however, the only route to truth or knowing? From a holistic perspective there are many routes to truth and knowing. Intuition, for instance, is considered to be as truthful as experiential learning or the logic reasoned by the powers of the intellect. For the dualist, on the other hand, the subjective realities of intuition and experience cannot be accepted as truths. On the contrary, only the objective reality of rational thought can be admitted as truth; truth is logic.

Axiology

The third dimension of philosophy is axiology, which is concerned with the study of values. Two types of questions are addressed by axiology: questions of value with regard to what is desirable or beautiful in the world (aesthetics), and questions of value with regard to standards or rules for right conduct (ethics). Most people would agree that a long life is a desirable thing, something that is valued. Some people might argue that a long life without a sense of quality is a life that is not worth living. Almost everyone would maintain that it is wrong to take a life, and yet there are those who believe that "a life for a life" might be justified in some instances.

Conflicting values and standards often produce dilemmas that are not easily resolved. If life is valued, for example, is it right or moral to disconnect the support systems maintaining the life of a person who has been certified as "brain dead?" Is it right or moral to prolong a life that may not be a worth living? These are difficult questions of value of what is desirable or beautiful in the world and of the standards that will be applied in pursuing that which is valued.

Each profession has choices to make with regard to what it considers beautiful and desirable in the world and the ethical principles that it will follow in achieving its goals. For medicine, the preservation of life is the first priority, and perhaps this is as it should be. But is this the highest priority of the other health care professions? Should it be the highest priority? A profession that claims to be holistic cannot be satisfied with saving lives. Instead, a holistic profession would maintain that a life worth saving must be a life worth living.

Given this brief glimpse of metaphysics, epistemology, and axiology, each dimension can be discussed as it relates to the philosophy of occupational therapy. Specifically, four questions need to be addressed:

1 The metaphysical question of "what is man?"
2 The epistemological question of "how does man know what he knows?"
3 The aesthetic question of "what is beautiful or desirable in the world?"
4 The ethical question of "what are the rules of right conduct?"

Two approaches will be taken in responding to these questions. The first is to examine the philosophy of Adolph Meyer, who was primarily responsible for providing occupational therapy with a philosophical foundation for practice. The second approach is to explore the extent to which this philosophical base has survived the test of time.

The Evolution of Occupational Therapy

Occupational therapy evolved from the moral treatment movement that began in the early 19th century.[3] If there was a single purpose to which the champions of this movement were committed, it was to humanize and provide more humane forms of treatment for the mentally ill incarcerated in the large asylums in this country and abroad. Marching under the banner of humanism, the leaders of this movement sought to defend and preserve the dignity of all human beings, particularly the sick and the disabled.

Among these humanists who carried the movement into the 20th century was the psychiatrist Adolph Meyer whose paper on "The Philosophy of Occupation Therapy"[4] laid the foundation for the practice and promotion of occupational therapy. Meyer's philosophy was based on his observations of everyday living, and from his beliefs about the nature of man, about life, and about a life worth living the pioneers of the profession emerged to chart its course. Although Meyer has been quoted frequently in the literature of recent years, a more extensive discussion of his philosophy is provided here because, to date, his thoughts have not been examined within the context of metaphysics, epistemology, and axiology.

A Retrospective Glance at The Philosophy of Adolph Meyer

What is man?

Meyer's perspective of man was holistic. "Our body is not merely so many pounds of flesh and bone figuring as a machine, with an abstract mind or soul added to it. (Rather it is a live organism acting) with its own nature and the nature about it."[4] For Meyer, three characteristics distinguished man from all other organisms: his sense of time, his capacity for imagination, and his need for occupation.

Man's sense of time—past, present and future—was the central theme of Meyer's philosophy. It is man's sense of time, and particularly time past (experience), that provides man with an advantage over other living organisms in terms of adapting in the present and manipulating the future. This capacity to learn from experience, when blended with man's capacity for imagination or creativity, allows man to alter his environment. The squirrel, for example, is totally dependent on its environment for food and shelter during the winter months. Man, on the other hand, through his experience and imagination, has been able to alter his environment to ensure survival through food preservation techniques and heat producing systems.

The need for occupation was regarded by Meyer as a distinctly human characteristic. He defined occupation as "any form of helpful enjoyment,"[4] which clearly transcends the notion of occupation as being limited to work. On the contrary, the meaning of occupation was extended by Meyer to include all of those activities that comprise a normal day, particularly work and play. He considered occupation important to all, the sick as well as the healthy. Each individual must achieve a balance among his occupations, a balanced life of not only work and play, but also of rest and sleep.[4]

How does man know what he knows?

Man learns not only from his experience but also from "doing": engaging mind and body in occupation. It is in doing that man is able to achieve. Fidler and Fidler, in reiterating this theme in the 1970's, maintained that doing is linked to becoming, to realizing one's potential.[5] Fundamental to achieving and becoming is doing. In doing, man comes to know about himself and the world. In doing, man knows that he knows.

What is desirable or beautiful in the world?

For Meyer, man is not content simply existing in the world. Instead, man seeks a sense of quality to his life that comes from the pleasure in achievement.[4] It is in engaging the total self that man comes to experience the pleasure in achievement which Reilly, in her Eleanor Clarke Slagle lectureship, articulated so beautifully:[6]

> "Man, through the use of his hands as they are energized by mind and will, can influence the state of his own health." It is in doing that man achieves and is able to acquire a sense of quality in his life.

What are the rules of right conduct?

Meyer, in outlining the guiding principles for the practice of occupational therapy, maintained that the occupation worker should provide opportunities, not prescriptions.[4] Prescriptions tend to constrain the development of one's potential, while opportunities nourish it. To apply prescriptions is to treat the patient as an object; to offer opportunities is to regard the patient as a person. Inherent in this principle of right conduct is a belief in the type of relationship that the occupation worker should maintain with the patient a helping, caring relationship in which patients are indeed treated as persons and not as objects.

To summarize, Meyer's perspective of man was holistic. He emphasized doing as the primary route to truth and to achieving a sense of quality in one's life. Prerequisite to doing, however, is opportunity. Lacking the opportunity to do, man, like the squirrel, cannot control his own destiny. On the contrary, man becomes nothing more than a squirrel, controlled and manipulated by his environment.

The Test of Time

Has the philosophy of Adolph Meyer, which provided the direction for the practice and promotion of occupational therapy, survived the test of time, or has the profession, as it matured, changed its direction based on a different set of values, beliefs, truths, and principles? The answer is reflected in the report to the American Occupational Therapy Association Project to Identify the Philosophical Base Of Occupational Therapy, which was submitted to the Executive Board of the AOTA in 1983.[7] This report does not represent "an official position" of the AOTA with regard to the philosophy of occupational therapy, but is the documentation of a 6½ year project that was designed to trace the philosophical beliefs of the profession historically and to interpret those beliefs within the context of more modern times. In reviewing the degree to which the beliefs of Adolph Meyer have withstood the test of time, the four philosophical questions addressed earlier are once again discussed in the sections that follow.

What is man?

The belief in holism has persisted in the profession.[7] Indeed, one of the unique aspects of occupational therapy is its integrating function, where mind and body are activated to promote the patient's total involvement in the treatment process. To lose sight of this function is to lose sight of one of the major contributions of occupational therapy, attending to the "whole person."

One might speculate that it is the profession's commitment to holism that has attracted people to occupational therapy, in contrast to some of the other health professions that appear to be less holistic. Even in occupational therapy, however, the concept of holism, though universally professed, is not uniformly applied in practice. Action is not always consistent with intent. When practice takes the form of dealing only with the mind, only with the body, or worse yet, only with certain parts of the body, the commitment to holism has been compromised and there is a contradiction between what one believes and what one does.

For example, hand rehabilitation has become a highly specialized area of practice. Unquestionably, there is a significant contribution to be made to health care in this area. However, when some of the practitioners in rehabilitation begin to refer to themselves as "hand therapists" versus "occupational therapists," there is an implicit shift away from holism. The belief in holism may remain, but the explicit actions that follow are sometimes not holistic. Only when hand rehabilitation focuses on the whole person can the therapy retain its holistic function.

Another example of a contradiction between belief and action can be found in the area of mental health. Probably one of the first signs indicating the shift away from holism in mental health is when the practitioner in this area uses the title "psychiatric occupational therapist" or "psychiatric occupational therapy assistant.""Psychiatric occupational therapy" personnel tend to focus only on the mind of the patient to the exclusion of the patient's body. Furthermore, when the practitioner's actions are directed primarily toward the unconscious mind, as in providing activities for the sublimation of innate drives, attention is not even focused on the whole mind, much less the mind and body. Again, the belief in holism may be contradicted by the actions of the practitioner.

Surely these examples are not characteristic of most practitioners in mental health, nor is "hand therapy" necessarily limited to the treatment of the hand. The point, however, is that when the broad concerns of occupational therapy are narrowed, the patient is somehow cheated in the process.

Also surviving the test of time is the belief in those distinguishing characteristics of man identified by Adolph Meyer. Indeed, in responding to the needs of "man the patient," occupational therapy has placed a high priority on time as a continuum in the life of a patient, designing programs of treatment within the the context of the patient's past, present, and future. In implementing these programs, the patient's capacity for imagination or creativity is challenged in the interest of serving his or her need for occupation.

Occupation, as defined in the report from the AOTA Project to Identify the Philosophical Base of Occupational Therapy, is "goal-directed behavior aimed at the development of play, work, and life skills for optimal time management."[7] If, as Reilly proposed, man's need for occupation is a vital need which is served by occupational therapy,[6] then to reduce the concept of occupation to the level of exercising bodily parts with weights and pulleys or occupying the patient's mind with activities that bear no relationship to the nature of his or her occupation, another unique aspect of the profession is somehow lost in the transformation of belief into action.

In contrast, by drawing upon the patient's past experiences in work and play and in exploring the patient's values, capacities, and interests, experiences that will serve the patient's need for occupation should be provided. Also, in tapping the creative potential of the patient in areas such as problem-solving and decision-making, his or her capacities for altering the environment are expanded, thereby expanding the patient's potential for adapting in the present and for controlling his or her own destiny into the future.

How does man know that he knows?

From the beginning, occupational therapy has taught the active versus the passive involvement of the patient in treatment. But, as Adolph Meyer believed, doing is but one way of knowing. There are multiple routes to truth—experience, thinking, feeling, and doing—which the modern day practitioner also accepts as reality.[7] One knows, for example, what happiness means because it has been experienced and/or because it can be felt. Happiness cannot be measured, but this does not make it any less real.

Among the many ways of knowing, however, doing is emphasized in the profession as the means for acquiring the skills for daily living and knowing one's capabilities in the present and one's potential for the future. Here again, the opportunities for doing must be framed within the context of the whole person. Consider, for example, the active engagement of the patient in sensory-integration activities. One of the major reasons for involving a patient in an activity of this type is because the ability to receive and process sensory information is one way of knowing. For example, one knows that it is cold and, therefore, that the body should be protected with warm clothing, because one is able to feel cold, process this input, and take the appropriate steps to protect oneself.

Lacking the ability to process sensory information, the person is denied an important, if not critical, source of information. In this case, doing in the form of involving the individual in sensory-integration activities is an important step in the process of knowing. On the other hand, if the benefits accrued to the patient by his or her involvement in occupational therapy are limited to those derived from applying the techniques of sensory-integration, occupational therapy has not served its holistic function, nor has it served the patient's need for occupation.

The practitioner takes a step away from this belief in doing when the action of "having the patient do" is replaced with the action of "doing to the patient." Another unique aspect of occupational therapy is obscured when the patient is denied the opportunity for doing.

What is beautiful or desirable in the world?

To subsist, according to Meyer, is not enough for man. Man seeks something beyond subsistence or survival: the "good life." In maintaining this position over the years, occupational therapy has focused attention in two directions, minimizing the deficits and maximizing the strengths of the patient.[7] Attending to one without attending to the other is incomplete and insufficient if the goals go beyond mere survival.

Traditionally, occupational therapy has minimized its contribution to the survival aspects of care and maximized its role in promoting a life of quality for its patients. Consider, for example, the patient who has not learned the techniques of wheelchair mobility. The patient will not survive, at least as a self-sufficient being. Consider also the patient who cannot dress himself or organize time to meet the demands of daily living. He or she will not be able to survive with any degree of autonomy and self-respect. Furthermore, as Shannon stated, "bodies and minds that are not active will atrophy from disuse, they will die."[8] Also, "people who lack quality in their lives sometimes engage in self-destructive behaviors, such as alcoholism, that lead to deterioration and death."[8] Does occupational therapy contribute to the preservation of life? Surely, as these examples suggest, occupational therapy contributes to the survival of the patient directly if survival is interpreted to mean the ability to care for self, and indirectly by adding a sense of quality to the lives of those served by the profession.

Reilly stated that "the first duty of an organism is to be alive; the second duty is to grow and be productive."[6] If survival is the first priority of the organism, then perhaps the position of the profession can be strengthened by developing an argument for the practice and promotion of occupational therapy that includes a commitment to the survival of the patient as well as to the quality of his or her life.[8] In developing this argument, it must be made clear that the first priority of the profession is to teach the patient skills that will ensure survival. The second priority is to guide the patient toward the realization of his or her potential and social worth as a member of society as evidenced by the ability to perform an occupational role, according to Heard.[9] Indeed, it is for these reasons that man engages in occupation, and it is also for these reasons that occupational therapy exists.

Occupational therapy has expressed its commitment to the second priority, but its actions are often directed to the first.[7,8] As Heard maintained, it is in addressing the second priority, and particularly the social worth of the patient, that occupational therapy has been most negligent.[9] Yet, in attending to the social worth of the patient the profession is making a major contribution to a more healthy society. Certainly in making this contribution, as Yerxa argued that it must,[10] the profession's value is increased and its survival guaranteed.

What are the rules of right conduct?

Adolph Meyer's principle of providing opportunities, not prescriptions, for patients has been one of the distinguishing characteristics of the profession. In applying the rule of non-prescription, the patient becomes an active partner in treatment. Why is this important?

First, the skills and habits necessary for the performance of occupational roles cannot be administered to the patient; the patient must be given opportunities to acquire these for himself or herself. Second, prescriptions tend to foster pawn-like (externally controlled) behaviors, while opportunities encourage origin-like (internally conrolled) behaviors, as defined by Burke.[11] In applying prescriptions the patient is treated as a pawn, externally controlled by those responsible for his or her care. If taking charge of one's own life is important and assuming control for one's own destiny is valued, providing opportunities and not prescriptions is a necessary first step.

In offering opportunities for patients to take charge of their own lives, two ethical principles guide the actions of the practitioner. The first of these is the principle of *nonmaleficence*, which states that not only should one do no harm, but also that one should promote the good. The second is the principle of *beneficence*, or the rule that one should show kindness and caring.[12] Perhaps no profession can lay greater claim to applying these principles than the occupational therapy. In showing kindness and caring, however, the issue of patient versus client has raised questions about the meaning of caring. The major question is: which is more legitimate, a therapist-patient relationship or a therapist-client relationship?

In a therapist-client relationship the client is perceived as an object, an "it," because only one aspect of the client becomes the focus of attention. This approach is similar to that of a used car salesman has only one goal: to sell his client a used car regardless of whether the client can afford gasoline or has the financial resources to insure and maintain it.

In a therapist-patient relationship the patient is perceived not as an object, but as a person. Patients expect that their total well-being will somehow be improved when seeking health care.

Reilly argues that there is a special bond in the therapist-patient relationship, similar to the bonding relationship of teacher-student, that is not present in a therapist-client relationship. Like teacher-student, the therapist-patient relationship is reciprocal, one involving mutual loyalities, obligations, and caring.[13]

Over the years occupational therapy has prided itself on the fact that it cares. In caring about its patients, the profession has demonstrated that it is holistic and humanistic. If a different type of caring evolves, as implied by the use of the term "client," then any future claim of being a holistic, humanistic enterprise may have to be altered.

Future Directions

Guided by its belief in holism, occupational therapy has grown and prospered over the years. The price that it has had to pay for adopting this holistic position is complexity. Among the health care professions, occupational therapy is probably one of the most complex in terms of the knowledge and skills required for certification as a practitioner. On the other hand, it is also one of the most challenging and rewarding professions in the world today. The possibilities for continued growth dazzle the imagination.

What happens in the future is dependent upon how future generations use the dowry of philosophical values, beliefs, truths, and principles provided from the profession's past. This is a responsibility of some magnitude. In accepting this responsibility, one is subordinating one's personal life to the lives of those less fortunate. In the process of helping others, however, one's personal life is also somehow enriched. One only needs to open the door to discover the rewards that lie beyond.

Summary

The philosophical bases of the profession of occupational therapy provide the context in which the COTA acts. From its inception, occupational therapy has been founded on considerations from the philosophical dimensions of metaphysics, epistemology, and axiology. Adolph Meyer's belief in the importance of the "holistic" approach to treatment has persisted to the present day as crucial to the profession.

References

1. Thomas CE: *Sport in a Philosophic Context*, Philadelphia: Lea and Febiger, 1983, p. 19.

2. Randall JH and Buchler J: *Philosophy: An Introduction*, New York: Barnes and Noble, Inc., 1960, p. 5.

3. Bockhoven JS: Legacy of moral treatment 1800s to 1910, *Am J Occup Ther*, 25:223-225, 1971.

4. Meyer A: The philosophy of occupation therapy, *Am J Occup Ther*, 31:639-642, 1977.

5. Fidler GS and Fidler JW: Doing and becoming: Purposeful action and self-actualization, *Am J Occup Ther*, 32:305-310, 1978.

6. Reilly M: Occupational therapy can be one of the great ideas of 20th century medicine, *Am J Occup Ther*, 16:1-9, 1962.

7. Shannon PD: Report on the AOTA Project to Identify the Philosophical Base of Occupational Therapy, January 1983. Condensed under the title: *Toward a Philosophy of Occupational Therapy*, August 1983.

8. Shannon PD: From another perspective: An overview of the issue on the roles of occupational therapists in continuity of care, *Occup Ther in Health Care*, 2:3-11, 1985.

9. Heard C: Occupational role acquisition: A perspective on the chronically disabled, *Am J Occup Ther*, 31:243-247, 1977.

10. Yerxa E: The philosophical base of occupational therapy, In: *Occupational Therapy: 2001 AD*, Rockville, MD: American Occupational Therapy Association, 1979, p 26-30.

11. Burke JP: A clinical perspective on motivation: Pawn versus origin, *Am J Occup Ther*, 31:254-258, 1977.

12. Beauchamp TL and Childress JF: *Principles of Biomedical Ethics*, New York: Oxford University Press, 1983, pp. 106-107, 148.

13. Reilly M: The importance of the patient versus client issue for occupational therapy, *Am J Occup Ther*, 38:404-406, 1984.

Bibliography

Sharrott GW, and Yerxa EJ: The Issue Is: Promises to keep: Implications of the referent "patient" versus "client" for those served by occupational therapy, *Am J Occup Ther*, 39:401-405, 1985.

CHAPTER 4

Theoretical Frameworks and Approaches

Sally E. Ryan, COTA

Introduction

The theoretical foundations, frameworks, and approaches for the practice of occupational therapy have been drawn from many areas, including the biological sciences, medicine, psychology, sociology, humanities, and the arts.[1] Because so many different disciplines have contributed to the profession, compound words such as "biopsychosocial" are often used.

Unless otherwise noted, the theoretical frameworks and approaches which follow were developed by occupational therapists, and they are discussed from general to specific. Very basic information is provided to acquaint the reader with some of the primary principles that are used as a foundation for the practice of occupational therapy.

Theory is used to describe the relationships or basic principles of certain observations which have been verified to some degree.[2] For example, we are all familiar with the theory of gravity; we have observed its effects in our daily lives but it remains a theory because science has not yet completely uncovered or fully verified why it works. A theory is also a scheme or collection of abstract or basic fundamental principles which provide a foundation for science and the arts.[3] A *framework* may be defined as a structure, plan, or specified arrangement.[2] It is a way of putting ideas together into a meaningful whole. An *approach* is a method of treating or dealing with something.[2]

In the late fall of 1984, the author sent a survey to all occupational therapy assistant program directors to determine which theories should be included in this text. There was a 50% return of questionnaires, a number less than valid for research purposes. However, since an exhaustive review of the literature did not yield any additional information on this topic, it was decided to use the survey results as a guide for the inclusion of the most appropriate theories and approaches.

Occupational Behavior

The occupational behavior theoretical framework builds on the beliefs of Meyer regarding daily living patterns that were discussed in Chapter 1.[4] The framework was developed in the late 1960s by Mary Reilly, and is based on biopsychosocial and developmental models. This framework emphasizes the continuum of work and play and focuses on the many activities of daily living for patients receiving occupational therapy treatment. Occupation is defined broadly here to include the full range of activities that occupy a person. It requires the active engagement of the person. Reilly, in her Eleanor Clarke Slagle address in 1960, stated that "Man through the use of his hands, as energized by mind and will, can influence the state of his health."[5] Loukran wrote that Reilly stressed the need for looking at members of society in terms of the many life roles that they assume. Questions about the skills necessary to support and carry out the roles, and how this activity assists in adapting to the community need to be addressed. Once the answers are known, an environment can be created to allow individuals to practice necessary skills and roles.[6]

Occupational Behavior Framework

The occupational behavior framework was initially developed for treatment of psychiatric patients. It can be used with physically disabled persons, and has been used on a limited basis with children. The framework is based on three major components: patient achievement, play and work, and roles.[4]

Achievement

Matsutsuyu, in discussing Reilly's work, has stated that achievement is developmental and centers on abilities, interests, skills, and habits. She elaborates that cooperation and competition are important elements in the drive for achievement.[7]

Play and Work

Competence and achievement are built and enhanced through active participation in play and work occupations. Activities from simple to complex develop patterns of organization for the patient. The skills of exploration, acquisition, and adaptation are gained through play and assist in establishing behaviors that transfer to the work role.[7]

Roles

Preschooler, student, worker, homemaker, and retiree are the roles that are focused on in occupational behavior theory. These roles should relate directly to activities of daily living in meeting individual occupational therapy treatment objectives. People fulfill many roles during their lifetimes and, according to Matsutsuyu, the resulting skills and habits are interdependent. They assist the patient in moving to new roles and in gaining competence.[7]

Human Occupation

Gary Kielhofner and Janice Burke have developed their theoretical framework of human occupation in part on the occupational behavior principles stated by Reilly. They also use general systems theory principles of input, output, and feedback (see Figure 4-1) and draw from a number of theorists in the areas of play, work, competence and human development.[4] The framework is made up of three major parts:[8]

Volition

Volition may be defined as exercise of the will or willpower.[2] It guides choices of the individual and is influenced by values and interests.

Habituation

Habituation refers to the individual's habits and internalized roles. It helps the individual to maintain activity and action.

Performance

Performance in this context refers to actions produced through skill acquisition.

The three parts should be viewed as interactive and dynamic. They all work together to produce motives for the individual to explore, gain skills, and develop habits and achievements that eventually result in the acquisition of a variety of roles.[4]

Kielhofner and Burke view the environment as an open system consisting of objects, people, and events. They also see the human as an open system interacting with the environment in the occupations of work and play.[8] Kielhofner views the occupation of human beings as a dominant activity which is the result of evolutionary development. It is reflected in the individual's need for both productive and enjoyable behavior.[9] Roann Barris has also contributed to the development of this

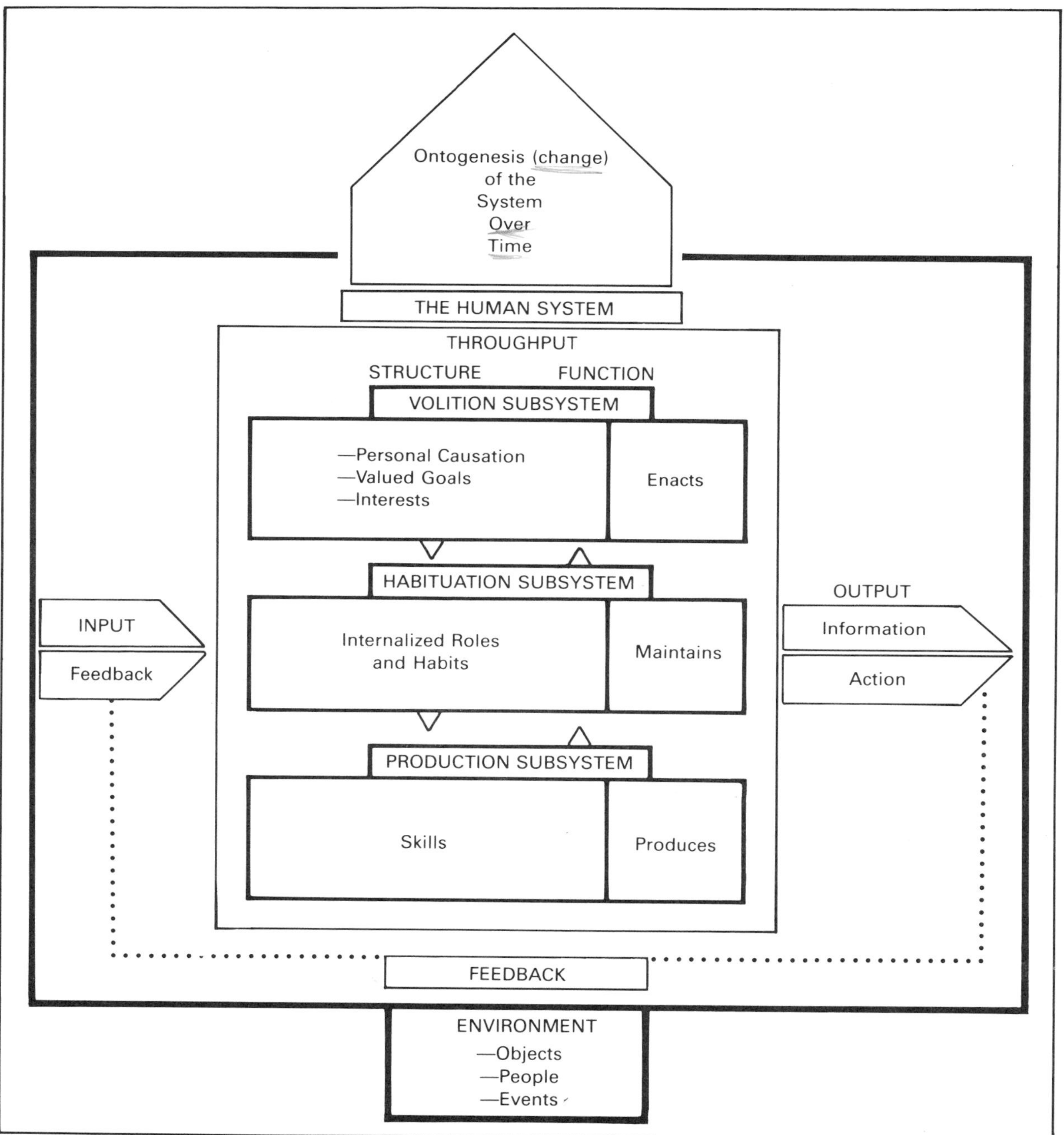

Figure 4-1. Developed by Kielfhofner and Burke. Reprinted with the permission of the American Occupational Therapy Association, AJOT, 1980.

model, particularly in relation to its environmental aspects.

Adaptive Responses

Lorna Jean King's theoretical framework of adaptive responses is founded on the biological principles of adaptation. Developed in the 1970s, it was presented as an Eleanor Clarke Slagle lecture in 1978. This framework stresses that an adaptive response is a means of assessing a specific activity in which a patient is engaged.[4] The individual's ability to adapt, and the level of his or her adaptive responses have a direct impact on interpersonal relationships and performance of life tasks.[10] Other points which King discusses include the following:[4]

1. The adaptive response is the core of occupational therapy.
2. Adaptive responses are organized below the conscious level.
3. Adaptive responses must be active, not passive.
4. Environmental challenges bring about adaptive responses.
5. Adaptive responses can produce higher level interaction.
6. Sensory loss and changes in the environment can have a negative impact on a person's ability to make an adaptive response.

Kleinman and Buckley have expanded King's concepts and presented a graphic continuum of adaptation which follows a progression from: (a) basic reactions to maintain homeostasis to (b) adaptive responses to (c) adaptive skills, arriving at (d) adaptive patterns of behavior.[12] This framework has applications to all areas of occupational therapy practice.[4]

Adaptation Through Occupation

Introduced in the early 1980's by Kathlyn Reed, the model of adaptation through occupation presents occupation as the core concept of occupational therapy. Occupation is viewed as being "fundamental to human existence and health because it maintains and provides for the life support systems and because it gives meaning to life."[4] According to Reed, occupation is a dynamic, changing process performed in a holistic manner that is influenced by the individual's biological, physical, and sociocultural environments.[4]

Adaptation to and manipulation of the environment can be facilitated through occupation. Conversely, an individual's health and well-being can be impaired owing to problems in his or her ability to perform such adaptive occupations as self-maintenance, productivity, and leisure. Reed states that these adaptive occupations can be further classified in terms of orientation, order, and activation, as well as by the specific occupation performance categories of motor, sensory, cognitive, intrapersonal, and interpersonal.[4] Through occupational therapy intervention, the patient can learn problem solving methods which will assist in occupation performance and effective adaptation.

Facilitating Growth and Development

Based on principles of biopsychosocial development and mastery of tasks,[4] the facilitating growth and development framework was presented in Lela Llorens's 1969 Eleanor Clarke Slagle address, in which the following points were made:[13]

1. Human development occurs horizontally (e.g., encompassing physical and psychosocial growth, language, and skills of daily living).
2. Human development occurs longitudinally in all of the above areas; as an individual ages, development takes place as a continuous process.
3. Occupational therapy is a process of facilitation of development.
4. Facilitation assists the patient in developing coping skills and mastery of life tasks.
5. Development of coping skills and mastery of life tasks require practice in appropriate environments.
6. Attention to the developmental level of the patient is the key to effective treatment.
7. Activities used and relationships established must relate to the first level of need before others are introduced.

The facilitating growth and development framework is used primarily with children and with adult psychiatric patients.[10]

Doing and Becoming: Purposeful Action

Gail Fidler, OTR, and her husband Jay Fidler, a psychiatrist, introduced their framework in the

1970s. Their concepts center on the role of doing and purposeful action as a means of helping the individual to achieve the necessary performance skills to satisfy needs and to be a contributing member of society.[4] In discussing this framework, Mosey stresses that purposeful activity involves those "doing processes" which have a definite end result, rather than random activities for which no goal is set.[3]

The Fidlers believe that "*doing* is a process of investigating, trying out, and gaining evidence of one's capacities for experiencing, responding, managing, creating, and controlling. It is through such action with feedback from both the non-human and human objects that an individual comes to know the potential and limitations of self and the environment." Through doing, the individual "achieves a sense of competence and intrinsic worth."[14]

Occupational therapy treatment focuses on the identification of the patient's doing and becoming problems. Doing and purposeful activities are selected to assist the patient in need satisfaction through the development of necessary skills. This framework has been used primarily in mental health.

Activities Therapy

The activities therapy framework, developed by Anne Mosey, is based on the assumption that many individuals who are unable to learn to function in the community have mental health problems.[4] These problems are due to basic skill deficits in planning and carrying out activities of daily living and limitations in expressing feelings in a socially acceptable way.[15]

Activities therapy takes place in a therapeutic community; both individual and group methods are used in treatment. The treatment focuses on the patient's future needs and the knowledge and skills necessary to meet these needs. Individual values are also considered in planning the treatment activities, which emphasize learning by doing.[15] Examples include how to plan meals, shop for and prepare nutritious food, read a bus schedule, and take a bus to and from a specified location. This model is used primarily in adult mental health.

Sensory Integration

The sensory integration approach to occupational therapy intervention was introduced by A. Jean Ayres in the 1960s based on her earlier work with perceptual motor deficits.[4] Sensory integration may be defined as the ability to develop and coordinate sensory information, motor responses, and sensory feedback.[16] Deficits are identified through the the administration of the Southern California Sensory Integration Tests (SCSIT) which include visual, kinesthetic, tactile, and motor areas. Test scores are viewed as a "total picture" rather than individually.[17] They provide information on how the human brain receives and processes sensory messages and organizes a response to this information.[4]

Sensory integration treatment procedures might include rubbing the skin with terry cloth to provide tactile stimulation or having a child lie prone on a scooterboard and move about in a specific way to provide vestibular stimulation.[4] This approach has been widely used with children and with adult schizophrenics. Lewis indicates that some applications have also been successful with elderly patients.[18]

Spaciotemporal Adaptation

Spaciotemporal adaptation is a model developed by Elnora Gilfoyle and Ann Grady that is based on the human development milestones and learning sequence of Gesell and Piaget, respectively, as well as on biopsychosocial perspectives[4] and the Bobath approach. The model focuses on adaptation to space and timing of movements to build postural and movement strategies which are adapted to achieve purposeful behaviors such as creeping, crawling, and walking. The behaviors are a foundation for development of skills and the performance of purposeful activities.[4] Gilfoyle and Grady view the behaviors in a spiraling continuum in which adaptation begins prior to birth. When considering the present status of a child, past behaviors are called upon to improve the present situation and enhance future skill acquisition and adaptation. Figure 4-2 illustrates the sequence of the model and the relationship of sensory input, motor output, and sensory feedback. The follow-

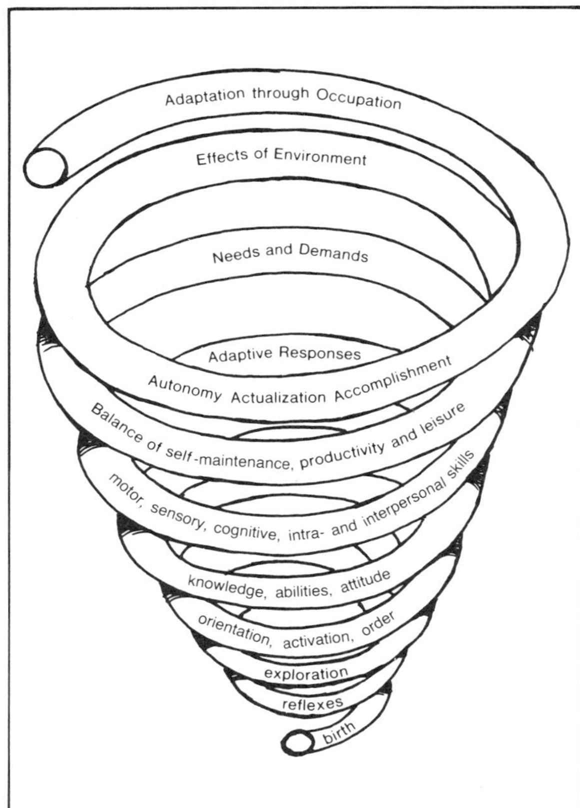

Figure 4-2. From Gilfoyler, Grady, and Moore: *Children Adapt,* Thorofare, NJ: SLACK, Inc., 1981.

ing are brief definitions of the terms used in the continuum to achieve spaciotemporal adaptation:[2]

1 *Assimilation* refers to the ability to absorb information and make it a part of one's thinking.
2 *Accommodation* refers to the ability to modify or adjust in response to the environment.
3 *Association* refers to the ability to relate factors from the past to experiences in the present.
4 *Differentiation* refers to the ability to determine what differences exist between objects and events.

To provide further illustration, the following scenario describes a little boy who is just beginning to crawl. The child learns that reciprocal movement of the arms and legs will move him forward a given distance. He also learns that he can crawl that distance at a fast or slow rate. This information is *assimilated* and recalled the next time the child has an opportunity to crawl. The child is crawling on another occasion and becomes distracted. He crawls too close to the wall and hits his head. The child then crawls away from the wall, thus *accommodating* to this environmental barrier. He continues crawling about the room and touches a lamp cord. The mother responds by lightly tapping the child's hand and saying "no." He touches the cord again, and the mother responds in the same way. Eventually the child learns to *differentiate* what he may touch and what should not be touched.

The Rood Approach

Margaret Rood, physical therapist and occupational therapist, developed her neurophysiological approach to treatment while working with cerebral palsy and hemiplegia patients.[4,19] Her treatment centers on the the principles that sensory stimulation can assist in developing normal muscle tone and motor response, and that stimulation of reflex responses is the first step in motor control development.[20]

Sensory stimulation is a central focus for effecting the desired motor response. Treatment includes relaxation techniques such as slow stroking of the spinal column, slow side-to-side rolling, and neutral warmth which entails wrapping the patient or a part of the patient in a blanket. Sensory stimulation may be provided by using a vibrator, a brush, or through rubbing the belly of a muscle to facilitate the desired response.[2,21]

Rood was a strong advocate of purposeful activity, and promoted the use of her techniques in conjunction with such woodworking tasks as sanding a bread board. Through engagement in an activity, the patient's attention is focused on the task at hand and achievement of that task rather than the correct motor response.[21]

Proprioceptive Neuromuscular Facilitation

The *proprioceptive neuromuscular facilitation approach*, often referred to as PNF, was developed by a physician, Herman Kabat. It was later expanded by Margaret Knott and Dorothy Voss, both physical therapists. PNF is used with cerebral palsy patients as well as those with spinal cord injuries, orthopedic problems, or other disabilities affecting the neuromuscular system. The basic thrust of this approach is the stimulation of the proprioceptors. Proprioceptors are located in the muscles, tendons, and joints, and through movement provide the patient with awareness of position, balance, and equilibrium changes.

Mass movement patterns are developed first through such activities as washing a floor in a creeping position or finger painting on the floor on "all fours." Making a macramé project is an example of how fine motor coordination might be used. Diagonal patterns of motion are stressed as a means of facilitating the appropriate motor responses. The patient's active participation in the process is emphasized.[22]

Neurodevelopmental Approach

Karel Bobath, a neuropsychiatrist, and Berta Bobath, a physical therapist, both practicing in London, developed the *neurodevelopmental approach to treatment,* which is often referred to as NDT. This approach, used with cerebral palsy and hemiplegia patients, is based on the following concepts:[20]

1 Patterns of movement are learned and refined to enable the individual to develop skills.
2 Abnormal patterns of posture, balance, and movement occur when the brain has been damaged.
3 Abnormal patterns interfere with the individual's ability to carry out normal activities of daily living.

Basic treatment is centered on the inhibition or restraint of abnormal reflex patterns through handling and sensory stimulation. The goal is to help the patient produce the desired normal movement pattern. For example, the therapist might place a child on top of a large inflated ball and roll the ball from side to side. The desired response is that the child will extend his or her hands and arms to maintain balance and as a protection against falling off the ball.[20] As this activity is repeated, changes will occur in muscle tone that will promote normal movement.[21]

Movement Therapy

The movement therapy approach to treatment was developed in the 1950s by Signe Brunnstrom, a physical therapist, as a method for treating patients with hemiplegia. Based on the principles of neurodevelopment, she defined specific states of recovery of the hand, arm, and leg. She also developed related techniques to establish patterns of motion or synergies.[20] Some of these techniques include tapping the belly of a muscle, pressure on a tendon, and quick stroking of a muscle.

Primitive reflexes present in the early stages of normal development often reappear in a patient who has had a cerebral vascular accident. These reflexes are facilitated in occupational therapy treatment to promote the return of functional movement patterns. This might be accomplished by the use of activities that offer resistance, such as weaving and woodworking, which allow a neurological impulse to spread to other muscles in a group. Visual and verbal clues are also very important to the total treatment process.[20,23] Brunnstrom noted that the movement therapy patterns that primarily involve the lower extremities should be dealt with by a physical therapist.[20]

Summary

This chapter presented an overview of some of the theoretical frameworks and approaches that are frequently used in occupational therapy as a guide for practice. Some are general and have application to all areas of practice, while others deal with specific clinical settings, such as psychiatry. Theoretical approaches related to the application of definitive techniques (such as sensory stimulation and proprioceptive neuromuscular facilitation) were also addressed. Reference is often made to human development as a basis for many of these theories, but the profession has not yet identified or adopted a singular theoretical model.[24] As both the profession and society continue to grow and change, some frameworks and approaches will be discarded, others will be combined, and new ones will emerge.

References

1. *Webster's New Twentieth Century Dictionary*, 2nd Edition, New York: Simon and Shuster, 1979
2. *The Doubleday Dictionary*, New York: Doubleday, 1975.
3. Mosey AC: *Occupational Therapy, Configuration of a Profession*, New York: Raven Press, 1981.
4. Reed KL: *Models of Practice in Occupational Therapy*, Baltimore: Williams and Wilkins, 1984.
5. Reilly M: Occupational therapy can be one of the great ideas of twentieth century medicine, *Am J Occup Ther*, 16:1-9, 1962.
6. Loukaran VH: Toward a model of occupational therapy for community health, *Am J Occup Ther*, 31:71, 1977.
7. Matsutsuyu J: Occupational behavior approach. In: Willard and Spackman: *Occupational Therapy*, 6th Edition, Philadelphia: JB Lippincott Co., 1983.
8. Kielhofner G and Burke JP: A model of human occupation. Part 1: Conceptual framework and content, *Am J Occup Ther*, 34:657-666, 1980.
9. Kielhofner G: Occupation. In: Willard and Spackman: *Occupational Therapy*, 6th Edition, Philadelphia: JB Lippincott Co., 1983.
10. Tiffany EG: Developmental approaches. In: Willard and Spackman: *Occupational Therapy*, 6th Edition. Philadelphia: JB Lippincott Co., 1983.
11. King LJ: Toward a science of adaptive responses, *Am J Occup Ther*, 32:429-437, 1978.
12. Kleinman BL and Buckley BL: Some implications of a science of adaptive responses, *Am J Occup Ther*, 36:15-19, 1982.
13. Llorens L: Facilitating growth and development: The promise of occupational therapy, *Am J Occup Ther*, 24:93-101, 1970.
14. Fidler GS and Fidler JW: Doing and becoming: Purposeful action and self-actualization, *Am J Occup Ther*, 32:306, 1978.
15. Mosey AC: *Activities Therapy*, New York: Raven Press, 1973.
16. *Uniform Terminology for Reporting Occupational Therapy Services*, Rockville, MD: American Occupational Therapy Association, 1979.
17. Vezie MB: Sensory integration: A foundation for learning, *Academic Therapy*, 10:348, 1975.
18. Lewis SC: *The Mature Years*, Thorofare, NJ: Charles B. Slack, Inc., 1979, p 93.
19. Cromwell FS: In memoriam, *Am J Occup Ther*, 39:54, 1985.
20. Trombly CA and Scott AD: *Occupational Therapy for Physical Dysfunction*, Baltimore: Williams and Wilkins, 1983.
21. Huss AJ: Overview of sensorimotor approaches, In: Willard and Spackman: *Occupational Therapy*, 6th Edition, Philadelphia: JB Lippincott Co., 1983.
22. Voss DE: Proproceptive neuromuscular facilitation: Application of patterns and techniques in occupational therapy, *Am J Occup Ther*, 13:193, 1959.
23. Huss AJ: Sensory motor treatment approaches, In: Willard and Spackman: *Occupational Therapy*, 4th Edition, Philadelphia: JB Lippincott Co., 1971, pp 379-380.
24. Hopkins HL: Current basis for theory and philosophy of occupational therapy, In: Willard and Spackman: *Occupational Therapy*, 6th Edition, Philadelphia: JB Lippincot Co. 1983, p 28.

Bibliography

Cynkin S: *Occupational Therapy: Toward Health Through Activities*, Boston: Little, Brown and Company, 1979.

Gilfoyle E, Grady A and Moore JC: *Children Adapt*, Thorofare, NJ: Charles B. Slack, Inc., 1981.

Acknowledgments

The author wishes to thank Miriam Joseph Cummings, MA, OTR, FAOTA, and Crystal Woodin, MS, OTR, for their content and editorial suggestions.

CHAPTER 5

Basic Theories of Human Development

Sister Miriam Joseph Cummings, OTR

Introduction

Human development is an essential basis for all occupational therapy practice. The subject of human development is vast and cannot be covered completely in this discussion. However, the elements that are most essential as a foundation for the practice of occupational therapy will be addressed. These areas are *motor, cognitive,* and *psychosocial* development. Language development, although important, will not be considered here. The basic theorists who will be discussed are Jean Piaget, Erik Erikson, Arnold Gesell, Robert Havighurst, and Abraham Maslow. There are, of course, many others who have contributed greatly to the field of human development.

Motor Development

Many investigators have contributed to the body of knowledge regarding motor development; among the most important is Arnold Gesell. Gesell studied and developed his theories first at Yale University and eventually at the Gesell Institute of Child Development. His important work is in the area of infant and child development.

Motor development occurs in a sequence that is relatively unvaried. The timing of the occurrence of each step in the sequence may be highly varied, however. Some of the principles recognized are the *cephalocaudal* development and the *proximal-distal* development, meaning that development proceeds from the head to the lower extremities (tail) and from the parts close to the midline to the extremities, respectively. Control of the head occurs before control of the limbs; control of the trunk and shoulder occurs before contol of the hand.[1] Through careful studies, Gesell determined milestones of development that the infant should accomplish at particular times. The major milestones are shown in Figure 5-1.[1,2,3]

Most children follow this sequence, although sometimes the sequence is altered or a stage is omitted. The actual time spent becoming stable in these tasks varies greatly. There is also a distinction between the time when the child is capable of performing these tasks given optimal conditions, and the time when the tasks appear spontaneously. How strongly the parents desire to have a child perform the particular task seems to influence development; children who are encouraged and given many opportunities to practice or perform may master a task sooner than those who do not receive that encouragement.

A second major area of motor development is that of hand function. This can be divided into the components of reach, grasp and release, and manipulation.

Reach and Early Manipulation

Reaching in the supine position using small incipient movements occurs from 8 to 12 weeks of age. Spontaneous regard of objects occurs at about 16 weeks, accompanied by greatly increased arm activity. Bilateral approach movements begin around 20 weeks, and at 24 weeks bilateral grasp of objects occurs. Beyond 28 weeks, the activity becomes more and more unilateral.

In the sitting position only passive and brief regard for reaching occurs from 12 to 16 weeks. At 20 weeks the child makes movements that are likely to cause contact with the object. At 24 weeks the child grasps the object and can do some manipulation of it. When the baby is about 28 weeks old he or she can move an object such as a rattle from hand to hand and manipulate it in a variety of ways. By 18 months the baby reaches for near objects easily and automatically, but reaches for distant ones more awkwardly. This reaching for distant objects gradually becomes smoother and more coordinated by 5 years of age.

FIGURE 5-1 Milestones in Gross Motor Development and Postural Control

Accomplishment	Age in months
Lift head to 45° when prone	2
Lift chest off floor when prone	3
Sit up when supported	4
Sit by self	7
Crawl	8
Pull self up on furniture	9
Creep	10
Walk when led	11
Stand alone	14
Walk alone, straddle-toddle (feet far apart, full sole step)	15
Toddle (longer steps, narrower width, lower step height)	18
Run	21

Grasp and Release

Grasp occurs as a reflex in the prenatal life of the baby. There are two aspects to this reflex action: finger closure and gripping. Light pressure or stroking on the palm is the stimulus that elicits closure. Stretching the finger tendons elicits gripping. The closure aspect of the reflex disappears

FIGURE 5-2. Milestones in Grasp, Release and Manipulation

Accomplishment	Age
Hands fisted	4 weeks
Hands open; scratches and clutches	16 weeks
Grasps cube in palm; rakes at pellet	28 weeks
Crude release	40 weeks
Prehends pellet with neat pincer grasp	52 weeks
Builds tower of 3 cubes; turns 2–3 pages at once	18 months
Builds tower of 6 cubes; turns pages singly	24 months
Builds tower of 10 cubes; holds crayon in adult fashion	36 months
Traces within lines	48 months

from 16 to 24 weeks after birth; the gripping aspect weakens and then disappears after 12 to 24 weeks.

Voluntary grasping, in contrast to reflex grasping, follows a relatively precise pattern. In the beginning of development of this function, the grasp is one in which the ulnar side of the hand is used in a raking manner. Objects are palmed, rather than handled precisely by the fingers. At 18 weeks the hand is open until it contacts the object; the thumb is in opposition.[2,3]

At 24 weeks the squeeze grasp is normally achieved. By 28 weeks the hand grasp is accomplished, and a palm grasp usually is performed by 32 weeks. At 52 weeks the baby shows improved ability to use a four finger grasp. Other milestones which may be termed predrawing include the abilities to hold a crayon or object of similar size at 12 months, to "scribble" at 18 months, and to follow a horizontal line with a crayon at 30 months.

When the baby is 8 weeks old a swiping movement is used to reach an object, but the baby does not come into contact with it. At the age of 3 months, swiping results in some contact. By 4 months, the child is using a palmar grasp, which means that all fingers and the palm are in contact with the object. At 6 months there is a mitten pattern of grasp present, whereby all of the fingers are together and the thumb is in opposition. When the baby reaches the age of 7 months, the fingers, particularly the middle finger, are used as a rake to get an object into the palm with the thumb in opposition. At 8 months, there is beginning palmar prehension, with thumb, index, and middle fingers in opposition to each other. By 1 year the child can use more advanced palmar or fingertip prehension.[4]

Releasing is a more difficult motor activity than grasping. At 9 months the child begins to release objects voluntarily. At this age, the child will drop things spontaneously or will release an object when an adult takes hold of it. At approximately 11 to 12 months the child will let go of things upon request.[5] Figure 5-2 presents a table of grasp, release, and manipulation milestones.[1]

Cognitive Development

The principal formulator of the theory of cognitive development was Jean Piaget, who was born in Switzerland in 1896. His early work was in biology, but he eventually became interested in normal child development, particularly in the cognitive area. He used a clinical method of careful observation of children, beginning with his own, to study and analyze behavior and thinking. He did not use control groups, random sampling, or other research techniques of that type, but instead studied children in their natural environment doing their normal activities. He later developed a series of tasks to be presented to children as a basis for observation and analysis. Piaget died in 1983.[4,6,7,8]

Piaget's theory of intellectual development includes the concepts of organization and adaptation. Organization refers to a person's tendency to develop a coherent system. Adaptation is the tendency to adjust to the environment. As new knowledge is attained, it must be brought into balance with previous experience. This balance is called equilibration.[4,6]

Organization and adaptation are two tendencies within each person. Experiences are changed into knowledge through two complementary processes: assimilation and accommodation. Assimilation is a process by which an experience is incorporated into existing knowledge; accommodation is a process by which what is known is adjusted to the environment.

Knowledge is gained when experiences are organized, systemized, and related to previous experiences. This knowledge is adjusted according to the outside environment, the reality of things around the individual. A dynamic balance is being sought between what is known and what is objectively present. "Accommodation and assimilation, which are two complementary aspects of adaptation, are perpetually in action, are trying to maintain an equilibrium which is perpetually disrupted."[9]

Piaget described four stages of cognitive development. The order of acquiring the skills in each period is constant, but the timing is not. Piaget emphasized the integrative nature of stages: the structures of each stage become an integral part of the next stage. Each stage includes a period of preparation and a level of completion.[10] The four stages are the *sensory-motor* period, the *pre-operational* period, the *concrete-operational* periods, and the *formal-operational* period.

Sensory-Motor Period

This period extends from birth until the appearance of language at about two years of age.

It is a period that begins with reflex activity, particularly sucking, eye movements, and the palmar reflex. Through the use of reflexes the baby brings information in and begins the process of assimilation. As the child reacts to objects through reflex activity, he or she gradually develops habits of response. These habits become organized as the baby learns to perceive and identify objects. The child learns to relate actions to objects and to see objects as things outside self. As children move through this stage, they learn the names of objects but do not name them, since this is a preverbal stage. A child will search for objects that are not visible, try out different means of securing objects, and experiment with different properties of objects. At this point the child begins to relate the means (his or her actions) to the end (achieving what he or she wants).

Pre-Operational Period

The pre-operational period is the time from approximately two to seven years of age. An operation is defined as a mental action that can be reversed; pre-operational refers to the period in which the child is unable to reverse mental actions. The child's reasoning is from the particular to the particular.[9] Generalization is not possible, and neither inductive nor deductive reasoning is present. The child is not able to distinguish between what is real and what is fantasy. One strong characteristic of this period is animistic thinking. The child regards inanimate objects as living and gives feelings and thoughts to inanimate objects. The child is aware of past and future, as well as present, but only of short durations in each direction. Concepts of time are limited, but an awareness does exist.

Concrete-Operational Period

The concrete-operational period is from about seven to eleven years of age. In this stage the child is able to use logic in thinking and is able to reverse mental actions. He or she is able to analyze, to understand part and whole relationships, to combine or separate things mentally, to put things in order, and to multiply and divide. This stage is concrete because the mental processes are limited to those objects that are present and deal with the concrete. The child is not able to generalize. Abstract thinking begins to occur at the end of this period.

Formal-Operational Period

Toward the end of elementary school age and into high school age, the young person develops the ability to reason hypothetically. The person in the formal-operational period is able to think about thinking. He or she is able to think abstractly; objects do not need to be present. Logical thinking and the ability to reason with syllogisms (a form of reasoning involving three propositions) are present. Theories can be developed and understood.

The development of the abilities in this stage leads to adult thinking patterns. Experience has shown that many adults do not think with adult thinking patterns, but may be using concrete-operational patterns. It is also apparent that the development of cognition is closely related to sensorimotor development. Lack of normal development in the sensorimotor area will limit the child's ability to experiment with and explore cognitive skills. When a disability or condition interferes with the active exploration of the environment, it will be necessary to make such exploration central in treatment.

Psychosocial Development

Erik Erikson is usually classified as a neo-Freudian. He contributed greatly to the development of theories relating to psychosocial development, and provided a framework for looking at development throughout the life span. He defined "eight ages of man," first described in his book, *Childhood and Society*. For each of the eight ages he identified a pair of alternative attitudes toward life, the self, and other people. The person must resolve each of the issues identified. Ego strength develops from this at each age, and these strengths continue throughout life; this development is cumulative.[11,12]

First Stage: Trust Versus Mistrust

Erikson's first stage centers on the polarity between trust and mistrust. It is the time of infancy and complete dependence upon others who provide care. How this care is given determines the basic outlook of the infant. If the quality of the care is good and loving, then the infant develops a sense of expecting the good. If the child's needs are not fulfilled in a caring manner, a sense of expecting the worst develops. Trust, then, is the result of the relationship between feeling comfort and having that feeling relate to the world. This does not mean that mistrust does not occur or is not appropriate in some situations. Part of the balance is the recognition of when to trust and when not to do so.

The quality that results from the appropriate resolution of trust-mistrust is that of hope. This refers to an expectation that needs will be met. As growth and development proceed, a basic attitude of hope will mean that the person will expect the good and will have an optimistic approach to all aspects of life. If mistrust is emphasized, the person will lack this expectancy, be pessimistic, and usually look at the dark side of any situation. This stage corresponds to Freud's oral stage of development.

Erikson points out that it is not the quality of food and basic care that influences this feeling of trust, but the quality of the relationship between the provider, usually the mother, and the infant. The mother-child relationship is crucial.[11]

Second Stage: Autonomy Versus Shame and Doubt

The second stage involves autonomy versus shame and doubt. This stage is the beginning of independent action on the part of the child. As the child begins to move independently by standing and walking, develops control over bodily functions, and clearly distinguishes self from others, he or she begins to establish control over self and the environment. How the parents react to these efforts at independence and how much control they feel they must exert will determine the balance between autonomy and shame. Again, this is a dynamic balance, not a matter of all or none.

The quality resulting from the resolution of this stage is will or free choice, the ability to choose to behave in a certain manner because it is the best way to behave under the circumstances. A person who successfully resolves this conflict will be able to accept the law and act independently within it as an adult.[11,12]

Third Stage: Initiative Versus Guilt

The third stage focuses on the balance between initiative and guilt. At this stage the child is highly active, is able to use language effectively, and is learning to control the environment. The balance needed is between having confidence to try new activities and fearing the consequences of behavior. Questions of what others will think, how they will react to behavior, and what will happen as the result of the behavior are factors. This balance may result in a person who is confident to strike out on new things, explore possibilities, and work for goals, or a person who is fearful, feels guilty about doing or not doing, and is overly concerned about what will happen as a result of behavior. This ability to establish goals and act to reach them is purpose, the quality that is the resolution of this stage.

Play, particularly the use of toys, is of great importance in the development and resolution of this stage. Often this is a means the child uses to try new behaviors to learn of the reactions of others. Toys and play can help to develop initiative and confidence at this stage.

Fourth Stage: Industry Versus Inferiority

As the child reaches school age, which in most societies is approximately five years of age, the world becomes a wider arena. Play becomes the child's work. Tasks take on a greater degree of importance; how the child relates to these tasks will determine the balance within this stage. Industry versus inferiority is the focus of this fourth stage. If the child succeeds and gains confidence from the tasks attempted, the ability to take on new tasks and the feeling of being able to achieve whatever is desired will be fostered. If the child feels a failure in comparison with other children, a sense of inferiority results. This can interfere with the ability to experiment and enjoy new activities. The use of tools, generally the same tools used by adults, is an important task at this stage.

The resulting quality of the dynamic balance in this stage is competence. This is described by Erikson as the ability to use dexterity and intelligence in the completion of tasks, which implies a sense of satisfaction in the completion. This developmental stage covers elementary school: approximately five to thirteen years of age.

Fifth Stage: Identity Versus Role Confusion

The fifth stage is that of identity versus role confusion, and is the stage of adolescence. Erikson describes this as the stage in which youths are concerned with how they appear in the eyes of others rather than how they appear to themselves.[11] It is a time of great physiological change. It is also a time of solidifying the skills developed in earlier stages and focusing these on the adult world of work. Knowing who they are and how they will relate to the world is an essential task. Peer relationships are highly important. Casual observation of adolescents confirms that being a part of a group, experimenting with all aspects of behavior, being different from those of any other age, and at the same time seeking acceptance are all characteristics of this time.

Role confusion is the other end of this dynamic balance. This means that the youth is unable to identify with the adult world of work and cannot clearly define what his or her role will be in the environment. Much of the behavior of adolescence is an attempt to avoid this role confusion and to seek out and establish appropriate boundaries.

The quality that develops in the successful fulfillment of this stage is fidelity. This is the ability to maintain loyalties in spite of differences. This loyalty is the result of strong peer identification.

Sixth Stage: Intimacy Versus Isolation

Young adulthood, the early twenties, focuses on the development of the capacity for intimacy. Erikson defines intimacy as "the capacity to commit oneself to concrete affiliations and partnerships and to develop the ethical strength to abide by such commitments, even though they may call for significant sacrifices and compromises."[11] Sexual relations are an important part of achieving this intimacy. The achievement of unity with another person and the development of a new identity that includes that person within it are the purpose and the result of a sexual relationship. Previous sexual relationships may have had the different purpose of establishing and solidifying self-identity.[12]

The opposite pole is isolation: avoiding contacts which might lead to intimacy.[11] Love is the result of the successful resolution of this stage. Although marriage is often the societal expression of this stage, marriage itself does not necessitate true intimacy.

Seventh Stage: Generativity Versus Stagnation

Generativity refers to the concern for the establishment and guidance of the next generation. It does not necessarily include the bearing and rearing of children, although that is a common way for this stage to be expressed, but centers on a concern that what is important to human beings and society be passed on to the next generation. Erikson indicates that productivity and creativity are facets of this, but cannot replace generativity itself.[11] Older, more mature persons need to be able to share and to give. Generativity implies giving without expecting in return. Care (concern for what has been generated) is the quality that emerges from the resolution of this stage.

The opposite pole of generativity is stagnation. Without sharing or giving, the person becomes preoccupied with self, without concern for growth or change. Erikson likens this to having self as a child or pet. People may turn in on themselves and lavish the love and care they would give their children or pets on themselves.

Eighth Stage: Ego Integrity Versus Despair

Ego integrity includes an acceptance of self, nature, and one's life. It means that the person recognizes the value of the particular life led and does not grieve over what might have been. Such a person has inner satisfaction and is not compelled to try desperately to "live life to the fullest" or to make up for lost time. No time is regarded as "lost."

The opposite pole is despair, in which the person fears death with a feeling of unfulfillment: "There's so much left to do and no time to do it." This is characterized by agonizing concern and penetrating dissatisfaction.

The quality of the resolution of this stage is wisdom. A person who is wise has knowledge of what is true and has the necessary judgment to act on what is right. This is a culmination of all the qualities described. As indicated, these qualities are cumulative, each being incorporated into the next and surviving in the subsequent stage. Thus, a fully developed person has a sense of hope, determines options by free choice, establishes purpose, is competent, is faithful to self and to others, is capable of loving and caring, and is able to know and act on the truth.

Erikson made a major contribution to the field of development by the exploration of psychosocial development throughout the life span. He has pointed out that each of these stages presents a crisis or critical choice. This does not mean that it is catastrophic, but rather that what emerges is particular to each stage. The way in which each polarity is resolved serves as the basis for development in the next stage.

Developmental Life Tasks

The concept of developmental life tasks was enunciated by Robert Havighurst. His book, *Developmental Tasks and Education*, is the primary source of information on this concept.[13] This approach is based on the idea that living and growing involve learning. There are inner and outer forces that influence the development of life tasks. For instance, a child does not have the life task of walking until his or her physical condition and nervous system development allow for it. These are inner forces. The fact that the child is expected, encouraged, and helped to walk at a certain age is an outer force. In addition, there are forces that come from personal motives and values. These three types of forces combine to create the need to accomplish tasks.

Developmental life tasks must be accomplished by each person for successful living. It is also necessary that tasks be learned at the time most appropriate for them. It is useless to try to teach a developmental task before the combined physical, psychological, and personal forces are present to make the task appropriate.

Havighurst divides development into six age periods and discusses six to ten developmental tasks for each period. He emphasizes that this is an arbitrary presentation of the tasks and that there may be additional tasks within each period. Each set of developmental tasks needs to be accomplished for adequate development and to form the basis for development in the next period.

Infancy and Early Childhood

Havighurst lists nine developmental life tasks of this period, in which the age range is from birth to about six years of age. He indicates that many of these could be broken down into a number of separate tasks. However, the principal tasks are:

1 learning to walk;
2 learning to take solid foods;
3 learning to talk;
4 learning to control the elimination of bodily wastes;
5 learning sex differences and sexual modesty;
6 achieving physiological stability (the only one of these tasks that appears to be purely biological);
7 forming simple concepts of social and physical reality;
8 learning to relate oneself emotionally to parents, siblings, and others; and
9 learning to distinguish right from wrong and developing a conscience.

Middle Childhood

This is the period from about 6 to 12 years of age, and is equivalent to Erikson's school age (industry versus inferiority). Havighurst points out that there are three "great outward pushes" on the child during this period: into the peer group, into games and work requiring neuromuscular skills, and into adult concepts and communication. Nine developmental life tasks relate to these three outward thrusts:

1 learning physical skills necessary for ordinary games (throwing, catching, handling simple tools);
2 building wholesome attitudes toward oneself as a growing organism (habits of self-care, cleanliness, ability to enjoy using the body, wholesome attitudes toward sex, etc.);
3 learning to get along with peers;
4 learning an appropriate masculine or feminine social role (the cultural basis of this is the most important, since there appears to be no basis for sexual differences in motor skills, and since role expectations are changing);
5 developing fundamental skills in reading, writing, and calculating;
6 developing concepts necessary for everyday living ("The task is to acquire a store of concepts sufficient for thinking effectively about ordinary occupational, civic, and social matters");
7 developing conscience, morality, and a beginning scale of values (which develops slowly during this period);
8 achieving personal independence (developing the authority to make choices for oneself); and
9 developing attitudes toward social groups and institutions (religious and economic groups).

Adolescence

This period extends from 12 to 18 years of age. The principle developmental life tasks during this period, according to Havighurst, are as follows:

1 achieving new and more mature relations with peers of both sexes (the goal is to "become an adult among adults"; working with others and leading without dominating are the most crucial parts of the adolescent's life);
2 achieving a masculine or feminine social role (a changing phenomenon in our society—it is now more difficult to define the appropriate and acceptable sex role, or to be certain that there is one, than when Havighurst considered these tasks);
3 accepting one's physique and using the body effectively (physiological maturity affects the chronological age at which this becomes an important task);
4 achieving emotional independence of parents and other adults (the important task is development of affection and respect for parents and older adults);
5 achieving assurance of economic independence (feeling able to make a living—today most adolescents begin some type of work early in this period, but are not financially independent until later);
6 selecting and preparing for an occupation;
7 preparing for marriage and family life (there is a great deal of variation in how adolescents view marriage and their own desire for it);
8 developing intellectual skills and concepts necessary for civic competence (direct or vicarious experiences in government, economics, politics, and psychology are the bases for the development of concepts necessary for civic competence);
9 desiring and achieving socially responsible behavior (older adolescents often develop altruism and want to be able to "make a difference" in society); and
10 acquiring a set of values and an ethical system to guide behavior (solidifying present values, developing new ones, and becoming aware of values held are aspects of this task).

Early Adulthood

This a period from 18 to 30 years of age. For most individuals a great many things happen during this time. It is usually the period in which marriage takes place, having children begins, full-time career-oriented employment is begun, and independence in living arrangements is achieved. Havighurst feels that this is a time when the person is most able to learn, but in which there is little effort made by others to teach.[13] The eight developmental tasks are:

1 selecting a mate (the most interesting and disturbing of the tasks, usually considered almost totally the responsibility of the persons involved);
2 learning to live with a marriage partner (success is built upon successful fulfillment of the previous life tasks);
3 starting a family (both mother and father must assume new roles and adapt psychologically to the changes that this brings);
4 rearing children (meeting the physical and emotional needs of the child, adapting to new circumstances, and taking on responsibilities for another person);
5 managing a home physically (furnishing, repairing, decorating, cleaning, and providing an atmosphere conducive to living), psychologically (providing an environment that allows those living in the place to feel comfortable and to be themselves), and socially (providing for relationships between the persons who reside there) - Havighurst indicated that much of this was the responsibility of women, although men also contributed;[13]
6 getting started in an occupation (Havighurst first related this task to men, and noted that it is so important that a young person may delay fulfilling other tasks, such as choosing a partner, until this has been accomplished;
7 taking on civic responsibility (this is less important early in this period; young adults begin to see the advantages of belonging to and influencing organizations of all kinds once the other tasks have become more solidified); and
8 finding a congenial social group (the group of friends from adolescence is often psychologically and/or geographically distanced, so new friendships must be established.

Middle Age

From about 30 to 55 years of age the individual is exceedingly active in fulfilling what are perceived as life goals. It is a time of great productivity. For those who are married and have a family the life tasks have a different focus from that for those who have not married. For family members the tasks will be reciprocal as individuals react to each other.[13] Havighurst lists seven developmental tasks for this period:

1 achieving civic and social responsibility by taking part in organizations and taking on responsibilities in effecting change (middle age is the period in which most people are able to make their best contributions in this area—they have the greatest interest, the most energy to give, and the most time available);
2 establishing and maintaining an economic standard of living (this is the most important task of the period for many people, with social and even psychological needs sacrificed to economic necessity);
3 assisting teenaged children to become responsible and happy adults (being a good role model—the middle-aged parent has the task of facilitating the adolescent in maturing and becoming independent);
4 developing adult leisure-time activities (due to increases in leisure time and changes in the kinds of leisure activities that appeal to the person);
5 relating to one's spouse as a person (husbands and wives relate to each other in different ways as parenting becomes less demanding and securing economic stability is of less concern);
6 accepting and adjusting to the physiological changes of middle age (the gradual aging which went unnoticed earlier is replaced by more dramatic changes which can no longer be ignored, particularly the stress of female menopause); and
7 adjusting to aging parents (taking on the care of parents and working out new psychological relationships, which reflect the way developmental tasks were handled early in life, the socioeconomic realities, the ages and physical and mental conditions of both parents and adult children, and a host of other factors).

Later Maturity

This later time of life is still a period of learning. Many new circumstances require adaptation by the older person. Usually retirement from the occupation that has sustained the person for decades will occur. There will often be marked economic changes during this period, as well as major changes in interpersonal relationships. The life tasks are many. Havighurst lists the following six:

1. adjusting to decreasing physical strength and health (the rate of decrease is different for each person, but all must adjust to a loss of vigor and independence in action, and many older persons have health problems affecting the cardiovascular system, the nervous system, and the joints);
2. adjusting to retirement and reduced income (work is often intimately related to feelings of self-worth, although some people look forward to retirement and enjoy it immensely);
3. adjusting to the death of a spouse (probably the most difficult life task faced by individuals, often including a change of living arrangements, learning to do things that the spouse always did, dealing with loneliness, and handling changes in financial stability);
4. establishing an explicit affiliation with one's age group (receiving social security payments, moving to a retirement village, requesting a senior citizen discount, joining a senior citizen group, etc.);
5. meeting social and civic responsibilities (as the population ages it becomes increasingly more important for older people to maintain their interest and concern with the political and social climate); and
6. establishing satisfactory living arrangements (preferably making housing decisions themselves, keeping the physical condition of one's home in satisfactory repair and cleanliness, moving into smaller quarters while remaining independent, living with relatives, becoming acclimated to some form of congregate living, or accepting skilled nursing care).

These are the life tasks as described by Havighurst, whose original work was published in 1948. Society has changed in many ways since that time, but most of the life tasks remain valid for most people. One of the areas to which he did not refer is adjustment to divorce by both parents and children.

Havighurst's work has formed an important basis for occupational therapy. When completion of life tasks is disrupted by illness or disability, an essential role of therapy is to provide opportunities for those life tasks to be accomplished.

Psychosocial Needs

Another approach to the consideration of human development was formulated by Abraham Maslow. Maslow described a hierarchy of needs which must be fulfilled to achieve full development as a human being. Maslow feared the misapplication of his theories, and emphasized the flexibility of this hierarchy and the importance of other motivating factors.[14]

Maslow's theory centers on the idea that the individual has basic needs which are never completely satisfied, but which approach satisfaction to varying degrees. These needs are in a hierarchy: usually the most basic must be partially met before the next set emerges. This is in many ways cyclical: one always moves back to more basic needs and then further up the hierarchy before coming back to the basics. There are five sets of needs: physiological, safety, belongingness and love, esteem, and self-actualization.[14]

Physiological Needs

The physiological needs are the basic drives to attain what is necessary to maintain homeostasis in the body. The needs related to homeostasis usually are needs for food and water to supply nutrients to the body. However, there are other basic physiological needs that do not appear to relate closely to homeostasis, such as the needs for sexual activity, sleep, and activity.[14] These must be met to some extent before other needs emerge. Maslow points out that if these needs are seriously unfilled, no others will exist; a person who is starving is unable to appreciate any other needs. Gratification of the basic physiological needs will lead to the emergence of the next level of needs (safety), while deprivation of these needs will lead to an all-encompassing concern for their fulfillment.

Safety Needs

Safety needs include the needs for security, protection, structure, law, and similar components that create a feeling of safety. Maslow indicates that this can be seen more clearly in infants and young children, but that the needs are also important in the adult. All people appear to have a need for routine, predictability, and protection from danger. The infant reacts strongly to any threat to security; adults have learned to be more controlling of reactions.

The need for adequate housing is a prominent safety need which is often lacking in society. Many elderly people feel that they are in danger whenever they leave their own homes. People also seek to give themselves structure and routine if they are not present. This is one means of meeting safety needs.

Belongingness and Love Needs

The needs to experience love and affection, to have deep relationships with people, to have friends, and to feel a secure place in one's family or group are some of the aspects of this level of Maslow's hierarchy. When physiological and safety needs are met, these needs for belongingness become prominent.

Maslow points out that the mobility in our society creates problems in relation to these needs. Adjusting to new neighborhoods, making new friends, leaving old friends, establishing new roots, and relating to a totally new set of persons cause upheaval in the fulfillment of these needs. Developing loyalties to country, city, neighborhood, employer, and family are ways in which this need is demonstrated. Persons who are alienated do not feel a sense of belonging; their needs on this level are thwarted. The great interest in tracing family history may well be a response to the difficulties people in our mobile society are experiencing and a strong expression of the need to belong.

The more severe psychological disorders may be traced to the person's lack of fulfillment of these needs.[14] One of the major problems of aging is the gradual loss of relationships with spouse and friends, and the consequent isolation.

Esteem Needs

These needs are divided by Maslow into those related to the concept of self (feelings of adequacy, sense of competency, self-esteem, and self-respect), and those related to other people's estimation of the person. Reputation, status, attention, and recognition come from outside the person, and may or may not be correlated with the person's own perceptions. A person with an excellent reputation and high status and recognition in his or her profession may still feel inadequate and incompetent. Maslow also includes the needs for independence and freedom in this category.

Self-Actualization Needs

This is the highest level of need. It is the desire to feel fulfilled, and to be all that one is capable of being. This includes the ability to most capably carry out that for which one is most fitted. Many people search for a number of years yet never find their real place in their world. For these needs to emerge, it is usually necessary for the physiological, safety, belongingness and love, and esteem needs be at least partially filled.

Although these five levels of needs are described as a hierarchy, there is a great deal of flexibility. For some people the need for self-actualization is so strong that it overrides hunger or the need for status. Maslow also points out that one's values may change the relative importance of the levels of need. The framework of the hierarchy, however, is valid for most people.

Conclusion

It is essential that all occupational therapy personnel be knowledgeable in the areas of human development. Development occurs over the entire life span. There are a number of areas of development (motor, social, speech and language, psychological, cognitive, and sensory) but a person should be thought of as a whole person. It is desirable to think of the patient as *person* and consider all of the areas of development at the particular stage of that individual. To facilitate the correlation of some of the developmental data from birth through adolescence, Mary K. Cowan, MA, OTR, FAOTA, has developed a useful chart, which is shown in Appendix L.

Disability, whether physical, psychological, or both, affects development at all ages. Understanding the appropriate aspects of development will help to direct the formation of occupational therapy treatment goals and assist in the selection of suitable treatment approaches and media.

Summary

Basic theories of human development have been presented. These include motor development from birth through five years of age, primarily as described by Gesell and associates; cognitive development as studied by Piaget; psychosocial development throughout the life span according to Erikson; the developmental tasks first discussed by Havighurst; and the basic needs hierarchy of Maslow.

References

1. Knoblock H and Pasamanick B, Eds: *Gesell and Amatruda's Developmental Diagnosis*, Hagerstown, MD: Harper and Row, 1974.

2. Gesell A: *The First Five Years of Life*, New York: Harper and Row, 1940.

3. Ames L, Gillespie C, et al: *The Gesell Institute's Child from One to Six*, New York: Harper and Row, 1979.

4. Biehler RF: *Child Development*, Boston: Houghton Mifflin, 1976.

5. Barclay LK: *Infant Development*, New York: Holt, Rinehart and Winston, 1985.

6. Ginsberg H and Opper S: *Piaget's Theory of Intellectual Development*, Englewood Cliffs, NJ: Prentice Hall, 1969.

7. Flavell JH: *The Developmental Psychology of Jean Piaget*, Princeton, NJ: D. Von Nostrand, 1963.

8. Rosen H: *Pathway to Piaget*, Cherry Hill, NJ: Postgraduate International, 1977.

9. Wursten H: *Jean Piaget and His Work*, unpublished paper presented at the American Occupational Therapy Conference, Los Angeles, 1972.

10. Gruber H and Coneche JJ: *The Essential Piaget*, New York: Basic Books, 1977.

11. Erikson EH: *Childhood and Society*, New York: WW Norton, 1963.

12. Stevens R: *Erik Erikson*, New York: St. Martin's Press, 1983.

13. Havighurst RJ: *Developmental Life Tasks and Education*, New York: David McKay Company, 1952.

14. Maslow AH: *Motivation and Personality*, New York: Harper and Row, 1970.

CHAPTER 6

Individualization of Occupational Therapy: Environment, Society, Change, and Prevention

Bonnie Brooks, OTR

Introduction

One of the foundations of occupational therapy theory is that humans have a need to be active and participate in various occupations. Occupation is essential for basic survival and optimal mental and physical health. Occupation is also an integral part of survival and a basic drive of man. It is within this individual frame of reference that a person's activities and occupations enable him or her to function as a central part of a larger whole. This makes the difference between just existing and actively participating. Participation and optimal functioning within the environment provide an individual with feelings of purpose and self-esteem throughout his or her life span.

What does the word "occupation" mean? To those in occupational therapy, it means engaging in purposeful activity. Occupations are effective in preventing or reducing disability and in promoting independence through the acquisition of skills, as the following examples illustrate:

1 The occupation of a disabled preschool child is learning the motor skills necessary to enter school.
2 The primary occupation for a young adult may be planning for a career or vocation.
3 Occupation for others may be providing for financial security through employment, which may require a variety of activities.
4 Occupation for an individual with serious cardiac problems may include learning to conserve energy while performing daily activities.
5 An occupation for the elderly may be prolonging participation in rewarding activities and maintaining personal independence.

An occupation may require a variety of activities and skills. For example, the occupation of self-care includes the activities of bathing, shaving, dressing, and feeding, each of which requires varying degrees of skill in gross and fine motor coordination and judgment.

Occupational therapy is the art and science of directing an individual's participation in selected tasks to restore, reinforce, and enhance performance. Occupational therapy facilitates learning of skills and functions essential for adaptation and productivity, for diminishing or correcting pathology, and for promoting and maintaining health. The word "occupation" in the professional title refers to goal-directed use of time, energy, interest, and attention. Occupational therapy's fundamental concern is developing and maintaining the capacity to perform, with satisfaction to self and others, the tasks and roles essential to productive living and to the mastery of the environment throughout the life span.[1]

* Three main types of occupation are necessary for the achievement of optimal performance and quality of life: self-care, work, and leisure. These areas are discussed in greater depth in Chapter 7. Acquiring and maintaining skills in these areas enable a person to interact successfully with the environment. Activities and skills also enable a person to engage in a variety of occupations that result in the establishment of the individual's life style.

* Occupational therapy provides service to those individuals whose abilities to cope with tasks of living are threatened or impaired by developmental deficits, the aging process, physical injury or illness, or psychological and social disability.[2]

* Intervention programs in occupational therapy are designed to enable the patient to become adequate or proficient in basic life skills, work, and leisure, and thereby feel competent to resume his or her place in life and interact with the environment effectively.

Case Studies in Individuality

The profession of occupational therapy recognizes that the level of optimal functioning to which a patient may aspire is highly individual and determined by all of the circumstances of the individual's life.[3] No two patients are alike, even if they are the same age and have identical problems or disabilities. Intervention programs should be individualized. To understand the multitude of factors that create an individual life style, a description of John and Darlene follows. They will be referred to later in this chapter to illustrate various content areas.

Case Study: John

John is a 24 year old obese male. He smoked two packages of cigarettes a day for 4 years and recently quit. He appears in good health.

Family Information

John is the oldest of three children. His sisters, aged 19 and 21, are away at college. The mother is 53 years old and in good health. The father is 57 years old and has high blood pressure. Three years ago the father experienced two severe heart attacks and was hospitalized both times. The following year the father had three minor attacks. He had generalized weakness and has been very depressed; however, he has exhibited significant improvement recently.

Vocational Information

John graduated from college two years ago. He returned home to manage the farm owing to his father's illness. The crop farm is located 25 miles outside a rural town in southern Minnesota. Employment opportunities were very limited for John in that particular region of the state, and he had just accepted a job to work as an accountant in Duluth. He plans to move there in four months.

Leisure and Socialization

During the winter, John watches television a great deal and plays cards. Recently he decided to take half-hour walks twice a day to lose weight. In the summer, John plays softball on a local team, goes swimming, and meets socially with friends.

Case Study: Darlene

Darlene is a 35-year-old female in good health. She is slightly underweight because of constant dieting.

Family Information

She is an only child. Darlene was married for five years, lived in California, and divorced two years ago. She had no children. Her mother is 62 years old and her father is 65 years old and retired. They are healthy and travel extensively, spending most of their time in Florida. Darlene lives in her parent's home in a wealthy suburb of New York City.

Vocational Information

Darlene worked for a short time prior to her marriage at age 27. Before that time she took classes at a local college periodically and worked in her father's office part-time. Darlene completed a computer course three years ago and now works as a full-time programmer for a moderate salary. She pays no expenses while living in her parent's home; however, she does buy groceries and presents for her parents periodically. Her parents recently decided to sell their home and move to a condominium in Florida.

Leisure and Socialization

Darlene is very active. She goes out every evening and frequently takes weekend trips. She is very fashion-conscious, often attending fashion shows, and identifies shopping as a major interest. After shopping sprees she and her friends frequently go to art galleries or the theater. Darlene belongs to a health spa, racquetball club, and country club. She enjoys golf and swimming.

John and Darlene have been discussed to provide a context to examine some of the factors that have impact on the development of their present life styles. These include effects of the environment, sociocultural aspects, local customs, and economic implications. All these factors must be considered to gain an understanding of a person's current life style, who they are, what roles they have, what they want and expect, and what they need.

Environment

A person's environment is comprised of all of the factors that provide input to the individual. The environment includes all conditions that influence and modify a person's life style and activity level. Environmental considerations vary significantly in complexity. They can be as simple as climate, geographic location, or economic status, or as complex as the sociocultural aspects of traditions, local customs, superstitions, values, beliefs, and habits.

Every individual has two environments that constantly provide input: internal and external. These are so closely integrated in an individual's life style that it is often difficult to consider them separately. Both internal and external environments must be considered in designing treatment intervention which will allow a person to function at maximum capacity. This coordinated approach is the essence of total patient treatment in occupational therapy.

Internal Environment

One method of separating the internal and external environments is by considering the physiological feedback provided by the various body systems. This feedback is the body's way of informing a person of his or her ability to respond to the daily requirements of the external environment.

Some common examples of this feedback occur when an individual has not had enough sleep the night before, or has eaten something that was not agreeable. Often there is a generalized feeling of unresponsiveness of the body. This commonly occurs prior to the development of a cold or flu. It can be a temporary condition (such as muscle cramps, indigestion, or premenstrual syndrome), or it can be a warning signal or early symptom of disease, such as diabetes or ulcers.

Moods and emotional states can be considered parts of the internal environment which influence the way a person responds to the external environment. Depressed persons frequently respond more slowly to their environment and may decrease social activities. Some may further restrict the external environment by remaining at home. Mood is often the direct result of something that has occurred in the external environment. Grief is an internal reaction that can result from the loss of a loved one through death, divorce, or the termination of a relationship. Euphoria and states of elation and happiness can result from a promotion, salary increase, falling in love, or inheriting money, for example. These moods affect an individual's ability level and daily occupations.

Moods and emotional states can also be totally unrelated to the external environment. Some people complain of loneliness. These feelings can persist even when a person is with a group of people he or she knows. Such individuals complain of shallowness in relationships and interactions, and can feel lonely even in a crowd.

Self-image is another example of previous feedback from the external environment that creates an internal "set" or environment. These internal environments can exist long after the external environment has changed. One can encounter a person who has lost a significant amount of weight and yet still feels "fat" and dresses to camouflage weight that no longer exists. Conversely, others may gain weight and dress as they did when they were thin. Persons who have been demoted from high authority positions or who have changed jobs to assume lesser positions may still present themselves as authority figures and dress accordingly. They maintain the same nonverbal body language as they did in their previous status. Periodically one encounters an individual who graduated from college 30 years ago and still wears a Phi Beta Kappa key in an effort to maintain a self-image that was appropriately achieved three decades before.

Phobia Case Study: Mrs. A

Phobias are yet another example of adverse internal environments, as illustrated in the following case.

Mrs. A is 45 years old, married, and the mother of two children, aged 13 and 17. Her husband's job as an industrial consultant requires periodic travel for up to four consecutive weeks at a time. He is generally at home one week at a time between trips.

Approximately eight years ago Mrs. A began to decline social invitations from friends when her husband was at home. She would excuse herself for some minor or nonexistent complaint or say that their time together was so limited that they needed to be alone as a family. Eventually, she reached the stage where she encouraged her husband to attend events without her, because of headaches.

Mrs. A no longer liked driving the car. She complained about heavy traffic, crowded grocery stores, and rude clerks in department stores. She located a small grocery store that would deliver orders, and began buying mail-order clothing. Cosmetics and other items were ordered through door-to-door distributors. Her family became concerned and began encouraging her to go for rides or have an occasional dinner out. Mrs. A was very uncomfortable and obviously in a state of anxiety when she did go out. Finally she simply refused to leave her home.

Mrs. A was exhibiting the symptoms of the condition known as agoraphobia, a Greek term meaning fear of the marketplace. In all probability her agoraphobia had occurred as a result of previous environmental feedback; however, once the condition developed, it became an internal environment affecting her occupation and effectiveness as a member of her family unit.

External Environment

One of the most obvious external environmental factors is the climate. Some climates are warm or cold for most of the year and offer extremes in temperatures and weather hazards during several months. Many regions experience four seasons. In general, spring and fall are periods of transition, while winter and summer exhibit extremes in weather, such as floods, hurricanes, tornadoes, or blizzards. Individual responses to climates and weather conditions vary. Many people dislike the winter months and restrict their activities at that time. It is very common for some people to gain weight during these months and then lose the added pounds when the weather permits them to resume their outdoor activities.

The Effects of Climate on John and Darlene

The impact of winter weather is greater for John than for Darlene. Darlene's work and leisure activities occur within a much smaller geographic area than those of John. Her suburban environment offers a variety of transportation options. The winter months impose more restrictions on John. This period of snow storms and icy conditions usually limits his transportation, which in turn restricts his opportunities for socialization. During severe weather, John restricts his leisure activities to watching television and playing cards, and he frequently gains weight during this period.

Summer also affects John more than Darlene. While Darlene experiences some changes, these have minimal impact on her activity level. John's farm work requires heavy labor as soon as the soil is workable, beginning with the first sign of spring and continuing well into the fall. He completely changes his leisure, recreation, and social activities, which include playing on a softball team, swimming, and meeting with friends.

Special Splint Consideration: Case Illustration

A patient living in Georgia was required to wear a basic cock-up splint. During his monthly visits to the clinic, his splint always needed significant adjustments. It was discovered that he would frequently leave the splint on the back shelf of the car. The internal temperature of the closed car in a hot climate was excessive. The splint had been fabricated from a low temperature material which tended to change shape in the high heat. A new splint was made from a heavier material that would withstand high temperatures, thus solving the problem.

Severe cold can also affect the selection of splinting materials. Some are made of plastic that can become brittle and shatter on impact in extreme cold. It also should be noted that metal braces and splints can be very uncomfortable in extreme temperatures. Special attention needs to be given to lining the splint to protect the skin which comes into contact with the device.

Community

Another important environmental consideration is the type of community in which a person lives. There are three basic types of communities: urban, suburban, and rural. Each type has different characteristics that can affect an individual's occupations, activities, and life style.

Rural communities have small populations distributed over large geographic areas, with a somewhat denser population near the town center. Resources can vary greatly in rural communities. Public transportation is often extremely limited or nonexistent. Social activities often revolve around community groups (such as Rotary and Lions Clubs), socials, and dinners sponsored by churches and schools.

Urban communities contrast sharply with rural areas. They are densely populated within small geographic areas. There is usually a variety of public transportation, such as buses, taxis, and subways, and a wide range of resources is available. Material goods (such as groceries, clothing, and furniture) and services (such as car repair and medical care) must be selected from a wide variety of options. Urban areas may still offer activities designed by community members and groups; however, these represent a much smaller component of the overall offerings. There is usually a wide variety of leisure activities to choose from, including theater, museums, galleries, concerts, and sporting events. Crowding affords individuals anonymity and privacy, in contrast to rural communities in which individuals seem to know each other and come into contact with one another more frequently.

The Effects of Community on John and Darlene

John is well known in his small farming community. His neighbors know that he completed college and returned home to help his father. John knows his grocer, auto mechanic, drug store clerk, dentist, and physician personally.

Darlene shops and receives necessary services in a variety of places, and therefore does not know many of these people personally. She knows the names of two women who work in her favorite boutiques. Personalized service and recognition in elite situations can be status symbols if deliberately developed.

Economic Environment

The economic environment of the community and the economic status of individuals must also be considered. Values and standards vary greatly, and these affect occupational therapy treatment, as shown by the three examples which follow.

Case Study: Susan

Susan was 16 years old when she was diagnosed as having juvenile arthritis, which was affecting her right hand. The rheumatologist referred her to occupational therapy to have a splint fabricated which would block metacarpophalangeal (MCP) flexion of all four fingers. A variety of splints were presented to the patient and her family. All were visually unacceptable. The patient agreed to wear the "ugly" splint when she was at home, but adamantly refused to wear it in public. Her family supported her in this decision, even though they understood the medical benefits that could be achieved by a regular wearing schedule. The parents requested that the occupational therapist work in collaboration with their local jeweler to design something more attractive.

Working with the jeweler, the OTR designed rings for each finger which were connected by chains to a large medallion on the back of the hand. The medallion was then connected by chains to a snug, wide bracelet. The design proved to be highly workable, although not ideal medically. The final product was made of 14-carat gold and studded with rubies and pearls. The patient wore it constantly and several of her friends requested similar jewelry. It seemed that the "splint" had become a status symbol in her social group.

Case Study: Mrs. K

A diagnosis of rheumatoid arthritis had far reaching implications for Mrs. K, a 36 year old woman employed as a bank clerk in a small community. Weight bearing had become very painful, and a total hip replacement and bilateral knee surgery had been recommended.

Several months before the diagnois was made, persistent pain and stiffness had forced Mrs. K to give up her job in the bank, even though her salary was important in maintaining the family's modest standard of living. She had allowed her health insurance coverage to lapse and was in the process of applying for coverage under her husband's policy when her condition was diagnosed. As a result, she was denied coverage.

Mrs. K was referred to occupational therapy for homemaking training and self-care activities prior to surgery. The evaluation revealed the need for a variety of adaptive equipment, including a wheelchair and a ramp to provide access to her home. She also needed a commode, as the only bathroom was upstairs. A utility cart was needed for basic kitchen activities.

When these recommendations were presented, Mrs. K began to cry. She explained that the family had already remortgaged their home in order to pay for her medical bills and the planned surgery. There was no money for the necessary equipment. She felt that in less than a year she had gone from being a contributing member of society to becoming a burden on her family. She was worried about the effects of financial stress on her husband and her inability to care for their two small children. The mere mention of possible sources of community assistance brought a fresh flood of tears.

The COTA working with Mrs. K had grown up in a small community and knew how important it was for people to maintain their pride and sense of self-worth. She also knew that friends and neighbors would welcome the opportunity to help Mrs. K and others like her who might need assistance. She suggested to the occupational therapist that they contact the local Kiwanis and Lions Clubs to propose the development of a community adaptive equipment bank. She also recommended that Mrs. K be asked to serve as coordinator of the equipment bank, receiving requests from physicians and family members, arranging for purchase and delivery of equipment, and maintaining records and inventory. The occupational therapist approved the plan, which was put into action within two weeks. Mrs. K was pleased to have an opportunity to utilize her office and managerial skills and to have the use of the equipment until she recovered from her surgery.

Case Study: Mr. J

Mr. J had recently experienced a stroke, with resultant right sided hemiparesis and severe disarthria. He also exhibited overt personality and behavioral changes and was very hostile. Mr. J was a very wealthy, prominent public figure. Once he had been medically stabilized he refused to stay in a hospital room and instead rented a penthouse suite in a hotel across the street from the hospital.

A referral was received by an occupational therapist to evaluate the patient's functional level and begin remediation treatment and self-care activities. When seen for the initial evaluation Mr. J was being fed a sandwich by a male companion. Although eating a sandwich is a one-handed activity, he preferred to be fed.

The evaluation began with a discussion of Mr. J's functional level with his companion. The companion explained that he had signed a two-year contract to see to all of Mr. J's basic needs. While providing neuromuscular and other remediation treatments, occupational therapy intervention also included treating the patient indirectly by advising and training the companion in transfer techniques, dressing techniques, and identifying one-handed activities. The occupational therapy assistant was primarily responsible for carrying out this aspect of the program.

Sociocultural Considerations

Many communities contain diverse ethnic groups. People from the same cultural background have common traditions, interests, beliefs, and behavior patterns that give them a common identity. Frequently these individuals tend to cluster in geographic areas to preserve their customs, values, traditions, and (at times) their native language. The ethnic neighborhood can be viewed as a society within a society. These clusters or environs provide individuals with opportunities for perpetuation of their culture and life styles.

Some cultures are *matriarchal*, or female controlled, while others are *patriarchial*, or male controlled. The roles and performance expectations of the oldest, middle, or youngest child can also vary among cultural groups. In some societies the number of male children may determine the financial security of the parents in later life.

Customs

A custom is a pattern of behavior or practice that is common to many members of a particular class or ethnic group. Although rules are unwritten, the practice is repeated and handed down from generation to generation. Cultural implications can have a significant impact on designing occupational therapy intervention techniques that enable a person to function at his or her maximum in the specific environment, as shown in the following example.

Case Study: Mrs. F

Mrs. F is a 61-year-old Italian woman who had recently had a stroke. Her primary residual deficit was mild right-sided hemiparesis. Mrs. F was also slightly disarthric and difficult to understand, as her native language was not English.

When she returned home from the hospital, Mrs. F was depressed, unmotivated, and not interested in beginning any of the activities of daily living. When cooking activities were suggested, she became very upset and burst into tears. This behavior was discussed with one of her sons, and it was discovered that the entire family routinely gathered at the parents' home for Sunday dinner. Mrs. F greatly enjoyed this custom. She made all of her own pasta and canned home-grown tomatoes for sauce. She did not want her daughters-in-law to bring food or assist too much in meal preparation. Convenience foods and ready-made pastas had never been used, and the suggestion was totally unacceptable to the family.

In occupational therapy at the rehabilitation center, Mrs. F was encouraged to regain her cooking skills, which required some minor adaptations. Her family bought her an electric pasta machine, since she was no longer able to knead and roll her own pasta. Her heavy cooking pots were replaced with new, light-weight styles. Once Mrs. F regained her cooking skills and resumed a role that was important to her, she became receptive to relearning other aspects of daily living skills.

Traditions

Traditions are patterns of thought or action that can be handed down through generations or can be developed in singular family units; they also may be perpetuated through future generations. Many families develop their own special traditions during holidays, birthdays, or vacations, as well as on other occasions.

Customs and traditions may also occur on a day-to-day basis and can be highly individualized. Their origin may be unknown and not related to any particular sociocultural custom or event, as illustrated by the following case.

Case Study: Mr. W

Mr. W, who is 50 years of age, was admitted to the Veterans Hospital with a diagnosis of multiple sclerosis. He was confined to a wheelchair and exhibited severe weakness of the upper extremities. His wife was 45 years old, and they had six children living at home who ranged in age from 4 to 16 years.

In occupational therapy Mr. W participated in dressing activities, bathing, and transfer techniques, and actively experimented with a variety of adaptive equipment that would assist him in returning to his previous employment. Although he was a quiet, nonverbal person, he seemed highly motivated and always carried through on any requests made as part of his treatment.

When the occupational therapy assistant suggested that he begin shaving techniques, Mr. W said that it simply wasn't necessary and told the assistant not to worry about it. The COTA reminded him of the accomplishments he was making in independent living skills and pointed out that this was one more activity in which he could achieve independence. He acquiesced and went along with the program to please the COTA. One day, when Mr. W had successfully shaved himself, the COTA asked him if he didn't feel better shaving independently. Mr. White replied that "it felt okay;" however, in his family it was a tradition for the wives to shave their husbands. Mr. and Mrs. W felt that this daily activity reaffirmed their commitment to each other and was a daily declaration of their devotion.

Superstitions

Superstitions can be difficult to identify and define. They can be customs, traditions, and beliefs of a very small population that may be geographically localized. They can also be highly individualized and border on mental or emotional pathologic states. Webster defines them as "beliefs and practices resulting from ignorance and fear of the unknown."[4] They are also viewed as a statement of trust in magic. Superstitions are further defined as irrational attitudes of the mind toward supernatural forces.

It can be very difficult for occupational therapy personnel to deal with superstitions. It may be easy for a therapist or assistant to point out how "ridiculous" superstitions are and to present facts that disprove such "ignorant" notions. The personal environment, standards, values, traditions, and beliefs of the COTA and OTR can, at times, be in direct conflict with those of the patient. Occupational therapy personnel must realize that the ultimate goal of occupational therapy is to return the individual to his or her life style with all of its implications. The following example illustrates this point.

Case Study: Mrs. C

Mrs. C is an 82-year-old woman who was admitted to the hospital with severe circulatory disturbances in her left leg. This condition resulted in surgical amputation of the lower left extremity.

The patient was referred to occupational therapy for generalized strengthening activities, cognitive stimulation, and reality reorientation. Altough she frequently did not know where she was, past memory appeared to be intact. Mrs. C presented herself as a very pleasant person with a warm, personable manner.

During one of her initial treatment sessions it was noted that she wore a small bag of coins tied tightly around her right thigh with several strips of gauze. When the occupational therapist questioned her about this, she explained that the bag of coins "kept evil spirits away" and made a person happy. She elaborated further and said that she had always worn the bag on her left leg, but since the doctors had to remove that leg, she would now have to tie it to the right one. This situation had not been noted during prior medical examinations, since Mrs. C always removed the bag when she disrobed.

Occupational therapy intervention consisted of introducing a six inch wide cohesive, light woven, elastic bandage, applied lightly on the thigh, with the small bag of coins attached with a safety pin. This solution was acceptable to Mrs. C. When the patient was asked whether other family members also observed this practice, it was learned that all of them did. Therefore all 12 family members were also instructed in this new method.

Life Styles, Values, Standards, and Attitudes

Values, standards, and attitudes are other aspects of an individual that develop through environmental transaction and influence life style. These usually result from feedback received from other people within one's work and leisure environments, as well as from the individual's sociocultural and economic status and self-image. They are very personal and become an important part of a person's internal environment. The presence of disease or injury can be very disruptive and require reassessment of all aspects of an individual's life and life style, requiring some temporary or permanent adaptations. It is important for occupational therapy personnel to use intervention techniques which can be adapted to minimize the stresses that occur when the patient's values, standards, and attitudes are in jeopardy or must be compromised to some extent. Two examples are presented to elaborate on these points.

Case Study: Mr. H

Mr. H, a 50-year-old farmer living in a rural community in Indiana, had sustained a nerve injury to his left wrist. When his wrist was maintained in 50° hyperextension he could perform most prehension patterns and his hand was functional.

All standard splints were unacceptable to Mr. H, who stated that he would "feel like a sissy" and wouldn't wear any of them in front of his friends. The solution was to fabricate a splint from a tablespoon which was bent and angled to the correct medical alignment. The spoon was then riveted to a wide leather wrist band. Mr. H wore the splint daily and enjoyed joking with his friends that he was "always looking for a meal." This adaptation made the difference in whether the patient wore the appliance or not.

Case Study: Mrs. B

Mrs. B was 60 years old when she had a stroke which resulted in left hemiparesis. She had slight subluxation of the left shoulder. Shoulder subluxations are very common, as the pull of gravity on the paralyzed or weakened limb frequently causes the ligaments surrounding a joint to stretch and the head of the humerus to pull out of the socket. Hemiplegic arm slings are almost always recommended to prevent this condition. These slings are very noticeable and not very attractive.

The patient was a very well-dressed, fashion conscious woman of financial means. She frequently met with friends for luncheons and other social gatherings at her country club. Wearing the sling was an embarrassment for her. A solution was found which involved using a leather shoulder bag which was adapted for her to wear on these occasions. The bag was strong and large enough to support her forearm, and the strap was adjusted to a length that would support the humeral head in the shoulder joint. A wooden handle was attached to the bag which maintained Mrs. B's wrist in hyperextension and held her thumb in opposition.

Consideration of these individual values and self-images enabled the occupational therapist to use everyday objects to fabricate necessary medical appliances in a form that was acceptable to the patients and compatible with their life styles.

Each occupational therapist and assistant has values, standards, and attitudes that may be in direct conflict with those of the patient, thus making it difficult to work with some individuals, as noted in the example which follows.

Case Study: Mr. S

An occupational therapist was working one-half day per week in a small, rural general hospital. When she reported for work, she found four treatment requests for one patient, Mr. S. Two were referrals from physicians requesting immediate initiation of feeding and toileting activities. There were also memoranda from the Director of Nursing and the Hospital Administrator requesting the same services. Mr. S had been admitted for prostate surgery. He refused to use the toilet in his room, preferring a small, rectangular, plastic-lined wastepaper basket instead.

The patient was seen for an initial evaluation during the lunch hour. The meal consisted of cube steak with gravy, mashed potatoes, carrots, and a dish of sherbet. Mr. S used no utensils; he ate with his fingers and licked up some foods. This behavior, together with his lip-smacking and belching noises, was in total violation of the therapist's standards and values, as well as those of two female aides who cleaned up the food scatterings on the bed.

Limited information was available in Mr. S's medical record. In addition to the problems noted above, nursing notes indicated that his behavior was that of a very hostile and angry person. It was difficult to determine whether Mr. S was experiencing mental changes that required psychiatric intervention, whether his behavior was a reflected form of his personal life style, or whether a combination of both was involved. Intake records revealed that Mr. S refused to state his age or financial status.

Since there was no social worker available, the occupational therapist was requested to gather additional information from neighbors and the community. Mr. S was described by his neighbors as an antisocial recluse. He had lived for at least 40 years in a large tool shed on the back acres of a farm which was a long distance from town. There had been windows in the building; however, he had covered them with roofing material many years ago. His home had no electricity or running water. He was always piling up wood and rubbish, so the neighbors felt certain that he had some sort of stove for cooking and heating.

The therapist visited a small grocery store nearby to see whether Mr. S bought food there. It was learned that he had indeed shopped there as long as the elderly owners could remember. Mr. S would slip a grocery list under the door and specify when he would pick up the items. He always paid in cash and requested that no females be present when he came to the store. He would talk with the male owner and periodically try new products that he recommended. If the owner's wife or other females were present, Mr. S would slip in the back entrance, grab his groceries, pay, and leave hurriedly. With this information, the therapist made the following changes when she returned to the hospital:

1 A male orderly was assigned to the patient.
2 Mr. S was informed that he could eat in any manner he chose; however, he would

have to change his own linen. He began to cover himself with a large towel when eating and fold it neatly when finished.

3 A portable commode was placed in his room. Mr. S liked it and stated that he had disliked the coldness of the toilet seat and the loud rushing water. He also had disliked two females taking him to the bathroom.

If Mr. S had recently developed this life style, intervention techniques might have been different. When a therapist or an assistant encounters a life style that has existed for over 40 years, however, it requires different consideration. At times it can be difficult to understand how persons living in the same general environment respond in such highly individualized manners.

Change and Its Impact

Changes in life styles, roles, and activity levels occur throughout the life cycle. Normal changes are expected at various ages. For example, a child is expected to walk and talk at a certain age, and a young adult is expected to begin a career when he or she has completed the necessary education.

Changes can be self-imposed or superimposed on an individual. Self-imposed and superimposed changes and their resulting influence on the individual can occur over a prolonged period or be very sudden. The length of time and timing of such change have an impact to varying degrees on life styles, roles, self-image and activity levels.

Retirement, whether self-imposed or superimposed, is a change that affects most aspects of a person's life. Many professionals are becoming involved in preretirement planning programs. These programs are designed to help people consider the various aspects of their lives and plan ahead. The emphasis is on all of the important aspects of life.

Stress

The potential for stress is inherent in any change. Individuals react differently to what appear to be similar stress situations. People who have explored different environments and adapted to change may have some sense of mastery over the environment. They can recall and apply previous actions and thoughts that worked successfully or were ineffective. This provides them with more resources and information to plan actions and respond appropriately.

John and Darlene: Follow-up

Both John and Darlene will be experiencing significant changes in their environments. These changes will affect their activities, roles and life styles. John's decision to relocate in Duluth is a self-imposed change. He has given a lot of thought to this decision to move and start a new career. This cognitive planning has prepared him for the changes in his environment, new roles, and a markedly different life style from the one he has established on the farm.

Darlene's future change has been superimposed on her by her parent's decision to move. She must now identify and evaluate alternatives and make a decision. She could locate a place of her own or move to Florida with her parents. These two alternatives offer very different considerations in terms of finances, employment, social status, and activities, as well as the total physical environment.

As changes occur, they will create stress for both John and Darlene. Individuals who have made significant changes in the past often find that they can draw upon these past events in terms of future decision making and adjustment.

Severe Disruptions

Disruptions are sudden changes in a person's environment which require immediate attention and response. They are usually superimposed on an individual. Disruptions can be as simple and temporary as a common cold or loss of a job, or as complex and permanent as a stroke or the death of a loved one. Most disruptions are high stress situations for the individual directly affected, and they can also cause stress for other persons in the individual's environment.

Case Study: Michael

Michael, a mentally retarded young man functioning at about a five-year-old level, had a severe disruption when his parents were in an automobile accident. Owing to the multiple injuries they both sustained and the length of time needed for rehabilitation, it was necessary to move Michael from his home to an institution. Michael's reaction to this abrupt change was evidenced by withdrawal and frequent tantrums. The OTR at the facility visited the parents in the hospital to gain information that might assist in helping Michael to adjust to his new environment. She learned that Michael had particular food preferences, favorite television programs, and enjoyed hearing short bedtime stories. Other details of his daily routine were discussed. The therapist then made the appropriate changes in Michael's daily regimen, and Michael discontinued his tantrums and began relating to others again.

Case Study: John

John was recently discharged from the hospital following his involvement in a tractor accident. The tractor had overturned and his left arm was almost completely severed. He also experienced a head injury and was comatose for 5 days.

The patient was seen in occupational therapy for reality orientation, daily living skills, and instruction in stump care. When first seen, John was confused, his speech was slightly impaired, and his left arm had been surgically amputated just above the elbow. John is right-handed.

John was pleasant, highly motivated, and exhibited a good sense of humor. Several of his friends came for regular visits, as did his family. He showed them some of his one-handed activities and talked about what he would do when he got his new prosthesis.

He exhibited much improvement during his five week hospitalization. John was no longer confused and his speech was almost normal. His stump had healed well, and a prosthesis had been ordered. He became independent in most self-care activities and used minimal adaptive equipment. John and his mother were instructed in stump massage and wrapping techniques. At the time of discharge John needed minimal assistance with these activities.

John's accident had a profound effect on his parents. His father had difficulty accepting the appearance of his son's missing arm and seemed to blame himself for the accident. He became very depressed and cried about his son's being disabled for life. John's mother appeared exhausted from the daily drives to the hospital. She seemed to feel burdened with the needs of her son and her husband, who both required so much help and attention.

As John developed his ability to perform self-care activities, his parents were encouraged to attend occupational therapy sessions. They soon began to realize that he would be independent again. John's mother observed some of her son's struggles to learn to perform various self-care activities. As a result, she decreased the amount of assistance she had been providing, offering verbal encouragement and praise instead. After watching John engage in various activities, his father seemed more accepting of his son's disability. He became intrigued with adaptive equipment and spent hours with John discussing devices he could invent. His depression began to subside.

The family minister visited John and also attended a treatment session. He said that the neighbors were working the farm while John's parents were at the hospital. The occupational therapist explained that John would need to be seen as an out-patient three times a week for an extended period of time. She indicated that this was very difficult and exhausting for the parents, since the hospital was 60 miles from their farm. The minister said that other church members would be happy to provide transportation twice a week so that John's parents could return to their work at home.

Case Study: Darlene

Darlene had been admitted to a hospital several months previously. She had been cooking when grease caught fire and exploded. She had first degree burns on the lower left side of her face and neck, the dorsum of her left hand, and the distal third of her left forearm. There were possible second degree burns on the anterior portion of the left glenohumeral area and upper arm.

The patient received occupational and physical therapy on an out-patient basis for exercises and activities to maintain range of motion at the shoulder. The first degree burns healed very quickly, and the skin was only slightly pink, which was barely noticeable. The second degree burn areas healed and did not require skin grafting.

When seen in occupational therapy, Darlene was wearing a scarf draped across the lower third of her face and a long-sleeved blouse. She adamantly refused to remove the scarf because of her disfigurement. She also refused to believe that there were no visable markings on her face and neck. This situation was discussed with her parents, who indicated that Darlene was seeing a counselor.

The accident had occurred about six weeks after Darlene had moved to Florida. She was just beginning to explore the area and establish new relationships. Since her release from the hospital she had refused to go anywhere and stayed in her room when her parents entertained guests. Darlene's parents felt guilty whenever they went out and left her alone. It was also awkward for them to have friends at their home.

The occupational therapist contacted the counselor and recommended a referral to vocational rehabilitation. Eventually, Darlene was encouraged to work part-time and assist a boutique in opening a central office. Darlene convinced them to purchase a computer. She is now a partner in the firm, has her own apartment, and no longer wears scarves or feels deformed.

Case Comparison of Change

In comparing the cases of John and Darlene it is important to note that John was still at home when the disruption occurred, whereas Darlene had just changed her environment. Darlene had no friends, no job, and was not familiar with the area when her accident occurred. The only constant element in her environment was her parents, who were also in the process of change and adjustment to their new surroundings.

John and his parents had a strong support system in their community. The people knew of their problems and offered their help in a variety of ways. Fortunately, John was comfortable with his role in the family, the community, and working on the farm. He had been apprehensive about moving to the city and working regular hours on a new job. He knew what was expected of him in his home environment, where he could work toward achieving familiar roles, life styles, and activity levels before exploring a new environment.

On the other hand, Darlene was not only adjusting to a new environment, but was also entering a new role with her parents. When she had first moved back home, her parents traveled a great deal. Her presence at home was quite independent of them. They appreciated the fact that her presence made the home look "lived in," and she was also available if anything went wrong. This arrangement had been mutually beneficial. Now she was simply living with them.

Darlene's disruption occurred at a time when her stress was paramount in relation to the external environment, and the potential disfigurement was an assault on her self-image and her relationship with the external environment.

John's body image and internal environment were also disrupted. While he was concerned about his appearance, his values and standards placed a priority on performance. He had made achievements while in the hospital, and knew he would be independent again with the prosthesis.

While the changes brought about by John's disruption seemed more severe than Darlene's, both individuals required therapeutic intervention in order to resume successful performance in their environments and successfully adjust to change.

Prevention

Humans strive to achieve a balance between their individual internal and external environments. This is an ongoing process occurring throughout an individual's life span. The same principle can be applied to the structure and function of the human body. No body part, system, or organ functions in isolation. Physiologically, the body works to achieve a homeostatic balance among all of its parts. It is essential to remember that any change in the structure or function of a part results in a corresponding impact or change of other parts.

At times the change in the structure or function of a part may have a healthy and positive influence on another part. For example, a person who begins an exercise program may increase the strength and range of motion of a muscle group, improve vital capacity, and increase heart rate, general circulation, and activity tolerance. Changes in the structure and function of a part can also result in pathological responses in other areas. Such responses are usually referred to as misuse or disuse syndromes. Health care personnel need to be aware of these syndromes in order to include prevention techniques in their treatment programs.

Prevention may be defined as taking measures to keep something from happening.[5] It is a global subject which has numerous components that must be considered. In health care fields these include adequate environmental shelter and safety, preventative health care (such as inoculations and regular medical checkups), a diet that provides adequate nutrients, moderation in the use of alcohol, abstinence from tobacco, regular exercise, and (particularly in occupational therapy) a healthy balance between work, play/leisure, self-care, rest, and sleep activities.

Many studies have confirmed that activity is necessary to the well-being of an individual. Activity enhances health and promotes mental abilities while reducing stress. It provides individuals with a feeling of self-control and mastery of the environment, which is necessary for self-satisfaction.

Studies have also documented the impact of inactivity on an organism. Complications arising from inactivity are called hypokinetic diseases, and are a direct result of inactivity or lack of use of a part. Hypokinetic diseases are more commonly referred to as disuse syndromes.[6]

Disuse Syndromes

Many disuse syndromes are preventable and reversible; however, some become irreversible. Prolonged inactivity without preventive intervention can create disuse syndromes or secondary complications which can lead to morbidity. When prevention measures are not initiated, these common disuse syndromes frequently become secondary complications that can be more disabling and life threatening than the primary diagnosis or disability.

A primary disability is the presenting diagnosis and the direct result of pathologic change or injury. Secondary complications are frequently created by the primary disability. These can be the result of superimposed activity restrictions that occur as a direct result of the disease process or injury. Examples include the patient who must spend weeks in traction owing to a back injury, or the depressed, suicidal patient who must be kept under constant surveillance in a small locked unit.

Prolonged disuse is inherent in a multitude of different diagnostic categories. It is important for health care team members to recognize this problem and initiate appropriate prevention and health promotion techniques. For example, an individual presents with a primary diagnosis of a stroke with paralysis on one side of the body. If preventive techniques are not initiated within a few weeks, secondary complications can develop such as bed sores (decubitus ulcers), contracted joints, deformities of upper and lower extremities, urinary tract infections, and incontinence. Mental health may also deteriorate as evidenced by withdrawal, dependence, and depression.

The health problems that result in inactivity or disuse of a part are caused by a variety of conditions and demands. Some of these include the following:

1 pain resulting in a protective response;
2 loss of sensation;
3 enforced bed rest;
4 restricted activity due to a primary disability, such as cardiac precautions or recent surgery;
5 immobilization of a part due to casts or braces;
6 mental disorders that result in activity level changes or self-imposed decreases in range of motion; and
7 limited activity due to cultural or vocational requirements.

Some restrictions are temporary and resultant complications can be reversed in a short period of time. A broken arm or leg which is immobilized in a cast may restrict a person's activity level until the cast is removed. Normal function usually returns after a short period of generalized weakness and decreased range of motion. Physical therapy and occupational therapy personnel frequently treat such individuals and assist in reversing any disuse limitations as quickly as possible.

Prolonged restrictions and permanent changes require specific, ongoing intervention techniques to prevent the ten most common disuse syndromes.

Ten Disuse Syndromes

1. Decubitus Ulcers

These are areas of tissue necrosis (cell death) due to prolonged pressure. The ulcers frequently occur in bedridden and paralyzed patients. They usually occur around large bony prominences, such as the trochanter, when the patient is in a sidelying position. It also can occur around the ischial tuberosity from prolonged sitting, and the sacrum from maintaining a supine position for prolonged periods.

Prolonged pressure in these areas results initially in a red or blistered area. These areas become discolored or black and eventually the necrotic tissue sloughs off, leaving a deep open ulcer. Decubitus ulcers can be prevented by frequent changes in position and special mattresses and chair pads.

2. Muscle Atrophy

Muscle atrophy is the diminution of muscle mass due to disuse. The two major types of atrophy are *denervation* and *disuse*. Denervation atrophy occurs when a muscle has lost its nerve supply. This is a normal physiological reaction to some conditions and is not preventable or reversible. In contrast, disuse atrophy is preventable and usually reversible. This type of atrophy takes place when a muscle has not been contracted for a period of time. The muscle fibers gradually diminish in size and maintain whatever length is required in their position. They lose their elasticity. Volitional contractions can occur as well; however, the involved muscles are usually very weak.

3. Joint Contractures

Contractures of the joints are brought about when the soft tissue surrounding the joint shortens owing to a decrease in range of motion. If a joint is not moved through its full range of motion for a prolonged period of time, the contracture can be irreversible or require surgical intervention. These are usually referred to as "frozen" joints. Complete contractures do not exhibit an increased range of motion, even when the area is anesthetized.

4. Orthostatic Hypotension

This condition is caused by a rapid fall in blood pressure when assuming an upright position. It is usually caused by blood pooling in the abdominal area and the lower extremities, which is a result of the loss of elasticity of the blood vessels. Persons who have been confined to bed for three or four days frequently experience dizziness or weakness when they first stand up. However, if a patient is maintained in an upright position after prolonged recumbency, brain damage and death can occur. Quadriplegics and other patients are frequently placed on tilt tables, and the upright position is assumed by degrees over a period of time.

5. Phlebothrombosis

This disuse syndrome most frequently occurs in the lower extremities owing to lack of motion or prolonged positioning. The stasis of blood in the circulatory system can allow the development of a venous thrombosis (vascular obstruction). This can become a pulmonary embolism, which is often fatal.

6. Pneumonia

Another complication of prolonged disuse is pneumonia, which is frequently seen in persons who are bedridden. The decrease in vital capacity leads to an accumulation of fluid in the lungs, causing congestion. Many persons die of pneumonia as a secondary complication of enforced or prolonged bed rest.

7. Osteoporosis

This metabolic disturbance can occur with immobilization. When the muscles do not pull on their origins or insertions, the bones begin losing their matrix and excreting minerals, and become porous and brittle. Osteoporosis can be painful and render a person susceptible to fractures. Calcium is the most common mineral excreted by the bone. The abundance of calcium in the system can also lead to the development of stones in the urinary tract.

8. Kidney and Bladder Stones

These conditions can be brought about as the result of disuse syndromes. One causative factor is the overabundance of calcium circulating through the body. This problem is frequently compounded by the high calcium content of hospital diets. The patient who is in a prolonged supine position may have urine pooling in the kidneys and bladder, which encourages the development of stones.

9. Incontinence

This is a common complication of disuse from a prolonged supine position. It can be a result of decreased gravitational "push" against the sphincters of the urethra and colon which, under normal circumstances, elicits sphincter contractions that permit control of elimination of body wastes.

10. Psychological Deterioration

The condition of psychological deterioration is perhaps the most devastating disuse syndrome. Prolonged inactivity can be catastrophic to some individuals. These persons frequently exhibit loss of appetite, decrease in communication, and lethargy. It can seem as though they have "lost the will to live." The many personality changes that lead to psychological deterioration depend on the individual and range from withdrawal to aggression.

Most of the disuse syndromes discussed can be prevented by three simple, physical intervention techniques: active exercise, passive exercise or range of motion, and frequent changes in position. These physical intervention techniques will be effective only when combined with psychological considerations.

In the area of psychosocial dysfunction, it is important to provide a variety of activities within the interest area and ability of the patient. Efforts must be made to provide opportunities for decision making and control over elements of the environment. Maintaining communication with family and friends is another important factor. More specific information on the diagnostic categories and techniques outlined may be found in the case studies which appear in Section Three.

Misuse Syndromes

Any change in the structure or function of a part can result in the misuse and abuse of other parts. While disuse syndromes affect other body parts and systems, misuse syndromes usually occur at the primary site of assault or abuse. Some misuse syndromes develop as a result of leisure activities, some are work related, and some develop in response to a change in another body part.

Complications from leisure activities were observed during the sudden popularity of video games, which resulted in a medical condition commonly referred to as "Atari thumb." This is actually the development of tendonitis of the thumb due to excessive use. Tennis elbow is another example of a misuse syndrome.

Work related conditions are very common. People who install carpet frequently have one enlarged knee. This is due to the accumulation of calcium in the knee that is used to strike the carpet stretch hammer. The quadriceps of the same leg may also be more developed than those of the other extremity.

Functional changes require special consideration. Occupational therapists and assistants frequently work with persons who have difficulty in reaching a standing position from a seated position. This can be due to the normal aging process, arthritis in the hips and knees, or pain and other medical problems in the lower extremities. Many of these individuals have a "favorite" chair in their home. These chairs are frequently large, overstuffed, and have a bottom cushion that provides support from the sacrum to just behind the knees. These chairs may also support the calves of the lower legs and maintain the knees in 90° flexion. This position makes it difficult, if not impossible, for most people to easily assume a standing position. Persons experiencing this difficulty usually put excessive strain on their upper extremities. It is common for these individuals to form a tripod pattern with their thumbs and first two fingers and then push on these small joints to lift their body weight. Prevention of this misuse syndrome in the hand can be accomplished by providing instruction in using the entire length of the forearms to bear body weight. If grab bars are available, it is important for occupational therapy personnel to instruct these individuals not to grasp the bars with their hands, but rather to loop the entire forearm around the bar and then pull up.

In addition to analyzing self-care and other daily activities, the OTR and COTA may need to investigate the patient's daily use of tools, appliances, and accessories. It may be necessary to check on something as simple as a handbag or purse that the individual routinely carries, as these vary greatly in style, size, weight, and types of closures.

Mrs. B, the stroke patient discussed previously, agreed to use an adapted shoulder bag instead of a sling. When she was seen in the occupational therapy clinic on an outpatient visit, the COTA asked her about the adapted purse. Mrs. B stated that it was effective and added that her husband also appreciated the added convenience of having her carry such extra items as his camera, extra film, maps, and tour guides when they went on their frequent day trips. The occupational therapy assistant instructed Mrs. B to keep her purse as light as possible, and suggested that Mr. B purchase a separate carrying case for his equipment.

The examination of the type of purse carried by a person with arthritis can be critical in preventing damage to the joints of the upper extremity. Unfortunately, this consideration is frequently overlooked.

There is no existing list of common misuse syndromes comparable to those for disuse syndromes. Existing misuse and abuse problems and the potential for development of misuse syndromes need to be identified on an individual basis. These problems and preventive measures are identified through the therapists' and assistants' knowledge and understanding of the interrelationships of the various body parts and the components of task and activity analysis as they relate to the individual's values and life style.

Summary

It is much easier for health care personnel to treat arthritis, hand injuries, personality disorders, suicide attempts, or amputees than it is to treat *whole* people. The latter requires knowledge and insight regarding the individuals' development, values, life styles, environments, self-images, roles, and activities in planning and implementing purposeful and meaningful therapeutic intervention programs.

The goal of occupational therapy is to return the person to his or her environment with the skills necessary to resume previous occupations. Occupational therapy is concerned with the quality of life, and this is determined by the individual and his or her environment. The relationship between humans and their environs goes far beyond simple stimulus and response theory. A total transaction occurs between the individual and the external and internal circumstances that make up the person's unique environment.

In order to effectively treat a person and not a disability, all members of the profession must know the sociocultural, economic, physical, and psychological aspects and view them in relation to the standards, values, and attitudes of the patient's total environment. Occupational therapists and assistants are performance specialists who must design and implement highly individualized developmental, remediation, and prevention programs.

References

1. The Philosophical Base of Occupational Therapy. American Occupational Therapy Association Resolution #531, April 1979.

2. Reed K and Saunderson S: *Concepts of Occupational Therapy*, 2nd Edition, Baltimore, MD: Williams & Wilkins, 1983.

3. American Occupational Therapy Association Council on Standards: Occupational therapy: Its definition and functions, *Am J Occup Ther*, 26:204-205, 1972.

4. Guralnik DB: *Webster's New World Dictionary*, 2nd College Edition, New York: Simon and Schuster, 1982.

5. *The Doubleday Dictionary*, New York: Doubleday, 1975.

6. Kielhofner G: *Health Through Occupation*, Philadelphia: FA Davis, 1983, pp. 98-99.

Bibliography

Freeman J: *Crowding and Behavior*, New York: Viking Press, 1973.

English O and Pearson G: *Emotional Problems of Living*, 3rd Edition, New York: WW Norton, 1963.

Opler M: *Culture and Social Psychiatry*, Part II, New York: Atherton Press, 1967.

Knutson A: *The Individual, Society and Health Behavior*, New York: Nussel Sage Foundation, 1965.

CHAPTER 7

Daily Living Skills

Doris Y. Witherspoon, OTR, with
Joyce L. Packer, OTR

Introduction

Daily living skills are those things done each day which sustain and enhance life. Everyday life presents few problems to individuals who have "good" physical and emotional health. Occupational therapy personnel work with patients with health problems brought about by such causes as birth defects, injury, or illness. These impairments can affect a person's ability to meet needs and fulfill desired life goals.[1]

Early occupational therapy practice was founded on the idea that activity promotes mental and physical well-being and that, conversely, absence of activity leads to deterioration or loss of mental and physical function.[2]

Occupational therapy assumes that daily activities play a central part in everyone's life. This assumption grew out of knowledge and concern that people must be able to perform certain tasks at prescribed levels of competence.[3] In recent years Reilly and Johnson, among others, have identified these activities as occupation.

The three major categories of occupation are self-care, work, and play/leisure activities. Healthful living and self-esteem depend on the balance established among these three types of occupational performance. Individuals who fail to develop balanced living routines or whose routines have been disrupted may learn to regain their occupations through participation in occupational therapy.[3] Balanced occupational performance results in a state of equilibrium in self-care, work, and leisure activities.

Self-care in one situation may be considered work but may prove to be a leisurely activity in another set of circumstances. An example of this contrast can be found in the situation where a woman does house cleaning in client's homes and considers her tasks gainful employment. When she cleans her own home in preparation for guests, however, the same activity could be described as leisurely.

The relationship between self-care, work, and leisure activities changes markedly as individuals progress from infancy to adulthood. Consequently, the daily living routines of infants and adults are dissimilar.[4] One's cultural environment and related social status help in defining the balance among activities. Routine activity for blue collar workers will differ substantially from the regular activity of executives and homemakers.

A lack of balance in healthful activity can cause withdrawal, depression, or deterioration in the individual's capacity to meet daily needs. Occupational therapy assists in developing, redeveloping or maintaining necessary activity skills which lead to productive and satisfying life styles. Skill acquisition allows the impaired individual to return to independent, wholesome living in the community.[3]

Everyone needs balanced activity to adapt to societal living. An important goal of occupational therapy is to correct deficiencies that interfere with the exercise of independence by teaching self-care, work, and leisure activity skills.

The Occupational Therapy Process

The essential focus of the occupational therapy evaluation is on the occupational skills and roles of the patient which consist of self-care, work and play/leisure responsibilities. Occupational therapy personnel study these skill levels, roles, and responsibilities and determine how the patient's normal patterns of dealing with them have changed. Both the family and the patient are involved in determining the specific discrepancies between past and present activities and the level of performance, and discovering what level of function is necessary and acceptable to the patient in his or her particular personal environment and social/cultural setting. An objective assessment of the patient's needs and potential is essential for the registered occupational therapist and the certified occupational therapy assistant to plan and implement a treatment program that will allow the patient to gain or regain as many functional abilities as possible. Daily living skills are a primary focus of the occupational therapy process.

Occupational therapy assistants must understand and appreciate the roles of self-care, work, and play/leisure activities in order to provide the most effective therapeutic intervention strategies in meeting the individual patient's needs. They can assist patients in determining their present status and the additional skills or attitudes they may need to acquire in order to achieve their goals.[5] Additional detailed information on the occupational therapy process may be found in Chapter 10.

Self-Care

While play/leisure and work activities are equally important daily living skills, the area of self-care is presented first because it is a prerequisite to work and play/leisure and is paramount to independent survival.[6]

An individual is expected to perform routine tasks such as dressing, feeding, and grooming before he or she is considered to be well-adapted to community life.[7] These tasks are referred to as activities of daily living (ADL) in more traditional professional language, but are currently referred to as independent living/daily living skills.[8] Occupational therapy personnel are responsible for assessing the patient's basic potential and teaching primary skills in self-care. Such assessments are based on mental as well as chronological age, and the goals for children and adults differ greatly. Moreover, the methods for teaching these two groups vary considerably.

Self-help and daily living skills training are critical in dealing with attitudes patients have formed about their conditions. If they receive adequate instruction and support, routine life may be less burdensome, and self-care skill may be a motivating force for pursuing work and leisure activities.[7]

Self-care skills are developed in three essential ways. First and foremost is the ability to perform self-care tasks independently. Secondly, assistive devices may be developed to aid the physically impaired in accomplishing such tasks. Finally, other persons within an individual's environment may be trained to assist the patient in the performance of certain tasks. Many disabled persons learn to achieve daily living skills through a combination of these three methods.

Adaptations in Physical Daily Living Skills—Definition and Purpose

Physical daily living in self-care is defined as grooming and hygiene, feeding/eating, dressing, functional mobility, and object manipulation.[8] Without such skills it would be difficult to fulfill daily needs. In every aspect of life—play, leisure, or work—daily living needs act as both prerequisites and corequisites to accomplishing everyday routines.

The certified occupational therapy assistant, under the supervision of the registered occupational therapist, evaluates patients' abilities to perform daily living activities and identifies deficiencies and strengths. The COTA may assist the OTR in the establishment of goals for the treatment plan and the methods that will be used to accomplish these goals through acceptable levels of activity. Patients and their families are informed about the occupational therapy treatment plans and are encouraged to participate in the rehabilitation/hablitation process. A variety of methods are used to teach skills, including verbal instruction, demonstration, and visual or verbal cues.[9]

The need for independence in daily living skills is often more acute for the physically disabled population. Though individuals may be limited in physical abilities, the need to eat, dress, work, recreate, and manipulate the environment generally remain undiminished. The disabled person learns to perform necessary daily living tasks through adaptation. He or she must alter the surrounding environment by manipulating those elements which are within his or her control. This manipulation may take many forms, including:

1 assistive aids;
2 adaptive equipment;
3 energy conservation techniques;
4 work simplification skills;
5 effective time management;
6 positioning;
7 designs to eliminate barriers; and
8 job analysis and placement.

These techniques entail using the environment in creative ways to fulfill tasks which appear simple to the physically able.

Beyond environmental concerns, a patient's functional impairments may contribute to his or her inability to perform daily living tasks. These include the impairments shown in the table below.

These functional impairments are attributable to various pathological diseases and disorders. The combination of functional impairment and environmental barriers causes a need for change in the patient's daily routine through adaptation. They compel the patient to rethink or relearn otherwise simple activities commensurate with the changes in his or her abilities.

Assessing the Need for Assistive/ Adaptive Equipment

Several important factors should be considered prior to recommending, constructing, or ordering adaptive aids for patients. Cost, design, and maintenance are three of the primary considerations.

Spasticity	Rigidity
Joint motion limitation	Contractures/deformities
Muscle weakness/paralysis	Decreased physical tolerance/endurance
Motor ataxia/sensory ataxia	Sensory impairment
Lack of trunk control/balance	Impaired visual perception
Athetoid/tremorous movements	Impaired coordination
Impaired cognition	Motor/sensory/kinetic apraxia
Concentration/attention span	Pain/edema

Cost

The following questions must be answered: Is the recommended item covered as reimbursable in the patient's insurance plan? If so, what percentage of the cost will be covered? If not, what is the maximum amount the patient can afford? Is it less expensive and more feasible for the occupational therapist or assistant to construct the item than to purchase it?

Design

The following questions must be answered: Will the recommended item serve more than one purpose? How durable is the item, especially if it will be used frequently? Is it attractive as well as functional? Is the item easy to use or wear, or is it too cumbersome? Is the patient embarrassed about using the device? (If so, it may not accomplish the intended purpose.)

Maintenance

The following questions must be answered: If the item requires repair or replacement, is there a local vendor who can fulfill this need? Can the patient make minor repairs or adjustments? Can the device be cleaned easily?

Assistive/adaptive equipment is often the key to independence for the disabled person. Not only can it assist in improving the quality of life for the patient, but it can often help to restore the patient's sense of dignity and self-esteem through newly found independence.

Evaluating Physical Daily Living Skills

The first step in any rehabilitation plan is to evaluate the patient's abilities and dysfunctions. Figure 7-1 provides an example of a form that may be followed.

Independence is the focus of daily living skills; therefore, the COTA must observe and analyze each action. It is not enough merely to identify skills that the patient is unable to perform. How the patient performs the task is equally important, since this determines the level and quality of the skill performance in carrying out selected tasks. It may be possible for the patient to complete some tasks independently, but the evaluator needs to study the "how" very closely and answer the following questions:

1 How much time was necessary to perform the activity?
2 Did the activity take twice the time an average person would use to complete the same task?
3 Did the patient complain of fatigue and need frequent rest periods?
4 Was the patient, despite working steadily, still unable to complete the task because movements were too slow?
5 Which motions are functional, and how do they function? Did the patient make uncoordinated movements?
6 When did the patient first require assistance, and what kind of assistance was needed? The COTA may choose to grade the need for assistance in various areas.

Although terminology may vary, COTAs may report patient needs in terms of the following observations:

Stand-by Assistance (SBA)

The patient is independent in completing the activity, but may lack confidence. The patient may require verbal or physical assistance in completing the activity.

Minimal Physical Assistance (Min. PA)

The patient requires physical assistance in completing the activity.

Moderate Physical Assistance (Mod. PA)

The patient requires physical assistance in continuing and completing the activity.

Maximal Physical Assistance (Max. PA)

The patient requires physical assistance in initiating, continuing, and completing the activity.

Mechanical Assistance

The patient is independent in activity with the use of an assistive or adaptive aid.

FIGURE 7-1. Daily Living Skills Evaluation

Name: ______________________________ Age: __________

Address: ______________________________

Diagnosis: ______________________ Occupation: ______________________

GROOMING	Date	Needs Equipment	Needs Assistance	Needs Minimal Assistance	Needs No Assistance
Comb/brush hair					
Wash hair					
Set hair					
Shave					
Apply make-up					
Trim nails					
File nails					
Manage feminine hygiene					
Brush teeth					
Manage toothpaste or powder					
BATHING					
Shower					
Turn on/off faucet					
Bathe					
Dry self					
DRESSING					
Over shirts					
Button shirt/blouse					
Ties					
Jacket/coats					
Hats/gloves					
Zipping					
Putting on shoes					
Tying shoes					
Lace shoes					
Putting on socks/hose					
Pants					
Skirts/slacks					
Dress					
Secure clothes from drawer					
Hang up clothing					

FIGURE 7-1. Daily Living Skills Evaluation (continued)

Name: ______________________ Age: ________

Address: ______________________

Diagnosis: ______________________ Occupation: ______________________

COMMUNICATION	**Date**	**Needs Equipment**	**Needs Assistance**	**Needs Minimal Assistance**	**Needs No Assistance**
Dial phone number					
Read book or magazine					
Write/type					
Speaks coherently					
Comprehends spoken words					
TRANSPORTATION					
Bus					
Drive					
Walk					
COOKING					
Peel					
Measure basic ingredients					
Mix					
Follow simple directions					
Follow complex directions					
Prepare cold meal					
Prepare hot meal					
Convenience foods					
Boxed					
Frozen					
Canned					
CLEANUP					
Wipe counters					
Sweep floors					
Scour sink					
Wash pots/pans					
Dishes/silver, glasses					
Put away supplies					
Dishes, bowls, spoons					
Find supplies (memory)					

FIGURE 7-1. Daily Living Skills Evaluation (continued)

Name: ______________________ Age: ________
Address: ______________________
Diagnosis: ______________________ Occupation: ______________________

CLEANING	Date	Needs Equipment	Needs Assistance	Needs Minimal Assistance	Needs No Assistance
Dusting					
Mop floor					
Make bed					
Change bed					
Wash clothes					
Vacuum					
Clean tub					
Clean toilet					
Windows					
TIME MANAGEMENT					
Planning day					
Planning meals					
Coordinating schedules					
Manage watch					
MONEY MANAGEMENT					
Making change					
Checks					
Paying bills					
EATING					
Eat with fingers					
Pick up utensils					
Use fork/spoon					
Cut food					
Spread butter on bread					
Use salt and pepper					
Drink from glass/cup					
Open milk container					
Pour from container					
Stir liquid					
Open screw top bottles					

FIGURE 7-1. Daily Living Skills Evaluation (continued)

Name: ______________________________ Age: __________
Address: ______________________________
Diagnosis: ______________________ Occupation: ______________________

MOBILITY	Date	Needs Equipment	Needs Assistance	Needs Minimal Assistance	Needs No Assistance
Get on/off toilet					
Sit balanced on edge of bed					
Get in/out of bed					
Turn over in bed					
Sit in straight chair					
Rise from straight chair					
Open doors					
Stand unsupported					
Walk					
Walk carrying objects					
Pick up objects from floor					
Independent transfers					
MISCELLANEOUS					
Manage keys					
Manage glasses					
Operate radio or TV					

Wayne County Community College
Occupational Therapy Assistant Program

During the evaluation it is important that the COTA remember to actually observe the patient in the performance of each task. This gives the assistant an opportunity to monitor the patient rather than rely on the patient's descriptive statements regarding how the activity was or will be performed. This also provides a more accurate assessment of how the patient will function in the performance of daily self-care needs once he or she no longer is receiving direct care.

The COTA, in collaboration with the OTR, determines the underlying reason or reasons for lack of independence in self-care activities, such as muscle weakness, lack of coordination, poor balance, or visual perceptual deficits. Short- and long-term goals are then formulated. Short-term goals should focus on improving the functional impairment, while long-term goals should emphasize independence of function in self-care.

Case Study

A patient is unable to dress himself. He lacks trunk balance and has limited shoulder range. Short-term goals would center on improving balance, thus freeing the upper extremities for functional activities, while allowing trunk range and "righting" and increasing range at the shoulder joints. This will allow more reaching and extending movements. The end result will be improved physical function, thus allowing the patient to focus on the long-term goal of improving self-care skills.

Self-Care Adaptations in Treatment Implementation

There are a number of items on the market to assist the patient with various functional impairments, such as muscle weakness, paralysis, joint limitation, or poor grasp. Although too numerous to list in detail, the more common items are illustrated in Figures 7-2 and 7-3.

Grooming and Hygiene

Grooming and hygiene include the skills of bathing, toileting, hair care, shaving, application of cosmetics, and other health needs.[10] When the patient is unable to perform tasks without assistance, an assessment for use of the adaptive equipment should be made. The following aids are commonly used to improve independence in grooming and hygiene: long handled bath brush, hair brush, scrub sponge, hand mirror, shaver, built up handle on toothbrush and comb; tube squeezer, electric razor holder, deodorant/shaving cream dispenser handle, suction denture brush, toilet tissue dispenser holder; raised toilet seat, toilet and bath safety rails, bath seat/chair lift, tub chair; hand held shower nozzle, and rubber tub mat.

Feeding and Eating

Feeding includes the skills of chewing, sucking, swallowing, and the use of feeding utensils.[10] The patient must be alert, and proper body positioning is critical. It may be necessary to instruct the patient in sucking, chewing, and swallowing. Some of the more common types of adapted equipment used to increase functional use of feeding utensils include: long handled, lightweight, or swivel spoons; forks with built-up handles or triangular finger grips; plastic handle mugs with pedestal cups and other modified drinking utensils; splints with palmar clips; straw holders; scoop dishes; plate/food guards; suction plates; rubber mats; weighted utensils; rocker knives; ball bearing and offset suspension feeders; and universal cuffs and splints.

Dressing

Dressing instruction universally begins with dressing the disabled side first and undressing it last.[10] Clothes that are loose-fitting and open are recommended for easy wear. Some of the common adaptive equipment used for dressing tasks includes: long handled shoe horns, sock aids, dressing sticks and reachers; stabilizing button hooks; velcro or clip shoe fasteners and elastic laces; one handed belts, zipper, and trouser pulls; and velcro fasteners, elastic waistbands and suspenders.

Mobility

Mobility includes the ability to move physically from one position or place to another. Such movement includes bed mobility; transfers to and from bed, chair, toilet, tub, and automobile; wheelchair mobility; and ambulation.[10] Some of the common adaptive equipment used to facilitate mobility includes: manual and electric wheelchairs, motorized scooters, mechanical and hydraulic lifts, trapeze bars, walkers with or without bag attachments, canes and cane seats, crutches, transfer boards, elevated chair and toilet seats, and modified vans, cars, and public transportation vehicles.

Communication

Communication includes the ability to receive and transmit information verbally or nonverbally. Adapted devices used to enhance communication skills include: telephones, talking books, tape recorders, computers with printers and Braille writers, typewriters, radios, televisions, prism glasses, page turners, clip boards, and mouth sticks.[10]

Object Manipulation

Object manipulation includes the skill and performance of handling large and small objects such as calculators, keys, money, light switches, doorknobs, and packages. To assist the patient in manipulating common objects, positioning splints and other types of adaptive equipment are useful. These include: tweezers, mouth stick holder/wands, light switch extensions/levers, key holders and markers, and doorknob extenders and turners.

Psychological/Emotional Daily Living Skills

While this section focuses on the patient with psychosocial/emotional problems, it is important for the reader to note that these problems may also be seen with a physically disabled patient. Conversely, the psychiatric patient (possibly owing to medication) may experience problems with gross motor, fine motor, and coordination skills.

Self-care for the psychiatric patient is also centered around self-concept, self-identity, and coping with life situations in organizational and community involvement. Unlike the physically disabled patient, the psychiatric patient has the motor ability to perform the tasks in most cases, but may not have the desire or motivation to carry out tasks because of emotional conflicts. The patient may not attend to personal hygiene and grooming without assistance or verbal prompting from others. Occupational therapy provides patients with a structured setting in which to learn how to take charge of their lives and be responsible for personal actions. Through therapy, the patient is guided in decision-making activities with the assurance that behaviors exhibited *can be acceptable*. With the contemporary emphasis on community mental health, the COTA is an important team member responsible for contributing to program planning and carrying out day-to-day activities.

The occupational therapy program in psychiatry provides service to the individual whose ability to meet psychosocial needs is impaired. This inability may be demonstrated through socialization, personal self-care, or play. For example, an individual may become disorganized or preoccupied, resulting in an inability to perform some task. The person may be very demanding and hostile, resulting in upsetting relationships with family and peers. The person may withdraw, become fearful, and reject communication with those close to him or her.

Treatment begins with a psychosocial evaluation to assess the individual's self-concept, orientation to reality, ability to communicate with others, and ability to perform life tasks. The patient's level of motivation, maturity, socialization, interpersonal relationships, and ability to cope with frustration and conflicts are also essential factors that must be considered in an evaluation. Evaluation tools, techniques, and methods used by occupational therapy personnel include:

1 observation;
2 interest checklists;
3 anecdotal notes;
4 cumulative records;
5 rating scales;
6 self-report forms;
7 sociometric devices;
8 psychological tests;
9 standard tests;
10 interviews; and
11 history taking.

Patients who are referred to occupational therapy in psychiatry may have problems with self-care for a number of reasons; for example, depression may leave them with little energy to cope with routine activities. The patient who is out of touch with reality may be unable to cook and eat because of fear that the food is poisoned.

Teaching self-care tasks to psychiatric patients can be very challenging and offer opportunities for creativity on the part of the therapist. The most common areas of self-care addressed by the COTA practicing in psychiatry are grooming, cooking, time management, and organizational skills. Helping patients learn or relearn skills in these areas can result in their heightened awareness and self-esteem.

Case Study

A creative therapist responsible for treating chemically dependent adolescent patients recently learned of the latest fad for painting striped fingernails. The therapist taught this skill to a female patient, and the patient proceeded to teach the technique to her peers. Through teaching the patient a new skill, the therapist developed a closer relationship with her that helped them discuss problems more openly. The patient's relationships with peers were also improved through this activity.

Case Study

A male patient who was in the midst of a divorce was admitted to a hospital for depression. He could not cope effectively because his wife had always taken care of so many of his daily needs. Occupational therapy personnel taught him basic cooking, washing, and cleaning skills. Following discharge, the patient informed the staff of his successes, one of which included cooking dinner for six guests.

Program Planning

The reduction in in-patient hospital insurance coverage for psychiatric care influences decisions about the nature of treatment and changes in the therapist's role. These budgetary constraints have caused a rethinking of traditional occupational therapy rehabilitative services and new planning

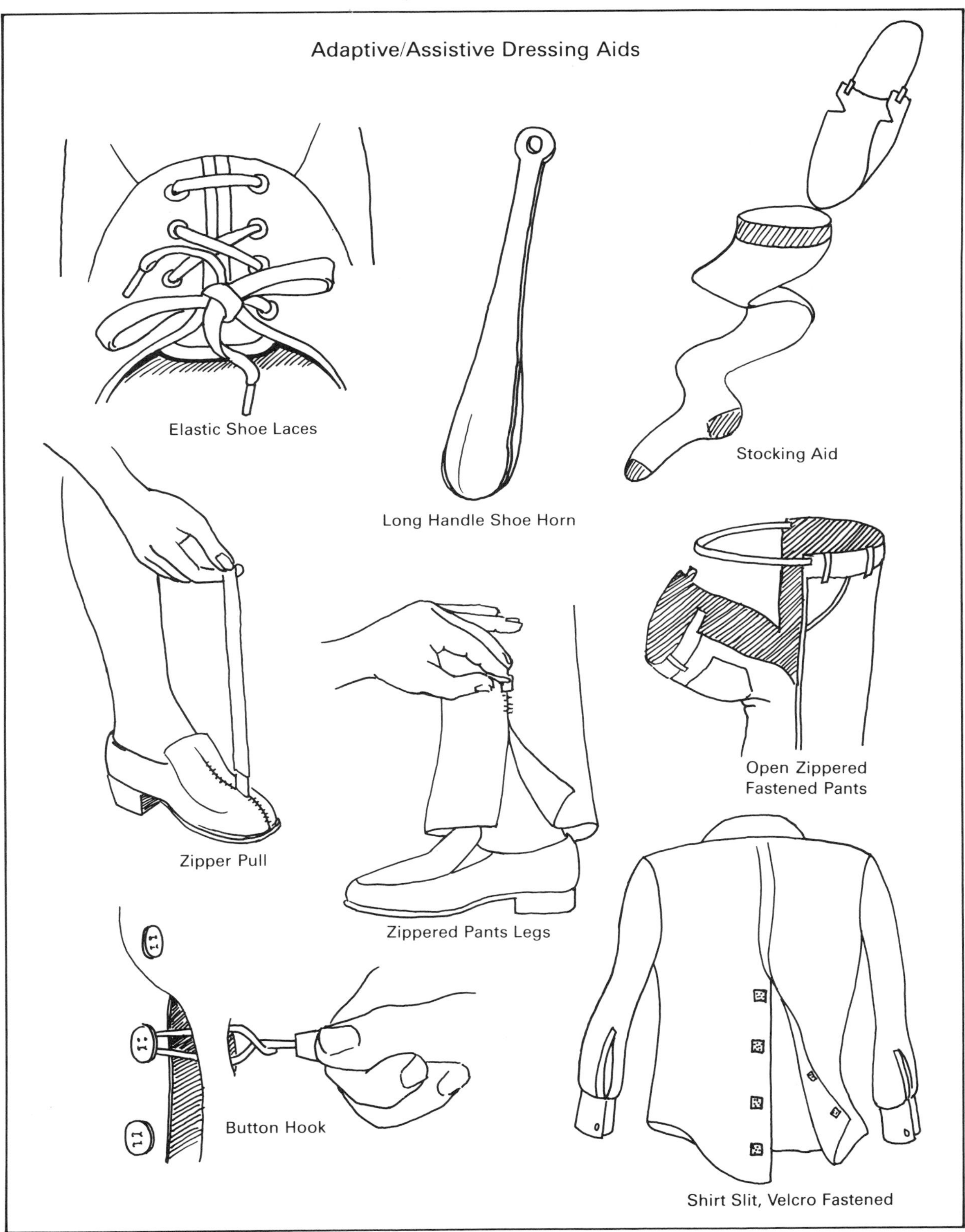
Adaptive/Assistive Dressing Aids
Elastic Shoe Laces
Long Handle Shoe Horn
Stocking Aid
Zipper Pull
Zippered Pants Legs
Open Zippered
Fastened Pants
Button Hook
Shirt Slit, Velcro Fastened

Figure 7-2

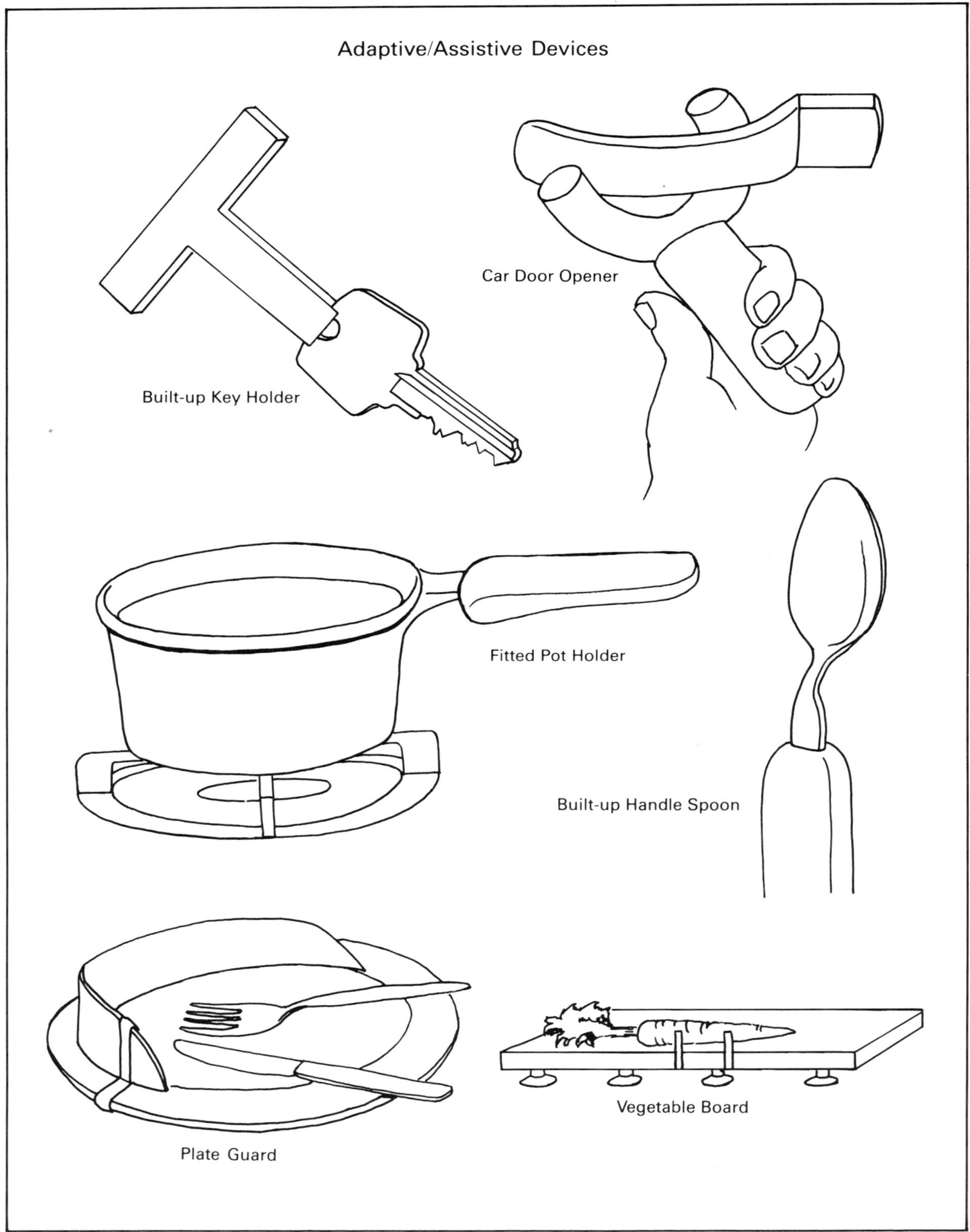
Adaptive/Assistive Devices
Built-up Key Holder
Car Door Opener
Fitted Pot Holder
Built-up Handle Spoon
Plate Guard
Vegetable Board

Figure 7-3

and structuring to assure the most cost effective delivery of services.

Occupational therapy personnel frequently plan and implement a group approach to patient treatment. Task oriented groups which focus on a particular self-care skills are often referred to as daily living groups. The foci includes the following topics:

1 personal hygiene and grooming;
2 laundry care;
3 budgeting;
4 personal care shopping;
5 menu planning;
6 grocery shopping;
7 cooking and table setting;
8 kitchen and household safety;
9 home management and housekeeping; and
10 seasonal dressing.

Within the structure of such a group the leader may use specific methods to assist patients in developing skills. These include behavior modification using a token reward system, individual patient contracts regarding goal achievement, and shaping which uses prompts to promote desired behavior.

Group experiences are also used to provide opportunities for patient interaction while activities are performed. A primary goal is to enhance social interaction skills relative to the patient's potential and the conditions of the home and community environments. This overall goal may also include reinforcement of socially acceptable behavior, fostering of effective communication skills, encouraging self-awareness, and strengthening interpersonal confidence. For example, a patient may be assigned to participate in a group where the members must cooperate in planning a holiday party. Through the planning and decision making experience, each member learns to recognize the ways his or her behavior affects the achievement of tasks and the other members of the group. Greater awareness of these facts is often gained after the task has been completed and members discuss their observations and feelings openly. Such discussions are often termed "processing the group." Occupational therapy personnel are skilled in using activities and group process as structures to develop healthy interpersonal relationships. This topic is discussed in more detail in Chapter 9.

The patient experiencing problems in reality orientation is an ideal candidate for task and activity experiences. Persons who are unable to distinguish reality are given concrete examples through activities that require the use of the five senses: sight, hearing, smell, touch, and speech. The occupational therapy program helps work toward recognizing and reacting to reality in both work and social relationships.

Community Involvement

The profession of occupational therapy is committed to patients returning to their communities and successfully managing life tasks at the end of hospitalization or rehabilitation. The occupational therapist and the assistant may visit the patient's home or work place to assure that these environments provide adequate safety and sufficient functional freedom.

Many patients do not progress smoothly through mental health care. In some cases it is necessary to provide the patient a longer adjustment period for successful re-entry into the life of the community. Community involvement causes the patient to interact with others and to understand the social norms. Activities must be planned to introduce the patient to more complex scheduling, organizing, and executing personal daily life activities. These activity experiences may include budgeting time, social role management, independent housing arrangements, and assessing and using community resources. The latter is encouraged by teaching techniques such as taking a bus, using an instant cash machine, and understanding the rules of organized meetings and the ways to participate in such meetings.[11]

Occupational therapy plays an important role in re-establishing community support systems for patients. Support groups such as family, friends, church members, and day program and community center participants are important links in the patient's total rehabilitation. The recognition and positive responses furnished by the patient's support systems are crucial to the resumption of life tasks and roles.

Play

In medieval Europe, there was no concept of childhood as it is conceived today. Even among some contemporary societies, nearly all community resources are devoted to the business of survival, and little time is allotted to children. Play as a concept has evolved considerably in the last 20 years. The earlier neglect of play as meaningful activity is perhaps attributable to the perception that it was thought peripheral to the mainstream of individual development. The modern individual views play as an activity engaged in primarily by children.[12]

Play is a concept which is difficult to define because it is so broad in scope and includes many forms of behavior. It may, however, be classified in several meaningful ways including simple to complex, evolutionary, and developmental. There are also a number of play dichotomies which include:[8]

1 social or asocial;
2 cooperative or competitive;
3 imitative or original;
4 repetitive or novel;
5 overt or covert;
6 active or passive;
7 organized or spontaneous; and
8 peaceful or boisterous.

Scholars define play in various ways. As a process, play lies at the core of human behavior and development. Play is an intrinsic activity done purely for its own sake rather than as a means to an end. It is spontaneous and voluntary, undertaken by choice and not compulsion. Play involves enjoyment and activity which lead to fun.[12] One author suggests that play is what children do when they are not eating, sleeping, resting, or doing what parents tell them to do. The preschool child's play is "serious business." It is his or her work; it is a means of discovering the world.[13] In 1916 a Swiss scientist, Karl Goes, proposed that play is the way children rehearse roles they are destined to fill in adult life. Play gives us permission to make mistakes.[12] Scholars emphasize life preparation, recapitulation, and surplus energy in explaining play activities. Although these notions have changed in recent years, they are still considered important features of play. Contemporary researchers focus on the spontaneous, voluntary, active, and pleasurable aspects of play.[14]

It is generally accepted that play makes a substantial contribution throughout the life span and affects every aspect of human behavior. This view presumes that adults play and that such activity involves both work and recreational activity. These activities serve both conscious and psychological purposes.[14]

How Play Contributes to Development

Play makes an important contribution to personal and social development throughout the life span, as noted in the following examples:

Physical Development

Play is closely associated with physical development at all ages. Infants respond by squirming and wiggling their bodies when adults play with them. As toddlers their play involves gross motor activities such as climbing, running, and jumping. Sports become important during middle childhood, with football, basketball, and swimming being common activities. Physical ability finds an outlet in play, and such activities lead to further refinement of physical ability.

Intellectual Development

As a form of symbolic expression, play can be a transitory process that takes the child from the earliest form of sensory-motor intelligence to the operational structures that characterize mature adult thought. Since play is cumulative, it has both immediate and long-range effects on development. Play leads to more complex, sophisticated cognitive behavior which affects the content of play in a continuous upward spiral. In the cognitive domain play functions in four ways:[14]

1 providing access to more avenues of information;
2 serving to consolidate mastery of skills and concepts;
3 promoting and maintaining effective functioning of intellectual abilities through the use of cognitive operations; and
4 promoting creativity through the playful use of skills and concepts.

Language Development

Language and play are mutually reinforcing. Where play preceded the advent of language play, it formed a language embodying symbolic representation. Hence some scholars suggest that the ability to represent objects, actions, and feelings in symbolic play is paralleled by a corresponding ability to represent those phenomena in language.[12]

Social Development

The primary goal of childhood is to allow socialization into active and productive adult roles in society. When social relationships pose problems for children, play is often a way to prevent frustration and act out possible solutions without fear of reprisals. In learning and practicing socially desirable behavior, such as cooperation and sharing, the child uses play as a foundation for adult behavior.

Emotional Development

Much of the social learning occurring in childhood involves a balance between individual needs and the demands of social behavior. Play is an important medium for learning this balance, and children deprived of play find it difficult to adapt to social demands in the future.

Types of Play

Play can be classified primarily as *physical* or *manipulative*. In physical play, action and boisterousness is the focus. The child attempts to gain control over the environment in manipulative play. Two additional types of play are *symbolic play* and *games*. Symbolic play includes pretending, make believe or fantasy play, and nonsense rhymes. Pretend play is exhibited as early as 18 months of age. It increases steadily with age into middle childhood and then disappears. Children rarely engage in pretend play after puberty; instead, they daydream.[12] When play is governed by rules or conventions, it is called a game. There are two important characteristics of games: 1) they involve mutual involvement in some shared activity; and 2) the interactions are identified by alternating opportunities to play, repetition, and succession in chances to play.[12]

In a classic study in 1932 Mildred B. Parten observed the play of children in nursery school settings. She identified the following six types of play, based on the nature and extent of the children's social involvement:[15]

1 unoccupied play: children spend time watching others;
2 solitary play: children play with toys, making no effort to play with others;
3 onlooker behavior: children watch other children play but make no effort to join in;
4 parallel play: children play alongside other children but not with them;
5 associative play: children interact with each other, borrowing or lending material; and
6 cooperative play: children integrate their play activities, and group members assume different roles and responsibilities.

Psychologists believe that play contributes to childhood development. In 1952 Piaget emphasized the importance of exploration and play behavior as vehicles of cognitive stimulation. Ultimately play allows children to develop a sense of self-identity and objectivity. More information on the work of Piaget may be found in Chapter 5 and Chapter 8.

Play is an essential phase in childhood. It is critical to health development and useful to the individual and society in explaining roles. Play activities are a key to developing sound minds and bodies. Figure 7-4 shows some of the play activity behavior patterns from ages six months to six years.

Different developmental disabilities (such as mental retardation), cerebral palsy, or disorders which are characterized by difficulties in organizing and interpreting incoming stimuli (such as learning disabilities) may result in the level and proficiency of the child's play skill being directly related to his or her mastery of a specific domain. A child may be unable to become involved in all of the many social interaction skills of play, such as sharing, taking turns, asserting self, recognizing the feelings of others, and showing awareness of rules. Without the acquisition of these social skills, many forms of play (such as competitive play, small group play, and social play) cannot occur.

The relationship of psychomotor skills to play skills is also interdependent. Without the devel-

FIGURE 7-4. Play Activity Behavior Patterns

Typical play activity behavior patterns of children from 6 months to 6 years are indicated in the following chart.

AT SIX TO SEVEN MONTHS

He holds toys and plays actively with a rattle.
She looks at herself in a mirror, smiles, vocalizes, and pats the mirror.
He watches things and movements about him.
She can amuse herself and keep busy for at least 15 minutes at a time.

AT NINE MONTHS

He bangs one toy against another.
She imitates movements such as splashing in the tub, crumpling paper, shaking a rattle.

AT TWELVE MONTHS

He responds to music.
She examines toys and objects with eyes and hands, feeling them, poking them, and turning them around.
He likes to put objects in and out of containers.

AT EIGHTEEN MONTHS

She purposefully moves toys and other objects from one place to another.
He often carries a doll or stuffed animal about with him.
She likes to play with sand, letting it run between her fingers and pouring it in and out of containers.
He hugs a doll or stuffed animal, showing affection or other personal reaction to it.
She likes picture books or familiar objects.
He scribbles spontaneously with a pencil or crayon.
She plays with blocks in a simple manner—carrying them around, fingering and handling them, gathering them together—but does not build purposefully with them. It takes many trials before she can make three or four stand in a tower.
He imitates simple things he sees others do, such as "reading" a book or spanking his doll.

AT TWO YEARS

She likes to investigate and play with small objects such as toys, cars, blocks, pebbles, sand, water.
He likes to play with messy materials such as clay, patting, pinching and fingering it.
She likes to play with large objects such as huggies and wagons.
He can snip with scissors but is awkward.
She imitates everyday household activities such as cooking, hanging up clothes. These are usually activities with which she is closely associated and things she sees rather than remembers.
He plays with blocks, lining them up or using them to fill wagons or other toys.
She can, with urging, build a tower of six or seven blocks.

AT THREE YEARS

He pushes trains, cars, fire engines, in make-believe activities.
She cuts with scissors, not necessarily in a constructive manner.
He makes well-controlled marks with crayon or pencil and sometimes attempts to draw simple figures.
She gives rhythmic physical response to music: clapping or swaying or marching.
He initiates his own play activities when supplied with interesting materials.
She likes to imitate activities of others, especially real-life activities.
He likes to take a toy or doll to bed with him.
She delays sleeping by calling for a drink of water or asking to go to the bathroom.

FIGURE 7-4. Play Activity Behavior Patterns (continued)

AT FOUR YEARS

In playing with materials such as blocks, clay, and sand, the four-year-old is more constructive and creative. Such play is often cooperative.
He uses much imagination in play and wants more in the way of costumes and materials than formerly.
She draws simple figures of things she sees or imagines, but these have few details and are not always recognizable to others.
He can cut or trace along a line with fair accuracy.

AT FIVE YEARS

She plays active games of a competitive nature, such as hide-and-go-seek, tag, and hopscotch.
He builds houses, garages, and elaborate structures with blocks.
She likes dramatic play—playing house, dressing up, cowboy, spaceman, war games—and acts out stories heard. This is more complicated and better organized than at age four.
He uses pencils and crayons freely. His drawings are simple but can usually be recognized.
She enjoys cutting out things with scissors—pictures from magazines, paper dolls.
He can sing, dance to music, play records on the phonograph.

AT SIX YEARS

The six-year-old can learn to play simple table games such as tiddly-winks, marbles, parchesi, and dominoes.
He likes stunts and gymnastics and many kinds of physical activity.
She wrestles and scuffles in a coordinated manner with other children.
At this point the play interests of boys and girls are different.

Wayne County Community College
Occupational Therapy Assistant Program

opment of certain gross motor, fine motor, and coordination skills, a child would have difficulty engaging in midline hard play, object play, frolic play, or exploitive play. Perceptual skills are needed to fully participate in imaginative play, pretend play, dramatic play, means-end play, or creative play.

Children's play skills are related directly to behavior they have learned. Their proficiency, interaction, and understanding of how and why to carry out play activities are based upon mastery of developmental stages.

Leisure

As individuals progress from childhood to adulthood, activities once described as play become leisure activities. Leisure is an integral part of a balanced American life style. Just as children learn about themselves and the world through structured activity (play), so do adults. Through work and leisure individuals learn about themselves and their environments. This learning process is perpetual, and continues throughout the life span.

By the year 2,000 life expectancy is anticipated to increase by five to ten years. Flexible alternative work patterns are being proposed to provide greater worker flexibility and improve the quality of life. The quality of one's life is determined by, among other factors, the combination of work and non-work activities. Numerous studies have shown that repressive working conditions and impoverished social environments create a meager existence for many workers.[16] The quality of life is greatly influenced by leisure activities.

Leisure is a subjective term which can mean different things. Individuals define leisure by their perceptions, taking into consideration their values and cultural orientation. One commonly used conceptualization in sociological literature is leisure of discretionary time. That is, leisure is the time remaining after the basic requirements of subsistence (work) and existence (meeting daily needs) are met.[17] Leisure may also be viewed as "non-work activity" engaged in during free time.[18] Actually, leisure is not a category but rather a style of behavior which may occur in any activity. For example, one can work while listening to music, thus providing a leisure aspect. Leisure is free time where content is oriented towards self-fulfillment as an ultimate end. This time is granted to the individual by society when he or she has complied with occupational, family, spiritual, and political obligations.[19]

Leisure is progressive rebirth, regrowth, and reacquaintance with one's self, renewing, refulfilling, and recreating.[20] It should be compatible with physical, mental, and social well-being. Most scholars agree that leisure is characterized by a search for a state of satisfaction. This search is the primary condition of leisure. When leisure fails to give the expected pleasure, or is uninteresting, "it is not fun."[21]

There are two dimensions of leisure: the satisfaction inherent in the activity itself, and the relations of the activity to external values or social well-being.[20]

In 1960 Dumazedier identified periods of leisure, including the end of the day and during retirement. During such times leisure covers a number of structured activities connected with physical and mental needs defined as artistic, intellectual, and social pursuits within the limits of economic, political, and cultural conditions in each society.

Purposes and Functions

The fundamental purpose of leisure is to provide an opportunity to develop talents and interests. Leisure also meets the following needs:[20]

1 belonging;
2 individuality (through interests and abilities that distinguish the individual);
3 multifunctional purposes in behavior (some activities offer a wide dimension of function);
4 multidimensional effects of behavior (some activities serve additional persons in society at the same time they serve the participant); and
5 activities and created objects as projections of the person (providing expression for feelings and projection of self-knowledge and objects for future pleasure).

Classifications

There have been many attempts to classify leisure. In a study of leisure in Kansas City in 1955 Havighurst distinguished eleven categories:[22]

1 participation in organized groups;
2 participation in unorganized groups;
3 pleasure trips;
4 participation in sports;
5 spectator sports (excluding television);
6 television and radio;
7 fishing and hunting;
8 gardening and country walks;
9 crafts (sewing, carpentry, and do-it-yourself);
10 imaginative activities, music, and art; and
11 visits to relatives and friends.

In another study Kaplan suggested six major types of leisure connected with six foci of interest, as shown in Figure 7-5.[20]

Developmental Aspects

Leisure patterns are also related to developmental tasks and issues individuals face at different stages in the life cycle. In many cases these will be shaped by their preoccupations, culture, and needs at each stage.[23] Since infants cannot distinguish between obligatory and non-obligatory activity, it is doubtful whether the concept of leisure is relevant to them. Socialization through play, however, influences the child's ability to cope in interpersonal relationships and is the beginning of adult leisure behavior.[24] Leisure activities help to socialize male and female adolescents to adult attitudes and roles.[46] During adolescence leisure time activities are an important preoccupation. Activities represent an extension of a school subject, or may be extracurricular. Among young adults leisure is important for marital satisfaction as it provides an environment for personal communication, sharing of experiences, and family cohesiveness. These joint activities encourage interaction and shared commitments.

Work and family continue to be the dominant themes in early maturity (ages 30 to 40). Leisure activities in this category are often home and family centered and provide a means of increasing the growth and stability of marriage and the family. At full maturity (ages 45 to retirement) leisure activities may become less home and family centered, as there are fewer family responsibilities in many instances. There often are increased economic resources to provide opportunities for more evenings out, travel, and other less home-oriented forms of leisure.

FIGURE 7-5. Connection of Leisure and Interests

Types of Leisure	Focus of Interest
1. Sociability	People
2. Association	Interest
3. Play	Rules
4. Arts	Traditions
5. Exploration	Going into the world
6. Immobility	Receiving the world

Leisure and Retirement

Individuals sometimes need to rediscover or develop new leisure interests as work diminishes and retirement approaches. Retirement can result in a relinquishment of social involvements. Leisure can provide a context for autonomous decision making and social integration with meaningful other persons whose support and encouragement is very important to life cycle transition at old age.[23]

Because of improved medical science and social welfare, more people are living past retirement age and longer. Prime predictors of retirement adjustment are adequate retirement income and retired friends with whom to share leisure time. The loss of income, rather than employment, accounts for the negative retirement effects for many. Activities that build skills and interests of preretirement should provide a foundation of personal adjustment and life satisfaction after retirement.[23]

How do elderly people employ the time freed from work? Time budget surveys have demonstrated that leisure takes most of the spare time enjoyed by the elderly, even more than personal, household, and family care activities. The amount of leisure activity increases with age. Eighty percent of those age 65 and over have at least five hours of leisure time per day, according to Dumazedie.

Retired persons often face the problem of what to do with extra time. This problem affects men more because women may find that retirement from their responsibilities is replaced, to some extent, by activities related to their grandchildren.

The impact of retirement is considerably different in various social classes and cultures. Men in professional occupations are often able to continue some form of work after official retirement. This is less possible for those in "blue-collar" or service occupations. Middle class women who reach retirement status are more likely to be members of voluntary organizations than working class women. Among American blacks church is an important and approved medium of social activities and entertainment for the elderly. The church is a place to meet and relate with friends. In addition to ministering to spiritual needs, the church sponsors such activities as bazaars, dinners, bowling teams, travel clubs, special lectures, picnics, and other activities which constitute a rich offering of social opportunities.

The influence of pre-retirement leisure activity patterns on retirement planning and attitudes toward retirement was investigated by two occupational therapists. Sixty male retirees were surveyed to determine the degree of pre-retirement planning and the type and extent of leisure participation before and after retirement. The results showed that a high degree of pre-retirement leisure participation correlates with a high degree of pre-retirement planning.[25] If the patterns that predict satisfaction among retirees can be identified, they can be used in activity planning to structure the healthful use of time for retirees. Further, if one or more characteristic activity patterns can be associated with retirement satisfaction, then occupational therapy personnel can implement preretirement programs accordingly.

Recreation

Recreation is a term often used to suggest leisure. In its literal sense re-creating is seen as one of the functions of leisure, that of renewing the self or preparing for work. Thus recreation is characterized by the attitude of a person when participating in activities that satisfy, amuse, direct, relax, or provide opportunities for self-expression. It is generally associated with arts and crafts, outdoor activities, hobbies, literary activities, culture, clubs, and other organized groups.[26]

Leisure and Sexuality

Sexual activity is an important component of leisure activity. Although there is overwhelming evidence that sex-related activity constitutes an increasingly important use of leisure, sex is rarely studied from the standpoint of leisure activity.

Changing values and beliefs, more effective contraception, and the increasing equality of the sexes have contributed to the use of sex as a leisure activity in contemporary society. Sex today has three primary uses, according to Alexander Comfort: 1) sex as parenthood, 2) sex as total intimacy between two people (relational sex); and 3) sex as physical play (recreational sex).

Leisure Activities for the Physically Disabled

Physically disabled persons have a need for leisure. Today these individuals participate in nearly every sport and craft activity and engage in other forms of leisure, such as drama, dance, and music. Participation in these activities is both enjoyable and therapeutic. In addition, persons with physical disabilities are recreating more and more with with the nondisabled, thus integrating into the mainstream of society. Yet the need for adaptation, speed, and strength dictates that many disabled train and compete with others of similar functional abilities. This is particularly true in sports.

Occupational therapy personnel are not recreation specialists; however OTRs and COTAs are adaptation specialists and are often called upon to evaluate the need for adaptation with a particular leisure activity. In many instances the patient is more skilled at the activity than the OTR or the COTA; however, as adaptation specialists occupational therapy personnel can adapt equipment and teach compensatory movements so the patient can engage in the leisure task as independently as possible. This could range from instructing the visually impaired in threading a needle to adapting a tripod for a photographer in a wheelchair. The following questions should be considered in making adaptations:

1 *Cost*: How much can the patient or family afford for the adaptation needed?
2 *Use*: How frequently will the equipment or aid be used? Does the frequency of use justify the cost?
3 *Expense*: What expense will be required each time the patient engages in the activity?
4 *Maintenance*: Will the adaptation be primarily maintenance free? Are replacement parts readily available?
5 *Location*: Will the leisure activity be easily accessible? and
6 *Appearance*: Is the adaptation so prominent that the patient will be embarrassed to use it, or is the activity so altered that it no longer resembles its original form?

Goals of Leisure Activity

Leisure activity can assist in developing both psychomotor and affective skills, both of which can lead to helping the patient re-establish his or her role in society. Possible goals include the following, as shown in Figure 7-5A.

Leisure Activities for Psychiatric Patients

Individual activity patterns are often lost with the onset of mental illness. Since these activity patterns are the expressions of the individual's proper use and appreciation of time, the loss of these patterns can result in reality disorientation with others, the environment, and time.[27]

Consequently, many patients have difficulty engaging in play and leisure activities. There is also an inability to identify satisfying leisure-time interests. Fidler notes several possible factors which may contribute to these deficits:[27]

1 limited self-awareness concerning one's strengths, skills, present and past accomplishments, personal goals, beliefs, and values;
2 lack of adequate planning skills;
3 pragmatic barriers to participation, such as locked wards, insuffcient finances, lack of transportation, lack of equipment, and lack of opportunity;
4 limited knowledge of resources and how to use them; and
5 lack of underlying competencies in sensorimotor skills, cognitive skills, and/or interpersonal skills needed to participate and experience pleasure.

The activity histories of many members of the patient population receiving psychiatric occupational therapy generally reveal a sparse repertoire of childhood play experiences on which to base adult leisure experiences. Play is widely recognized as the child's arena for learning and practicing rules and social skills necessary for subsequent roles in school, work, and recreation. Play and leisure competencies are developed along with other daily living skills and may, in fact, facilitate the development of other functional roles, such as work.[27]

The patient's use of leisure time can be measured by having the individual complete a schedule of a typical day and a leisure questionnaire. An example of the latter is shown in Figure 7-6. It may be found that a patient's television viewing consumes 90 percent of his or her leisure time. Exploring patient talents and interests and providing opportunities to experiment with and experience some of them might lead to more gratifying activity patterns.

Case Study

A "hard driving" professional man who rarely had any time for leisure was admitted to a psychiatric treatment center with the diagnosis of major affective disorder. While in occupational therapy he developed an interest in making clay pots on a potter's wheel. The occupational therapy assistant who was responsible for carrying out his treatment encouraged him to continue his work following discharge. She maintained a resource file of community leisure resources and drew on this material to locate a nearby art association that held classes and periodic exhibits. By sharing this information with the patient, an avenue was provided for him to continue to pursue his interest and develop a new area of leisure. A knowledge of activities and interest groups within the community is essential for all occupational therapy personnel who treat patients.

Leisure Task Groups

The use of task groups is a common way to treat patients in occupational therapy. Examples of the types of patients, treatment goals, attitudes and approaches, and tasks used in typical groups follows:

Psychomotor:	**Affective:**
Improve visual perception	Improve self-esteem
Improve range of motion	Improve interpersonal skills
Improve muscle strength	Improve social skills
Improve balance	Improve communication skills
Improve physical tolerance and endurance	Aid in acceptance of disability
Improve coordination	Develop friendship/comradeship
Increase attention span	Improve self-discipline

Figure 7-5A

Types of Patients

1 males and females of all ages (except the very young);
2 those having neurological disorders, physical, or mental impairments;
3 those needing to increase their levels of independence;
4 those having inadequate social skills;
5 those unfamiliar with community resources;
6 those who make poor use of free time;
7 those who are unable to identify leisure interests; and
8 those who have poor leisure planning skills.

Treatment Goals

1 to provide exposure to the community and its resources;
2 to develop new leisure and interest options;
3 to increase independent functioning;
4 to provide transition between the hospital and the community;
5 to further develop the ability to make decisions and follow through; and
6 to improve the use of free time.

FIGURE 7-6. Leisure Interest Questionnaire*

Name ______________________ Date __________

Ward or Room ______________________ Age _____ Sex __________

INSTRUCTIONS: Put an X before the activities you know and would like to do.
Put an O before the activities you do not know, but would like to learn or take part in.
Write, under "Other," any activities not listed that you would like to do.

QUIET GAMES

_____ Bridge
_____ Canasta
_____ Checkers
_____ Chess
_____ Pinochle
_____ Dominoes
_____ Rummy
Other:
_____ ______________________
_____ ______________________

ACTIVE GAMES

_____ Ring toss
_____ Billiards
_____ Horseshoes
_____ Darts
_____ Croquet
_____ Bowling
_____ Basketball
_____ ______________________
_____ ______________________

SOCIAL ACTIVITIES

_____ Game nights
_____ Bingo
_____ Parties
_____ Folk dancing
_____ Square dancing
_____ Dancing
_____ Picnics
_____ Trips and tours
Other:
_____ ______________________
_____ ______________________

ENTERTAINMENT

_____ Amateur nights
_____ Variety shows
_____ Puppet shows
_____ Quiz programs
_____ Plays
_____ Pageants
_____ Festivals
Other:
_____ ______________________
_____ ______________________

_____ Baseball
_____ Boccie
_____ Football
_____ Golf
Other:
_____ ______________________
_____ ______________________

DRAMA

_____ Acting
_____ Stagecraft
_____ Script writing
_____ Costuming
_____ Makeup
Other:
_____ ______________________
_____ ______________________

NEWSPAPER

_____ Writing
_____ Reporting
_____ Artwork

FIGURE 7-6. Leisure Interest Questionnaire* (continued)

Name ______________________________ Date ____________

Ward or Room ______________________ Age ____ Sex ____________

INSTRUCTIONS: Put an X before the activities you know and would like to do.
Put an O before the activities you do not know, but would like to learn or take part in.
Write, under "Other," any activities not listed that you would like to do.

MUSIC

_____ Community singing
_____ Quartet
_____ Choir
_____ Chorus
_____ Instrument instruction
_____ Instrument playing
_____ Rhythm band
_____ Orchestra
_____ Listening
_____ Music appreciation
Other:
_____ ______________________
_____ ______________________

ARTS AND CRAFTS

_____ Drawing and painting
_____ Leathercraft
_____ Woodcarving
_____ Ceramics
_____ Jewelry making
_____ Shellcraft
_____ Basketry
_____ Weaving
_____ Needlework
_____ Party decorations
Other:
_____ ______________________
_____ ______________________

HOBBIES AND CLUBS

_____ Photography
_____ Discussion groups
_____ Magic
_____ Nature lore
_____ Stamp collecting
Other:
_____ ______________________
_____ ______________________

_____ Creative writing
_____ Model building
_____ Gardening
_____ Reading
Other:
_____ ______________________
_____ ______________________

List other special interests: ______________________

What kinds of books do you like to read? ______________________

What kind of movies do you like to see? ______________________

What kind of music do you like to hear? ______________________

What kind of songs do you like to sing? ______________________

How do you spend your leisure time? ______________________

____

*Wayne County Community College
Occupational Therapy Assistant Program

Attitudes and Approaches of Leader

- reassuring
- supportive
- friendly
- open
- flexible
- creative
- resourceful, and
- fair

Sample Activity Tasks Used

Trips to places of interest, such as art and historical museums, zoos, theaters, parks, cider mills, shopping centers, and movies, can be planned. Ideas for trips may be suggested by either the group leader or the participants. A decision may be made by consensus or majority vote. Once a decision has been made, additional procedures or rules may be established by the task group, depending upon the nature of the activity. For example, if the activity agreed to is that of going to a particular movie, the following rules could be established:

1 Each patient must sign up on the van transportation form in the occupational therapy office.
2 Each patient must be dressed appropriately for the outing.
3 Each patient must be at the van pick-up site at the designated time.
4 Each patient must purchase his or her own ticket and count the change.
5 Each patient must purchase his or her own refreshments.

Outside Meals

Meals can be planned at restaurants. If the task group decides on this activity, rules 1, 2, and 3 above would apply. The group may also wish to establish additional requirements, which might include learning proper use of a menu, how to place an order, correct table manners, paying the bill, and tipping.

Table Games

A number of suitable table games can be chosen. When task group members determine a game or games to be played, a member may volunteer or be appointed to be responsible for obtaining the needed supplies and equipment. Another group member could be in charge of explaining the rules of the game. Depending upon the specific nature of the particular game chosen, additional tasks might include awarding prizes to winners or teaching the game to nongroup members.

Kitchen Activities

Kitchen activities can involve many tasks depending on the scope of the activity. Some of these might include planning the menu, obtaining the necessary supplies and equipment, making copies of the recipes to be used, inviting guests, cooking, table setting, serving, and clean-up. Some of the rules that could be established include the following:

1 All patients will wash their hands thoroughly.
2 Patients working with food will wear hair nets.
3 Everyone in the group will be responsible for carrying out at least one task.

Following each group activity the group leader or leaders can discuss the event with the patients in the task group. Topics should include positive and negative aspects, with patients being given constructive feedback on their behaviors. All members should also have an opportunity to discuss their personal feelings. More information on task groups may be found in Chapter 9.

Case Study: John

John was 30 years old when he was referred to the occupational therapy department following surgical removal of a brain tumor. He had been living in a group home prior to the surgery, and had worked as a factory foreman up until the previous year. He began having seizures which ultimately interfered with his job responsibilities, and he was terminated from his position.

Family members reported that John withdrew from social and physical activities upon learning of his tumor and losing his job. He became extremely depressed. Following an occupational therapy evaluation, the following goals were established in collaboration with the patient:

1 develop social skills necessary for active community participation upon discharge from the hospital;

2 encourage independent functioning in self-care and productive activities;
3 improve self-esteem and feeling of self-worth;
4 increase personal involvement in leisure activities;
5 increase ability to structure leisure time; and
6 utilize resources to aid in transition from hospital to community.

The COTA responsible for supervising John's treatment activities in relation to leisure goals used an approach which was supportive and flexible, offering John encouragement and reassurance as appropriate. Among other activities, the patient participated in a number of trips, very reluctantly at first. He enjoyed the parks and particularly the beautiful fall colors of the trees. The COTA provided him with a city map and assisted him in locating parks near his home. She also pointed out the availability of guided nature hikes. John took his family on one of these hikes during a weekend leave from the facility.

As John became involved in meaningful activities, including leisure, his depression disappeared and his self-esteem improved. He became interested in community activities again and expressed a desire to return to the cider mill as well as a museum he had visited with a patient group.[28]

Included in Appendix B is a list of recreational organizations for disabled individuals located throughout the United States. Many organizations can provide the names and addresses of individual contacts near the patient's community.

Work

In 1909 R.C. Cabolt, a professor of medicine at Harvard University, wrote an article entitled "Work Cure," suggesting that work is the best of all psychotherapies. In a later book, *What Men Live By*, he discussed the relationship between work, play, love, and religion and called for a balance among them. He believed work caused greater physical and emotional health. The relationship between a healthy body and work is also suggested throughout occupational therapy literature. Work can provide a source of satisfaction and emotional well-being.

Occupational therapy views work as skill in socially productive activities. These activities may take place in the home, school, or community and include homemaking, child care/parenting, and employment preparation.[8]

Public opinion surveys reveal that work, in addition to its economic function, structures time, provides a context in which to relate to other people, offers an escape from boredom, and sustains a sense of worth. Moreover, work affects the individual's freedom, responsibility, social position, attitude, mental capacities, achievements, friends, self-concept, and "chances in life."[20] As one writer suggests, work is not a part of life; it is literally life itself.

Studs Turkel wrote that "the job" is a search for working Americans to find daily meaning as well as "daily bread" for recognition. Turkel clearly recognized the linkage between mental health and meaningful work, pride in accomplishment, recognition, hunger for beauty, and a need to be remembered by "the job."[29]

Significance of Work

Work provides an opportunity to associate with others. It is through membership in work organizations that individuals are provided with a fundamental index of status and self-respect. The relationship to work influences one's use of time and leisure, the nature of the individual's family, and the state of one's mental health.[30]

The importance of work is pervasive; it determines what is produced, what is consumed, how individuals live, and what type of society is created and perpetuated.[30] Human motivation ranges beyond the drive for satisfaction of essential and discretionary materialistic needs. It is assumed that there are higher needs which must be satisfied in order to approach the fullest potential of human existence through the activity of work.

Parker categorized life space as the total of activities or ways of spending time. In considering the various definitions of work and leisure, to allocate all the parts of life space either to work or to leisure would be a gross over-simplification. It is possible to use the exhaustive categories of work and non-work, but this still does not enable a line to be drawn between the two categories. Analyzing the 24-hour day in five main groups is suggested by Parker:[21] 1) work, 2) working time, 3) sold time, 4) semi-leisure time, and 5) leisure.

When analyzing life space, work is usually identified with earning a living, even though work has a wider meaning than employment. Homemaking, parenting and child care, as well as the student's work of achieving an education are examples.

Apart from actual working time, most people have to spend a certain amount of time traveling to places of work and preparing for work. At least part of the traveling time may be regarded more as a form of leisure than as work related, such as time spent reading the newspaper or a book, knitting, or chatting with fellow travelers. Other activities related to working time involve husbands and wives sharing in household tasks that were considered to be solely "women's work" in the past, voluntary overtime or having a second job, reading related to one's job while at home, and attending work-related conferences and meetings.

Parker's use of the term *sold time* refers to meeting the person's physiological needs. The satisfaction of these self-care needs includes sleeping, eating, bathing, eliminating, and sexual activities. Beyond the time necessary for reasonably healthy living, extra time spent on these tasks may become a leisure activity, such as eating for leisure, or taking extra care with one's appearance prior to attending a party.

Domestic work such as making beds, caring for a pet, gardening, and odd jobs in the home are examples of semi-leisure tasks. Semi-leisure arises from leisure, but represents the character of obligations in differing degrees. These obligations are usually to other people, but may be to pets, homes, or gardens as well.

Leisure is free time, spare time, uncommitted time, discretionary time, and choosing time .[21] It is time free from obligations either to self or others, a time to do as one chooses.

Analysis of life space based on the majority, those who are employed full time, would be incomplete. Those who do not work at full-time, paid positions must be considered as well. People in these groups include housewives, prisoners, the unemployed and, in some instances, the rich.

For example, the life space of a prisoner is much more constricted than that of the average citizen in terms of both time and activity dimensions. Although some prisoners are employed outside the prison, the choice of work is severely restricted, and the motivation for it is rather different. Insofar as some prison work may be more or less voluntarily undertaken to relieve boredom or satisfy a physiological or psychological need to work, it may resemble the "work obligation" of the average citizen.

Doing housework is often the housewife's work. When compared with the husband's paid employment, it usually offers less scope for interest and less social contact. There is no real difference between work obligations and the responsibilities of the household.[21]

Many unemployed individuals develop feelings of uselessness and may be driven to occupy themselves with trivial tasks and time filling routines. They lose the companionship and social support of co-workers. Lack of money produces a restriction on the range of leisure activities, thus narrowing the scope of life experiences. The retired are similar to the unemployed, except that absence of employment is normally planned and permanent.

Worker Satisfaction

The highly productive economy of the 1970s reduced the moral value of work. There is much discussion today about worker dissatisfaction. While the degree of job satisfaction differs, studies reveal that substantial numbers are dissatisfied with their job because the job does not meet their need for self-actualization, that is, the chance to perform well, opportunities for achievement and growth, and the chance to contribute something personal and unique.[31] Scholars have identified six elements which bring satisfaction on the job:

1 creating something where the individual is reflected in the product;
2 using skill;
3 working wholeheartedly;
4 using initiative and having responsibilty;
5 mixing with people; and
6 working with people who know their job.

It appears that the most desirable work-related outcomes are as follows:

1 to feel pride and craftsmanship in one's work;
2 to feel more worthwhile;
3 to be recognized and respected by others;
4 to require little direct supervision; and
5 to have contact with others in the same type of work, both on and off the job.

Women and Work

The American family has changed in recent years in that the percentage of working wives has increased significantly. Women represent nearly 46 percent of the national labor force.[31] If one spouse must stay home to care for the children, however, it is almost always the wife who does so.[21] In interviews with housewives in one community study, some women thought that leisure came when all the household chores were done and children were in bed.[20]

Growth of the female work force can be traced to many factors which include the increasing availability of contraceptives, a preference for smaller families, inflation, a rising divorce rate, an increasing number of equality-oriented college women, expansion of the service-oriented economy, and changing attitudes toward careers for women outside the home.[31] While a greater number of women are employed outside the home, a majority are in low paying occupations. Many women work in service industries. Like homemakers, they teach children, care for the sick, and prepare food.[32]

Types and Phases of Work

Aristotle believed that there were two types of work: bread and labor, or work for the purpose of subsistence; and leisure work, or labor which is interesting in and of itself. In today's society, individuals do not work solely for economic self-interest, but also because work is psychologically necessary. Work is important to human dignity. The majority of the poor do not want to remain idle and accept welfare. Eighty percent of the labor force state that they would work even if they did not need the income because work keeps them occupied and healthy. Without it, they would feel lost, useless, and bored.[33]

Sociologists and psychologists identify five work phases in life:

1 preparatory - usually school;
2 initial - first employment;
3 trial - a period of job changing as the worker tries to find work which is attractive;
4 stable - usually the longest period, when there are relatively few changes in occupations; and
5 retirement.

One test of the importance of work in the lives of individuals is found in the activities of retired persons. Less than 20 percent of males drawing Social Security benefits retire to enjoy leisure. Almost three-fourths of these retirements are involuntary due to the employer retiring the worker or the worker being forced to retire because of poor health.

Occupational Therapy and Work

In occupational therapy, work and related skills and performance may be defined as the functional ability and proficiency needed to carry out the task of productive activity. Nelson has said that the concept of activity includes "activity as form" and "activity as action." Action is that part of the activity concerned with one's actual performance of the activity, that is, the specific operations needed to carry out the activity, whether it be work, play/leisure, or self-care. Activity as form denotes the cultural expectations or general procedures an individual would follow in order to do the activity well. The term function describes activity of form.[6]

Since skill and performance are functional abilities, occupational therapy personnel must concentrate their efforts on a thorough analysis of the patient's functional abilities, along with his or her affective skills. Such an analysis could assist in determining the feasibility of the patient's chosen work.

Function can be divided into the following categories: physical tolerance demands; motor, including perception and sensory; daily living skills; and affective skills. The sub-components of each of these categories are enumerated in Figure 7-7.

It is the responsibilty of the occupational therapy assistant in collaboration with the occupational therapist to relate each functional ability to the impact it will have on a patient's work, whether at home, in an office, or in the community. The interrelatedness of skill to the work task must be determined. Figure 7-8 shows a sample vocational evaluation report outline, and Figure 7-9 outlines the vocational evaluation process.

Relationship of Work to Daily Living

Where does work fit into the daily living routine? It would seem that, because of cultural dictates, self-care would be a precursor to work and work a precursor to leisure. This culture dictates that one's grooming and hygiene be completed before going to the work place. It is also generally accepted that leisure is a reward activity for one's hard work. In addition, many of the funtional abilities acquired through work activities and training are used in everyday leisure activities. The interrelationship of the primary components of independent daily living skills is shown in Figure 7-10 on page 112.

Relationship of Work to Physical Disability

Managing such tasks as homemaking and child care can be difficult for anyone, but for the individual with a physical disability, the need for good management and organization is essential for success. The evaluation and training for these skills can be done through formal and informal testing. Much valuable information can be obtained when the individual completes daily living skill tasks as well as through interviews with the patient and significant others, such as close family members.

Of concern to the COTA are the following questions which must be answered before planning and implementing an occupational therapy program to meet the patient's needs in relation to home making and child care:

1 What is the extent of the patient's handicap, and what is the subsequent functional loss?
2 What is the apparent cause of the functional loss (e.g., sensory, judgment, ROM limitation)?
3 What role in homemaking and child care did the patient have prior to the disability?
4 What financial resources are available to the patient for task assistance?
5 What are the patient's goals for homemaking and child care independence?

Other principles must also be considered in planning an occupation therapy program:

1 energy conservation—includes work simplification and time management needs for adaptive/assistive equipment including carts, chairs, utensils, etc.;
2 barrier free design—ranges from simple adaptations such as removing scatter rugs, to kitchen modification of shelves and cabinets, to use of a microwave oven, to re-designing doorways, entrances and bathrooms;
3 physical abilities—includes reaching, stooping, bending, balancing, walking, standing, sitting, pushing, pulling, lifting, coordination, and speed;
4 sensory awareness such as temperature, proprioception, and kinesthesia;
5 cognition—includes attention span, judgment, organization, and memory;
6 family expectations—total independence or independence with assistance; and
7 community resources—home delivered meals, catalog shopping, child care.

The COTA should stress to the patient the need for organized, planned activities. Every step saved and the amount of energy conserved are to the individual's advantage. Simulated homemaking tasks should be practiced in the occupational therapy clinic as frequently as possible prior to discharge. A detailed reference, giving step-by-step guidelines for many homemaking tasks, is the *Mealtime Manual: For People with Disabilities and the Aging*, compiled by Judith Klinger, OTR.

Psychosocial Implications

The emphasis in the area of homemaking with a psychiatric patient is quite different from that in physical dysfunction. Rather than stressing functional abilities from the psychomotor domain, the focus is on the affective domain. Goals may include some of the following:

1 developing interpersonal relationships, which the patient may have lost as a result of illness or never acquired;
2 improving self-esteem;
3 developing decision making skills by encouraging individual responsibility;
4 encouraging socialization; and
5 developing skills such as budgeting, time management, purchasing, and menu planning.

FIGURE 7-7. Work Behavior Skills*

Physical Tolerance and Demands	Sensory/Perception	Motor
Work pace/rhythm Standing tolerance Sitting tolerance Endurance Performance with repetition Muscle strength Walking Lifting Carrying Pushing Pulling Climbing	Color discrimination Form perception Size discrimination Spatial relationship Ability to follow visual instruction Texture discrimination Digital discrimination Figure-ground Form constancy Visual closure Parts-to-whole Shape discrimination Kinesthesia	Finger dexterity Manual dexterity Coordination: eye-hand eye-hand-foot fine motor gross motor bimanual bilateral Use of hand tools ROM: stopping kneeling crouching crawling reaching Balancing
Daily Living Skills	**Cognition**	**Affective**
Self care: personal hygiene grooming dressing eating/feeding object manipulation Mobility transfers travel (mode of) transportation Communication with peers with supervisor writing dialing phone talking on phone typing	Numerical ability Measuring ability Safety consciousness Care in handling work and tools Work quality Accuracy Neatness Attention span Planning/organization Ability to follow: verbal instruction written instruction Retention of instruction Work judgment Ability to learn new task Orientation	Attendance Punctuality Response to: praise criticism assistance frustrating situation Relationship with evaluator co-worker Work flexibility Attitude toward work Behavior in structured setting Ability to work independently Initiative (In psychiatry you would also observe for additional pathological behavior.)

*Wayne County Community College
Occupational Therapy Assistant Program

The hospitalized psychiatric patient may never have worked, may be temporarily unemployed or deprived of the work role due to the illness. The occupational therapy clinic offers a work area where the patient can learn new skills and develop existing ones. In work adjustment programs, tasks are chosen that will promote and teach work skills to allow the patient to function at the optimum level of his or her abilities. These skills might include the ability to follow written and oral directions, sustain attention to tasks, or organize work according to priority.[34] The structured activity or craft task group may be used to assist patients in learning skills as well as to assess their readiness to return to life activities such as work or school.

FIGURE 7-8. Vocational Evaluation Report*

NAME ______________________ DATE OF BIRTH ______________

EDUCATIONAL CLASSIFICATION ______________ DATES TESTED ______________

Tests Used
(List)

Areas Assessed
(List)

Section I: Referral Reason

Section II: Behavioral Observations
- A. Attendance/punctuality
- B. Communication skills
- C. Personal hygiene/grooming/attire
- D. Persistence
- E. Level of maturity
- F. Personal intervention (with others and environment)

Section III: Medical Concerns

Section IV: Special Work Factors (performance/test results)

Section V: Vocational Experience

Section VI: Self-awareness

Section VII: Situational Assessment

Section VIII: Summary
- A. Statement written
- B. Areas needing remedial activities
- C. Worker trait analysis
- D. Placement recommendations

The above categories are neither static nor all-inclusive.

*Wayne County Community College Occupational Therapy Assistant Program

Vocational Assessment Case Study: Tom

Tom is a 19-year-old mentally retarded male who was classified as trainable mentally impaired (TMI) according to the educational classification system. He was referred to occupational therapy for a vocational assessment and recommendations for placement.

A review of Tom's social history indicated that he had been orphaned at the age of 4 and adopted at the age of 14 years. He has a strong and loving relationship with his adopted parents and is their only child. The parents indicated that their goal was for Tom to be self-sufficient and possibly to live in a group home. They are in their early 60s and feel that soon they will not be able to care for Tom properly.

Tom attended special education classes on a limited basis for a number of years. School records indicated that he had never been employed.

The occupational therapist determined that the following areas were to be assessed:

1. gross and fine motor skills;
2. range of motion and movement patterns;
3. muscle strength;
4. general knowledge and comprehension;
5. vocational interest; and
6. vocational aptitude (handling, clerical, machines, manipulation).

A number of tests were administered over a five day period. Behavioral observations noted that Tom was alert and cooperative during this time. Throughout the testing, the patient was unable to retain directions and was disoriented to place. He was often distracted, looking at other people in the room and not attending to the task at hand. He seldom initiated conversation with others. On two occasions, testing procedures were interrupted as Tom complained of feeling ill and went home early. Tom's personal hygiene, grooming,

FIGURE 7-9. Vocational Evaluation Process*

SCREENING	Gather Background Data
EVALUATION	Assessment in Classroom/OT Clinic Situational Assessment in vocational training area or simulated activities in occupational therapy department
RECOMMENDATIONS/PLACEMENT	
FOLLOW-UP SERVICES	A) Adaptive or Assistive Devices Required for Effective Job Performance B) Assist in Designing More Effective Work Stations C) Demonstrate Work Simplification Techniques D) Perform Task Analysis E) Perform Job Analysis F) Provide Other Services to Improve Functional Performance G) Serve as a General Consultant to Other Members of the Interdisciplinary Team, or Family

REHABILITATION SETTING	SCHOOL SETTING	
Physician	Administrator (principal)	Social Worker
Psychologist	Classroom Teacher	Work Study Coordinator
Rehabilitation Nurse	Teacher Consultant	Job Developer
Voc. Rehab. Counselor	Psychologist	Family Members
Social Worker	Nurse	
Family Members		

*Wayne County Community College
Occupational Therapy Assistant Program

and attire were appropriate for a work setting.

The following test results were documented:

Range/Movement/Gross Motor

Range of motion is within normal limits for both upper and lower extremities. The patient is able to bend, stoop, reach and squat without difficulty.

Muscle Strength/Coordination

Muscle strength is left-hand dominant. Coordination is adequate for bilateral fine motor skills. The patient is unable to make rapid, skillful, controlled manipulative movements of small objects where the fingers are primarily involved. He is able to print his name in large, childlike letters. Cursive writing was not observed.

General Knowledge and Comprehension

Functional academic skills are quite low. The patient is unable to recognize most letters of the alphabet, recognize/read survival words, complete forms, add coin combinations, use a calendar accurately, or tell time without maximum assistance.

Vocational Information and Evaluation Work Samples (VIEWS)

Twelve of the 16 subtests were administered. Others were not given as they were too difficult for the patient to learn. Of those tests completed, work rhythm, coordination, speed, and accuracy of task were generally below average.

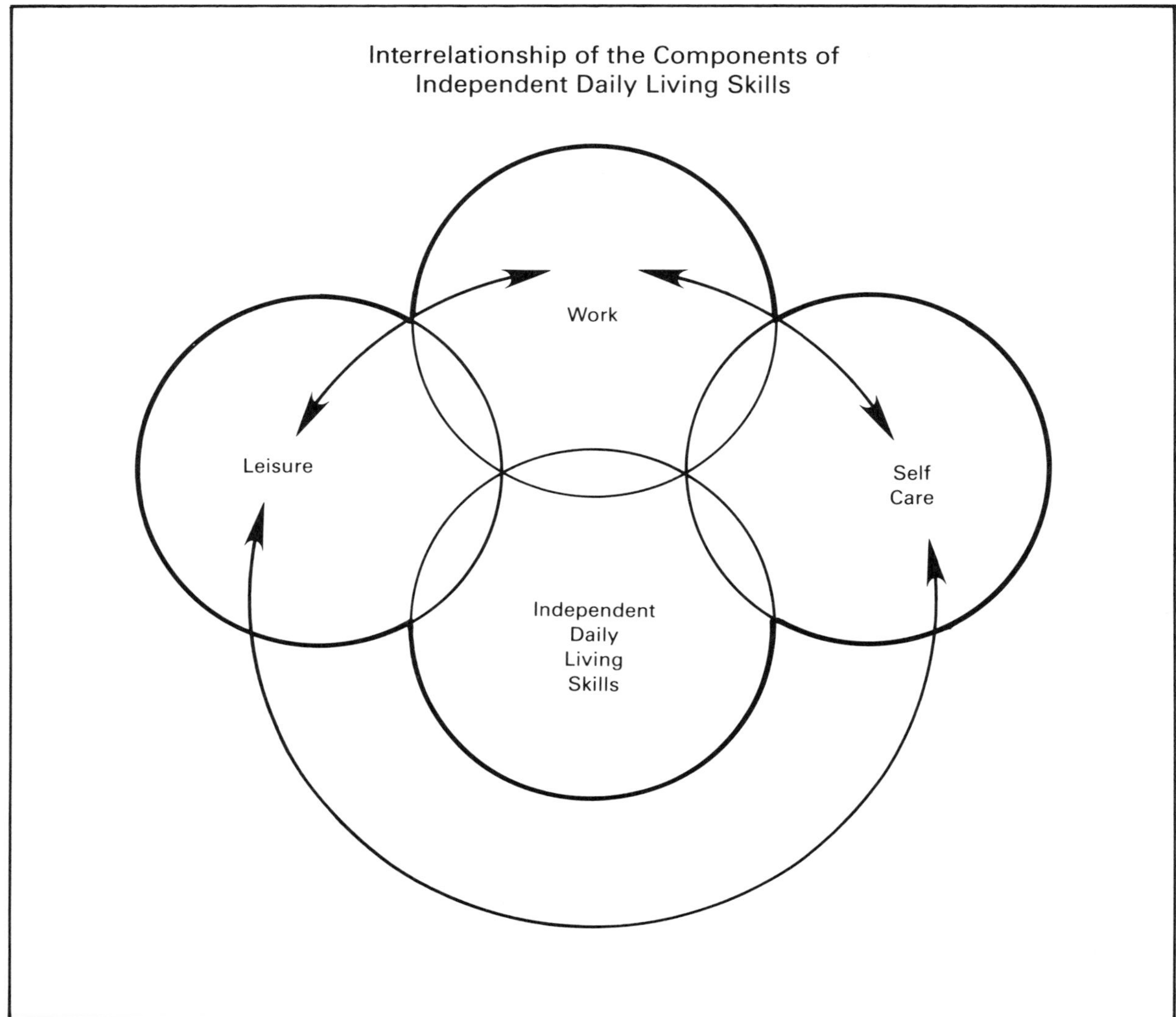

Figure 7-10

Becker Reading Free Vocational Interest Inventory

Test results were invalid as the patient made random choices without looking at all of the choices given.

Situational Assessment

The patient had been placed in an industrial skills and commercial housekeeping program. According to reports from area supervisors, his work production fell far below exit criteria. It was also stated that it is highly unlikely that he would reach the required vocational level.

Summary:

Tom is a 19-year-old, socially immature male in need of learning a number of work adjustment skills prior to any type of vocational training. Prevocational training and experiences should emphasize the following:

1 improving task behavior;
2 increasing production;
3 developing appropriate social interaction skills with staff members and co-workers;
4 improving/increasing functional academic skills to highest level possible;

5 developing appropriate job-related behaviors; and
6 increasing career awareness.

After one year of intensive work adjustment training, Tom had made progress in most areas. He was able to attend to a task for 30 minutes. His production rate was still below the norm, at 80 percent of the competitive rate. He was able to interact with his peers appropriately and often intiated conversation during coffee breaks. Coping skills had improved and he no longer reacted negatively when corrected. Functional academic skills remain unchanged. Tom had begun to think about his future and expressed an interest in working in the janitorial field someday.

It was recomended that Tom be gradually integrated into the maintenance training program offered by a local vocational agency. The occupational therapist would work with the staff to do a task analysis of each required activity.

More information on work and related topics may be found in Chapter 23.

Activity Analysis

Activity analysis is extremely important in the occupational therapy process. This process involves the "breaking down" of activity into detailed sub-parts and steps. This topic is an important foundation for all self-care, play/leisure, and work activities used in occupational therapy. It is an examination of the therapeutic characteristics and value of activities that fulfill the patient's many needs, interests, and abilities. Without such analysis, it may be impossible to use the proper application of activity or to obtain the best treatment results. Skill in activity analysis is critical in determining the validity of the use of activities in occupational therapy treatment.

There are many approaches used by occupational therapy personnel to analyze activities. The type of activity analysis used will be determined, at least in part, by the individual therapist's or assistant's frame of reference.[35] Such analysis will also be influenced by the use of particular techniques and variations in the use of equipment. While there is no universally accepted method of activity analysis, it is useful to consider the general categories of motor, sensory, cognitive, intrapersonal, and interpersonal skills, as well as adaptations.[3] Other considerations should include such factors as the supplies and equipment needed, cost, the number of steps required for completion, time involved, supervision required, space needed, precautions, and contraindications. It is also helpful to think of several aspects of experience or functional requirements of the activity, and then to analyze these in terms of gradability.[36]

The activity analysis yields the kind of data needed for determining therapeutic potential of a particular activity in relation to established patient goals, interests, and needs. As specific techniques and equipment vary considerably for many activities, so will the results of an activity analysis. Once an activity is thoroughly analyzed, it can be adapted for therapeutic purposes. The following example of an activity analysis for donning a shirt is provided as an example:

Donning a Shirt Activity Analysis

Reprinted with permission of the Occupational Therapy Assistant Program, Wayne County Community College.

1 *Name of Activity*: Donning a shirt with front buttons
2 *Type of Program*: Daily living task
3 *Type of Patient Indicated*: Variable
4 *Number of Patients Involved*: One or small group
5 *Materials and Equipment Needed*: Shirt or shirts with front buttons
6 *Cost*: Variable; patients can have shirt brought from home if not available in setting
7 *Preparation Required*: None
8 *Time Involved*: Depends upon patient; usually about three minutes
9 *Space Needed or Physical Setting Required*: May be done at bedside or in clinic
10 *Qualities of Activity*: Quiet, clean, practical; problems may occur in buttoning shirt incorrectly
11 *Amount of Supervision Required*: Minimal once demonstrated and learned; practice may be independent
12 *Directions Required*: Oral and demonstration
13 *Procedure*
- Unbutton shirt
- Position shirt
- Pick up shirt
- Put arm in shirt sleeve

- Pull shirt over shoulder
- Put other arm in shirt sleeve
- Pull shirt together
- Fasten buttons on shirt front
- Straighten shirt

14 *Physical Functions or Requirements*: May be done sitting or standing, if patient has adequate balance; may also be done in a supine position; dexterity and coordination are needed for buttoning buttons. Motions involved include: shoulder flexion and abduction when picking up shirt; elbow flexion and extension when pulling the shirt over the shoulder; and forearm pronation and suppination, wrist hyperextension, finger flexion, and neck flexion.

15 *Cognitive, Sensory, Perceptual Motor Functions*: Ability to comprehend simple verbal and demonstrated instructions; ability to cross the midline in bringing the shirt over the shoulder; vision and hearing not required.

16 *Psychological Functions*: Not frustrating; short-term; some judgment needed to avoid putting shirt on inside out or buttoning incorrectly; may be done independently.

17 *Potential Therapeutic Goals*:
- Increase daily living independence in area of self-care (dressing)
- Aid in adjustment to residual abilities
- Improve tactile abilities (buttoning) and motor coordination
- Increase reality orientation (appropriate shirt for weather or season)
- Build self-esteem (success provides gratification)
- Aid in assuming responsibility (patient encouraged to dress daily)

18 *Gradation*: Learn to button buttons first; then don shirt.

19 *Potential for Adaptation*: Use of a button aid or velcro fasteners; pull-over shirt can be used to eliminate buttons

20 *Relationship to Experience*: Necessary in life activities

21 *Precautions and Contraindications*: Activity not limited to any particular diagnosis; maintain proper posture

22 *Comments*: Should be initiated early in the patient's treatment

An activity analysis of a cooking activity follows. It is presented as a contrast to the dressing activity to point out the great variety of ways an activity may be analyzed and also to contrast a simple activity with one that is quite complex. It should be noted that this example, while detailed, tends to explore more general aspects of the activity in five rather than 22 categories.

Rosette Cooking Activity Analysis

Reprinted with permission of the Occupational Therapy Assistant Program, Wayne County Community College.

1 *Materials Needed:*
- Rosette iron molds (80 different ones available)
- Rosette iron handle
- Deep fryer or heavy saucepan
- Paper towels
- Oil for frying
- Metal tongs
- ½ cup evaporated milk
- ½ cup water
- ¼ teaspoon salt
- 1 teaspoon sugar
- 1 egg, beaten
- 1 cup flour
- garnishes: powdered sugar, cinnamon, whipped cream and/or fruit

2 *Directions:*
- Prepare batter in order listed; slowly stir in flour and beat until smooth
- Place approximately 2 inches of oil in deep fryer or heavy saucepan
- Heat oil to 365° F
- Attach rosette iron mold to mold handle
- Immerse iron mold in hot oil until thoroughly heated
- Lift mold out and blot excess oil with paper towel
- Dip mold into batter until it is ¾ covered; do not cover the entire mold
- Hold the mold in the bowl for a few seconds; lift it out and shake off any excess batter

- Dip the batter coated mold into the hot oil
- Once the rosette begins to brown slightly, lift the mold and let the rosette gently drop into the hot oil
- Using metal tongs, turn the rosette over and cook for a few more seconds
- Use the tongs to lift the finished rosette out of the oil and drain it on paper towels
- Sprinkle with powdered sugar, cinnamon or other garnishes

3 *Type of Group or Individual Patient Indicated*: This activity is appropriate for a lower functioning patient group, with close supervision and some assistance, owing to its immediate gratification and success assured qualities. Patient groups functioning at a higher level would also benefit from this type of activity, requiring minimal supervision and encouragement. It would provide a means of moving to higher level task skills required in many areas of daily living. The activity can be structured to enhance group cohesiveness by delineating various tasks and having small groups or individuals carry them out. In this way, all members are able to make a contribution to the end-product of the project group.

4 *Precautions*: The hot oil presents the main safety hazard and should be closely monitored at all times. Ingredients may need to be substituted to accomodate special diets.

5 *Goals*:
- Upgrade both basic and higher level daily living task skills
- Increase self-esteem
- Increase attention span and concentration
- Increase motivation to carry out a single project to completion; provide immediate, basic gratification and fulfillment
- Increase group cohesiveness (may also be used with individuals)

Summary

This chapter provides an overview of the daily living skills of self-care, play/leisure and work, skills which are the primary foundations of the profession of occupational therapy. Each section focuses on theories, principles and adaptations; illustrative case studies are provided to explain the importance of these activities in the individual's life. Self-care is a prerequiste for the other areas. These basic skills must be mastered before the individual can be well adapted to community life. The focus is on independence as well as improving the quality of the patient's life, and to assist in restoring a sense of dignity and self-esteem for many through new-found abilities.

Play as a process lies at the core of human behavior and development. It is an intrinsic activity done purely for its own sake rather than a means to an end. It is activity that is spontaneous and pleasurable, voluntarily selected and actively engaged in. Play activities lead to more complex and sophisticated cognitive behavior. They promote creativity, enhance social and emotional development and make a valuable contribution to the growth of the individual.

Though we live in a work-oriented society, leisure, a natural outgrowth of play, fulfills many significant human needs. It can relieve tensions, strain, and boredom that have become so much a part of modern technological society. Leisure or discretionary time greatly influences the quality of life.

Work is presented as skill in socially productive activities and, in addition to full-time employment, includes homemaking, child care/parenting and employment preparation activities. It provides the individual with a source of satisfaction and emotional well-being.

Activity analysis is highlighted as an important aspect of the profession. The process of determining the specific components and tasks inherent in particular activities aids occupational therapy personnel in using activities therapeutically in patient treatment.

Skills in self-care, play/leisure, and work activities, coupled with a healthy balance among these activities, assist individuals in adapting to society, in assuming occupational roles, in receiving gratification, and in reaching self-actualization.

References

1. Havighurst R: Social roles, work, leisure, and education. In: Eisendorfer C and Lawton MP, ed: *The Psychology of Adult Development and Aging*, Washington, DC: American Psychological Association, 1973, p. 805.

2. Cynkin S: *Occupational Therapy: Toward Health Through Activities*, Boston: Little, Brown, 1979, p. 6.

3. Reed K and Saunderson S: *Concepts of Occupational Therapy*, 2nd Edition, Baltimore, MD: Williams and Wilkins, 1983.

4. Rogers J: Why study occupations? *Am J Occup Ther*, 38:47, 1984.

5. Mosey AC: *Activities Therapy*, New York: Raven Press, 1973, p. 7.

6. Nelson D: *Children with Autism and Other Pervasive Disorders of Development and Behavior: Therapy Through Activities*, Thorofare, NJ: Slack, 1984, p. 38.

7. Deloach C and Greer B: *Adjustments to Serve Physical Disability: A Metamorphosis*, New York: McGraw-Hill, 1981, pp. 94-109.

8. *Uniform Terminology for Reporting Occupational Therapy Services*, Rockville, MD: American Occupational Therapy Association, 1979.

9. Shillam L, Beeman C, and Loshin M: Effect of occupational therapy intervention on bathing independence of disabled persons, *Am J Occup Ther*, 37:744, 1983.

10. Hopkins H and Smith H, ed: *Willard and Spackman's Occupational Therapy*, 6th Edition, Philadelphia: JB Lippincott, 1983.

11. Bradlee T: The use of groups in short-term psychiatric settings, *Occup Ther In Mental Health*, 3:47-57, 1984.

12. Chance P: *Learning Through Play*, New York: Garner Press, 1979.

13. Stone J and Church J: *Childhood and Adolescence*, New York: Random House, 1966, pp. 108-12, 150-56.

14. Yawkey T and Pellegrin A: *Child's Play, Developmental and Applied*, Hillsdale, NJ: Lawrence Erlleaum Assoc., 1984.

15. Parten MB: Social participation among pre-school children, *J Abn Soc Psychol*, 27:243, 1932.

16. Cherrington D: *The Work Ethic, Working Values and Values That Work*, New York: Amacom Press, 1980, p. 262.

17. Murphy J: *Concepts of Leisure*, Englewood Cliffs, NJ: Prentice-Hall, 1981, p. 26.

18. Kraus R: *Recreation and Leisure in Modern Society*, 2nd edition, Santa Monica, CA: Goodyear Publishing, 1978, p. 40.

19. Dumazedier J: *Sociology of Leisure*, Amsterdam: Elsevier Publishing, 1974.

20. Kaplan M: *Leisure in America, A Social Inquiry*, New York: John Wiley and Sons, 1960.

21. Parker S: *The Future of Work and Leisure*, New York: Praeger, 1971.

22. Havighurst R: The leisure activities of the middle-aged, *Am J Sociol*, 63:152-162, 1957.

23. Teaff J: *Leisure Services with the Elderly*, St. Louis: Times Mirror/Mosby, 1985, pp. 43-56.

24. Yoesting D and Burkhead D: Significance of childhood recreation experience on adult leisure behavior, *J Leisure Res*, 5:25-36 1973.

25. Orthner D: Leisure activity patterns and marital satisfaction over the marital career, *J Marriage Family*, 37:91-102, 1975.

26. American Association for Health, Physical Education and Recreation: *Guidelines for Professional Preparation Programs for Personnel Involved in Physical Education and Recreation for the Handicapped*, Washinton, DC: Bureau of Education for the Handicapped, U.S. Office of Education, 1973, p. 5.

27. Fidler G: *Design of Rehabilitation Services in Psychiatric Hospital Settings*, Laurel, MD: Ramsco, 1984.

28. Berry J: *Activity Therapy Services*, North Billera, MA: Curriculum Associates, 1977.

29. Turkel S: *Working*, New York: Patheon Books, 1974.

30. Best F: *The Future of Work*, Englewood Cliffs, NJ: Prentice-Hall, 1973.

31. Zander J: *Human Development*, New York: Alfred A. Knopf, 1981.

32. Gross E: *Work and Society*, New York: Thomas Y. Crowell, 1958.

33. Evans R: *Foundations of Vocational Education*, Columbus, OH: Charles H. Merrill, 1971.

34. Minnesota Occupational Therapy Association: *Description of Occupational Therapy Services*, Minneapolis, MN: Minnesota Occupational Therapy Association, 1972, pp. 15-23.

35. Hopkins HL, Smith HD, and Tiffany EC: Therapeutic application of activity. In: Hopkins H and Smith H, eds: *Willard and Spackman's Occupationl Therapy*, 6th Edition, Philadelphia: JB Lippincott, 1983, p. 225.

36. Tiffany EC: Psychiatry and mental health. In: Hopkins H and Smith H, eds: *Willard and Spackman's Occupational Therapy*, 6th Edition, Philadelphia: JB Lippincott, 1983.

Bibliography

American Occupational Therapy Association: *Entry-Level OTR and COTA Role Delineation*, Rockville, MD: AOTA, 1981.

Berger B: The sociology of leisure: Some suggestions. In: Smigel ED, ed: *Work and Leisure: A Contemporary Social Problem*, New Haven, CT: New Haven College and University Press, 1979.

Broderick T and Glazer B: Leisure participation and the retirement process, *Am J Occup*, 37:15-22.

Cheek N and Brunch W: *The Social Organization of Leisure in Human Society*, New York: Harper and Row, 1976.

Childs E and Childs J: Children and leisure. In: Smith MA et al, eds: *Leisure and Society in Britain*, London: Allen Lane, 1974.

Clayre A: *Work and Play, Ideas and Experience of Work and Leisure*, New York: Harper and Row, 1974.

Comfort A: *Future Sex Mores, Sexuality in a Zero Growth Society*, London: Current, February 1973.

Degrazia S: *Of Time, Work and Leisure*, New York: Doubleday, 1962.

Dumazedier J: *Toward a Society of Leisure*, New York: Free Press, 1967.

Friedman E and Havighurst R: *The Meaning of Work and Retirement*, Chicago, IL: Chicago Press, 1954.

Fuch, VR: Womens earnings: Recent trends and long-run prospects, *Monthly Labor Review*, 97(May):22-26.

Havighurst R: The nature and values of meaningful free time. In: Kleemier R, ed: *Aging and Leisure: A Research Perspective into Meaningful Use of Time*, New York: Oxford University Press, 1961.

Hinojosa J, Sabari J, and Rosenfield M: Purposeful activity guidelines and position paper, *Am J Occup Ther*, 37:805, 1983.

Huizinger J: *Homoludens: A Study of Play Element in Culture*, Boston: Beacon Press, 1951.

Kimmel D: *Adulthood and Aging*, New York: John Wiley and Sons, 1974.

Klinger J, Friedman F, Sullivand R: *Mealtime for the Aged and Handicapped*, New York: Simon and Schuster, 1970.

Llorens L: Changing balance: Environment and individual, *Am J Occup Ther*, 38:29-31, 1984.

Mitchell E and Mason B: *The Theory of Play*, New York: AS Barnes and Co., 1934.

Neulinger J: *The Psychology of Leisure: Research Approaches to the Study*, Springfield, IL: Charles C Thomas, 1974.

Pebler D and Rubin K: *The Play of Children: Current Theory and Reasearch Contributions to Human Development*, New York: Tanner and Basshardt, 1982.

Piepus J: *Leisure: The Basis of Culture*, New York: Partheon Books, 1952.

Reilly M: *Play as Exploratory Learning*, Beverly Hills, CA: Sage Publications, 1974.

Thackery M, Skidmore R, and Farley W: *Introduction to Mental Health Field and Practice*, New York: Prentice-Hall, 1979.

Trombly CA and Scott AD: *Occupational Therapy for Physical Dysfunction*, Baltimore, MD: Williams and Wilkins, 1983.

Willard HS and Spackman CS, eds: *Occupational Therapy*, 4th Edition, Philadelphia: JB Lippincott, 1971.

CHAPTER 8

The Teaching/Learning Process

M. Jeanne Madigan, OTR
with B. Joan Bellman, OTR

Introduction

Occupational therapists and assistants teach every day. They teach the "whats," the "hows," and even the "whys" of everyday living. They have an additional task in that they must teach persons who have cognitive, emotional, or motor problems, or a combination of all three. In addition to identifying the assets and limitations of patients and evaluating whether the patients have accomplished goals of independent functioning, occupational therapy personnel use teaching/learning principles. These principles enable their patients to accomplish tasks they were not able to perform owing to birth defects, social problems, illnesses, or injuries.

For example, consider the case of Lottie, a 29-year-old female who is mentally retarded. She was institutionalized all her life, but has been discharged to a sheltered home situation with a court-appointed guardian. Assessment findings indicated that she was ambulatory and cooperative but highly distractable. Lottie held a spoon awkwardly, spilling food on herself and the table. She could don clothes but could not button small buttons or tie a bow. She was able to manage toileting independently, but needed assistance in hand-washing in terms of turning the faucet on and off and drying her hands. Hand function patterns were normal only for gross cylindrical grasp; thumb opposition and wrist stabilization were poor. After discussing the patient with the guardian, the registered occupational therapist indicated that the first goal to be addressed in occupational therapy treatment was to improve independent feeding. The certified occupational therapy assistant was assigned to work with Lottie on achievement of this task.

In this scenario, the COTA can be identified as the instructor or teacher and the patient as the learner. The teaching/learning problem then becomes threefold:

1. What is the best way to teach the patient to use eating utensils?
2. What methods will best facilitate this learning process?

3 What is the process called learning?

Learning has been defined as a relatively permanent change in behavior resulting from exposure to conditions in the environment.[1] Although this definition implies observable events, learning cannot be observed directly, and it is difficult to know what has happened within the learner. However, one can find out whether the learner has acquired the knowledge or understanding in question by posing a problem which requires an individual to use the knowledge, and by then observing whether the learner can accomplish the task at hand.

The teacher's role is to help the learner to change behavior in specified directions. To do this effectively, the teacher must know not only what is to be taught, but also the methods which will facilitate the desired changes. The first section of this chapter briefly discusses theories of learning; the second section presents some conditions which aid or impede learning; and the final section outlines steps in the teaching process which will be helpful to consider when planning to work with patients.

Theories of Learning

There are two main theoretical approaches to learning: connectionist and cognitive. A brief overview of these two positions will be given to provide better understanding of the various techniques associated with them. Information for this section has been drawn from the writings of Travers, Biehler, Hilgard, and Hill.[1,2,3,4]

The Connectionist School

Connectionism is also known as *reductionism*, *associationism*, and *behaviorism*. In this school, learning is considered to be a matter of making connections between stimuli and responses. A response is any item of behavior, and a stimulus is any input of energy that tends to affect behavior. A simple illustration would be a child who eagerly reaches for a cookie upon seeing the cookie jar. An earlier "handout" from the jar brings forth memories of delectable tastes.

Ivan Pavlov was the first man to study learning under highly controlled experimental conditions. One of his earliest experiments was to give a dish of food to a dog a few seconds after a bell was rung. After many repetitions, the dog salivated upon the sound of the bell even though no food was given. This process was referred to as *classic conditioning*, that is, tying a reflex to a particular stimulus so that a desired response can be triggered at will. It should be noted, however, that if the bell was rung too many times without food being presented, the response tended to disappear (become extinct). Once conditioned, the dog tended to salivate to almost any similar sound. To prevent indiscriminate salivating, Pavlov repeatedly rewarded the dog with food only after the bell sound but never after similar sounds.

John B. Watson popularized Pavlovian theory in the United States by conducting experiments demonstrating that human behavior could be conditioned. He also did much to establish the tradition of objectivity and the concern with observable behavior in psychology, and thus became known as the founder of behaviorism.

Edward L. Thorndike conducted experiments using a hungry cat in a cage that had a door with a release mechanism and food outside the cage. After repeated attempts to get at the food, the cat hit the opening mechanism by chance. After repeated trials, the cat learned to make the correct response (hitting the release mechanism) almost immediately. Thorndike concluded from this trial and error process that learning consists of making connections between stimuli and responses, and that repetition is essential.

Following these traditions, B.F. Skinner conducted experiments with rats and pigeons in which he shaped their behavior by reinforcing the action he wanted with a reward. This process, the learning of voluntary responses, is termed *instrumental conditioning* and is highly dependent on the consequences of the response. Skinner referred to it as *operant conditioning* to emphasize that a person can operate on his or her environment to produce an event or cause a change in an event. Instrumental conditioning involves trial and error during the learning process, but the response must be rewarded if it is to be repeated. If a response produces positive reinforcement or removes negative reinforcement, it will be strengthened; if negative reinforcers are produced or if positive reinforcement is removed, the response will not be repeated and behavior will be extinguished. Secondary reinforcement (such as gold stars or smile stickers) will also strengthen the behavior.

Reinforcing a desired response every time it occurs is described as following a schedule of *continuous reinforcement*. When the number of responses between reinforcement varies, a schedule of *intermittent reinforcement* is being used. It has been found that the fastest, most efficient learning occurs with continuous reinforcement, but that learning is less readily extinguished when intermittent reinforcement is used.

Shaping is the process of changing behavior by reinforcing responses that approximate the desired response. At first, any behavior that is close to the desired response is rewarded. Gradually, only those responses that more and more nearly resemble the desired response are rewarded.

Behavior modification consists of reinforcing desirable responses while ignoring undesirable ones. Reinforcers may be food, praise, opportunities to perform a favorite activity, or tokens to be traded in for prizes or privileges.

Skinner applied what he discovered to the field of teaching by inventing teaching machines and programmed instruction methods. He maintained that to promote effective learning a teacher must divide what is to be learned into a large number of very small steps and reinforce the successful accomplishment of each step. By making the steps as small as possible, the frequency of reinforcement is high and the possibility of errors is low. The basic techniques of deciding terminal behavior and then shaping behavior have been used by some educators as the foundation for the development of instructional objectives that are used to structure learning experiences, the mastery learning approach, and performance contracting. Thus, it can be seen that many educational practices in use today are derived directly or indirectly from operant conditioning techniques based on Skinner's and other behaviorists' research and theories.

The Cognitive School

Cognitive theories, also known by the terms *gestalt*, *field theory* and *discovery approach*, are concerned with the perceptions or attitudes that individuals have about their environments and the ways these cognitions determine behavior. This school of thought was developed as a counter against researchers who accepted only measurable behavior as experimental evidence and who were preoccupied with physiological concepts. Early cognitive theorists emphasized whole systems in which the parts are seen as interrelated in such a way that the whole is more than a sum of its parts. They also studied the ways in which cognition is modified by experiences.

About the same time that Thorndike was developing his laws (1920s), a group of German psychologists began experimenting with chimpanzees. Wolfgang Kohler put a chimpanzee named Sultan in a large cage with a variety of objects, including sticks. Sultan discovered he could use a stick to rake things toward himself. One day, he discovered he could use a small stick to reach a long stick which, in turn, he used to rake a banana that was outside his cage and too far away to reach with the short stick. This "learning" involved a rearrangement of a previous pattern of behavior. It was a new application of a previous activity. This example is the essence of learning as viewed by a cognitive or field theorist: the perception of new relationships. Rather than learning by conditioning or trial and error, the problem was solved by gaining insight into the relationships between the objects. However, it should be recognized that Sultan's previous experience with the essentials of the problem was necessary in order for the insight to occur.

Kurt Lewin provided an important link in the development of cognitive-field theory. He used concepts from mathematics and physics to devise a system of diagramming behavioral situations which he called the *field of forces*. He also defined life space, which he said consists of everything that influences a person's behavior (objects, goals, and barriers to those goals, for example). He and his followers believe that individuals behave not only because of external forces to which they are exposed, but also as a consequence of how things seem to them, or what they believe them to be.

Edward C. Tolman's "cognitive map" or *sign theory* forms a bridge between strict behaviorist and gestalt theories. He said that human learning depends on the meaning individuals attach to situations or objects in their environment. While concerned with observable evidence, Tolman hypothesized that numerous intervening variables existed between the situation and the resultant behavior; learners vary their responses according to conditions as they know them. Thus, experience is the underlying factor in insightful and cognitive learning.

Jean Piaget believed that a person organizes and adapts sensory information through two basic mental operations: assimilation and accommodation. In assimilation, incoming information is perceived and interpreted according to existing schema that have already been established through previous experience. Accommodation is the changing of existing schema as a result of new information. Piaget described four stages of cognitive development. During the first, sensorimotor, which begins at birth, children form the most basic conceptions about the material world. They learn the relationships of objects to each other and themselves. The pre-operational stage, beginning at approximately two years of age, is when children are conscious of their existence in a world of permanent objects that are separate from themselves, and they realize the causal effects between them. Behavior is still directly linked to what the child perceives and does at the time. During the concrete operations stage, beginning at seven years, children's thinking is no longer restricted to physical objects. They are able to make inferences from verbal information that is linked with movement or other information. In the final stage, beginning at eleven years, children develop adult abilities and characteristics. They can deal with words and relationships, solve problems involving manipulation of several variables, intellectually examine hypothetical ideas, and evaluate alternatives. (See Chapter 5 for more information.)

Jerome Bruner, who regards learning as a rearrangement of thought patterns, stresses the importance of structure and of providing opportunities for intuitive thinking. He believes that emphasizing structure in teaching makes the subject more comprehensible, more easily remembered, and more able to be transferred. Believing that knowledge is a process rather than a product, Bruner's techniques for teaching by the discovery method include the following components:

1. emphasizing contrast;
2. stimulating informed guessing;
3. encouraging active participation; and
4. stimulating awareness.

Proponents of the *discovery* or *reflective* method of teaching also believe that too much exposure to lectures, texts, or programs tends to make a student dependent upon others and minimizes the likelihood that he or she will seek answers or solve problems independently.

Thus, learning can be considered to be either an accumulation of associations or the perception of new relationships.

Depending upon which theory one adheres to, the teacher would use quite different techniques to instruct another person. It should be noted, however, that some theorists feel that rigidity in adhering to a single theory is wrong and that the individual should make selected use of the techniques based on different theories.

D.O. Hebb proposed that there are two basic periods of learning: primary learning and later learning. *Primary learning* begins at birth and continues until about age twelve. It consists of sensory events which impose new types of organization through classic and instrumental conditioning. *Later learning* is conceptual in nature and involves patterns whose parts are familiar and have a number of well-formed associations. Following this line of reasoning, one could conclude that much of adult learning requires few trials unless one is confronted with situations in which there has been no past experience. Somewhat along this same line, Robert Gagne identified eight progressively complex types of learning:[5]

1. *Signal Learning* — an involuntary reflex is activated by a selected stimulus;
2. *Stimulus-Response Learning* — voluntary actions are shaped by reinforcement;
3. *Chaining* — individual acts are combined and occur in rapid succession;
4. *Verbal Association* — verbal chains acquired by connecting previously acquired words and new words;
5. *Discrimination Learning* — varying responses to verbal associations as what is known becomes more numerous and complex;
6. *Concept Learning* — response to things or events as a class;
7. *Rule Learning* — combines or relates chains of concepts previously learned; and
8. *Problem Solving* — combines rules in a way that permits application to new situations.

Gagne believed these kinds of learning to be hierarchical and, therefore, the more advanced types of learning can take place only when a person has mastered a large variety of verbal associations based on a great deal of stimulus-response learning.

Another quite different classification of learning was proposed by Benjamin S. Bloom and his associates. They classified all learning into three domains: cognitive, affective, and psychomotor. Categories of the cognitive domain are:[6]

1 *Knowledge* — remembering ideas, material, or phenomena;
2 *Comprehension* — understanding material and being able to make some use of it; includes translation, interpretation, and extrapolation;
3 *Application* — being able to use the correct method, theory, principle, or abstraction in a new situation;
4 *Analysis* — breaking down material into its constituent parts and detecting relationships of the parts and the way they are organized;
5 *Synthesis* — putting together elements and parts to form the whole in such a way as to constitute a structure not previously there; and
6 *Evaluation* — making judgements about the value of ideas, methods, and materials.

Although the cognitive domain deals with remembering, using something which has been learned by combining old and synthesizing new ideas, the affective domain deals with a feeling, tone, awareness, appreciation, and the like. Categories in the affective domain include:[7]

1 *Receiving* (attending) — being aware, willing to receive, and attending to certain phenomena;
2 *Responding* — actively attending to a phenomenon by acting, which implies willingness and satisfaction in the response;
3 *Valuing* — internalizing a phenomenon and accepting it as having worth; preferring it and being committed to it;
4 *Organization* — building a value system which is interrelated; and
5 *Characterization by a value or value complex* — acting consistently in accordance with internalized values and providing a total philosophy or world view.

Bloom and his associates identified the psychomotor domain as including muscular or motor skill, manipulation of materials and objects, or some act which requires neuromuscular coordination. However, they did not go on to develop a classification or taxonomic system for it. A number of individuals have proposed schemes which have not received the wide acceptance accorded to the two previously outlined taxonomies. However, since the psychomotor domain is of great importance in occupational therapy, it is important to consider some classification of this domain. Harrow classifies the psychomotor domain as follows:[8]

1 *Reflex Movements* — include segmental, intersegmental, suprasegmental, and postural reflexes or movements which are involuntary in nature and are precursors of basic fundamental movements;
2 *Basic Fundamental Movements* — include locomotor, nonlocomotor, and manipulative movements;
3 *Perceptual Abilities* — include kinesthetic, visual, auditory, and tactile discrimination, as well as coordinated abilities;
4 *Physical Abilities* — include endurance, strength, flexibility, and agility;
5 *Skilled Movements* — include simple adaptive skills, compound adaptive skills, and complex adaptive skills; and
6 *Nondiscursive Communications* — include expressive and interpretive movements.

These taxonomic classifications could aid in planning learning experiences for teaching skills and activities to patients by identifying levels of ability and specifying graded objectives in one or more of the three domains.

Conditions Affecting Learning

What individuals bring to the learning situation in terms of personality traits, motivation and general background has an important influence on what they are willing to learn, what they can learn, and how efficiently they learn.[9]

The basic motivation for learning is found in the human organism's normal tendency to explore and make sense of its environment. Gradually, this general exploratory tendency is differentiated in terms of specific needs, interests, and goals, so that individuals are motivated to learn some things but remain relatively uninterested in learning other things. If curiosity is disapproved or punished, as it may be by some parents or societies, the natural inclination for learning is greatly dulled. If what is to be learned bears little relationship to the learner's immediate interests and purposes, motivation may have to be induced by manipulation of rewards and punishments.

An individual's frame of reference (assumptions and attitudes) determines in large part what one sees and learns. The range of information that will be meaningful, the way new material will be interpreted, and whether the learning task is perceived as a challenge, a threat, or of no importance will depend on the individual's picture of self and the world.

Usually an individual is eager to tackle learning tasks when they are seen as related to needs and purposes and appropriate to his or her competence level. On the other hand, an individual usually tries to avoid those tasks which appear of little value or with which he or she feels unable to cope. For some people, a vicious cycle may develop in which, feeling inadequate, they force themselves into a learning situation with anxiety and trepidation; they expect to do badly and do. The resulting negative feedback then reinforces their concept of being inadequate.

A learner must also be able to tolerate immediate frustration in the interest of achieving long-range goals. Preoccupation with inner conflicts, a high level of anxiety, feelings of discouragement and depression, and other maladaptive patterns can also seriously impair the ability to learn.

Characteristics of the Learning Task

Coleman outlined four characteristics of the learning task itself that influence how it should be approached and how easily it can be mastered.

Type of Task

Motor skills usually require time and practice to train the muscles to function with the desired skill and coordination. Meaningful verbal information results from intensive sessions, with a focus on relationships leading to quickest learning and best retention. Unrelated data often require a spaced drill for material that must be memorized.

Size, Complexity, and Familiarity

Generally, more material needs more time, though less time is needed for meaningful material than for unrelated data that must be memorized. Added complexity tends to increase the time required for study and understanding, but may be offset if the learner is familiar with the material in a general way and has adequate background for organizing and understanding it. (In this case, the teacher should try to relate new concepts to what the learner already knows.)

Clarity

The less clear the task, the more time and effort the learner will have to spend in mastering it. (Here, the teacher should point out the essential elements of the task to be learned.)

Environment

Things that make learning more difficult include disapproval by one's peers, unfavorable study conditions, lack of essential tools or resources, severe time constraints, and other distracting life demands. Ways to enhance learning include a well lighted, well ventilated place which is free of distractions, an overall view of the task, and an organization in terms of key elements. Long-range retention is encouraged by distributed study, periodic review, and tying new material in with previous learning and real life situations.

Little is known about how previous learning affects the ease with which individuals can understand and master later learning. The available evidence seems to indicate that some transfer will occur if there are identical elements in the two learning situations or if they can be understood in terms of the same general principles. Transfer of learning seems to depend upon the learner's ability to perceive the points of similarity between the old and the new.

The return of information individuals receive concerning the progress or outcome of their behavior (feedback) not only tells them whether or not they are proceeding satisfactorily, but also serves as reward or punishment. Learners can modify or adjust responses on the basis of feedback. Motivation, self-confidence, and learning efficiency (not having to unlearn errors) are all facilitated by frequent feedback. Praise and progress toward desired goals reinforce what has been learned and motivate further learning.

The Teaching Process

Once the patient has been evaluated and the goals of treatment specified, it will be necessary to identify what is to be taught and how to teach in order to best accomplish these goals. With principles from the theories discussed in the previous sections of this chapter, the steps in the teaching process are outlined and applied to specific patient treatment situations.

Teaching Process Steps

State learning objectives

Identify what it is that the patient needs to learn to do. This can be done with a great deal of specificity or in more general terms. In the case of Lottie, whose case study was discussed earlier in this chapter, the learning objectives could be stated as follows:

1 "The patient will be able to scoop applesauce with a spoon from a bowl and place it in her mouth without spilling any sauce on herself, the table, or the floor, in seven out of ten trials;" or
2 "The patient will be able to feed herself without spilling."

It is fairly obvious that the first objective leaves no room for guessing what exactly is to be accomplished and how the outcome is to be evaluated. A new therapist or assistant may find it useful to explicitly state all objectives in similar detail until it becomes second nature to think in these terms. If one is using a behavior modification approach, it is necessary to be even more specific in identifying what the present behavior is and the incremental steps between that and the target behavior. This will allow reinforcement to be applied for each small behavior that represents movement toward the desired behavior change.

Determine content

What exactly is to be taught? In the specific objective stated in the preceding section, the motor skills of grasping, bringing the spoon to the mouth, and removing food from the spoon with the mouth must be taught. Activities that are related but not included in the objective as it is stated are: selection of the proper eating utensil, cutting food, drinking from a glass, and using proper table manners.

Identify Modifications Necessary for the Particular Patient or Group

In planning this step, it is important to refer to the history and assessment of the patient to determine whether any physical, mental, or sociocultural findings require adjustment of methods or adaptation of equipment that will be used. The most basic consideration to assist in determining what to teach and in selecting appropriate methods to use is the patient's developmental level. One will have little success teaching a 2-year-old an activity which requires the neuromuscular coordination of a 4-year-old, or, in the case of Lottie, using abstract reasoning with a retarded adult who is still in the pre-operational stage.

It is also important to consider physical limitations, such as loss of mobility, coordination, sight, and hearing. The presence of pain or medications which affect the patient's functioning must also be taken into account. Educational and socioeconomic levels may require the teacher to adapt the general language and the technical terms used.

Lottie is functioning at a preschool level in many ways. It would be important to use simple words and short sentences when giving her directions. Because of her grasp and prehension difficulties, a spoon handle could be built up to facilitate grasp strength and control. Using a spoon, a bowl, and applesauce at first is desirable because it is easier to get the applesauce onto the spoon and less likely to spill than peas on a fork. Use of the applesauce will provide a greater chance for success early in the process. As Lottie gains skill, more difficult foods and utensils can be introduced.

Break Activity/Process into Small Units of Instruction

In the learning objective stated above, there are numerous steps that will need to be learned, which include:

1 Grasping the spoon;

2 Scooping the food onto the spoon;
3 Bringing the food to the mouth;
4 Holding the spoon so the food does not fall off;
5 Inserting the spoon in the mouth without knocking the food off the spoon;
6 Removing the food from the spoon with the teeth and lips;
7 Closing the mouth so that food does not dribble out; and
8 Chewing food with the mouth closed.

What seemed like a very simple activity is actually one with at least eight separate skills that will need to be taught and combined to accomplish the original objective.

Assemble Materials

To prevent delays in the process, it is important to gather all equipment and supplies that will be needed to complete the activity being taught. If the teacher is planning to use learning aids, such as diagrams, printed instructions, samples, and the like, they should be prepared in advance. The same precautions should be kept in mind when modifications are devised.

Since the learning objective in Lottie's case consists of psychomotor skills, and since she is functioning at the pre-operational stage of development, visual aids would probably only serve to confuse her. The materials needed for this activity are few. However, if one were teaching a patient copper tooling, it would be important to think through all of the steps and ensure that the necessary supplies were on hand so that the project could be carried through.

Arrange Work Space

Set up the table or area to be used so that needed materials are conveniently located. However, if the patient is very distractible, anything that is not being used at the moment should be kept out of sight. Ensure that the patient is comfortable, with good posture for performing the activity and minimizing fatigue. Lighting that illuminates the work area but does not shine in the patient's eyes is important. This is a critical concern for someone with failing eyesight. The person instructing must assume a position in relation to the patient that will be the most advantageous to demonstrate, assist, and observe, being careful that the patient's view of the task or activity is not obstructed. Usually, sitting next to the patient is preferable. In this way the work will be at the proper height, angle, and perspective. When teaching a group, one must be sure that all participants can see what is being shown.

Lottie is highly distractible; therefore, it would be important to try to reduce visible objects and eliminate sounds that may divert her attention from what is being demonstrated or displayed.

Simulate as closely as possible the conditions under which the patient will have to carry out the activity. If circumstances between the learning situation and the "real" one are very different, the patient may not be able to transfer the learning even though he or she can accomplish the task perfectly in the treatment setting.

Prepare the Patient or Group

Try to determine whether the patient is ready to learn by asking the following: Is the patient alert? Is the patient paying attention to the person in the teaching role? Does the patient appear interested in what is to happen? There may be concerns, anxieties or other emotions which will divert the patient's attention and make it difficult to concentrate on what is being taught. It may be necessary for the therapist or assistant to deal with these matters or to make a referral to a person from another discipline to attend to them before the patient is fully ready to learn.

Are there basic skills or knowledge that the patient needs to have before learning can proceed? Learning will be more successful if it can be tied to some familiar elements. Does the patient know what is going to happen and the purpose of the activity? Instruction will be more easily grasped and retained if the patient knows why he or she is doing the activity and feels that it is something needed or wanted.

For example, Lottie wanted to be like "other people," which included not having to wear a bib. This was her ultimate aim — no spilling, no bib!

Present the Instruction

Once the activity has been broken into small component steps, the next phase is presentation of the first step. Begin by securing the patient's attention. Tell the person what you are going to do and what you expect him or her to do. If diagrams or other visual aids are being used, point out the salient features. Demonstrate the first step accompanied by a verbal explanation which emphasizes a few key words that provide "word pictures," cues to the action or important signals for which to watch. In this way the instructor is providing input through two senses, sight and hearing. Repeat the step and observe whether the patient seems to understand. Ask questions that will indicate the level of comprehension. Point out precautions or common errors to be avoided.

Have the Patient Do a "Tryout"

Ask the patient to proceed with the activity independently. If working with an object, give it to the patient and do not assist in the task at hand. If help is needed, repeat the verbal cues. Have the patient repeat the step several times, gradually decreasing the cues until he or she is doing it independently. Correct any errors immediately so that the patient does not learn the incorrect method, as it will be difficult to unlearn the wrong way before relearning the correct way to proceed.

In Lottie's case, self-feeding had been accomplished in a very sloppy manner, so it will be difficult for her to overcome a set habit pattern and to learn a new way of eating.

Watch for nonverbal clues that the patient understands or does not; the individual may not want to admit confusion. Invite questions. Allow the patient to perform independently several times so that assurance is provided that the individual knows the correct procedure and did not just do it correctly by chance. Offer sincere praise for correct work. Look for indications of fatigue, pain, or waning attention. A rest or redirection may be necessary.

Lottie was eager to please others and so responded well to praise when she accomplished one of the component skills. Good performance was also rewarded by adding new foods which she liked, especially ice cream.

Evaluate Performance

Decide how many times, how far apart, and in how many different circumstances the correct performance should be observed to assure that the patient has mastered the skill or skills that have been taught. The carry-over when the instructor is not present will be greater if the patient has repeated the activity and made it a habit.

If the activity is composed of several steps, the instructor will need to present each, being sure the patient has learned that step before going on to the next. Retention will be aided if each previous step can be practiced repeatedly as a new step is added.

Questions the therapist and assistant need to ask themselves are:

1 Does a caretaker need to be instructed in the particular process so there will be more likelihood that the activity will be done correctly when the patient returns to the ward or home?
2 Does the patient have a sense of accomplishment?
3 Is the activity accomplishing the desired effect or goal?

Case Study — Mildred

The following brief case study is presented as a contrast to the profile of Lottie; it presents quite a different teaching/learning situation.

Mildred is a 57-year-old female with a diagnosis of degenerative joint disease. She complains of low back pain when performing many household chores. She lives at home with her husband, who is receiving disability benefits owing to a heart condition. He is unable to assist with heavy housework. Mildred is of average intelligence but has a high level of anxiety about keeping her home neat and clean. She is also fearful of pain. The occupational therapy goal was to enable Mildred to perform household work within a tolerable level of discomfort.

In this particular case, the COTA identified the learning objective: "The patient will apply principles of body mechanics and energy conversation to carry out household tasks." The content includes, for example, the correct method of lifting heavy objects to reduce bending and stretching. Because this patient has a high school education, is of average intelligence, and has no limitations other than the arthritis for which she is receiving treatment, no special modifications will need to be considered in the COTA's selection of teaching methods.

The occupational therapy assistant prepared charts illustrating each principle. The principle was printed at the top, and a stick-figure diagram showed how the principle applied in a particular cleaning or cooking task. The COTA discussed each principle with Mildred, pointing out how the illustration of the figure in the diagram made use of the principle. She then demonstrated several times how to perform the task correctly, noting precautions. Next, she asked Mildred to perform the same task, correcting errors as soon as they occurred. Mildred was asked to repeat the task until she could carry it out in the correct manner three consecutive times.

Because the objective was to have the patient apply the principles rather than just learn specific techniques, the occupational therapy assistant could not conclude her instruction at this point. She continued by asking Mildred to identify a chore she did in her home that could be accomplished by using the principle she had learned. At first, Mildred was at a loss to associate the principle with another task she did at home, so the COTA asked her to describe how she washed clothes. When Mildred described carrying the clothes basket from the bedroom to the washing machine, the COTA suggested that she could use the principle of lifting objects by keeping her trunk erect, bending at the knees, and holding the object (the clothes basket) close to her body. Mildred showed recognition that this task used the principle. The COTA again asked Mildred how the same principle could be used with another, closely related task. Mildred identified carrying a scrub bucket of water. A similar process was used in identifying chores which require the patient to bend and stretch and, as a result, Mildred altered how she carries out many household tasks. For example, she rearranged her cabinets and cupboards so that commonly used items would be within easy reach. She now uses a long handled feather duster to dust her bookcases and china cabinet, and cleans the kitchen and bathroom floors with a sponge mop which has a squeeze attachment at midshaft on the handle.

Once Mildred had mastered a principle (by correctly doing the task during the treatment session and identifying another task that used the same principle), she was directed to incorporate it into her home routine. She was also asked to look for ways to use the same principle with other chores. During the next treatment session, the COTA asked Mildred to list the tasks she had identified since the last treatment session and to demonstrate how she applied to the principle taught during the previous session. In this way, the occupational therapy assistant determined that the patient had understood the principle and could easily apply it to her everyday functioning. As she demonstrated that she understood and was using a principle, the COTA introduced additional ones. The COTA made up a little booklet with principles and diagrams so that Mildred could refer to it and continue to modify tasks in the future.

It should be noted that the occupational therapy assistant used some of the same teaching principles with Mildred as she did with Lottie (e.g., immediate correction of errors), but other techniques were not necessary. Praise of work well done and use of extrinsic rewards were not necessary because Mildred understood what was being accomplished, and the ability to keep up her house according to her standards while suffering less pain was reward enough. The COTA was able to use the modified discovery approach by having Mildred reason out how she could use the principles she had learned. This meant she would be able to apply the principles daily and not have to rely on the COTA to teach her the modified method for every task she needed to carry out.

Summary

Much of what occupational therapy assistants hope to accomplish through their treatment relates to patients actively carrying out certain activities as independently as their condition permits. Because the patient must do the activity himself or herself, rather than having occupational therapy personnel do it for the patient, it is necessary for the patient to learn/relearn how to do it. Thus, the COTA becomes a teacher, the patient must become a learner, and the treatment planning process must include consideration of the most effective and efficient methods to facilitate the learning process.

Knowledge of how learning occurs and which conditions aid or impede learning will improve the COTA's ability to help patients change their behavior in specified directions identified through evaluation and goal selection. Two main approaches to learning are correctionist theory and cognitive theory. The former, growing out of Pavlov's classic conditioning experiments, proposes that learning is a matter of making connections between stimuli and responses: careful attention to reinforcing desired responses will result in accomplishing behavioral changes. Cognitive theorists, on the other hand, regard learning as a perception of new relationships. Emphasis is on providing the basic knowledge and structure of a subject and motivating the learner to actively explore and discover concepts related to the subject at hand.

These monistic views are shunned by some individuals, who maintain that neither adequately explains all learning and propose a hierarchical progression of learning. They call for the use of different teaching methods for different levels and domains of learning. Other important considerations include the learner's previous experiences, motivation to learn, and personal and environmental conditions which aid or hinder the learning process.

References

1. Travers RMW: *Essentials of Learning*, 4th Edition. New York: Macmillan, 1977.
2. Biehler RF: *Psychology Applied to Teaching*, 2nd Edition. Boston: Houghton Mifflin, 1974.
3. Hilgard ER, Bower GH: *Theories of Learning*, 4th Edition. Englewood Cliffs, NJ: Prentice-Hall, 1975.
4. Hill WF: *Learning*, 3rd Edition. New York: Thomas Y. Crowell, 1977.
5. Gagne RM: *The Conditions of Learning*, 3rd Edition. New York: Holt, Rinehart and Winston, 1977.
6. Bloom BS, Ed: *Taxonomy of Educational Objectives Handbook I: Cognitive Domain*. New York: David McKay, 1956.
7. Krathwohl DR, Bloom BS, Masia BB: *Taxonomy of Educational Objectives Handbook II: Affective Domain*. New York: David McKay, 1964.
8. Harrow AJ: *A Taxonomy of the Psychomotor Domain*. New York: David McKay, 1972.
9. Coleman JC: *Psychology and Effective Behavior*. Glenview, IL: Scott, Foresman, and Co., 1969.

CHAPTER 9

Interpersonal Communication Skills and Group Dynamics

Toné F. Blechert, COTA
Nancy Kari, OTR

Introduction

Understanding oneself and learning how to live and work with others in satisfying relationships are goals for healthy living. Occupational therapy personnel teach skills which lead to improved interpersonal relationships. The teaching and reinforcement of these skills can happen within a one-to-one relationship or within a group setting. The registered occupational therapist makes this choice on the basis of the needs and skill levels of the patient.

Working effectively with people, whether on a one-to-one basis or within a group, requires that the occupational therapist and the certified occupational therapy assistant develop specific intrapersonal and interpersonal skills. Intrapersonal skills are those related to developing a clear and accurate sense of self. These skills allow the individual to cope effectively with the emotional demands of the environment. Interpersonal skills are communication skills which help occupational therapy personnel to interact effectively with a variety of people. One must be able to identify, assess, and strengthen his or her skills in both areas. These skills are prerequisites to group work.

Group work is an effective and powerful medium for planned change in occupational therapy treatment. The group creates an environment that enhances the individual's abilities to gain new insights and increased self-awareness. Within a therapeutic group, a controlled environment is carefully designed to provide opportunities for patients to identify and practice specific skills. Members establish peer relationships which can support and strengthen self-confidence and encourage risk taking. Members can experience conflict and personal struggle in a supportive setting. When resolution occurs, a heightened sense of affiliation with others emerges. In this way, the occupational therapy group becomes a "living laboratory" where members learn about themselves in relation to others.

It is strongly recommended that all entry-level occupational therapy personnel begin group work under the supervision of an experienced therapist.

Co-leading a group provides an opportunity for the beginner to learn and refine group facilitation skills. Team leading is also a benefit to group members, as it provides role models of appropriate interaction.

Abraham Maslow and Anne Mosey present two useful frameworks which help clarify the context for the description of communication skills and group dynamics as they relate to patient treatment. These frameworks can assist the therapist and the assistant to assess their own needs and skill levels and to identify those of the patient. The COTA works under the supervision of the registered occupational therapist to determine the patient's needs and skill levels. Goals are then set in collaboration with the patient.

Adaptive Skills and Basic Needs

Adaptive skills are abilities that enable the individual to satisfy his or her basic needs and function satisfactorily in the performance of life tasks. Sometimes these skills have never been learned by an individual because of physical or emotional illness, abnormal development, poverty, or lack of culturation. In other instances, skills have been acquired but lost because of physical injury or illness, psychological illness, or the aging process.[1] Adaptive skills permit satisfaction of basic needs. Figure 9-1 presents a table of adaptive skills.

Basic needs are inherent in every human being. Need is the lack of something required for the welfare of an individual. The best known classification of basic needs is that of Maslow who arranged human needs in an ascending hierarchy.[2] As the lowest level needs are satisfied, the higher level needs become apparent and influence a person's behavior. Maslow's work is discussed in more depth in Chapter 5. Mosey, in her review of basic needs has added an additional level: *mastery*.[1] A table of basic needs is shown in Figure 9-2.

Activity	Skill or Skill Component
Self-Care	Skills required to keep appearance, personal belongings, and surroundings in neat and appropriate order
Work	Skills required to be a productive worker as a student, homemaker, or paid employee
Play/Leisure	Skills necessary to engage in meaningful activities such as games, sports, and hobbies
Motor Skills	Use of muscles
Sensory Integration Skills	Use of senses
Cognitive Skills	Comprehension, concentration, communication, and problem solving
Psychological Skills	Intrapersonal
Social Skills	Interpersonal

FIGURE 9-1. Adaptive Skills[1]

Need	Characteristics
Physiological	Most basic and powerful of needs—the requirements of human survival: food, water, shelter, sleep, and air
Safety	Needs relating to environmental security and predictability
Love and Belonging	Desire to affiliate with others, to be valued and accepted within a group
Mastery	Need to understand and demonstrate competency in functioning within the environment
Esteem	Need for affirmation from others
Self-actualization	Need to do something of particular importance for oneself to attain and express individual uniqueness; recognition from others is not required

FIGURE 9-2. Basic Needs[1,2]

Intrapersonal and Interpersonal Skills

The establishment of a relationship between the therapist, the assistant, and the patient is the first step in the process of facilitating any change in a therapeutic setting. There are specific skills in effective communication and skills related to forming helping relationships, which will be discussed in following sections in detail. These are prerequisites to effective group leadership. Their importance cannot be overemphasized.

A COTA must first develop the skills to relate to others on a one-to-one basis. This level of interaction is defined as a *dyad*. People are "relating" when each is responding to the other as a person instead of an object. An example of the latter would be to say, "Hello, how are you?" when passing someone on the street, but then continuing on without stopping to hear the reply. Relating to another individual as a person involves time, interest, energy, and interpersonal skill. The ability to effectively relate to another is an art that can be learned and improved with experience and practice.

There are four characteristics that an effective occupational therapy assistant is able to demonstrate: self-awareness, self-acceptance, awareness of others, and the ability to communicate that awareness.[3] A person need not develop these competencies in sequence; they are singled out as important attributes. An occupational therapy assistant needs to achieve and integrate all four areas. One cannot become self-aware and accepting in isolation. These abilities are developed and refined simultaneously through interaction with others.

Self-Awareness

The ability to recognize one's behaviors and emotional responses is self-awareness. As one plays and works with other people, personal strengths and weaknesses emerge. Feedback is received from others and from the environment. Self-concept emerges from this dynamic, continuously developing process of interaction. Self-concept refers to the overall picture the individual has of self. Both positive and negative qualities are a part of this self-concept. The more experience one has with others, the more clear the picture becomes. Accompanying these pictures is a set of judgments and evaluations of self which have been accumulated over a long period of time. Examples of these judgments include: competent or incompetent, effective or ineffective, intelligent or dull. Feelings about self come from these evaluations and judgments. These feelings help to form self-esteem, which can be influenced by many feelings, including guilt, confidence, shame, security etc. Self-concept and self-esteem usually remain relatively stable but can fluctuate at times. For example, one may feel basically good about himself or herself but feel embarrassed or shameful about a specific action taken.[4]

The important point here is that in order for the COTA to communicate and relate effectively with the patient, it is necessary to have an awareness of self and an acceptance of individual limitations or weaknesses.

Self-Acceptance

Acceptance of one's own feelings is an important step in gaining self-respect. When a person dislikes himself or herself, feelings of worthlessness may occur and interfere with personal growth. However, people often make their greatest strides in personal growth just when they begin to see themselves realistically and recognize their limitations.[3]

Part of self-acceptance is learning to understand the difference between self-concept and self-ideal. Self-ideal refers to the way one would most like to be seen by others. The self-ideal may differ considerably from one's true self-image. Self-acceptance does not mean that a person is resigned to his or her self-image. It means that one does not dislike oneself. There is a recognition and acceptance of strengths, limitations, and the feelings that accompany these.

Awareness of and acceptance of one's own feelings enable a person to express those feelings more openly to other people. Verbal expression of feelings helps to provide a fuller understanding of them, as well as emotional relief. Openness, when appropriate, is a positive signal to others that can create opportunities to develop more meaningful interpersonal relationships.

Awareness of Others

To be highly sensitive and responsive to another person's feelings is to be *sentient*. Sentience is a quality that is difficult to describe. The COTA who learns to be keenly aware of the feelings of other people is more likely to gain the trust and cooperation of patients as well as co-workers. Sentience enables the COTA to enter empathetically into the lives of others. This does not happen on an intellectual level; instead, it occurs on a feeling level. One must behave in such a way that the patient can feel the concern being expressed. When the patient senses this interest and caring, a bond is created.[5]

People are motivated to take action and make changes in many different ways. Healthy people have need-satisfying environments, supportive friends and family, and energy reserves. Those who are suffering from emotional or physical trauma are sometimes lacking these supportive elements. Through affiliation with a sentient individual, a patient may receive the support and energy that are needed to make positive changes.

Demonstrating Acceptance and Awareness

Although it is important to have a clear understanding of oneself and others, this alone is not sufficient to establish a therapeutic relationship. The effective COTA must be able to communicate awareness of others. In a therapeutic environment there are a variety of important roles assumed by the therapist and the assistant. For example, he or she may be a catalyst creating challenges for the patient; a solution giver; a resource person; or a process helper by assisting the patient to identify his or her own needs and choose appropriate solutions. These are all legitimate and necessary roles in facilitating change. In the initial phases of the relationship, however, the most important role is that of the listener. It is essential to clearly understand the patient's point of view and to be able to communicate understanding. This is done most effectively though active listening. There are a variety of listening responses; some are actually blocks to communication, while others enhance understanding. Following are four common responses which can become barriers to communication in initial patient relationships.

Giving Advice

One way that people try to be helpful is by *giving advice*. Many times people don't really need or want advice at all. They have already thought through options and may even have the problem solved. What they need instead is a listener who can demonstrate true understanding. Giving advice tells a person that the primary interest is in the content rather than in the feelings expressed. Here is an example:

Patient: "I'm worried about telling my friends I've been in the hospital for treatment. I don't know if I want to tell them I've decided not to use drugs anymore."

Assistant: "The way I would handle that is to be as clear about it as possible. I'd make an announcement as soon as you are back in school that you are through using drugs."

In this situation the assistant ignores the feeling of concern expressed by the young patient. The response might imply a lack of confidence in the patient's ability to find his or her own solution. Although COTAs may need to assist the patient by giving advice at some point, it is an ineffective response when the individual is trying to communicate a feeling.

Offering Reassurance

Another response that is common in conversation is *offering reassurance*. Reassuring another person is usually well intended but can limit further communication. When one gives reassurance, there is a tendency for the person talking to feel that he or she ought not to continue discussing the problem. This can minimize the uncomfortable emotion expressed by the patient. Here is an example:

Patient: "I feel so confused and overwhelmed now, I don't know where to start."

Assistant: "Don't worry so much; things always work out in the end."

In this example, offering reassurance is a kind of emotional withdrawal from the patient. It does not acknowledge the feelings expressed. Encouragement and assurance are often important verbal responses in a therapeutic relationship. Reassurance used as a response to another's expression of a feeling is not effective.

Diverting

A third response choice, referred to as *diverting*, involves relating what the patient has said to one's own experience.[6] This is sometimes done in an effort to communicate understanding, or can be used to change the subject when the topic of conversation becomes uncomfortable. Sometimes people find it difficult to talk about topics such as anger, death, divorce, or violence because it creates an inner tension. Changing the subject or shifting the focus of the conversation may serve to reduce tension, but it does not communicate to the patient that the message has been heard. Here is an example:

Patient: "One of my biggest problems right now is feeling so lonely. That is worse than going through the divorce itself."

Assistant: "I know how you feel. My sister just had a divorce, and she talks about that often. She's joined a ski club though, and is meeting all kinds of people. Do you like to ski?"

In this example, the focus of the conversation is shifted by the assistant to his or her own experience; therefore, the assistant is not making a clear response to the feelings the patient has shared. The patient may feel as though the message had not been heard.

Questioning

A fourth response which is sometimes used ineffectively is *questioning*. In an effort to understand the details of an individual's situation, the COTA might ask questions which relate more to the facts than to the feelings expressed. Although it is important to have a clear picture of the patient's situation, excessive questioning or responding with an immediate question can limit the patient's opportunity to clearly describe the experience. In this regard, questioning is not a useful response to another's expression of feelings. Here is an example:

Patient: "The doctor told us our daughter's problems are caused by rheumatoid arthritis. We were so hoping it was just growing pains."

Assistant: "How old is your daughter?"

The question asked by the assistant in this example does not respond to the emotion shared by the patient.

Active Listening — Nonverbal and Verbal Components

Active listening is a term given to a set of skills which allows an individual to hear, understand, and indicate that the message has been communicated. It is an effective listening response. Active listening is a necessary component in the relationship established between the COTA and the patient. It is fundamental to effective communication and basic to the occupational therapy process. Active listening enables the assistant to undertand more objectively and accurately the meaning of the verbal and nonverbal messages communicated by the patient. It is important and sometimes difficult to achieve a balance between too little and too much listening. However, if the therapist and the assistant do not understand the meaning of the messages communicated by the patient, inappropriate treatment goals and treatment activities may be chosen. If the interview or treatment session is entirely unstructured and the therapist or assistant "listens" to whatever the patient wishes to say, valuable and expensive treatment time may be lost. Active listening on the part of a COTA is a combination of the verbal and nonverbal behaviors and skills which communicate an attitude of acceptance. These are discussed in terms of the following nonverbal components. The nonverbal behaviors which communicate openness and indicate listener receptivity include the following: appropriate body posture and position, eye contact, facial expression, and a nondistracting environment.

Body Posture and Positioning

The most effective body posture includes facing the patient in an open, relaxed manner and leaning forward slightly. Arms should not be folded across chest; legs should not be crossed. Tightly crossed arms and legs can be interpreted by the patient as rigidity or defensiveness.[7] Extraneous body motions such as swinging legs or tapping fingers do not indicate a relaxed posture and should be avoided. It is better not to sit behind a desk but to position oneself directly across from the patient. In an occupational therapy clinic it is acceptable and often desirable to use a table during the interview. In this instance sit across from or beside the patient. Optimal communication usually occurs at distances between 3 feet and 5 feet.[8] Cultural differences may dictate variations. It is always useful to watch for and respond to nonverbal cues given by the patient regarding a comfortable distance for communication.

Eye Contact

An effective listener maintains good eye contact with the speaker. Eye contact is thought to be an effective way of communicating empathy.[9] Avoiding another's eyes in an interaction can communicate disinterest, discomfort, or preoccupation.[8] At the same time, staring intently can make the speaker uncomfortable. It is important to look directly at the patient without staring.

Environmental Considerations

In order to actively listen to another, the interaction must take place in a nondistracting, pleasant environment. It is important to hold group sessions or dyadic interviews in quiet, uncluttered areas. Avoid interruptions from others or the telephone. It is sometimes useful to use "Do Not Disturb" signs and to ask that telephone calls be held.

Paraphrasing and Reflection

Two verbal techniques related to active listening include paraphrasing and reflection. Paraphrasing is repeating in one's own words the verbal content of the message received. Reflection is a summary of the affective meaning of the message and may include the patient's verbal and nonverbal communication. These techniques are used to ensure understanding by checking the accuracy of the message received. A paraphrasing response might begin with "Do you mean that..." or "I understand you to say..." and then rephrasing the content of the message. Message content includes information about an event or situation: who, what, when, where, how. The affective meaning is the accompanying feeling or emotion which is stated verbally or implied in nonverbal cues. It is important to listen to both aspects of the message. The following patient statements are provided as examples:

Patient 1: "I haven't had time to get used to the idea that I'll soon be leaving, and I'm scared to death of this change."

In this example, "I haven't had time to get used to the idea that I'll soon be leaving" is the content because it provides information about the situation. "I'm scared to death" is the affective message because it describes the emotion.

Patient 2: "I'm disappointed with the way this turned out. I guess I didn't read the directions thoroughly."

In the second example, "I'm disappointed" is the feeling response and, therefore, the affective message." I didn't read the directions thoroughly" is the content because it describes the "what" in the situation.

When the patient does not directly state how he or she feels about the situation just described but expresses this nonverbally through body movements, facial expression, or tone of voice, the assistant can reflect what the patient may be feeling by naming an emotion. To practice using reflection as a listening tool when the patient does not directly state the feeling, one can (1) listen for the feelings implied by the overall tone of the message, (2) observe patient body language, or (3) ask, "How would I feel?" Putting oneself in another's place allows one to guess another's reaction. This is sometimes helpful but it must be remembered that each person's response is unique.[6] Following are examples of a COTA's response to the feelings implied by the patient:

Patient 1: An elderly woman who recently moved to an apartment shares this experience with the COTA. "When my husband was alive he did everything for me. Now not only do I have to take care of things myself, I have no one to talk to."

Response: "It must be an empty feeling to suddenly find yourself without your spouse."

Patient 2: The COTA is assisting a patient who is recovering from severe burns over the upper half of her body. The patient's hair is gone and she is trying on the wig for the first time. She adjusts and re-adjusts the wig. Finally she says, "There, I can almost stand to look at myself again."

The assistant observes the patient's frustration and depressed manner and thinks that the woman feels unattractive, anxious, and depressed.

Response: "This recovery period must be a very difficult time for you. I can tell your appearance is important to you and that you are anxious to look yourself again."

Patient 3: A woman tells the COTA that her 10-year-old daughter is having trouble in school. "Nancy has never had problems before. She seems discouraged, and her teacher appears disinterested in Nancy."

The COTA thinks the patient is expressing anxiety or concern about her daughter and anger or frustration with what she thinks is the teacher's disinterest.

Response: "It's worrisome to see your child struggle, and it's irritating when the teacher doesn't seem interested."

Other Important Communication Components

There are other components of effective communication which incorporate both verbal and nonverbal responses. These include communicating respect, warmth, and genuineness.

Communicating Respect

The COTA must be able to effectively communicate respect to the patient. Respect means believing in the value and the potential of another person. When respect is communicated, a person feels more capable of helping himself or herself. Attention must be focused on the patient's interests and needs instead of the therapist's concerns. The COTA attempts to help the patient meet his or her needs without dominating the situation or the patient.

Communicating respect involves the process of affirmation. To affirm means to reinforce the worth of an individual. This allows the patient to begin to value himself or herself. The COTA must develop the capacity to quickly recognize the strengths in the patient, and these must be communicated to the patient whenever possible. A sense of timing is needed for this, however, because sometimes patients are not ready to hear their strengths and the feedback may be threatening. Communicating respect is associated with the ability to communicate personal warmth and genuineness.

Communicating Warmth

Warmth is the degree to which the therapist and assistant communicate caring to the patient. Warmth by itself is not adequate for developing a therapeutic relationship or for assisting someone in problem solving; however, it can facilitate these positive outcomes.

Warmth may be demonstrated in tone of voice, facial expression, or other body language, as well as in words and actions. Touching, for example, is an effective way of communicating concern and empathy. Touching a patient's hand or shoulder may offer reassurance, approval or encouragement.

Communicating Genuineness

Genuineness, also termed authenticity, is a human quality which greatly enhances communication and the establishment of therapeutic relationships. Individuals who communicate genuineness respond in an honest, unguarded, and spontaneous manner. This means the therapist is willing to appropriately share reactions to what she or he experiences within a group or dyadic relationship. The ability to communicate genuineness as well as respect and warmth through effective use of listening skills, body language, and feeling-centered messages enables the COTA to give and receive feedback in a responsible manner.

Giving Feedback

Giving and receiving feedback are important interpersonal skills necessary for the COTA when working with groups. The purpose in giving another person feedback is to describe as specifically and objectively as possible one's perception of another's behavior. Receiving feedback is one way people learn how they are perceived. It is a valuable tool in making behavioral change. It is essential that therapists and assistants know the guidelines for responsible feedback, because they must frequently teach this skill or serve as role models when working with groups. Following are five rules for responsible feedback.[10]

1. One of the first things to remember is that the feedback given represents an individual perception. It is therefore necessary to own what is said by making "I statements."

Response 1: "I'm upset when I see you come late to work as you did this morning."

Response 2: "We're all getting frustrated with your frequent tardiness."

Note that the second response is general in that it tries to represent everyone's reactions. This kind of statement is not responsible and can leave the receiver feeling defensive. The message can also be distorted.

2. Be specific rather than general; give examples of the behavior described. It is often difficult to respond accurately to a broad, nonspecific statement.

Response 1: "When you came in the room just now you slammed the door. I feel upset when you express your anger that way."

Response 2: "You are always going around expressing your hostility by banging things and slamming doors. I'm tired of it."

Phrases such as "you always" or "there you go again" are too general and become blaming statements. It is difficult not to react defensively to feedback worded in this way.

3. Be descriptive rather than evaluative. This

means the behavior should be described rather than labeled. Avoid making judgments about another's behavior as this is also likely to elicit defensiveness.

Response 1: "I heard you speaking to your friend in an abrupt manner. I thought you were not responding to his question seriously and it bothered me."

Response 2: "I've always thought you were too flippant, and when I heard you speak to your friend like that I thought you were a fool."

The words "flippant" and "fool" are labels and imply a judgment in the second example.

4. Feedback should be given as soon after the specific situation as possible. This is called "immediacy." Giving feedback immediately avoids problems caused by built-up feelings which are often expressed out of proportion to the incident if they have been held back for a period of time.

Response 1: "I feel frustrated and uneasy today because I don't know where you stand. You said nothing during this session."

Response 2: "This is the third week you have sat here and not made a response. I'm getting frustrated with you, and I don't trust you at all."

Because giving feedback requires risk taking, group members are often reluctant to state how they feel at the time. The second response is much angrier than the first, and therefore harder for the receiver to hear. The assistant needs to help group members express feelings as they arise; this helps the group build trust.

5. After giving feedback, check to see that the feedback has been heard accurately. This is a critical part of the feedback process. To do this one might say, "I want to make certain you understand what I've said. Could you tell me what you've heard?"

Responding to Feedback

Knowing how to respond to feedback is also important. Because giving feedback to another person requires risk taking, it is necessary to avoid misunderstanding. When feedback is given, the receiver should indicate what message was heard. It is not necessary to decide immediately what to do about it, but the person giving the feedback needs to know the message was heard accurately. The receiver might say, "I don't know how I feel about what you've just said, or what I'll do. I need some time to think this over. This is what I heard you say to me..."

Giving and receiving feedback in a group can initially create tense situations because of the risk taking involved, and it is a skill many people do not have. It is a necessary part of learning about oneself and making change. COTAs can help facilitate this process by teaching the skill using the guidelines listed in the preceding discussion. It is useful to provide groups or individuals with specific activities which elicit and reinforce these skills.

Understanding How Groups Work

A group is three or more people who establish some form of interdependent relationship with each other. In occupational therapy groups the activity usually provides the common ground for these relationships. This definition, however, does not include that human quality which is brought to an effective group by the leader and group members. This quality helps provide each individual with a sense of belonging and sharing which in turn facilitates and reinforces learning. The word "community" is also used to describe the desirable outcome of member relationships. Implied in this definition is "union with others." At their best, groups form true communities in which members are able to give and receive support and insights which in turn encourage personal growth. In order to achieve this degree of group cohesion, the COTA must understand how groups work.

Group process is a term which refers to how members relate to and communicate with each other, and how members accomplish the task. Group process might be described in terms of the way the group solves problems, makes decisions, or manages conflicts which arise. This process perspective of group assumes an holistic view which describes how different group functions fit together to determine the ongoing development of the group. To better understand how groups work, the following will be considered: group role functions, group norms, and developmental group stages.

Group Role Functions

Analysis of individual roles assumed within the group is one of the most familiar ways people use to understand how groups work. Bales suggested two main areas present in all groups based on types of communication that describe the particular behavioral roles. These are "task roles" and "maintenance" or group centered roles.[10] Task roles refer to those behaviors which facilitate task accomplishment. Group centered roles refer to those behaviors which enhance relationships among members. The COTA needs to be versatile in the roles that he or she assumes during group work. Role flexibility refers to an individual's ability to take the action necessary to accomplish a task and, at the same time, maintain cohesiveness in the group. Balancing task and group centered roles is an important goal for effective group work. In examining a group with a definite leader, one finds that the leader initially assumes multiple roles. As groups mature, leadership is distributed among the members who are able to play the functional roles described below.

Task Roles

Task roles are concerned with the accomplishment of the group task. Following is a summary of group task roles.

1. *Initiator/Designer*:

This role involves starting the group and providing direction. The person who assumes this role will plan activities and suggest learning experiences.

2. *Information Seeker/Information Giver*:

This role is assumed by asking for or offering facts related to task accomplishment.

3. *Opinion Seeker/Opinion Giver*:

The member who does this asks for reactions from others or states his or her own beliefs and values.

4. *Challenger/Confronter*:

This role involves asking for clarification regarding what is communicated. A member who assumes this role will also raise issues that are being avoided in the group.

5. *Summarizer*:

The member who does this stops the group occasionally to state what is being accomplished. This role serves to keep the group on track.

Group Centered Roles

Group centered roles are concerned with keeping the group together by maintaining relationships and satisfying the members' needs. The most important of these are:

1. *Encourager*:

The member who assumes this role is meeting the esteem needs of individuals in the group by offering praise in response to what members do or say.

2. *Gate-keeper*:

This role involves facilitating and regulating communication by spreading participation among the members. It involves drawing out quiet members and managing conversation monopolizers.

3. *Tension Reliever*:

The member who assumes this role is sensitive to the frustration level of self and others. It is a harmonizing role involving the use of appropriate jokes, kidding remarks, or suggestions for compromise that dissipate anxiety or hostility in the group.

The roles just described are considered *functional* because they support task accomplishment and the people within the group. There are also roles that are considered *nonfunctional* because they interfere with the group process. These roles are termed *self-centered*.

Self-Centered Roles

Self-centered roles are common in groups and occur because an individual is primarily concerned with satisfying his or her own needs and lacks the adaptive skills to function effectively. It is necessary for the COTA to learn to recognize and deal with these roles that interfere with individual and group progress.[11] Some of the most common self-centered roles include the following:

1. *Withdrawer*:

This member does not participate in the activity or discussion at any time. A person may withdraw because of feelings of insecurity, fear of rejection, anger, or lack of interest. A distinction should be made between a withdrawer and an active listener. The listener may be quiet for a time while absorbing information. The active listener does not remain passive for the entire session. To help a member who is withdrawn, the COTA may sit next to him or her, ask open-ended questions, take time at the beginning of the session to establish a greater comfort level among members, or take the individual aside and try to identify the reason for the withdrawal.

2. *Blocker*:

This individual may consistently raise objections or insist that nothing can be accomplished. A common phrase used by a blocker is "We've already tried this," or "It won't work," and he or she repeatedly brings up a topic or idea after the rest of the group has disposed of it. To help a person who is blocking progress in the group, the COTA must let the individual know how this behavior is affecting other members and task accomplishment. Direct feedback is necessary and may be provided within or outside the group depending on the skill level of the group members.

3. *Aggressor/Dominator*:

This member tries to take over the group by interrupting when others are speaking, deflating the status of others, insisting on having his or her own way, or telling other members what to do. To help members deal with an aggressor-dominator one may provide and encourage feedback by directing the discussion to identify feelings or call for "time out" to discuss what is happening in the group.

4. *Recognition Seeker*:

A recognition seeker tries to get the attention or approval of other group members in inappropriate ways. He or she may make distracting jokes or comments, engage in "horse play," boast about accomplishments, or seek pity or sympathy. The COTA may be helpful to a recognition seeker by offering approval of the member's strengths and discouraging inappropriate behaviors.

Group dynamics research is clear regarding the outcome of self-centered behaviors. Initially, considerable leader and group effort is directed to the member who behaves in the manner(s) described above. If the leader or group perceives that there is a reasonable chance of changing the behavior, this effort may go on for some time. If, at some point, it becomes clear that the inappropriate behavior cannot or will not change, communication toward the individual declines. Group members may begin to exclude the member, and he or she may have to be asked to leave.[12]

Group Norms

Group norms are standards of behavior which can be stated or unspoken. They define what behaviors are expected, accepted, and valued by group members. Group norms serve several purposes. They allow groups to function in an organized manner; they define ways in which members respond to conflict, make decisions or solve problems; they help define ways in which members relate to each other and to the leader. They define "reality" for the group. Norms can change as the group evolves and as expectations of member behavior changes. It is essential for those attempting to understand how groups work to carefully examine group norms. Sometimes it is useful for the members to identify their own group norms and to determine whether or how these norms should be changed. In this way implicit norms, or those which influence member behavior but which are unspoken, can be made explicit. Some examples of implicit norms might include manner of dress, attitudes toward authority, or group response to change.

The group leader can influence group norms when the group is forming. The norms that the COTA encourages influence the behaviors that will lead to trust, group cohesion, and goal attainment. Norms that might be facilitated by the COTA include: each member is valued, expression of feelings is important, making mistakes is expected, and disagreement is desirable.

Group Growth and Development

A third consideration in learning about how groups work is understanding the developmental phases of group life. There is agreement among researchers who study groups that there are common, predictable, sequential, and developmental stages which emerge as the group matures. Group phases are best observed in closed groups in which membership is stable over time. These stages often overlap, and earlier stages may be repeated with the introduction of new tasks or change in membership. For this reason, some theorists describe group evolution as a developmental spiral.[13]

There are many theorists who have studied and described phases of group development. Bales, for example, describes three stages: "orientation," or defining the problem/task; "evaluation," or how the group feels about the task; and "control," or how the task will be completed.[14] Tuckman summarized the literature available on group development and determined four stages:[15]

1 *Forming* deals with orientation issues of coming together;
2 *Storming* represents conflict and power struggles which relate to the issue of control;

3 *Norming* is the stage in which members determine how they will relate to one another;
4 *Performing* represents how the task will be accomplished.

It is important to use a developmental frame of reference when working with groups. This can help give meaning to events occurring within the group and can assist the leader in choosing an appropriate intervention.

For the purposes of this discussion, two dimensions of group development will be examined. Mosey's developmental framework lists and describes levels of group interaction. Those groups are parallel group, project group, ego-centric cooperative group, cooperative group, and mature group.[1] The maturation process within each developmental level will also be described. These phases will be defined as initial dependence, conflict, and interrelatedness.

Initial dependence describes the first phase of group maturation. Members are concerned about their place within the group. Feelings can be manifested in different ways depending upon the developmental level of the group; however, each newly formed group, regardless of developmental level, experiences an initial dependency phase.

The second phase of maturation within each level is characterized by some conflict and struggle. The important issue in this phase is control — control of self, and control of others or of the environment. This struggle is a necessary and normal part of group development. It should be recognized and encouraged because learning usually requires some degree of labor. It is necessary for groups to experience and resolve this issue before interrelatedness is achieved.

The final phase, interrelatedness, emerges through successful resolution of control issues. This stage is characterized by a high level of affiliation. Members relate at a deeper interpersonal level. It is at this point, when members experience a sense of community with each other, that greater risk taking can occur, thus enhancing the opportunity for greater personal growth. The potential for learning and behavioral change may vary among patients, especially those with cognitive limitations. But even in low level groups the opportunity of this phase of interrelatedness is present.

Application to Developmental Groups

The Parallel Group

The first and most basic group in terms of independence and interpersonal competence of the members is the parallel group. There are usually five to seven members who work side-by-side but on individual projects. The leader assumes total leadership and responsibility for meeting the group members' needs for security, love and belonging, and esteem while assisting them with their activity.[1] The treatment goals of this group are to develop work skills, experience mastery over a simple task, and develop basic awareness of others. Craft projects are designed to offer opportunities to meet these goals.

At first, the group members will exhibit anxiety and total dependence on the leader(s). Members may express uncertainty about why they are together, appear passive, laugh nervously, or seem confused. The activity presented in the parallel group provides a means of focusing a person's attention away from self and onto other objects in the environment.

The conflict phase in a parallel group is seen in the patient's struggle for control over the materials, tools, and the process of the task. For mastery to occur, the COTA must make certain that activities provide a manageable challenge. To do this, the occupational therapy assistant serving in this role must have a clear understanding of each person's limitations. Mastery must be strongly reinforced as the patient works.

Interconnectedness or community can occur even at this group level if the COTA helps to create the connections among members. One way to accomplish this is to have individuals work on similar kinds of projects.[1] As the assistant helps the patients recognize their success, self-esteem begins to build. A reinforced sense of self enables a person to begin to experience others.

Another means of providing individual identity to group members in a parallel group is through *sentient role recognition*. The COTA, serving as a group leader, learns to observe members carefully and to recognize and reinforce personality qualities that may have brought the individual recognition at one time. The leader may notice evidence of nurturing qualities, sociability, or a sense of humor in particular members. Once identified, the personality quality may be described to the patient in positive terms and its use directed. For example, a patient with nurturing qualities may be asked to sit next to a new member and told that his or her warmth and manner would make the new person feel more comfortable. If this quality is recognized by the patient and has given meaning and uniqueness to his or her self-concept, it will be strengthened by providing a special role for that person in the group.

It is ideal to work with an occupational therapist, sharing leadership responsibility and providing members with a "parental team." OTRs and COTAs, working together as a complementary team, model appropriate and caring interaction skills.[16]

Leader Preparation, Attitude, and Approach

Before the group arrives, it is important for the COTA to attend to the following:

1. Know as much as possible about the individuals in the group in order to provide members with meaningful activities; and
2. Preplan and organize the activities and instructions carefully so that energy is used most efficiently during the group itself.

After group members arrive, the leader is responsible for carrying out the following tasks with particular attention to affect and attitude.

1. Greet each member individually and use names frequently (name tags are visual reminders);
2. Project warmth, friendliness, and calmness through facial expression, words, and actions to promote comfort and trust;
3. Provide consistency in approach and routine through assignment of permanent seating and storage space for each individual;
4. Explain the purpose of the group and the activity;
5. Give clear and structured directions;
6. Sit down and spend time with each individual;
7. Stimulate members to perform at their highest level by offering activities which provide a manageable challenge with help from the leader;
8. Offer approval and recognition of members' efforts as well as their completed projects;
9. Establish a nurturing milieu by serving snacks and beverages;
10. If members become disruptive, take them aside for feedback or remove them from the group;
11. Encourage interaction among group members by expressing and modeling concern if individuals are absent or ill; and
12. Direct positive use of personality strengths to create opportunities for interaction.

The following are important activity qualities and examples that must also be given consideration by the group leader:

1. Activity length is dependent on the attention span of the members (from 15 minutes to 45 minutes, in most cases);
2. Structure activities to minimize the need for personal decision making and to assure success;
3. Activities should be meaningful and have a recognizable end product or provide a sense of identity; and
4. Provide projects that do not require heavy concentration, as this allows the opportunity for participants to develop an awareness of others in the group.

Most crafts can be adapted to meet the needs of the parallel group. The following are examples which the authors have found useful:

1. textile stenciling;
2. mosaics;
3. simple leather work;
4. needlecraft;
5. papercraft;
6. simple weaving;
7. copper tooling; and
8. ceramics.

Project Group

A project group requires higher level social and work skills. The larger group is broken down into subgroups of two and three people and a short-term task requiring some interaction and sharing is provided. Member interaction is secondary to the activity, and primary interest is in task completion.[1]

The dependence phase of the group presents itself in much the same way as the parallel group. Members will view the group leaders as protectors and authorities who define limits and goals and satisfy needs. The COTA allows this dependence but begins to encourage reliance on others.

The conflict emerges as dependency shifts from the leader to peers in the subgroup. Members may struggle as they attempt to establish trust in other members and cooperate in the shared activity. Members may seek out the leader for help instead of working with their partners. Some individuals may express dissatisfaction with the activity and the ability of peers. Members may appear overwhelmed by the task.

Interrelatedness begins to occur as the patients' sense of community encompasses the small work group. Patients are now able to share completion of the task, but this group level still will rely on the group leader or leaders to create connections or at least strengthen them through questions, comments, and summarizing activities. For example, after completion of a subgroup activity, a sharing session may be used to display completed projects. Members could be asked to name those with whom they worked. Each subgroup could be given a symbol or name to help members identify themselves as a member of a team. A short and competitive game between "teams" could be encouraged at the end of each session to reinforce the concept of belonging.[17]

Leader Preparation, Attitude, and Approach

1. Gently encourage members to rely on others in the group.
2. Answer some questions but re-direct questions to other members when possible.
3. Help members examine ideas and problems by asking pertinent questions.
4. Assist individuals in asking for help from partner or group by helping them to phrase questions.
5. Reinforce positive behaviors and relate them to *successful task completion*. (At this level the activity provides a concrete reference.)
6. If members appear overwhelmed, restructure a specific part of the activity and offer repeated contact and support.
7. If individuals in the group display negative behavior, intervene; help identify the problem and suggest possible solutions.
8. If negative behavior is persistent, and if it interferes with task completion, remove the person from the group to discuss the problem.

Activity Qualities and Examples

The projects should be short-term, lasting from 20 minutes to 1 hour. At first projects should have easily divided components so that cooperation and contact are not constantly required between members. The following are examples of activities that can be used at this level.

- menu planning
- "no bake" cookies
- stir and frost cakes
- simple dips for snacks
- pizza
- making holiday or other decorations
- assembling party favors
- shuffleboard
- decorating bulletin boards
- potting plants or planting a terrarium
- making collages
- making mobiles
- egg dying
- ice cream making
- games, including relays
- team bowling
- cards

Ego-centric Cooperative Group

The ego-centric cooperative group is one in which members work together on a long-term activity requiring substantial interaction, cooperation, and sharing. Members are primarily self-centered at this level and are able to recognize and verbalize their own needs. Members are beginning to identify the esteem needs of others because of a developing awareness of the effect of their behavior upon individuals in the group. The members begin to assume responsibility for selecting, planning, and implementing the activity.[1]

The dependence phase will be seen as ambivalence. Members may exhibit heavy reliance on authority at times and then shift to an attitude of disregard. Although this is sometimes difficult for the therapist or assistant to deal with, it may be regarded as a positive behavioral sign as it signals the members' growing sense of self.

Conflict occurs within individuals and externally among members as the group struggles with the increased complexity of the activity and the interpersonal demands of the expanded group. Competition will be evident. Some individuals may have difficulty following established norms and may arrive late or ask to take frequent breaks. This testing behavior is an attempt to identify boundaries, and the COTA must offer guidance, identify feelings, and stress each individual's value in the group. The group leader must avoid power struggles and yet reinforce cooperation and adherence to the agreed-upon rules as they pertain to successful task completion and interpersonal relations.

To help the group achieve interrelatedness or community, one must assist members in understanding what occurred as they worked together. Work time may be followed by discussion which focuses on the behavioral strengths that have enhanced group progress and also on the group norms that have been established.[1] A sense of community can be identified when individuals receive recognition from other members.

Leader Approach and Attitude

1. Reinforce autonomy by demonstrating respect and concern for the feelings and rights of each individual through direct verbal statements and acknowledgement of contributions.
2. Provide structure as the group begins by clarifying directions or plans for each session.
3. Assist the group in establishing implicit and explicit norms by clarifying behavioral expectations, modeling desired behaviors, and complimenting positive behaviors observed in peers.
4. Assist members to recognize the progress they are making by asking individuals to describe their own strengths and weaknesses after the activity is over.
5. Manage conflict between members by facilitating understanding of one another's perspectives.
6. Help members discuss whether they feel accepted and appreciated because they are learning to recognize esteem needs in others.
7. Model empathy and concern for the feelings of members.
8. Encourage members to provide support for each other.
9. Provide members with a decision making process that encourages participation by all. Brainstorming or taking turns can be used as procedures.
10. Provide constructive feedback within the group, because members are learning how their behavior affects others.

Activity Qualities and Examples

Activity time may be expanded to 45 minute to 60 minute periods, and the task may take more than one period to complete. Activities chosen should require consistent interaction among all members. The following are some examples:

newspaper lay-outs
party planning and implementation
picnic planning or outdoor cooking activities
furniture refinishing
mural painting
planning and presenting skits and videotaping the performance

Cooperative Groups

The cooperative group is most often homogeneous; that is, members share similarities of age, sex, values, and interests.[1] Because of these likenesses and the members' increasing ability to identify and articulate their own needs, they begin to recognize the multiple needs of other people as well. At this level the task becomes secondary and a vehicle for interaction. Interpersonal relationships become the primary focus.

Initially members will depend on the leader(s) for structure and support while establishing trust, and for guidance as new group roles are learned. Members will need help in identifying and responding to the needs of others as well as expressing positive and negative feelings. Members will also depend on the COTA to help maintain cohesiveness.

Conflict occurs as members attempt to learn the balance of task and group-centered roles. Some members will see conflict or disagreement as bad and will need help in understanding that disagreement is a positive element and a sign of growth.[18] Members must learn to deal with conflict as it occurs and then to give and receive feedback responsibly. At this level, members are capable of learning many new communication skills but may have difficulty as they practice new roles and behaviors.

Affiliation potential is very high as members experience a stronger belief in themselves. Individual strengths are validated by others, and members begin to feel accepted and understood. In this phase members are able to share leadership and a sense of equality which strengthens bonds between people. Members are able to identify problems, propose solutions, and have an improved sense of how the group as a whole functions. The group begins to deal openly with conflict, and members experience cohesion. Warmth and caring are evident even in disagreement.

Leader Attitude and Approach

The following steps should be utilized:

1. Assist members in establishing trust with one another by modeling accessibility and a willingness to be vulnerable (this means that the COTA should openly admit shortcomings and mistakes to the group);
2. Ask the group to decide what new skills members would like to learn;
3. Clarify the purpose of the group by emphasizing that although participation in the task is essential, the purpose of working together is to learn group and communication skills;
4. Offer skill building resources to the group and provide structure and information as necessary;
5. Monitor verbal and nonverbal communication to facilitate processing when the activity is over;
6. Encourage risk taking behavior;
7. Provide group with activities that teach group processes such as problem solving, decision making, and conflict management;
8. Assist members in taking on new leadership roles;
9. Provide activity choices that encourage the development of ability to give and receive feedback responsibly;
10. Provide encouragement and possibly activities or assignments for members to practice new skills outside the group.;
11. Teach members how to process their own group; and
12. Disengage self from the authority position as affiliation emerges.

Activity Qualities and Examples

A variety of suggestions may be offered to the cooperative group so that members may plan and implement an activity that could last through multiple periods. The process of choosing and planning the project provides an excellent opportunity for learning. It is useful to provide suggestions of shorter term tasks intermittently so that newly learned skills can be applied and gratification is immediate. This re-energizes the members. The following are some examples of long-term cooperative projects:

banner design and construction
quilt making
plays and talent shows
outdoor gardening
camping trips

Among the short-term cooperative projects that may be used occasionally are such activities as meal preparation, writing a group poem, designing a group symbol, and planning an outing.

Mature Groups

Mature groups function at the highest interpersonal level. They are heterogeneous, meaning that members vary in age, sex, values, interests, and socioeconomic or cultural background. Individuals able to function at this level are comfortable with a variety of people and are flexible in performing group roles. This is a skill level attained by healthy people and may be difficult to achieve in a hospital or rehabilitation setting. A COTA may more likely encounter a group at this level in a community setting, such as adult education groups, senior citizen centers, and neighborhood and special interest groups.

Dependency on occupational therapy personnel or any appointed leader will be minimal even in the initial meetings of this group. There may be an expectation that the COTA will make necessary physical arrangements for the meeting place or initiate discussion.

Members may experience conflict or ambivalence toward acceptance of increased responsibility and leadership roles. Issues related to the use of personal power may arise as members attempt to discover the extent of their influence over each other. Members struggle as they learn to draw upon their own assets more consistently and look inward for answers rather than relying upon others. Another phase of conflict may occur when the group loses members or comes to closure. This may cause the members to return to a brief dependency phase as they experience disequalibrium. These tensions usually last only briefly.

Members develop a strong social support system and experience a satisfying sense of community with others. Genuineness is evident in the sincere communication patterns. Openness and honesty become established group norms. Members respect and value each other. Each individual feels a sense of worth and importance in the group. Individuals feel deeply understood owing to empathetic communication. Risk taking occurs as members challenge each other and gain new personal insights leading to fuller awareness and social integration. Group members at this level not only accept diversity but seek it out and enjoy gaining new perspectives on self through understanding difference.

Leader Attitude and Approach

The following approaches are appropriate:

1. Facilitate formation of the group, and establish a conducive environment for meetings.
2. Relinquish leadership and allow the group to be self-directed.
3. Become an equal member of the group.

Activity Qualities and Examples

The group will determine its own direction and will choose activities related to the purpose of the group. As an activity specialist, the COTA will serve as a resource person to the group. Some possible activity categories include:

community service activities
academic/intellectual activities
creative thinking/problem solving activities
self-help activities, such as grief encounter groups and parenting.

Every group develops a process and profile unique unto itself. Occupational therapy personnel will seldom find a group that fits the developmental levels exactly as they have been described. These descriptions are intended as a guide in assessing individual and group levels and for planning appropriate activities to encourage growth.

A patient group is more likely to become cohesive and contribute to one anothers' growth if the members have been selected for their ability to function at a particular level. Too much variance in the members' abilities will interfere with individual and group progress.[18]

Many patients will never function at the cooperative or mature levels. However, it is important to recognize that through the effective use of interpersonal and group skills, the COTA can assist even low functioning groups to achieve a measure of interrelatedness or community. This sense of belonging will help satisfy basic needs, develop adaptive skills, and contribute to maintenance of physical and emotional health.

Groups which function at the higher developmental levels present more complicated patient issues, behaviors, and interactions. Entry-level COTAs need to work with groups over an extended period of time in order to develop and refine the necessary skills. Forms appropriate for use by a COTA in assisting with the assessment of patient social skills, as well as patient exercises, may be found in Appendices C and D.

Entry-level personnel are advised to seek supervision and guidance from advanced clinicians. Figure 9-3 provides an outline of the roles and functions of OTR and COTA team members involved in cooperative group work.

Summary

In this chapter, the need for certified occupational therapy assistants to be interpersonally competent was discussed. To become competent, one must gain an awareness of self and others and be able to demonstrate that awareness through the use of verbal and nonverbal communication skills. Active listening, a necessary communication skill used to help establish therapeutic rela-

FIGURE 9-3. Roles and Functions of Occupational Therapy Team Members in Group Work

Task	OTR	COTA
Screening	Determine appropriate screening information; initiate referrals; interpret findings; document recommendations	Collect information from patient, family, other resources; report findings to supervisor
Assessment	Determine patient's level of ability in cognitive, psychological, social, and sensory skill areas; determine appropriate group level	Determine dyadic and general work skill ability through interview, observation, and structured tasks
	Collaborative Roles	
Treatment planning	Plan patient's placement in a specific group, and examine profile of the total group, including such factors as ages, backgrounds, interests, and treatment goals. Collaborate with patients to set individual goals for each group member. Explore task and activity options. Analyze component parts of activity choice. Consider environmental factors in order to provide a meeting room and seating that satisfies the physical and security needs of the patients. Determine the role, attitude, and approach of team members, maximizing the use of personal strengths. Document the overall plan.	
Treatment	Introduce the activity; explain the purpose of the activity and reinforce individual goals. Engage the group; assume leadership roles as determined by the group level. Process the group; enable the members to achieve the maximum amount of learning from the group experience by providing time at the end of the session to discuss problems that occurred as members worked together; discuss progress the group is making, feelings related to problems and progress, and reaffirm or establish new group goals.[19]	
	Summarize and analyze each patient's progress; document response to program; reassess and modify program	Document patient performance as directed; assist in determining need for program change

tionships, was described.

A general knowledge of group leadership roles, group norms, and the maturation phases of small groups helps the COTA to develop a basic understanding of how groups work. This information can be applied to the use of groups in occupational therapy treatment. Groups used in this context can help the patient develop self-esteem, work skills, and interpersonal competence.

Mosey's developmental group levels identify group characteristics related to patient skill levels. Maturation phases of the group at each of the levels help the COTA recognize group and patient issues. This information allows the appropriate choice of an activity as well as structuring it to appropriately challenge group members. A skilled group leader will be able to help a group at any developmental level to work toward some form of community, also referred to as interrelatedness. The leader must allow for an initial dependency and help members to resolve the personal struggles and interpersonal conflicts as they arise within the group. From the successful resolution of these experiences, members are able to risk interaction on a deeper, more personal level. Group cohesion is strengthened, and members then have greater opportunities for insight and personal growth. Interpersonal skills are thus improved.

References

1. Mosey AC: *Activities Therapy*. New York: Raven Press, 1973.
2. Goble FC: *The Third Force: Psychology of Abraham Maslow*. New York: Grossman Publishers, 1970, Chapter 4.
3. *Basic International Relations: A Course for Small Groups*. Atlanta, GA: Human Development Institute, 1969, pp 15-21.
4. Miller F, Nunnally E, Wackman D: *Couple Communication: Talking Together*. Minneapolis, MN: Interpersonal Communication, 1979, pp 144-145.
5. Curran CA: *Counseling Learning*. New York: Grune and Stratton, 1979, pp 20-27.
6. Bolton E: *People Skills*. Englewood Cliffs, NJ: Prentice Hall, 1979.
7. Smith-Hannen SS: Affects of nonverbal behavior on judged levels of counselor warmth and empathy. *Journal of Counseling Psychology* 24:87-91, 1977.
8. Cormier WH, Cormier LS: *Interviewing Strategies for Helpers — A Guide to Assessment, Treatment and Evaluation*. Monteray, CA: Brooks Cole, 1979, p 44.

9. Hasse RF, Tepper D: Non verbal components of empathetic communication. *Journal of Counseling Psychology* 19:417-24, 1972.

10. *Basic Interpersonal Relations — Book 2: A Course for Small Groups*. Atlanta, GA: Human Development Institute, 1969.

11. Miles M: *Learning to Work in Groups*, 2nd Edition. New York: Teachers College, Columbia University, 1981, pp 241-245.

12. Bales RF: Task roles and social roles in problem solving groups. In TM Newcomb, EL Hartley, Eds: *Readings in Social Psychology,* 3rd Edition. New York: Holt, Rineholt and Winston, 1958.

13. Sampson DD, Marthas MS: *Group Process for Health Professions*. New York: John Wiley and Sons, 1977.

14. Bales RF: Adaptive and integrative changes as sources of strain in social systems. In AP Hare, EF Borgatta, RF Bales, Eds: *Small Groups*. New York: Alfred Knopf, 1955.

15. Tuckerman BW: Developmental sequence in small groups. *Psychological Bulletin* 63:384-399, 1965.

16. Napier R, Gershenfeld M: *Making Groups Work*. Boston: Houghton Mifflin, 1983, pp 108-109.

17. Hopkins HL, Smith HD: *Willard and Spackman's Occupational Therapy*, 5th Edition. Philadelphia: JB Lippincott, 1978, pp 293-295.

18. Loomis, ME: *Group Process for Nurses*. St. Louis: CV Mosby, 1981, pp 101-109.

19. Fidler G: The task oriented group as a context for treatment. *Am J Occup Ther,* 1:43-48, 1969.

Bibliography

Babcock PH: *The Role of the OTA in Mental Health*. Unpublished manual. Minneapolis, MN: St. Mary's Junior College, 1978.

CHAPTER 10

Therapeutic Intervention: An Overview

Sally E. Ryan, COTA

Introduction

The profession of occupational therapy has developed a specific plan for therapeutic intervention which is known as the *occupational therapy process*. It is made up of six distinct procedural categories that should be carried out in a particular order. (Exceptions are noted in the discussion of each category.) These sections are:[1]

1 referral;
2 assessment, which includes screening and evaluation;
3 program planning;
4 treatment, which includes periodic re-evaluation;
5 program discontinuation, which may include follow-up; and
6 service management.

General standards of practice for occupational therapy service programs and for occupational therapists providing direct service have been established by the American Occupational Therapy Association (AOTA). They were developed as guidelines to assist members of the profession. These standards have been reprinted in Appendix E-1, and they detail important aspects of the occupational therapy process in which the certified occupational therapy assistant serves an important role. In recent times, more specific standards of practice have been adopted in the areas of physical disabilities, developmental disabilities, mental health, home health and school settings. They are published in the *Reference Manual of the Official Documents of the American Occupational Therapy Association,* which is available from AOTA.[2]

Referral

Requests for occupational therapy services may come from many sources, including physicians, physical therapists, teachers, social workers and other health professionals as well as parents and patients themselves. Referrals may be initiated or received by the occupational therapist either before or after the initial screening of the patient. All referrals must be documented in writing and become a part of each patient's permanent record. The COTA may initiate patient referrals in the areas of independent living and daily living skills. In the event that a referral is received by a COTA, whether initiated or not, it must be given to the supervising OTR who is ultimately responsible for any action taken regarding the referral.[1]

The American Occupational Therapy Association does not require that a referral be received before services can be provided. In some instances, state laws or the requirements established by health care facilities will mandate the receipt of a referral.[3]

Assessment

The process of assessment includes both screening and evaluation and must take place before any individual program planning is done. A thorough assessment provides a comprehensive "picture" of the patient based on a complete analysis of all of the screening and evaluation data. It is a predictor of the need for occupational therapy or other services and the estimated duration of treatment.

Screening involves the collection and analysis of specific data and facts. Information is obtained through observation of the patient while performing tasks or engaging in social interactions; through interviews with the patient, the family or significant others such as a roommate or a close friend; and through a review of the patient's general history from sources which may include the a medical chart, a psychologist's report or a teacher's appraisal. The COTA collaborates with the supervising OTR in the screening process by collecting and reporting selected information as requested. For example, he or she may use a structured interview form to gather information about the patient's educational background, employment history, hobbies and self-care skills. If the occupational therapist's analysis of the screening information indicates that occupational therapy treatment would be of benefit to the patient, a comprehensive evaluation is done using the AOTA Uniform Evaluation Checklist as a guide.

The OTR is responsible for all aspects of the evaluation; however, the COTA may carry out some evaluative tasks under supervision. These might include administering an interest checklist or an activity configuration and summarizing the information in a written report, or observing the patient in a specific situation and reporting on interpersonal skills, coordination, strength, and endurance as they relate to daily living skills and tasks. Some of the areas which may be evaluated include:[1]

1 Physical Daily Living Skills: grooming, eating, dressing, mobility, communication, tools and common object handling;
2 Psychological Daily Living Skills: self-concept, situational coping, and community involvement;
3 Work Skills: homemaking, child care, and preparation for a job;
4 Play/Leisure Skills: awareness of needs and interests, participation in meaningful activities and use of community resources;
5 Sensorimotor Components: degree of reflex integration, range of motion, gross and fine coordination, strength and endurance, and sensory and body integration;
6 Cognitive Components: orientation, comprehension, concentration, attention span, memory and problem solving; and
7 Psychosocial Components: self-expression, self-control, and interaction with an individual or a group.

Evaluation is necessary to determine the patient's strengths and weaknesses, needs, and the degree of change possible through occupational therapy intervention. A variety of specific evaluations are used by occupational therapists.

Screening and evaluation data are analyzed and interpreted by the OTR to determine the total assessment results. Recommendations for continuance or dismissal from occupational therapy are made. Other services besides occupational therapy which may assist the patient are identified and referral may be made.

Program Planning

The active involvement of the patient and the family is essential for successful program planning. In this portion of the process, both long- and short-term goals and time lines are established. Specific activities are analyzed, selected, and sequenced to assist the patient in meeting the goals. Specific methods and approaches are also determined, and adaptations are planned. The patient's values, cultural identification, stage of biological and mental development, and interests and abilities are all carefully considered as an integral part of the process.

The COTA contributes to many aspects of the program plan; however, the OTR is responsible for the final plan that will best meet the patient's needs and will be acceptable to the patient. The long-term objectives of such a plan are to develop, improve, restore, or maintain the patient's abilities to enable him or her to lead a more productive and meaningful life. The short-term objectives must be stated in achievable outcomes and be met in a short enough time span that they can serve as a record of improvement.

Treatment

All occupational therapy treatment is based on the program plan. Effective treatment requires the patient to participate in selected, purposeful activities designed to achieve the established goals. The COTA, under close supervision, may implement a program for acutely ill individuals, such as a recent stroke patient or a depressed suicidal patient.[1] Close supervision is essential because of the complex problems and degree of change frequently seen, which may require a modified treatment approach or re-evaluation by the OTR. If the patient is in a more stable, nonacute, or controlled condition, the assistant may carry out treatment procedures with greater independence, as directed by the supervising occupational therapist. The COTA may also be responsible for monitoring the patient's performance and providing a summary report. It is the responsibility of the COTA to keep the supervising therapist informed of all changes in patient performance and any other pertinent facts. As treatment progresses, and changes are indeed noted, the assistant may contribute suggestions for program modifications or additions that will help the patient reach the established goals.[1]

In the event that the patient is not making satisfactory progress, the OTR will conduct a re-evaluation to determine necessary changes in the program plan and the treatment procedures. Specific aspects of the re-evaluation may be delegated to the assistant. Re-evaluation also takes place prior to discharge to determine discontinuation and discharge planning.

Program Discontinuation

Program discontinuation takes place when the patient has reached all of the established goals or when it is determined that he or she can no longer benefit from occupational therapy services. Among other tasks, the COTA may assist in this process by providing specific information on progress or lack of progress to be included in a summary report. Providing instructions for a home program and identifying community resources and personal or environmental adaptations that may assist the patient after discharge are other areas that may be the responsibility of the COTA.

While the standards adopted by AOTA do not specify that patient follow-up must occur, it is desirable to gather such information to determine the effectiveness of treatment, general adjustment outcomes, and the degree to which the patient is able to resume social, family, work, and leisure roles. This could be an OTR/COTA collaborative task, with the OTR determining the final conclusions. Follow-up also provides additional support to the patient in the transition from illness to health.

Service Management

Service management is a process that involves planning, structuring, developing, coordinating and evaluating the delivery of all occupational therapy services to insure quality, efficiency and effectiveness. It is the organizational framework and system that supports the occupational therapy process in therapeutic intervention. Service management is essential in the delivery of occupational therapy services. Because this area has so many specific components, it will be discussed in depth in Chapter 28.

Summary

Therapeutic intervention follows a specific plan which is called the occupational therapy process. This process includes sets of tasks that should be carried out in a particular order. Referral, assessment, program planning, treatment, and program discontinuation are the major categories. Service management is a system that allows the occupational therapy process to be carried out. The COTA may participate in all aspects of the process as directed by the supervising OTR.

Since this is indeed a brief overview, the reader is referred to the documents *Standards of Practice for Occupational Therapy* and the *Entry-Level OTR and COTA Role Delineation*, in Appendix E for more detailed information.

References

1. Entry-level role delineation for OTRs and COTAs, *Occup Ther Newspaper*, 35 (July):8-16, 1981.
2. *Reference Manual of the Official Documents of the American Occupational Therapy Association*. Revised edition. Rockville, MD: American Occupational Therapy Association, 1983, Chapter IV.
3. Commission on Practice Report. American Occupational Therapy Association, April 1981.

SECTION III

Intervention Strategies—The OTR/COTA Team Approach

This section provides the reader with specific, illustrative examples of the many ways the occupational therapist and the occupational therapy assistant can work together effectively in clinical practice. Eleven different case studies are presented that define the roles of occupational therapy personnel in the therapeutic intervention process. The selection of case studies represents a wide variety of different age groups, problems, intervention strategies, protocols, and treatment settings. Appropriate tasks and roles are presented, within the context of each case study, for both the entry-level and the experienced assistant. The *Entry-Level OTR and COTA Role Delineation,* published by the American Occupational Therapy Association, was used as the primary outline for each case presentation; however, some of the case examples illustrate intraprofessional roles beyond entry-level practice and the scope of this document. The role delineation has been reprinted in Appendix E of this text.

Many of the case studies are based on actual events, while others are a composite of several events and situations. Names, personal information, and other pertinent data have been changed to protect the identity of actual occupational therapy patients. Any similarities between the patients described and actual patients who have received occupational therapy services is purely coincidental.

Brief introductory material is provided for some of the case studies, particularly in those areas of practice where assistant roles are relatively new or changing or when the authors and the editor believed that additional background information would be useful.

It is very important for the reader to note that the case studies are examples, *not recommended standards,* for the intraprofessional team approach in the delivery of occupational therapy services. They are illustrations of how the occupational therapist and the occupational therapy assistant can work together with a particular diagnostic problem or within a specific area of occupational therapy practice. The authors have expressed their professional opinions based on actual experiences as well as hypothetical and ideal situations. The overall goals of the authors and the editor are to promote the profession of occupational therapy through the intraprofessional team approach and to provide quality health care services which are delivered in an efficient and effective manner.

CHAPTER 11

The Child with Cerebral Palsy

Teri Black, COTA
Toni Walski, OTR

History of School System Practice

Public education of handicapped youngsters has evolved in the 20th century. By 1918, all states had established compulsory attendance laws for school-age children, which indirectly prompted development of "special education" facilities for retarded children. In 1911, New Jersey pioneered in legislating educational programs for the retarded, and by 1955 most states had passed similar requirements.

The decades of the 1930s and 1940s witnessed organization of regional or city-wide schools educating physically handicapped children, while allowing them to remain at home. Occupational therapists were first employed in these orthopedic schools.

In 1961, President Kennedy established the President's Panel on Mental Retardation, and in 1966 the Bureau of Education of the Handicapped (BEH) was established as part of the U.S. Office of Education. The 1960s saw occupational therapy broadening its scope to serve students having developmental problems.

During the 1970s, Federal legislation revolutionized special education and greatly increased the need for school system therapists. Related education services such as occupational therapy were required by law to enable handicapped students to function more effectively in their school programs. Occupational therapists extended services to the learning disabled during this decade, and increased understanding of neurophysiology dramatically changed approaches for treating movement disorders. Neuromuscular techniques facilitated sensorimotor integration and normalization of movement and function, versus an earlier emphasis on developing compensatory movement patterns.

Occupational therapy has continued to evolve and diversify its school services. Practitioners collaborate with school team members in the mainstreaming of handicapped youngsters in regular education classrooms and in many specialized programs such as infant stimulation, preschool early intervention/prevention, elementary and secondary special education, and prevocational assessment.

Public Law 94-142: Education of All Handicapped Children Act

Major court cases from 1950 to the early 1970s, which dealt with racial segregation or exclusion of retarded and physically disabled individuals from public schools, supported a constitutional right to free and appropriate education. Beyond the courts, Federal laws, which included The Education of the Handicapped Act of 1970, The Rehabilitation Act of 1973, and The Right to Education Amendments Act of 1974, paved the way for PL 94-142, The Education of All Handicapped Children Act of 1975, which sought to "assure that all handicapped children have available to them a free appropriate public education which emphasizes special education and related services designed to meet their unique needs, to assure that the rights of handicapped children and their parents or guardians are protected, to assist states and localities to provide for the education of all handicapped children, and to assess and assure the effectiveness of efforts to educate handicapped children."[1]

Handicapped children were defined as: "children who are mentally retarded, hard of hearing, deaf, orthopedically impaired, other health impairments, speech impaired, visually handicapped, seriously mentally disturbed children with specific learning disabilities who by reason thereof require special education and related services."

Public Law 94-142 outlined six requirements for providing education services:[1]

1 *Zero Reject*: All handicapped youngsters must be given a free, appropriate public education. As of 1980, states were required to provide education services for ages 3 years to 21 years.
2 *Nondiscriminatory Evaluation*: Unbiased or culture-free assessment instruments for evaluating all areas of suspected disability must be provided through a multidisciplinary team of teachers and other specialists.
3 *Individualized Education Plan*: For each student whose evaluation indicates special needs, an Individualized Education Plan (IEP) must be written and updated yearly. Figure 11-1 illustrates the IEP process.
4 *Least Restrictive Environment*: Handicapped children must be mainstreamed to the fullest extent possible; therefore, placement in a regular classroom is preferred over special education, while the latter is preferred to an institutional setting.
5 *Due Process*: Procedures must safeguard the appropriateness of the educational plan. If needed, parents, guardians or surrogates appointed by public agencies can institute an impartial hearing process on behalf of the child.
6 *Parental Involvement*: Parents or guardians must participate in developing each student's Individualized Education Plan, and there should be an active parental role in public hearings and advisory boards which influence state educational plans for handicapped children.

States have also enacted laws which detail education of handicapped individuals within their purview. Rules governing Related Services are available through the State Department of Education. Professional policies for Certified Occupational Therapy Assistants relative to supervision, roles and functions are available from the American Occupational Therapy Association.

Case Study

Garfield Elementary School serves 315 neighborhood students. Children with special needs are transported to Garfield from other sections of the district. There are five special education classrooms: one for Learning Disabled (LD); two for Educable Mentally Impaired or Educable Mentally Retarded (EMI/EMR, approximate I.Q. 50 to 70); and two for Trainable Mentally Impaired or Trainable Mentally Retarded (TMI/TMR, approximate IQ 30 to 50). Also, several students

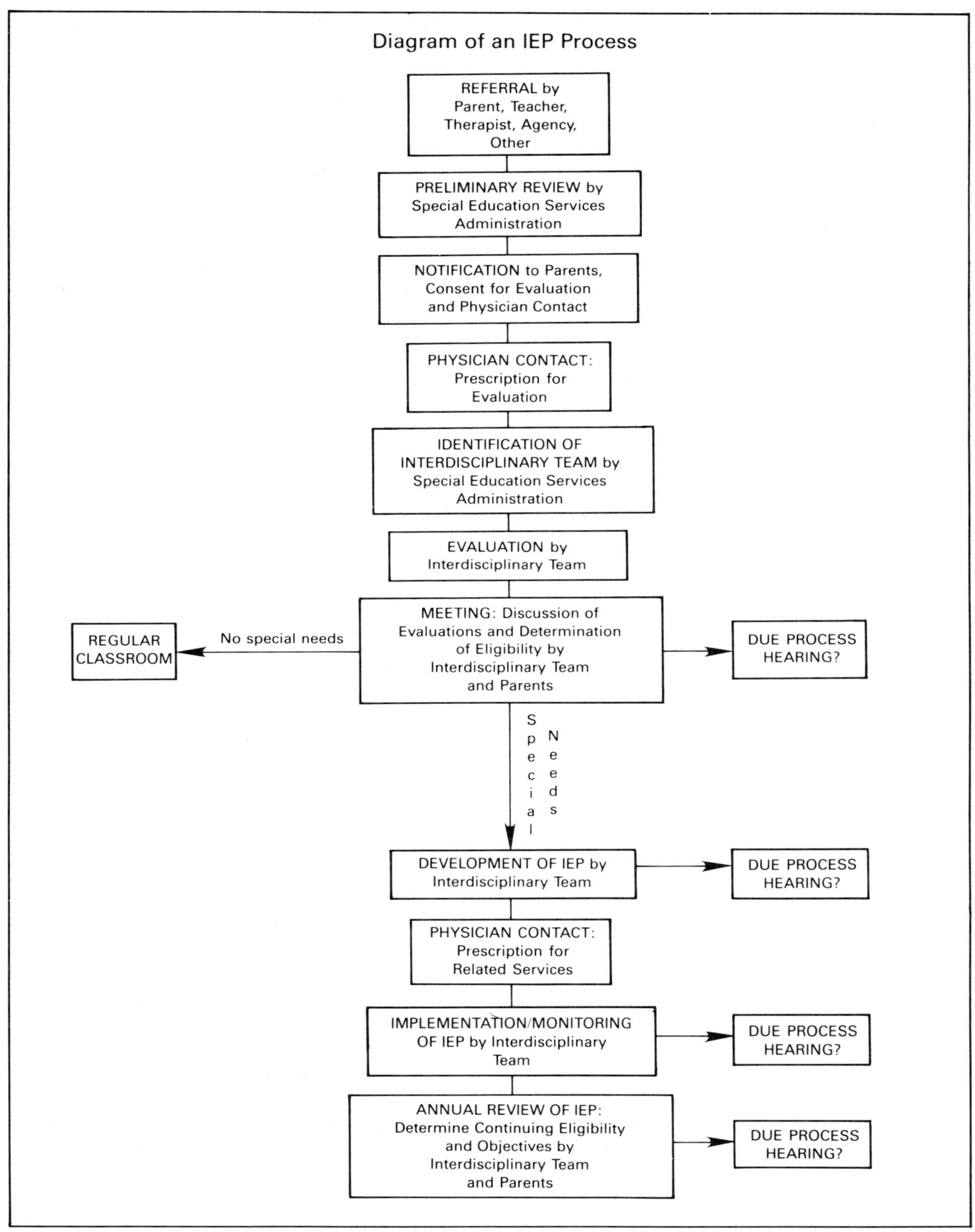
Diagram of an IEP Process
REFERRAL by Parent, Teacher, Therapist, Agency, Other
PRELIMINARY REVIEW by Special Education Services Administration
NOTIFICATION to Parents, Consent for Evaluation and Physician Contact
PHYSICIAN CONTACT: Prescription for Evaluation
IDENTIFICATION OF INTERDISCIPLINARY TEAM by Special Education Services Administration
EVALUATION by Interdisciplinary Team
MEETING: Discussion of Evaluations and Determination of Eligibility by Interdisciplinary Team and Parents
No special needs
REGULAR CLASSROOM
DUE PROCESS HEARING?
Special Needs
DEVELOPMENT OF IEP by Interdisciplinary Team
DUE PROCESS HEARING?
PHYSICIAN CONTACT: Prescription for Related Services
IMPLEMENTATION/MONITORING OF IEP by Interdisciplinary Team
DUE PROCESS HEARING?
ANNUAL REVIEW OF IEP: Determine Continuing Eligibility and Objectives by Interdisciplinary Team and Parents
DUE PROCESS HEARING?

Figure 11-1

with physical disabilities attend regular classes. Each of these classrooms is staffed by a special education teacher and an aide.

Related Services includes one half-time occupational therapist and one half-time physical therapist. A COTA and a health aide, the latter providing transportation and personal care assistance to students, are the only full-time Related Services personnel. A speech and language therapist provides services to Garfield as well as three other schools. In addition, a social worker, a psychologist, and special education consultants are available as needed. The part-time school nurse occasionally consults with Related Services regarding students' self-management of catheters, ileostomies, injections and such.

Referral

Jeff, an educable mentally retarded child with cerebral palsy, was referred by his classroom teacher who noted motor problems which limited the student's performance in academic and self-care activities. His age was 5 years, 7 months when he was first seen by occupational therapy personnel.

The referral was initially forwarded to an administrative office which coordinates services citywide. This office sent a notification of referral to the parents and a request for parental permission to evaluate the child and communicate with the physician was included. When the parents' consent form was received and the physician's prescription for an evaluation had been secured, appropriate school team members were contacted to evaluate the child, a process that required three weeks.

While the supervising OTR communicated with the doctor regarding specific aspects of the medical history, the COTA began compiling Jeff's occupational therapy (OT) file, including copies of the referral, parental consent, physician's prescription for evaluation, and any previous medical or therapy records. The COTA was responsible for maintaining the file throughout the student's involvement in OT.

Assessment

Initial Screening

An initial screening was done to judge Jeff's potential need for occupational therapy services and to determine what further evaluations would be necessary. Using an outline developed by the OTR supervisor, the COTA reviewed Jeff's file and recorded pertinent details of his educational background, clinical condition, and present level of functioning.

The COTA also compiled a mailing to Jeff's parents which included a cover letter, Related Services information pamphlet and a questionnaire. The questionnaire solicited information regarding home reinforcers (preferences in food and activities), parental priorities (functioning problems which concern parents), emotional adjustment, play patterns and preferences, and any behavior problems which bothered the parents such as tantrums, head banging or biting, and screaming during the night.[2]

Another aspect of the screening process involved gathering information from Jeff's teachers. The occupational therapy assistant used a structured interview/checklist form with behavioral descriptors noted to gather data which might indicate Jeff's potential problems in academic, gross motor, fine motor, tactile sensation, vestibular sensation, auditory language, visual perception, and emotional adjustment areas.[2]

These findings were then reported to the OTR who, following analysis and synthesis of all of the screening information, determined that Jeff could benefit from a more in-depth occupational therapy evaluation.

Evaluation

Jeff's evaluation was largely performed by the occupational therapist, as the complexity of the child's clinical condition and the particular evaluation instruments used required knowledge of sensorimotor development in making necessary observations and judgements. Several of the performance component evaluations were standardized, yielding normative comparisons of age equivalency.

Occasionally, the COTA assisted with Jeff's evaluation by positioning him for goniometric range of motion and standing by for added safety during the assessment of gross motor and locomotor functions such as balancing and jumping, thereby freeing the therapist to observe Jeff's movement more closely.

The COTA also contributed observations of Jeff's performance in classroom, playground, and lunchroom settings, which helped to confirm the functional effects of problems detected in the formal evaluation.

Jeff's dressing performance was evaluated by the COTA using a developmental skills checklist. The occupational therapy assistant also contributed greatly to the evaluation of Jeff's functioning in the areas of grooming and hygiene, object manipulation, emotional daily living skills, and play, integrating observations with relevant feedback from Jeff's parents and teachers. Because of Jeff's neuromuscular disability, the eating evaluation was conducted by the OTR.

Specific tests administered by the occupational therapist included the Milanni-Comparetti Test, Goodenough-Harris Drawing Test, Berry-Buktenica Test of Visual-Motor Integration (VMI), and Early Childhood Fine Motor Checklist.

Jeff was cooperative, though distractible during evaluation activities. His attention span was improved in a low stimulus environment. Muscular tone and body posturing increased as Jeff attempted motor tasks.

Following the three-week evaluation period, the OTR and the COTA met formally to review their respective assessments and observations and the OTR prepared the following report:

SEX:	Male	CLASS:	EMR
B.D.	2/15/79	TEACHER:	K W
C.A.	5.7 yrs.	D.O.E.:	9/27/84
DX:	Athetoid Quadriparesis, Mental Retardation, Multiple Congenital Anomalies	DR.:	M C, MD

Referral/Background

A brief narrative summary of the referral, Jeff's background and evaluation process, including dates, specific instruments and procedures used, appeared in this section and was followed by these findings:

Sensorimotor Components Neuromuscular

1 *Reflex Integration:* Jeff uses many postural fixations to compensate for instability in the trunk, shoulders, and hips. His arms make writhing motions distally. Righting reactions and equilibrium responses are delayed and unreliable.

2 *Range of Motion:* Joint range of motion (ROM) is generally within normal limits. Jeff exhibits slight tightness in right shoulder external rotation. Mild scapulohumeral fixation at the left shoulder can be disassociated with facilitation. Hyperextension at the metacarpophalangeal (MP) and interphalangeal (IP) joints is present bilaterally. Jeff may be at risk for spinal curves due to low muscle tone and unusual posturing. In addition, he tends to "W" sit to stabilize himself.

3 *Muscle Tone:* Jeff's overall tone is variable, but generally hypotonic. He often appears "floppy," but will stiffen his arms, legs, and mouth musculature when he becomes excited or performs motor activities. Bilateral upper extremity tone fluctuates between normal and mild spasticity, with slight resistance felt in shoulder adduction, internal rotation, and elbow flexion.

4 *Strength and Endurance:* Jeff shows limited strength and endurance in trunk, shoulders, and hips. Bilateral hand weakness interferes with classroom activities, while weak lateral grasp limits dressing. He shows poor endurance in most repetitive exercises or multistep tasks, though distractibility and increasing tone also interfere.

5 *Gross and Fine Coordination:*
- Muscle Control/Coordination: Jeff functions approximately at the three-year-old level of gross motor skills on the Milanni-Comparetti scale. He shows lack of proximal co-contraction and stability, and he is unable to perform any gross motor activities which require hip stability. When asked to stand from a squat position, Jeff exhibits tongue thrust and arm posturing. Generally he does not perform gross motor tasks in a smooth, coordinated manner; for instance, when pulling himself forward on a scooter board, his shoulders elevate to his ears. Jeff experiences difficulty isolating movements so that one arm can be used separately from the other in cutting with a scissors or holding clothing while dressing.
- Dexterity: Jeff performs at a three-year-old level on the Early Childhood Fine Motor Checklist. He has difficulty with quick release of objects and can isolate his index finger more easily on his right hand. He reverts to a primitive squeeze/raking pattern when his posture is stressed because of poor positioning in his chair. Repetitive hand movement results in a building of muscle tone and extraneous posturing. On the Goodenough-Harris Drawing Test, Jeff's production of a man was unrecognizable.

Sensorimotor Components: Sensory Integration

1 *Sensory Awareness*:
- Vision/Ocular Control: Visual acuity and field appear within normal limits. Jeff has difficulty isolating eye from head movements for smooth visual tracking and scanning.
- Tactile Awareness: There is some tactile hypersensitivity if touched unexpectedly or when agitated. Jeff shows some inability to locate light touch or two-point stimuli applied to his face and hands. He seems unaware when his chin is wet from drooling.

2 *Body Integration*:
- Postural Balance: Jeff's hypotonic trunk and lack of co-contraction at the shoulders and hips contribute to poor sitting balance. His balance is also jeopardized by increased muscle tone triggered by excitement, verbalization, or hand use; typically, Jeff's knees extend and elbows flex with athetoid movements distally.

• Bilateral Motor Coordination: Jeff is hesitant in using his left arm in bilateral activities such as catching a bouncing ball or stabilizing his paper when drawing. Again, postural instability, muscle tone increases, and weaknesses interfere with smooth use of two hands.

• Lateralization/Dominance: Jeff is right dominant and tends to neglect using his left hand assistively.

• Visual-Motor Integration (VMI): The VMI (Beery Buktenica Test) score is three years, two months. Since motor performance influences results, this score may not reflect his perceptual ability.

• Cognitive Components—Attention span: Jeff is able to attend to tasks for 10-minute intervals in a low stimulus room. He is highly distracted by environmental stimulation such as noise and touch, usually requiring verbal cues to bring him back to a task.

Independent Living/ Daily Living Skills

1 *Grooming/Hygiene*: Jeff requires moderate assistance in most tasks. He can brush his teeth once the toothpaste has been applied to the brush, but needs supervision for thoroughness. He manages his hair using a round bristle brush. He washes himself independently with a mitt-type washcloth. Jeff has good bowel and bladder control, but needs help pulling up his pants and handling fastners.

2 *Feeding/Eating*:
- *Oral Structure*: The palate is slightly high but stays clear of food while Jeff is eating.
- *Oro-facial Muscle Tone*: Musculature is hypotonic overall; however, abnormal

increased tone patterns of lip retraction and purse-string puckering are seen as associated movements in speaking and eating, especially when Jeff is excited or distracted.

- *Oral Movements*: Chewing action of the jaw is mostly vertical with slight rotary motion to the right and left. Lip closure is loose, but with increasing tone, lip retraction or purse-string action is seen, indicating emergence of a less controlled pattern. Jeff compensates for weakened lip closure by keeping his fingers to his lips. Tongue movements can be lateralized to the right, but are decreased toward the left. Drooling increases as tone rises.
- *Oral Patterns*: Jeff shows suckling and sucking patterns in drinking and consuming an ice lollipop. At times he doesn't swallow the last bit of liquid as promptly or completely as he did when in a suck-swallow sequence. A munching/tongue thrust pattern is seen in eating, and biting through hard or sticky foods is difficult.
- *Positioning*: During lunch, Jeff sits on a picnic bench with classmates. A footrest would allow him to plant his feet to compensate for trunk instability. His elbows rest on the table with shoulders in internal rotation.
- *Hand-to-Mouth Pattern*: Presently Jeff shows free forearm rotation on the right, holding a spoon loosely in a dagger or shovel grasp. He picks up and positions his spoon using his right hand only. He tends to bite off pieces of food versus cutting them to size, and shows inconsistent use of his left hand to assist in cutting food or stabilizing dishes. Trunk instability affects his ability to perform a smooth, controlled hand-to-mouth movement.

3 *Dressing*: Jeff needed assistance of varying degrees throughout the evaluation process. He was able to take clothes off with minor assistance in handling fasteners. Once started, he can pull on T-shirts. Given enough time he can pull on socks and pants.

4 *Functional Mobility:* Jeff walks with a shuffling gait and wide base of support. He can roll and crawl reciprocally, but cannot hop, skip, balance on one foot, or climb stairs. In two-foot jumping, he is barely able to clear the floor.

5 *Functional Communication:* Jeff has great difficulty articulating speech. Overall body tone, lip retraction, and drooling increase as Jeff tries to speak.

6 *Object Manipulation:* Using his right hand, Jeff holds a pencil in a loose lateral grasp and writes using gross arm versus finer wrist and hand motions. Repetitive hand activity results in increased muscle tone, and Jeff reverts to increasing shoulder movement and a more gross grasp of the pencil. Bilateral hand and finger weakness interferes with classroom activities such as cutting with scissors, squeezing a glue bottle, opening jars, manipulating door knobs, and operating faucets. Generally, objects should be larger or built up for adequate handling.

7 *Psychological/Emotional Daily Living Skills:* Jeff is reinforced by verbal praising of his accomplishments, interacting with favorite toys, or wearing his baseball cap. He adapts fairly well to new situations, but seems to prefer the same routine. Fast changes or stimulating environments trigger increased muscle tone and distractibility. Jeff communicates more readily on a one-to-one basis than in a classroom group situation. He tends to play with boys from his class, and he has a few other acquaintances, who assume helper rather than playmate roles.

8 *Play/Leisure:* Jeff tends to observe others on the playground. He will occasionally climb on lower equipment, but avoids swings and slides. During unstructured classroom time, he chooses eight to ten piece wooden puzzles and shape sorting toys. Jeff's mother has expressed concern with his tendency to watch television. She has asked whether a microcomputer might provide him with a more constructive outlet.

Assessment Summary and Recommendations

Jeff is functioning at approximately the 3-year level in gross and fine motor, visual motor and self-care skills. He has many motor delays which prevent maximal participation in his school program. Major interfering factors are:

1. Lack of proximal stability, co-contraction, and strength of the trunk, shoulders and hips, which limits his ability to steady his body for sitting or arm use.
2. Variable, but generally hypotonic or "floppy" muscle tone, resulting in poorly graded movements; increasing tone and associated stiffening of mouth, arm and leg musculature when stressed or performing motor tasks.
3. Lack of disassociated or isolated movements, so that using one arm separately from the other makes daily tasks difficult.
4. Generalized poor strength and endurance due to aforementioned factors and some unwillingness or inability to attend to tasks for a prolonged period.
5. Oral motor problems affecting eating, drinking, and speaking which increase when the student is excited or involved in motor activities.

Occupational therapy recommends direct and consultative services and environmental adaptations to promote proximal stability, normalize muscle tone, promote more coordinated and isolated movement patterns, improve arm and hand strength and endurance, develop better oral motor function, and build independence in daily living skills, especially dressing.

Program Planning

Using the assessment data, the OTR and the COTA collaborated in formulating a hierarchy of occupational therapy goals and corresponding measurable objectives. A specific intervention plan was developed which detailed techniques, media choices, and the sequence of particular activities. The COTA made numerous suggestions and provided specific recommendations on environmental modifications and adaptive equipment which would improve Jeff's level of functioning. The initial Individualized Therapy Plan (ITP) established for Jeff is reproduced in Figure 11-2.

The parents were then contacted by the OTR so that the rationale for treatment could be discussed as well as the need for mutual coordination, particularly in the area of daily living skills intervention. Plans for future communication were also established.

The OTR shared the occupational therapy plan with Jeff's classroom teacher, and they exchanged ideas regarding how the OT goals might be mutually reinforced through the Individualized Education Plan (IEP). For instance, having Jeff crawl on his palms in moving about the classroom could provide additional exercise to promote proximal stability. It was noted that several children in Jeff's class shared a common fine motor goal so activities were coordinated with the special education teacher to establish a fine motor group within the classroom.

The COTA forwarded a copy of the occupational therapy evaluation to the physician together with a request for a prescription for treatment. Once the prescription was received, the assistant was responsible for monitoring the prescription anniversary date so that a renewal could be secured if necessary. The COTA also made sure that copies of all current and subsequent evaluations and plans were forwarded to the central special education services office, the parents and the physician.

Treatment Implementation

The OTR and the COTA collaborated in implementing Jeff's treatment plan. Owing to the complexity of this child's clinical condition and the necessity for using certain neurodevelopmental modalities, the OTR assumed a primary treatment role. The following is a summary of the responsibilities assumed by the OTR/COTA team in relation to Jeff's specific objectives:

Objective 1: Increase stability of trunk, shoulders and hips. The OTR performed treatment in this area with the COTA assisting as needed. The COTA reinforced the treatment goal by correcting Jeff's positioning during school activities and advising his teachers and parents on appropriate positioning.

FIGURE 11-2. OT Individualized Treatment Plan

Annual Objectives	Programming and Assessment Procedures	Time Line	Progress to Date
Jeff will be able to: 1. Exhibit increased proximal stability at the hips, shoulders, and trunk across settings.	Provide weight bearing in a variety of positions—4-point, prone over the bolster. Promote weight bearing and inhibition through joint compression. Consult with classroom teacher to have her encourage weight bearing when possible.	School Year 1984-85	There is evidence that weight bearing is effective in decreasing extraneous movements; arm and hand flapping decreases after weight bearing on palms.
2. Demonstrate reliable righting and equilibrium responses when balance is challenged. 3. Demonstrate more coordinated, controlled fine motor skills, including the following: a. Maintain good sitting position. b. Demonstrate a finer prehension grasp on utensils (as opposed to lateral or shovel grasp). c. Perform bilateral activities. d. Practice voluntary release of objects.	Change positions from 4-point to kneel to side sit with facilitation at key points—shoulder girdle, hips. Use tilt board to challenge reactions. Have Jeff straddle bolster or lie prone lengthwise on bolster while tipping it. Have Jeff sit on therapist's lap, leaning side to side. Have Jeff participate in a fine motor group session once weekly, coplanned by OTR and classroom teacher. Complete a fine motor checklist to obtain baseline of functional ability. a. See Goal 6 and approaches. b. Provide functional activities, e,g, grooming tasks, hair/teeth brushing, dressing. c. Promote manual functioning—cutting paper with easy-grip scissors, zipping/unzipping, large bead stringing, opening wide-mouth jars. d. Practice release through bean bags, calls, cubes, peg board activities.	Fall 1984 and Spring 1985	He rolls in an uncoordinated way. When balance is challenged, Jeff's arms reach to the side and front. He is able to maintain a pivot prone position for several seconds. Checklist completed; will keep on practicing skills that Jeff has difficulty completing in a smooth, coordinated manner. Still uses a more lateral, shovel-type grasp, which is weak; has difficulty staying on task for multistep tasks. Will continue fine motor group one time weekly, and individual therapy two times/week.
4. Demonstrate lip closure and decrease drooling.	Provide oral facilitation 15 minutes before lunch every day. Use following techniques: inhibitory pressure-repeat 4-5 times; tongue pressure-broad handle of spoon-repeat 6 times; stretch pressure-quick stretch-3 times, upper and lower lip stretch from cheek to corner of mouth 3 times; sucking-suck on ice or popsicle-stretch pressure; straw drinking-tight fitting lid hole for straw.	School Year 1984-85	Jeff's active lip movements have increased slightly, but he still shows lack of active strong lip and cheek muscles in eating and drinking. Protrusion of tongue decreased slightly; not seeing good controlled sideward movements. Still exhibits some lip retraction when he is excited, but is able to close lips around spoon more consistently since facilitation techniques have been employed.

FIGURE 11-2. OT Individualized Treatment Plan (continued)

Annual Objectives	Programming and Assessment Procedures	Time Line	Progress to Date
5. Maintain a clean mouth at meals.	Provide verbal and sensory cues to remind when food is on mouth, so he will use napkin.		With verbal cues, Jeff will reach out, pick up napkin, and wipe face, but is not always consistent with this.
6. Assume an erect sitting posture with head up, chin tucked, and feet stabilized, for self-feeding and fine motor skills.	Consult with classroom teacher to choose chairs which will allow Jeff to maintain both feet on the ground or supply foot rest. Construct a portable foot rest to attach to lunchroom bench where Jeff eats, promoting more stability in sitting.		Jeff can assume correct position 75% of time during eating, with verbal reminders.
7. Demonstrate independent dressing skills. a. Practice a finer prehension grasp. b. Decrease the amount of assistance needed with fasteners.	Provide pre-dressing activities: buttons through plastic lids, peg board activities and such, to practice skills necessary for fasteners—*e.g.,* zipping, unzipping, buttons, snaps, untying shoes, practice taking on or off pull-over shirts, putting on shoes and socks.		Jeff has progressed in speed of putting on shirt and jacket and most other undressing skills; still needs minimal assistance in fasteners.

Objective 2: Develop reliable righting and equilibrium responses. Neurodevelopmental treatment was provided by the OTR on a one-to-one basis. Occasionally the COTA would assist when two people were needed to perform a particular technique. The assistant also reported relevent observations of Jeff's daily functioning.

Objective 3: Increase fine motor skills. A weekly fine motor group was planned collaboratively with the classroom teacher and conducted by the OTR and the COTA. The occupational therapy assistant also worked with Jeff individually twice a week, emphasizing the practice of bilateral self-care or academic related activities such as manipulating buttons, crayons, scissors, and related items.

Objective 4: Increase lip closure and decrease drooling during eating.

Objective 5: Maintain a clean mouth at meals. The OTR designed a feeding facilitation program, and she and the COTA alternated in performing neuromuscular facilitation of oral musculature prior to Jeff's lunch. The COTA supervised Jeff and other children with similar problems for positioning and self-feeding in the lunchroom.

Objective 6: Assume correct posture to improve arm and hand use. Jeff was instructed in the use of abdominal muscles and correct positioning by the OTR. The COTA monitored Jeff's posture in different school situations, giving him verbal reminders as necessary. The assistant also constructed two footrests of appropriate heights so that Jeff could sit more securely on regular classroom and lunchroom furniture.

Objective 7: Increase dressing independence. The COTA practiced dressing related skills with Jeff in therapy sessions twice weekly and provided adaptive equipment and clothing modifications as needed. Jeff's level of function was periodically reassessed by the assistant using the Dressing Skills Checklist. The COTA was also responsible for informing the family and classroom aides about the type and amount of assistance to offer Jeff in dressing and self-care.

Coordination of Jeff's home reinforcement program with the family was handled by the COTA. This involved teaching proper positioning, adaptive procedures, and adaptive equipment use.

The COTA frequently advises regular classroom teachers who may have little background in working with handicapped students. For instance, Jeff's physical education teacher tended to have him "sit out" during most class activities. Follow-

FIGURE 11-3. OTR/COTA Working Relationship

I. RESPONSIBILITIES OF OTR SUPERVISOR. The OTR supervisor is responsible for the development and utilization of staff in assuring quality and cost efficiency of OT services. The OTR supervises receipt of referrals, exercises professional judgment in delegating tasks to appropriate OT personnel, and oversees task performance in accord with accepted standards of professional practice.

II. STYLE OF SUPERVISION. To foster staff member growth and motivation, a collaborative style of supervision is developed, which involves technical personnel in sharing responsibility and decision-making regarding tasks they have been delegated.

III. ROLES OF OTR/COTA TEAM MEMBERS.

Independent Living/Daily Living Skills Intervention	Performance Component Intervention
Programs aimed at promoting health or adapting/teaching everyday living skills: 1. Physical daily living skills: Grooming and hygiene, feeding/eating, dressing, functional mobility, functional communication, and object manipulation 2. Psychological/emotional daily living skills: Self-concept/identity, situational coping, and community involvement 3. Work: Homemaking, child care/parenting, academics, employment preparation, and volunteer service 4. Play/leisure	Programs aimed at treating dysfunction—maintaining, developing or restoring the specific elements that underlie and permit performance of everyday activities: 1. Sensorimotor skills/performance components 2. Cognitive skills/performance components 3. Psychosocial skills/performance components
OTR or COTA with General Supervision	OTR or COTA with General or Close Supervision
COTA ROLE: OTRs and COTAs may work similarly in assessment, planning, and implementation of such programs	COTA ROLE: COTAs may perform assigned assessment, planning, and treatment tasks OTR's considerations of: 1. Condition of patient/client 2. Proficiencies of the COTA supervisee 3. Complexity of evaluation or therapy modality 4. Standards of government and regulatory agencies 5. Practice standards and guidelines of OT profession 6. Requirements of third party reimbursers

ing consultation with the OTR, the COTA met with the teacher to clarify Jeff's performance abilities and realistic precautions and made recommendations regarding ways the student could be included in regular gym activities.

Throughout the treatment program, the COTA shared observations, questions and suggestions with the supervising therapist. He maintained his own anecdotal notes on students receiving treatment and discussed them with the OTR in preparation for the spring ITP updates.

Summary

The certified occupational therapy assistant makes many valued contributions to Related Services and the delivery of occupational therapy services in a school setting. Employment of a COTA provides the additional manpower to extend OT services, thereby offering the benefits of more therapy time per child. A full-time, on-site assistant can greatly aid the therapist by maintaining communication with Related Services, teachers, and families, thus promoting continuity of care and facilitating mainstreaming. The COTA assures that Related Services and occupational therapy approaches are reinforced throughout the school day, so that functional gains made in therapy are better integrated into the students' daily routine of activities. Other areas of responsibility include maintaining the therapy room, ordering supplies and equipment, and supervising occupational therapy assistant students on field work assignment.

Figure 11-3 outlines the general roles and areas of mutual collaboration by the occupational therapy intraprofessional team members.[3]

References

1. Education for All Handicapped Children Act, 1975, P.L. 94-142. *Federal Register*, Tuesday, Aug. 23, 1977, sec. 601.

2. Gilfoyle EM: *Training: Occupational Therapy Educational Management in Schools*, Volume 2. Rockville, MD: American Occupational Therapy Association, Inc., 1980.

3. Practice Statement: COTA Supervision. Wisconsin Occupational Therapy Association, 1980.

Bibliography

Batshaw M, Perret Y: *Children with Handicaps: A Medical Primer*. Baltimore, MD: Paul H. Brookes, 1981.

Cerebral Palsy. Rockville, MD: Practice Division, American Occupational Therapy Association, Inc., 1983.

Colby IL: *Pediatric Assessment of Self-Care Activities*. St. Louis: C.V. Mosby, 1978.

Erhardt R: *Developmental Hand Dysfunction*. Laurel, MD: Ramsco, 1982.

Feeding and Dressing Techniques for the Cerebral Palsied. Chicago: National Society for Crippled Children and Adults.

Finnie N: *Handling the Young Cerebral Palsied Child at Home*, 2nd Edition. New York: EP Dutton, 1975.

Gilfoyle EM: *Training: Occupational Therapy Educational Management in Schools*. OSERS Grant G007801499. Rockville, MD: American Occupational Therapy Association, Inc., 1980.

Healy H, Stainback SB: *The Severely Motorically Impaired Student*. Springfield, IL: Charles C Thomas, 1980.

Howison M: Occupational therapy with children—cerebral palsy. In Hopkins H, Smith H, Eds: *Willard and Spackman's Occupational Therapy*, 6th Edition. Philadelphia: JB Lippincott, 1983.

Levitt S: *Treatment of Cerebral Palsy and Motor Delay*. Philadelphia: JB Lippincott, 1977.

Smith J: *Play Environments for Movement Experience*. Springfield, IL: Charles C Thomas, 1980.

Stainback SB, Healy HA: *Teaching Eating Skills, A Handbook for Teachers*. Springfield, IL: Charles C Thomas, 1982.

CHAPTER 12

The Mentally Retarded Child

Susan M. McFadden, OTR

Introduction

This chapter presents a case study of a mentally retarded child enrolled in a Head Start program who received occupational therapy services through a private practice. The case study illustrates a hypothetical example of one model of a collaborative relationship between a certified occupational therapy assistant and a registered occupational therapist. To better visualize the child and his situation, a brief description of the private practice and the Head Start program follows.

The Private Practice

In selecting a COTA for a private practice position, several factors must be considered. As with an OTR, private practice is not recommended for the new graduate. Since a private practice is a unique model for a collaborative COTA and OTR relationship, the COTA should have several years of experience, demonstrate maturity and independence, and have the ability to be self-directed prior to entering into such a model. Supervision of a COTA by an OTR in a private practice situation is often minimal. Circumstances generally do not allow for much direct observation of the assistant, and supervision cannot be conducted on a daily basis. Because of this indirect nature of supervision, good verbal and written communication skills are necessary for all involved in such a collaborative relationship. A private practice established by the author several years ago received contracts with a nursing home, a long-term care state psychiatric facility, a state institution for the retarded, and a private institution for the adult retarded. The occupational therapy services provided to these facilities included direct patient services of screening, evaluation, and program planning as well as indirect services, which included teaching aides or technicians, general inservice training, and program planning. Since the private practice was established, more and more facilities, including a Head Start program, have requested services from the occupational therapist. It became necessary to sub-contract with other occupational therapy personnel on a part-time basis owing to increasing needs for services.

FIGURE 12-1. Developmental Pre-Dressing Checklist*

Name: ______________________ Date: ____________

Approximate Age	Skill	Achieved Independently	Achieved with Help	Not Achieved
One year	Cooperates in dressing			
	Holds foot up for shoe			
	Holds arm out for sleeve			
	Puts hat on head and takes it off			
	Likes to pull shoes off			
	Pushes arms through sleeves and legs through pants			
	Removes socks			
Two years	Removes unfastened garment (coat)			
	Purposely removes shoes if laces are untied			
	Helps push down garment			
	Finds armholes in T-shirt			
Two and one-half years	Removes pull-down garment with elastic waist			
	Tries to put on socks			
	Puts on front-button type of coat, shirt, or sweater			
	Unbuttons one large button			
Three years	Puts on T-shirt, needing some assistance			
	Puts on shoes without fasteners (may be wrong foot)			
	Puts on socks with some difficulty turning heel			
	Independent with pull-down garment			

From Dunn, M. L.: Pre-Dressing Skills: Skill Starters for Self-Help Development. Tucsan, Communication Skill Builders, 1983.

Project Head Start

Project Head Start was launched in 1965 as a federally funded preschool summer program, part of the antipoverty campaign of the Johnson administration. The program is now administered by the Head Start Bureau, Office of Human Development Services, U.S. Department of Health and Human Services, and has expanded to a year-round service. Head Start was conceived as a child development program to provide comprehensive educational, social, and health services to preschool children of low income families. As a matter of policy, handicapped children have always been included in the program. Head Start began as an entirely center-based program, with children transported to a particular center to receive services. Home-based programming, with home visitation and some services provided in the home, was introduced in 1972. While there are federal guidelines which all Head Start programs must follow, individual programs vary widely regarding the services provided, staff utilized, and screening tools administered. Since Head Start programs cannot assume total responsibility for the hiring of full time staff for the many services needed,

FIGURE 12-2. Pretest of Dressing Skills Data Sheet*

Child's name: Date: Pretest of dressing skills	Independent	Verbal assistance	Physical assistance	Description of method child uses to complete the task
Undressing trousers, skirt 1. Pushes garment from waist to ankles 2. Pushes garment off one leg 3. Pushes garment off other leg				
Dressing trousers, skirt 1. Lays trousers in front of self with front side up 2. Inserts one foot into waist opening 3. Inserts other foot into waist opening 4. Pulls garment up to waist				
Undressing socks 1. Pushes sock down off heel 2. Pulls toe of sock, pulling sock off foot				
Dressing socks 1. Positions sock correctly with heel side down 2. Holds sock open at top 3. Inserts toes into sock 4. Pulls sock over heel 5. Pulls sock up				
Undressing cardigan 1. Takes dominant arm out of sleeve 2. Gets coat off back 3. Pulls other arm from sleeve				
Dressing cardigan flip-over method 1. Lays garment on table or floor in front of self 2. Gets dominant arm into sleeve 3. Other arm into sleeve 4. Positions coat on back				
Undressing polo shirt 1. Takes dominant arm out of sleeve 2. Pulls garment over head 3. Pulls other arm from sleeve				
Dressing polo shirt 1. Lays garment in front of self 2. Opens bottom of garment and puts arms into sleeves 3. Pulls garment over head 4. Pulls garment down to waist				
Undressing shoes 1. Loosens laces 2. Pulls shoe off heel 3. Pulls front of shoe to pull shoe off toes				
Dressing shoes 1. Prepares shoe by loosening laces and pulling tongue of shoe out of the way 2. Inserts toes into shoe 3. Pushes shoe on over heel				

*From Copeland, M., Ford, L., and Soloes, N.: Occupational Therapy for Mentally Retarded children. Baltimore, University Park Press, 1976.

they contract with other agencies to provide some services, such as occupational therapy. The child described in this case study was enrolled in a resource center program one day a week, and received home-based programming one day a week.

Referral

At the time of enrollment in the Head Start program Jason was three years old, the only boy and the second child in a family of three children. His sisters were six years and one year; the mother was a housewife with an eighth grade education. The father was unemployed, doing "fix-it" type work for individuals when possible, and also had an eighth grade education. Jason's family lived in a rural area, approximately 100 miles from a major city. The family income was estimated at $4,200 per year. Jason's parents reported that he had no major health problems, but they sensed that something was different about Jason when compared to his sisters.

As a part of its services, Head Start identifies families in need so that problems can be detected at an early age and services provided to help the children and families overcome adversities. Jason's sister came to the attention of Head Start when she was three years old, and the family was then enrolled in the Head Start program. Since the family had already been identified by the program, a screening process was initiated with Jason when he was three years old. The results of this screening indicated that Jason was significantly delayed in the areas of fine motor development, cognitive-verbal development, and gross motor development. The activities that Jason was not able to do when screened included: building a tower of seven blocks, buttoning one button, stringing four beads in two minutes, naming eight out of eleven pictures, repeating two-digit sequences of numbers, balancing on one foot for two seconds, walking on tiptoes when shown, and walking up stairs using alternating feet. The screening test used with Jason at 36 months indicated that he was functioning below 30 months of age, the lowest level of the screening tool. Because of the delay in fine motor, cognitive-verbal, and gross motor areas, a psychological evaluation was recommended for Jason and he was enrolled in a home-based Head Start program. The psychological evaluation revealed that Jason was moderately mentally retarded. The psychological examiner believed that an occupational therapy evaluation was necessary because Jason was not performing self-help skills appropriate to his mental age.

Assessment

Jason was evaluated by the OTR at the Head Start resource center. At the time of scheduling, Jason had just turned four. The occupational therapist's evaluation indicated that his reflex maturation was appropriate for his age, with no primitive reflexes present; his range of motion, strength, and muscle tone were normal. Jason's sensory awareness appeared to be normal since he responded to pinprick and rough and soft surfaces on his extremities.

As a part of the occupational therapy assessment, the Developmental Test of Visual Motor Integration by Berry and Buketnica was administered to Jason. On this design copying test, the child received a score of two years, eleven months. This score was within the range for a four-year-old, moderately retarded person. In explaining expectations to the parents as well as the COTA, they were reminded that moderately retarded children develop at about half the rate of nonhandicapped children. Therefore, Jason, a moderately mentally retarded child of four years of age, was developmentally similar to nonhandicapped children who are two years old.

Using the Gessell Developmental Scales as a guide, the OTR determined that Jason was able to perform most fine motor tasks for two-year-olds; however, the mother indicated that Jason was having difficulty undressing, dressing, and feeding himself. Since the home is a more natural environment, the COTA was assigned to visit the home and to assess Jason in these areas. The COTA gathered data on the activities of daily living skills of undressing, dressing, and eating by observing Jason perform these activities. Results were recorded on two different forms, which are shown in Figures 12-1 and 12-2. The combined use of these recommended forms included an approximate age level, as shown in the first, and a more detailed task analysis through use of the second.

A developmental type of checklist with age levels was not available for feeding; however, by using the information available in Copeland, Ford and Solon,[1] and the previously mentioned forms as a model, it was possible to gather similar information on eating skills.

To ensure that sufficient data were collected, the COTA made two home visits to observe Jason's performance of dressing, undressing, and feeding skills. The checklists previously described were used to record information observed on each visit. The assistant also noted the physical features of the home environment and assessed the parents' knowledge of Jason's developmental needs and their ability to manage his behavior.

Partial results of the COTA's assessment of Jason's dressing, undressing, and feeding skills are summarized in Figure 12-3.

An important aspect of the occupational therapy evaluation was determining Jason's need for occupational therapy services. Study of the COTA's observations, made it evident that Jason was not able to execute many of the skills expected for his mental age. The COTA's results showing that Jason was in fact functioning more like a one year old in dressing, undressing, and feeding were a key factor in determining the child's need for OT services. Also contributing to the recommendation for services was the COTA's impression that the parents did not understand that Jason should have been performing the dressing, undressing, and feeding skills equivalent to a two-year-old and performing other skills compatible with his mental age.

Program Planning

In collaboration with the OTR, the COTA developed a program to treat Jason in the home once a week. The therapist and the assistant agreed that approximately nine visits would be necessary for Jason to accomplish the following occupational therapy treatment objectives:

1 Remove an open front garment.
2 Put on an open front type garment.
3 Feed himself using a spoon with moderate spillage from the spoon.

An additional goal was to provide the Head Start resource teacher with information to assist Jason in meeting these objectives. After several home visits had been made, the COTA agreed to arrange for Jason's parents to visit the resource center. Involving the parents and the resource teacher in the program added to the day-to-day consistency and provided more opportunity for Jason to practice the skills in the occupational therapy program.

FIGURE 12-3. Dressing and Feeding Skills

Skills	Normal Developmental Age (Years)	Moderately Retarded Child (Years)	Jason
Removes socks	1	2	Yes
Likes to pull shoes off	1	2	Yes
Pushes arms through sleeves	1	2	Yes
Removes unfastened garment	1	4	No
Purposely removes shoes	2	4	No
Helps push down garment	2	4	No
Finds arm holes in T-shirt	2	4	No
Buttons large front buttons	3	6	No
Puts on shoes without fasteners	3	6	No
Independent with pull-down garment	3	6	No
Drinks well from cup	1.5	3	Yes
Handles glass with one hand	2	4	No
Moderate spillage from spoon	2	4	No
Likes to spear food with fork	3	6	No

Skill: Remove a Front-Button Shirt*

Objective:	Student will remove a front-button shirt.
Approximate Developmental Age:	Two years
Materials:	Use a front-button shirt, jacket, sweater, or pajama top that is too large or that fits loosely.
Note:	Start by unbuttoning or unzipping garment for student. Take same arm out first to help establish a routine.
Position:	Sitting or standing
Task Analysis:	Backward chaining. Trainer props student through entire process, leaving last part or parts for student to complete.

1. Student removes garment with one arm half-in.
2. Student removes garment with one arm in.
3. Student removes garment with one arm in and one half-in.
4. Student removes garment when pulled off shoulders.
5. Students removes garment.

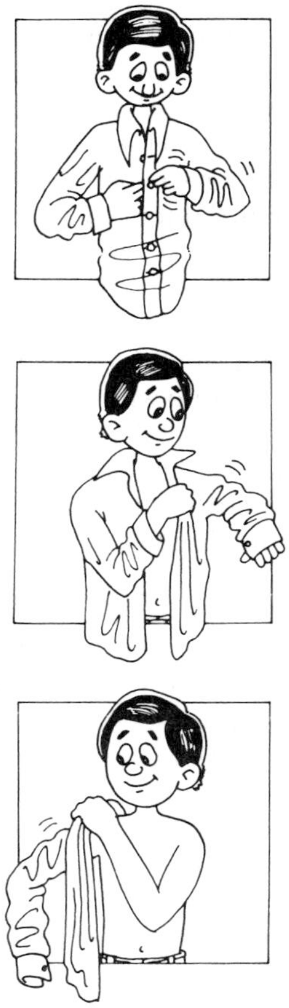

Figure 12-4.

From Dunn, M. L.: Pre-Dressing Skills: Skill Starters for Self-Help Development. Tucsan, Communication Skill Builders, 1983.

Treatment Implementation

Five of the nine occupational therapy treatments were directed toward attaining the undressing and dressing objectives. The COTA selected an initial activity of playing "dress up" using a variety of hats and shirts. The assistant had noticed Jason's interest in policemen and firemen and obtained their hats and shirts for Jason to use in practicing skills (Figure 12-4).

For an initial feeding activity, the COTA selected playing in the sand with a spoon to learn a scooping technique. The assistant noted that Jason was able to grasp the spoon while scooping and had adequate eye-hand coordination. The OTR concurred with the COTA's recommendation that a session of manual guidance in an actual meal setting was the next step in teaching Jason to feed himself. The COTA then requested that the mother prepare a meal for the next treatment session which

FIGURE 12-5. Feeding Task Analysis*

The student will feed himself with a spoon upon command after attaining five consecutive positive responses on each step of the task analysis below:

TASK ANALYSIS STEPS

The student will:

1. Let you use his hand to hold the spoon, scoop the spoon into the dish, lift the spoon to his mouth, and put the spoon in his mouth.
2. Put the spoon in his mouth from lip level after you have picked up the spoon using his hand, scooped it into the dish, lifted it to mouth level, and gestured for him to put it in his mouth.
3. Put the spoon in his mouth from lip level after you have picked up the spoon using his hand, scooped it into the dish, and lifted it to mouth level.
4. Put the spoon in his mouth from chin level after you have picked up the spoon using his hand, scooped it into the dish, lifted it to chin level, and gestured for him to put it in his mouth.
5. Put the spoon in his mouth from chin level after you have picked up the spoon with his hand, scooped it into the dish, and lifted it to chin level.
6. Put the spoon in his mouth from shoulder level after you have picked up the spoon using his hand, scooped it into the dish, lifted it to shoulder level, and gestured for him to put it in his mouth.
7. Put the spoon in his mouth from shoulder level after you have picked up the spoon using his hand, scooped it into the dish, and lifted it to shoulder level.
8. Put the spoon in his mouth after you have picked up the spoon using his hand, scooped it into the dish, lifted it above the dish, and gestured for him to put it in his mouth.
9. Put the spoon in his mouth after you have picked up the spoon using his hand, scooped it into the dish, and lifted it above the dish.
10. Put the spoon in his mouth after you have picked up the spoon using his hand, scooped it into the dish, and gestured for him to put it in his mouth.
11. Put the spoon in his mouth after you have picked up the spoon using his hand and scooped it into the dish.
12. Scoop into the dish and lift the spoon to his mouth after you have gestured for him to do so and after you have used his hand to pick up the spoon and put it into the bowl.
13. Scoop into the dish and lift the spoon to his mouth after you have used his hand to pick up the spoon and put it into the bowl.
14. Scoop into the dish and lift the spoon to his mouth after you have gestured for him to do so and after you have used his hand to pick up the spoon and take it to the dish.
15. Scoop into the dish and lift the spoon to his mouth after you have used his hand to pick up the spoon and take it to the dish.
16. Scoop into the dish after you have gestured for him to do so, and lift the spoon to his mouth after you have handed him the spoon.
17. Scoop into the dish and lift the spoon to his mouth after you have handed him the spoon.
18. Eat independently upon command.

*From Popovitch, D.: A Prescriptive Behavioral Checklist for the Severly and Profoundly Retarded. Austin, PRO-ED, Inc., 1981, Vol. II.

FIGURE 12-5. Feeding Task Analysis (continued)

IMPLEMENTATION

Materials

Spoon, bowl, mat to hold the bowl securely (built up handles or swivel spoon if needed)

Prerequisite Skills

The student must be able to grasp.

Procedure

A. Determine the student's reinforcement preference.

B. Be certain the student is seated properly with support provided if needed.

C. Determine the student's operant level.

This task is to be implemented during mealtime. For all three meals, serve food that can be eaten easily with a spoon (e.g., oatmeal, mashed potatoes, bite-size pieces of hamburger, thick stew, applesauce).

To determine the operant level, test on steps 3, 5, 7, 9, 11, 13, 15, 17, and 18. There will be a need for gradual fading between steps. When fading out your assistance in scooping, hold your student's hand with a looser and looser grip until you are barely guiding his hand through the scooping action. You will continue fading by putting your hand on his wrist and then his elbow, and guiding lightly as necessary.

The trainer should be standing behind the student during all steps. (All steps can be accomplished with the trainer sitting if standing is uncomfortable.)

Command: "(Student's name), eat."

would require Jason to use a spoon. During the meal, the COTA noticed that Jason had a good hand-to-mouth pattern as he attempted to eat using his fingers. The assistant provided manual guidance by placing her hand over Jason's hand as he filled the spoon and brought it toward his mouth. Whenever Jason attempted to use his fingers to feed himself, the COTA instructed him to use the spoon and followed this directive by guiding his hand toward the spoon. The assistant also pointed out to Jason's mother that she should tell Jason what to do instead of what not to do.

A detailed task analysis of the objective "student will feed himself with a spoon upon command after attaining five consecutive positive responses on each step" can be seen in Figure 12-5. This task analysis combines the use of manual guidance as indicated in the odd numbered steps and the use of gestures.

Jason's mother was present during all occupational therapy treatment sessions, and care was taken to ensure that the mother's questions were answered. The COTA concluded each session by asking the mother to continue modeling the demonstrated techniques during the coming week.

The COTA documented each weekly treatment session by noting the date, length of session, time of day, activities presented, and Jason's response to the activities. The assistant then discussed the results of each occupational therapy treatment session with the OTR and described the activities planned for the next week.

Program Discontinuation

Jason's progress toward meeting his occupational therapy objectives proceeded as had been anticipated. After nine sessions in the home and one visit to the resource center Jason had achieved all of the occupational therapy objectives. The OTR and the COTA discussed Jason's achievements and agreed that the occupational therapy program should be discontinued. In a final home visit, the assistant reviewed Jason's progress during the treatments with both parents. She explained developmental expectations in undressing, dressing, and feeding for Jason, and enumerated activities that the parents should continue to ensure Jason's maintenance of his newly learned skills.

Final notes were made regarding Jason's treatment's, and all progress notes were signed and turned over to the OTR. The therapist then informed the Head Start program of Jason's progress, skill achievement, and discontinuance of occupational therapy services. The OTR also forwarded the necessary documentation to the Head Start resource center.

While the role of the COTA in this case was hypothetical, the case itself was based on an actual experience and represents one example of how an experienced assistant can work in an advanced level of practice in a collaborative relationship with an OTR. It should be noted that in at least one state (as this text is being written), state law prohibits COTAs from practicing in a home setting without on-site supervision from a registered occupational therapist. It is understood that efforts are being made to change this supervisory regulation.

Reference

1. Copland M, Ford L, Solon N: *Occupational Therapy for Mentally Retarded Children*. Baltimore: University Park Press, 1976.

Bibliography

Clark PN, Allen AS: *Occupational Therapy for Children*. St. Louis: C.V. Mosby, 1985.

Dunn ML: *Pre-Dressing Skills*. Tucson, AZ: Communication Skill Builders, 1983.

Lederman EF: *Occupational Therapy in Mental Retardation*. Springfield, IL: Charles C Thomas, 1984.

Popovich D: *A Prescriptive Behavioral Checklist for the Severely and Profoundly Retarded*. Volume II. Austin, PRO-ED, Inc., 1981.

CHAPTER 13

The Depressed Adolescent

Linda Florey, OTR

Introduction

Ann, a short, attractive 15-year-old female, was admitted to the adolescent inpatient service with the diagnosis of post-traumatic stress disorder with depressed and anxious affect. Ann was born in Oklahoma, and shortly after her birth her mother and father separated. Her mother moved to Los Angeles and left Ann and her two older siblings, ages 3 years and 5 years, in the care of her father. Ann's father died when she was 4 years old, and from age 4 years to 7 years she and her older brothers were cared for by her paternal aunt and uncle. During this period, Ann's mother kept in contact with her family and brought Ann to live with her and her new husband and stepson when friends suspected that Ann had been sexually abused by her uncle.

At 10 years of age, Ann's 14-year-old stepbrother began to sexually abuse her. She became pregnant by him when she was 13 years old. Her mother assumed that Ann was "getting fat" and did not learn of her pregnancy until she took her to a doctor for a respiratory infection. Ann was afraid to tell her mother how she became pregnant as she feared her stepbrother might hurt her.

When Ann was 7 months pregnant, police were called by neighbors to stop a family argument. The police questioned Ann about her pregnancy, and she admitted to them that her stepbrother had abused her for several years. The stepbrother was arrested and convicted and began serving his sentence in jail. The Department of Public Social Services recommended that Ann attend a support group for victims of incest at a psychiatric facility.

Ann's baby was put up for adoption, and she continued to live with her mother and stepfather. Tension in the home became unbearable for Ann. Her stepfather continually blamed her for causing his son to be in jail and this led to several fights with Ann's mother. During a support group session, Ann said she was planning to kill herself and was then referred to the adolescent psychiatric inpatient service.

Assessment

As part of the interdisciplinary treatment plan, Ann was scheduled for an occupational therapy assessment. A screening process to determine the need for occupational therapy services was not performed. It is an expectation of the facility that all patients receive an assessment in order to determine the focus and frequency of occupational therapy intervention. The assessment is documented in the chart within the first 10 days of admission. This is referred to as the initial occupational therapy assessment. An additional evaluation may be done at a later time to probe deficit areas identified in the initial assessment.

The certified occupational therapy assistant reviewed the medical chart and reported the history to the occupational therapist as described in the introduction section. The first step in the assessment process was for both the COTA and OTR to meet briefly with Ann in order to explain occupational therapy services, prepare her for the evaluation process, and gain an impression of her willingness and ability to participate in the evaluation process. Because of Ann's ability to maintain eye contact, listen to information, and ask questions, the occupational therapy team determined that although the patient was shy, she was receptive to the evaluation process.

Initial Evaluation and Findings

The initial evaluation served as an indicator of level of function with respect to interests, time management, task performance, socialization, and vocational interests. Ann participated in five evaluations. The specific evaluation, its format, purpose, the responsible occupational therapy personnel, and findings follow.

Evaluation	Format	Purpose	Staff
"Typical Day Interview"	Semistructured interview	To determine patterns of daily living, school, leisure activities, chores, and time management	OTR

Findings: Ann spent most of her prehospital days in school. She devoted other time to self-care activities, chores, and homework. She was responsible for assisting with meal preparation and clean-up and household chores in addition to caring for her room. She spent a little time in the evenings reading or watching television. She reported that she had no close friends, but occasionally she would walk to and from school with a classmate. She did not engage in any hobbies or special interests. Ann said that she had never had any hobbies as she was "too busy with homework."

Evaluation	Format	Purpose	Staff
NPI Interest Checklist[1]	Structured checklist	To determine ability to discriminate interests, to identify clusters of interest	COTA

Findings: Ann was able to discriminate strengths of interests. Her strong interests were in the category of activities of daily living (e.g., sewing, housekeeping, cooking). Her secondary interests were in the category of social recreation. Her least preferred interests were in the area of culture and education.

Evaluation	Format	Purpose	Staff
Task performance using Westphal Decision Making Inventory[2]	Structured checklist	To determine decision making, problem solving ability, attention span	COTA

Findings: Initially Ann was unable to decide on a project and was given several suggestions. She then selected a simple structured task which required minimal problem solving. She required one-step verbal instructions with demonstration. She was able to recognize problems but initially required assistance in order to implement problem solving. She attended to her project for the full 50-minute session, completed it and verbalized enjoyment and satisfaction with the quality of her completed work. She stated that she wanted to learn how to do more "things" in future sessions.

Evaluation	Format	Purpose	Staff
Observation of socialization on unit, in OT workshop, in OT cooking group using observation guide	Semistructured guide	To determine frequency and content of interactions with peers and adults	OTR and COTA

Findings: In the occupational therapy workshop and on the unit, Ann sat with the group, watched what occurred but did not initiate conversation with peers. She approached staff when she had a question, such as "When do I have school?" When approached by peers and staff, she responded with short sentences.

Ann was observed in a cooking group with two peers that was conducted in a small kitchen adjacent to the workshop area. Ann listened to the conversation of her peers, occasionally laughed, responded to questions, but did not initiate any comments. When she was asked to measure some ingredient, she approached the COTA, asking, "What is one-third of a cup?" She said that she had never used a measuring cup, and she didn't know how to use one.

Evaluation	Format	Purpose	Staff
Adolescent Role Assessment[3]	Semistructured interview	To determine strengths/deficiencies in occupational choice process	OTR

Findings: The majority of Ann's scores indicated marginal behavior but no obvious student role dysfunction. She reported that she liked school but that her grades had dropped from B's to D's because she hadn't been able to concentrate for the past several months. She was enrolled in the tenth grade. Her favorite subject was typing. Ann said that she wished to finish high school and thought she might be a typist. She stated, "That's what my mom wants me to be." She also said that she had once thought that she wanted to be a policewoman or a model but now thought these ideas were "silly" because she wasn't strong enough to become a policewoman or pretty enough to be a model. Ann indicated that she had done some baby sitting but had never had any other work experience outside the home environment.

Summary of Assets and Deficits

With the findings of the initial evaluation, the OTR summarized Ann's assets and deficits as follows:

Assets:

Pleasant and cooperative.

Good attention span.

Eager to learn.

Learns quickly from verbal and demonstrated instructions.

Discriminates interests.

Deficits:

Difficulty initiating interaction with peers.

No reported friendships.

No diversified interests or hobbies.

Difficulty with measurement concepts in cooking.

Delayed occupational choice process.

Program Planning

Program planning for individual patients is done within the context of the existing occupational therapy program. The program is broadly designed to promote goals for most adolescent patients while addressing individual patient needs. The setting of treatment goals and the analysis, selection, and sequencing of activities to meet the goals are guided by two main dynamics: simple to complex and dependence to independence. Goals and activities are thought of as a continuum in which tasks and situations are paced to encourage increasing levels of difficulty and responsibility. Initial goals guide treatment intervention. They are usually broad in scope and become more focused in reaction to the patient's response to treatment.

Program planning is also done within the context of the interdisciplinary team. The members of different disciplines discuss the findings of their evaluations and goals of intervention and determine overall patient goals, anticipated length of hospitalization, and anticipated plans for discharge.

Ann's anticipated length of stay was three months. Depending on her family's response to family therapy, Ann would either return to her home or be placed outside of the home.

Short- and long-term goals for Ann as well as time frames were formulated by the OTR. The methods of intervention were formulated jointly by the OTR and the COTA as follows:

Short-Term Goals	Time Frame:
1. Initiate peer interaction in structured groups	3 weeks
2. Increase repertoire of interests	2 weeks
3. Select projects independently	4 weeks
4. Increase complexity of task skills	2 weeks
5. Increase measurement skills	3 weeks

Intervention

Ann was scheduled for the occupational therapy craft workshop with five peers three times weekly to increase interest and task skills, and independent selection of projects. The COTA was responsible for working with Ann to increase the complexity of task skills within her selected projects (e.g., moving from simple one-step projects to long-term projects requiring multiple steps). If Ann did not select a project independently, the

COTA would provide her with choices. The COTA would also engage Ann in simple conversation.

Ann was scheduled to attend the adolescent cooking group with three peers once weekly to increase her peer interaction, measurement skills, and skills in meal preparation. Once Ann initiated conversation with her peers, she would be placed in a social skills group with an increased focus on social interaction.

Long-Term Goals:	Time Frame:
1. Initiate peer interaction spontaneously	By the end of hospitalization
2. Increase awareness of interests and capacities and relate them to occupational choice	6 weeks and throughout hospitalization
3. Incorporate interest areas into leisure time on ward	1 month and throughout hospitalization

After Ann had begun to independently select and execute projects based on her interests, she would be placed in an occupational exploration group to discuss the occupational choice process and to learn job-related skills such as filling out an application for employment. After Ann had demonstrated ability to work independently at various levels of task complexity, she would be encouraged to bring projects to the ward to do in her spare time.

Treatment Implementation

Throughout her hospitalization, Ann was involved in the occupational therapy craft workshop and an adolescent cooking group. She was also part of a social skills group and an occupational exploration group for limited time periods. The occupational exploration group was conducted by the occupational therapist. The cooking group was led by the assistant, and the craft workshop and the social skill group were conducted by the OTR and the COTA. Ann's progress in the craft workshop and the cooking group is reviewed as these groups reflect the working relationship between the therapist and the assistant.

Craft Workshop

Ann was involved in the craft workshop three times a week with five other peers. In the first session, the COTA gave Ann an introduction to the workshop, explaining the type of project that could be selected. Initially Ann was unable to select a project. She seemed overwhelmed with the choices available, and uncertain of her capacities. She said "too many things" and "I've never done this." The COTA assured Ann that she would teach her and help her with whatever project she selected. She then presented Ann with three projects based on her strong interests.

Ann selected a simple three-step sewing project and learned quickly. In other sessions, the COTA suggested more complex projects, each of which built upon skills Ann had just acquired. Ann continued to learn quickly and began to work independently. Throughout the initial sessions, Ann was encouraged to sit next to her peers, and both the OTR and the COTA would initiate conversations revolving around the projects, different individual interests, and ward activities. When she encountered a problem, she was encouraged to ask for suggestions from her peers if they were familiar with the steps.

In subsequent sessions, Ann exhibited an increased interest in her peers and in the various projects on which they were working. She began to initiate contact and conversation spontaneously and to select projects independently. She continued to learn quickly and work carefully. Ann also asked to bring projects to the unit. This overall pattern continued throughout her hospitalization. Ann's interests, complexity of skills, independence, and social spontaneity increased. She seemed aware of her own capacities and was able to take risks in new learning situations. Her "I've never done this" set was replaced by an "I'll try it" set.

The occupational therapist was responsible for developing and monitoring the treatment plans for all of the patients in the group and was primarily responsible for implementing the plan with two patients in the group, one of whom was Ann. In this group the COTA and the OTR worked side by side and served to validate one another's observations of patient's response to treatment.

Cooking Group

Ann was involved in a lunch-time cooking group with three to four peers throughout her hospitalization. All members within the group were responsible for planning the menu and participating in meal preparation. On a rotating basis, one member of the group was responsible for the overall coordination of tasks.

Cooking was another of Ann's strong interest areas and one in which she had engaged at home. This combination of interest and skill in a smaller group may have made Ann more confident in this situation. In the third session she began initiating conversation and joking with her peers while engaging in a goal oriented activity. Ann's initial problems in using measuring cups decreased with specific teaching and practice. No problems with other measurements, as with a ruler, were noted in other areas.

During the third month of hospitalization, Ann became "bossy" with her peers and angry with them if something wasn't done the way she wanted it done. For example, Ann told one group member to "cut the onions smaller." Her peer responded by grating the onion into miniscule pieces. Ann responded, "You never do anything right," in an angry manner. After such an interaction, the COTA arranged time later in the day to talk to Ann to explore reasons for her behavior. In most instances Ann was usually angry at another peer for something that had happened outside of the cooking group. The COTA encouraged Ann to express her feelings in the context in which they occurred.

The cooking group was a positive experience for Ann. She enjoyed the group and continued to socialize spontaneously with peers and staff members invited to the group. She also began to assume a leadership role on the unit in the area of cooking. Ann took responsibility for baking birthday cakes and making evening snacks. Her skills and confidence in this area generalized to her daily ward routine.

The COTA was responsible for conducting the cooking group. The format of this group is more structured than the craft group in that it is focused on meal planning and preparation. The OTR and the COTA in consultation with the other members of the treatment team selected the patients for the group on the basis of their need to socialize, work cooperatively, increase independence and skill level or a combination thereof. Following each session, the COTA discussed the performance of the patients with the OTR. It was during these meetings that strategies were developed to deal with Ann's anger.

Program Discontinuation

Ann was hospitalized for a period of four months and was discharged to a group home for adolescent girls. One month prior to discharge, the OTR and the COTA began meeting with Ann to help her formulate plans for entering the home. Before her visit to the home was scheduled, they helped Ann formulate questions to ask about life in the home in order that she could enter the situation with as much information as possible. They involved Ann in a role play meeting with the housemother in which she asked questions about general living arrangements, proximity to public transportation, school and community resources, as well as the daily routine, responsibilities, and leisure time activities in the home. They also role played approaches for entering a new peer group.

Ann was excited when she returned from her visit. She said that the housemother and the six girls who lived at the home were "nice" and "friendly." She would have some chores to do, one of which was to help in meal preparation for dinner. She said, "It will be almost like the cooking group, and I love cooking." She also stated that her mother could visit her whenever she wished. The housemother had told her that all of the girls had privileges at the YWCA, which was located five blocks from the home. Ann noted that the YWCA had a swimming pool but no craft workshop. She felt, however, that she could buy some supplies for projects if she saved money from the allowance she would be getting.

All staff members who had worked with Ann were encouraged by her positive reaction to her new living situation. It was felt that she had benefited from the hospitalization. Ann and her mother had developed a good relationship and Ann's perception of herself had changed markedly. She no longer felt that she was at the "mercy" of the wishes and desires of others with no option on life but that she now had skills, abilities, and choices ahead of her.

References

1. Matsutsuyu J: The interest checklist. *Am J Occup Ther* 23:323-328, 1969.
2. Westphal M: A Study of Decision Making. Unpublished master's thesis, University of Southern California, 1967.
3. Black M: Adolescent role assessment. *Am J Occup Ther* 30:73-79, 1976.

CHAPTER 14

The Chemically Dependent Adolescent

Major Denise A. Rotert, OTR
Captain Frank E. Gainer, III, OTR

Introduction

Dependence on chemicals/substances to relieve pain, get "high," or reduce the effects of stress existed for as long as man. The medical profession identifies alcohol dependence (alcoholism), drug dependence, and cross addiction (addiction to a variety of chemical substances) as a disease. The disease is chronic, progressive and fatal, but can be halted through abstinence from abused substances.

The third edition of *The Diagnostic and Statistical Manual of Mental Disorders*, also referred to as DSM III, distinguishes between abuse and dependence on substances, whether alcohol, narcotics, or marijuana. Alcohol and drug abuse is defined as use in such a manner as to cause a substance-related disability. A substance-related disability is an impairment in social or occupational functioning due to a problematic pattern of use at least one month in duration. Dependence or addiction, however, adds significant tolerance or withdrawal to the substance-related disability. In most instances, tolerance is associated with experiencing blackouts, and withdrawal is associated with a rising level of symptoms from restlessness and shaking to hallucinations and delirium tremens (the DTs).

No other disease generates such an intensity of emotions and is so misunderstood as substance abuse. Biases toward the substance abuser include viewing him or her as an individual who lacks willpower, one who enjoys the situation and does not want to change, or as an individual who is antisocial and cannot be treated.

Adolescence is a time of change and turmoil. The adolescent undergoes a significant change in physical development. Rapid growth, poor posture, and physical and social awkwardness occur. The two primary developmental tasks of the age are achievement of independence and establishment of identity. Achievement of independence is characterized by conflicts with authority figures which develop as the adolescent struggles with emancipation from parents. Establishment of identity is characterized by a search for definition of one's own values. Peers become a primary support system as well as a basis for identity in that dress, actions, and behaviors are all associated with the peer group. Peer pressure becomes a more significant force than family relationships. The adolescent has feelings of ambivalence and frequently will test both limits and capabilities.

Drugs or alcohol can be used by adolescents to help overcome inadequate feelings, feel a part of the peer group, and get good feelings when "high." Typically, the adolescent withdraws from age appropriate activities because the heavy substance use interferes with the acquisition of skills and task achievement related to performance in general. When adolescents attempt to abstain, they often find themselves lagging behind peers in social, academic, and athletic skills. Difficulty in concentrating, recalling information, and interacting with others is made worse by the anxiety related to falling behind peers in achievement levels. Adolescents choose a "negative identity" because it is so difficult to fit in with their contemporaries who have developed competence in age related skills.

History has shown that it is not possible to separate drug and alcohol problems in adolescents. Evaluation of substance abusers illustrates the ease with which one drug may be substituted for another drug when the drug of choice is not available. Generally, once a problem with alcohol or another drug arises, there is an increased vulnerability to substance abuse problems of all kinds.

Case Background

Tom, a 17-year-old male, was admitted to the adolescent unit of a drug and alcohol recovery program. The precipitating events which led to his admission were his repetitive tardiness from school, being suspended twice for fighting and smoking marijuana, and decreased academic performance. In addition, he had been charged with driving while intoxicated (DWI) approximately four months prior to admission. When the school authorities confronted him with these incidents, Tom admitted to drinking and smoking marijuana heavily and feeling out of control. He requested help in dealing with his problems.

During an intake assessment for the program, Tom and his parents were interviewed. The following information was gathered: Tom was the oldest of three children and had a younger brother and sister. He lived in a small city and his family was middle class. His parents separated a year ago but had not divorced. The children lived with their mother but saw their father regularly. Tom's mother was a licensed practical nurse who worked full time on rotating shifts in a local hospital. His father was an alcoholic but had been abstinent for the past nine months. Tom reported that his mother was the disciplinarian in the family, and that "they got along fine." In addition, he stated that he and his father got along but had had difficulties in the past when his father had been drinking. The mother expressed some concern over Tom's legal and academic problems, deteriorating interactions with the family, and changing behavior. She stated that Tom used to be a good student, dependable, and a help around the house. This was in contrast with his current habits of staying out all night, being involved with a "bad bunch," and wanting to sleep all day.

Tom started drinking at the age of 13 years with heavy use over the past two years. His substance of choice was beer, although he would drink anything available, and he smoked marijuana. He had tried some other drugs but did not continue them because of inavailability, expense, or dislike. He drank three nights per week, primarily on weekends, and drank more when on vacation. He had one arrest for driving while intoxicated at which time his blood alcohol content was 0.12. Tom had experienced the following: loss of control, increased tolerance, increased preoccupation, sneaking drinks, gulping drinks, and had had three blackouts. His withdrawal symptoms included restlessness, loss of appetite, difficulty sleeping, and agitation. He had not made suicide attempts although he reported having had thoughts of suicide at the time his parents separated.

Evaluation

In conjunction with group therapy, individual counseling, family therapy, and educational sessions, Tom was referred to occupational therapy for an evaluation as a part of his treatment program on the unit. This decision was made at a multidisciplinary treatment planning meeting.

Appointments were arranged by the certified occupational therapy assistant for all new referrals to the department. At the time appointments were scheduled for Tom, the COTA provided him with a brief introduction to occupational therapy services and gave him a questionnaire to complete.

Prior to the evaluation, Tom's medical record was reviewed to gather any pertinent data. The occupational therapy evaluation consisted of a questionnaire, which Tom completed, concerning demographic information; an educational, work, leisure, and social history; and time clock figures representing an average school day and nonschool day prior to his admission to the program. After Tom completed the questionnaire, he was interviewed by the occupational therapist. The interview was directed at the information contained on the questionnaire. In addition to conducting the interview with Tom, the OTR made preliminary observations and assessed the data. Interview results included the following information:

Educational History

Tom was a junior in high school; therefore, his occupational role was as a student. His grade average was "C," which had consistently decreased over the past year. He was failing two courses.

Work History

He had a part-time job at a department store loading and unloading merchandise, and had worked there for a year. There had been no noticeable change in his work performance, and no one at work had spoken to him about his drinking or marijuana use.

Leisure History

Tom's leisure activities consisted of partying, chasing girls, auto repair, and going to movies. At school, he had been involved in the history and language clubs, the debate team, and varsity football, but had dropped all extracurricular activities except football.

Social History

He was fairly popular and had a number of school friends; however, this had decreased from the previous year. Five or six of Toms's friends also used alcohol and drugs. Tom stated that he had liked how he looked and was pleased with his potential and accomplishments before becoming heavily involved with alcohol and marijuana. He thought other people saw him as "nice and fun to be with." He disliked his shyness, difficulty in talking with girls, and his loss of self-confidence. The things Tom indicated he would like to change about himself were to be more responsible, get back to doing things he liked to do, and to cut back on his alcohol and marijuana use.

Time Utilization History

Tom's time records demonstrated that there was not a balance between school, work, leisure, self-care, rest, and sleep activities. After dropping some of his extracurricular activities, and starting to stay out all night, the times for sleep and constructive leisure were identified as primary problem areas.

The interview also included behavioral observations of Tom's social skills, his reactions to questions asked, his insight into the ways that substance abuse had interrupted his lifestyle, his ability to make decisions, and his self concept.

Tom appeared somewhat unsure of himself because he had difficulty answering some questions and maintaining eye contact. His social skills were appropriate during the interview, although Tom expressed that this was a problem for him in other social situations. His insight into how substance abuse had caused his problems in his daily living functioning demonstrated that he lacked the initiative to follow through with plans. Tom understood that his substance abuse had caused problems, but he had not made a commitment to totally stop substance use. He was cooperative during the interview and agreed to full participation in the occupational therapy program.

Treatment Planning

When the evaluation had been completed, the OTR met with the COTA to discuss the results. They developed the following treatment plan together:

1. Goal Achievement

Goal achievement in the areas of education, work, leisure, and social activities: Tom was unclear about what he wanted but knew that he had the potential to succeed. He was easily influenced by his peers. In addition, he had difficulty making a commitment and directing his attention and behavior to long-term goals.

Treatment Outcomes:

1 Complete a task utilizing the problem solving approach.
2 Establish a set of personal goals and an action plan for achievement of those goals.
3 Develop a life plan for use after discharge which does not include drugs or alcohol.

2. Time Management

Time management to include balancing activities for competent role performance: Tom became easily distracted when he was involved with school and extracurricular activities. He stated that he got bored, but upon further questioning, he indicated that he was feeling overwhelmed. This was related to his inability to recall facts and to follow directions.

Treatment Outcome: Develop a time management plan which includes a balance of school, work, leisure, self-care, rest, and sleep activities, and provides for need satisfaction.

3. Self-concept

Self-concept as related to assertiveness, communication, and socialization skills: Tom expressed some discontent about himself because of not being able to stand up for what he believed in, his shyness when talking to girls, and his loss of confidence.

Treatment Outcomes:

1 Identify realistic, personal strengths and weaknesses.
2 Demonstrate increased assertiveness, communication and socialization skills.

Emphasis on age-appropriate skills was the basis of the treatment outcomes. These skills were required to facilitate accomplishment of developmental tasks.

Prior to implementation of treatment, the plan was discussed with Tom. The discussion centered on the problems identified from the evaluation, treatment outcomes for resolution, and the occupational therapy media and methods that would be utilized to reach the treatment outcomes.

Treatment Implementation

On the basis of the treatment outcomes identified with Tom and an analysis of activities, the following occupational therapy media and sequence of activities were outlined:

Art and Craft Activity

A variety of activities were identified which would meet the specific outcomes for treatment. The activities had to require goal setting, organization, and time management and provide a success experience to help bolster Tom's self-concept. He was allowed to choose an activity from the identified list. This afforded him an opportunity for active participation in the treatment process, and would motivate and commit him to the task. Tom ultimately chose a woodworking project; however, he did have difficulty making the choice. To complete the project, he was required to utilize the problem solving method with guidance from the occupational therapy staff. The problem solving method had the following components: establishing a goal, step by step planning, and goal completion.

Tom's goal was the completion of a wooden cassette tape holder for his own personal use. He was required to draw plans for the holder, sequence the steps, select the materials, have the plans approved, and learn about tools and materials prior to beginning work on his project. Actual work on the tape holder included cutting out pieces of wood, sanding them, constructing the holder, staining and finishing it.

Three 50-minute treatment sessions were conducted weekly in the occupational therapy clinic. In addition, Tom was evaluated during each session for the following factors:

1 Attention span.
2 Frustration tolerance.
3 Motivation.
4 Decision/choice making.
5 Ability to make commitment and follow through.
6 Ability to follow written and verbal instructions.
7 Ability to handle constructive criticism and act accordingly.
8 Ability to delay gratification.

The COTA was responsible for monitoring safety and supervising Tom while he completed his project in the clinic. The assistant also ensured that Tom utilized the steps in the problem solving method. Tom was given assistance as needed, and the COTA provided him with feedback on the progress of his project.

Life Skills Development Group

Life skills development groups, geared to specific problem areas, were scheduled on the unit. Each patient was specifically placed in a group on the basis of the treatment outcomes identified. When patients were scheduled for a group, they were required to make a commitment to attend sessions, participate in the tasks and activities for that group, and provide input to other group members. The life skills development groups were task oriented, structured, learning groups with a purpose of skill acquisition through actual doing rather than discussion only.

The OTR and the COTA team co-facilitated the life skills development groups. Both were responsible for ensuring that the patients remained task oriented, and they elicited feedback from the patients regarding the topic of discussion.

Tom was scheduled for three of the life skills groups and attended the one-hour sessions on alternate days from clinical activities. In the goal setting group, Tom identified short- and long-term education, work, leisure, and social goals for himself. He initially wrote out his goals, shared them with the group, and received feedback from other group members. Once the goals were finalized, he prioritized them, developed a plan of action on how he was going to meet them, and shared his plan with the group. The final portion of the goal setting process addressed barriers to goal achievement and solutions to those barriers.

The final phase of this life skills development group was to develop a life plan for use following discharge. The primary purpose was for Tom to formally identify how he would manage a substance free lifestyle to include goals and a plan of action as well as a support system. His support system included an Alcoholics Anonymous (AA) sponsor, AA involvement, Narcotics Anonymous (NA) involvement, and Antabuse, if needed, and a plan for time utilization. Alateen involvement was also recommended in order for Tom to understand how his father's alcoholism had affected him. His plan would coincide with the aftercare plan which he developed as part of his treatment regimen.

Time Management Group

The second group Tom participated in focused on time management. Tom brought his time records to the group and shared them with the other members. He described problem areas and received feedback. Once the problem areas had been identified, Tom indicated those which he had control over, such as leisure time, and those which he did not, such as school time. He evaluated his records to see whether there was an imbalance between school, work, leisure, self-care, rest, and sleep activities. He then developed ideal time records and discussed the barriers that were keeping him from reaching his ideal, such as peer pressure. Methods for taking charge and overcoming those barriers were identified. In addition, occupational therapy provided assistance to Tom for planning unstructured time on the unit as well as his weekend passes.

Communication Skills

In the communication skills group, Tom completed a communication worksheet which included his own definition of communication, identifying what types of communication were the most difficult or easiest and why, identifying personal barriers to communication, such as no eye contact and communication enhancers, such as maintaining eye contact. He practiced assertiveness and socialization skills through role playing situations with peers in areas such as initiating and ending conversations, and he received group feedback. Following these exercises, Tom identified his personal strengths and weaknesses in writing and shared them with the group. Ways to capitalize on his strengths and to improve his weaknesses were also established.

Tom maintained a feelings journal throughout his treatment program. The journal included feelings that Tom experienced throughout the day and identification of the situations that were associated with those feelings. By using the journal, Tom had a cummulative source of information to share with staff and other patients.

Recreational Activities

Tom participated in structured physical activities, which included volleyball, bowling, and softball, twice a week. The intent of these activities was to promote physical fitness, encourage involvement in team sports and games, provide socialization, and explore alternate leisure activities. The COTA was responsible for supervising the physical activities and was also an active participant. Observations related to leadership qualities, competitiveness, cooperativeness, and sportsmanship were reported to the occupational therapist during their daily meetings.

Recreational outings were scheduled twice a month, and Tom participated on a regular basis. The purpose of these outings was for patients to learn how to have fun without the substance abuse. The outings also provided the opportunity for patients to identify community resources to use as alternatives to substance abuse and allowed for appropriate socialization. Examples of these outings included picnics at local parks, attending concerts and sports events, and visiting museums. Supervision of the recreational outings was rotated among the unit staff members. The occupational therapy assistant arranged for the logistical support, which included general scheduling, transportation, and lunches.

Family involvement was an intergral part of this drug and alcohol rehabilitation program. Tom's family was invited to participate in a group picnic and a family sports competition, and Tom was pleased that they agreed to come to these events. Efforts were also made to include his parents in other facets of his treatment program. They were scheduled to visit the occupational therapy clinic on several occassions to learn about Tom's treatment and progress and how they could continue to support his life plan when he returned home.

Documentation and Reporting

Throughout treatment, the COTA and the OTR were role models for Tom in terms of appropriate behavior. The occupational therapy assistant made behavioral observations of Tom's work skills, motivation, frustration tolerance, and level of socialization, and reported these findings to the occupational therapist at their daily meetings.

Occupational therapy services were documented in Tom's treatment record. The OTR was responsible for recording the results of the evaluation and treatment plan in Tom's medical record. In addition, these findings were discussed at the multidisciplinary treatment planning conferences, which both the COTA and the OTR attended. Continued observations were made and regular re-evaluations were completed and noted as they occurred. Program changes were based on Tom's participation and progress in treatment. Progress was discussed with Tom and his family, documented in the record by the OTR and the COTA, and shared with the multidisciplinary team. Treatment outcomes formulated by occupational therapy and the other disciplines were integrated into an overall treatment program for Tom that was a part of his treatment record.

Program Discontinuation

The drug and alcohol recovery program that provided Tom's treatment was a six-week, closed-ended program. Approximately two weeks prior to discharge, the COTA scheduled a meeting with Tom and his parents. The occupational therapist conducted this meeting and discussed the family's role in supporting Tom in his life plan and specific ways they could help in carrying out his aftercare plan, such as becoming involved in Al-anon.

References

Diagnostic and Statistical Manual of Mental Disorders, Third Edition. Washington, D.C.: American Psychiatric Association, 1980.

Diepenbrock EC: Handout:*Understanding Adolescents*, 1980.

Lorens LA: *Application of a Developmental Theory for Health and Rehabilitation*. Rockville, MD: American Occupational Therapy Association, 1976.

Acknowledgments

The authors wish to thank the following individuals and groups for their invaluable assistance in providing information and content and editorial suggestions: Elaine Diepenbrock, MEd, CCMHC, at Second Mile House, the Occupational Therapy Section staff members at Walter Reed Army Medical Center, and the Tri-Service Alcoholism Recovery Department at the Bethesda Naval Hospital.

CHAPTER 15

The Burned Young Adult

Bonnie E. Hoffman, OTR/L

Introduction

Bill was a 19-year-old college student who was burned when he lit a cigarette after filling a lawn mower with gasoline in his garage. He was able to put out the flames by rolling against the wall. Bill sustained a 26 percent total body surface area (TBSA) burn, 21 percent being second-degree burns of the head, chest, forearms, hands, thighs, and legs. Five percent were third-degree involving the neck, right forearm, and the dorsum of both hands. He was taken by ambulance to the hospital emergency room and admitted to the burn unit.

Over a period of two months, the patient underwent three surgical procedures for split-thickness autografting: (1) 14 days after injury for both arms and hands; (2) two and one-half weeks later for thighs and right arm; and (3) three weeks later for spots on the left thigh and right arm.

Occupational therapy personnel began following the patient immediately upon admission for prevention of contractures and deformity, preservation/restoration of functional abilities, and assistance with psychological adjustment. When the patient was discharged from the hospital two and one-half months after injury, the supervising occupational therapist referred him to another outpatient clinic where he was treated for one additional year, until he had returned to full functional independence and the burn scar had matured. Throughout treatment in this clinic, the occupational therapist, registered (OTR), and the entry-level certified occupational therapy assistant (COTA) collaborated closely because of the possible complications that can occur with a major burn patient.

Because the long-range effects of the burn injury can delay recovery and result in loss of function, it was the policy of the burn unit to refer the patient upon admission to each service of the burn team for screening and evaluation. This was an automatic referral by the physician in charge. As a result, Bill's treatment was initiated within three hours after arrival.

Assessment

Use of Screening Tools

Before the patient arrived on the unit, initial screening was accomplished by reviewing the emergency room referral information. This indicated that the upper extremities were involved. While the patient was undergoing initial debridement, the admission note was reviewed for historical data such as respiratory tract injury, fractures, and pre-existing disease which might affect edema or infection. The "Rule of Nines" figures and Lund-Browder tables were reviewed as soon as available for location, percentage, and degree of burn.

The injury was sustained from a flash burn. Since he was wearing only cut-off shorts, Bill had burns of most of the exposed anterior areas except his face, which he had protected with his hands. No complications were noted. The fact that both hands had areas of third-degree burns placed Bill in the critical burn category, and was an indication for occupational therapy intervention in order to preserve or restore his functional ability.

Use of Evaluation Tools

Evaluation was more detailed with each stage of recovery. Initial evaluation was done at the patient's bedside after triage. While he was appropriate in his response to questions, his medication was "wearing off" and the pain made concentration difficult. Hence, interaction was informal and brief, and data gathering was mostly observational. Although initial information was structured by the occupational therapy interview form, it was done in short segments scheduled between medical, nursing, and therapy procedures and was further limited by the patient's pain at the time.

It was noted that the patient had an intravenous line in his left arm for resuscitation fluids. There were also two heat lamps in use to help him maintain body temperature. He did not have a catheter. His hips and knees were flexed while arms were adducted and elbows flexed. Edema was noted, particularly in the upper extremities. Third-degree burns were present on the anterior neck and chest (1.5% TBSA), posterior right forearm (1.5%), and dorsum of both wrists and hands (1% each), and there was questionable third degree injury of the right index and long fingers. While shoulder and elbow joints had been spared, his chest burn extended close to the right axillary region, and the right forearm burn wrapped radially to within ½ inch of the antecubital fossa. Other burn wounds were second degree over muscle belly areas and were clear of joints. This visual assessment was the basis for determining the occupational therapy intervention to reduce edema in the upper extremities, and to maintain therapeutic positioning of the upper extremities and neck.

Later, Bill was able to demonstrate to the COTA that he had adequate bed mobility for nursing care and functional grasp for feeding. The physical therapy (PT) evaluation revealed full active range of motion (AROM) of upper and lower extremities except for the right hand, which lacked one finger's breadth of full flexion due to edema. This indicated that the patient had the capacity to perform other self-care activities such as dressing. However, since this burn unit used the open method of burn treatment, he was not specifically evaluated in this area until his wounds were closed.

From the time of admission, Bill was also observed for psychological adjustment by all staff for effects on his self-concept, his interaction with others (especially family), and his situational coping skills (to treatment in early stages and to resuming former activity/interaction later). Nonverbal signs such as change in affect, decreased activity level, and decreased appetite were also monitored and reported to appropriate staff members.

With completion of fluid resuscitation and beginning of diuresis (excretion of urine), about 72 hours after admission, the critical period was passed and Bill was assessed for the second stage of treatment. During this wound healing period, the OTR and COTA monitored edema and positioning, psychological status, orientation, and comprehension on a daily basis. An additional area of emphasis at this stage was the monitoring of AROM and normal movement patterns. Since the physical therapist had reported that Bill was unable to demonstrate full AROM at the beginning of exercise sessions and took some time to stretch out, Bill was evaluated for pregraft splinting to maintain range of motion and normal alignment patterns. As time for grafting approached, postgrafting splints were discussed with the physician. Since burns on both hands and the right forearm were over or near joints, splints were indicated for immobilization.

Sensation in noninjured areas was evaluated by the COTA, using two-point discrimination and temperature testing, 5 days after admission and 30 minutes after medication. Since the palms were not involved, responses were within normal limits.

As the burn wounds healed, the upper extremities were evaluated for protective sensation using sharp/dull discrimination, temperature, and light touch. Bill was found to be hypersensitive. The sensorimotor components of coordination, strength, and endurance were evaluated through combined efforts of the OTR, the COTA and the physical therapist. Each morning, the occupational and physical therapists met to review the patient's performance of the previous day. Initially, occupational therapy staff observed feeding skills and involvement in self-care to assess coordination, while the physical therapy department worked with the patient in active and active assistance range of motion exercise, observing the motion achieved to avoid infection. As endurance increased and wounds closed, the physical therapist could then use a goniometer and dynamometer for objective measurement. It was possible for the COTA to measure hand function objectively using such tools as the Minnesota Rate of Manipulation Tests, the Purdue Pegboard Test and the Bennett Hand Tool Assessment.

Other areas of skill such as self-care and communication were also assessed. His ability to perform hygiene and dressing tasks was observed. Bill was given writing and typing tests by the COTA, to establish a base line before treatment. Results indicated a decrease in fine dexterity and strength of the right upper extremity which affected speed on bilateral activities as well.

Program Planning and Goal Development

The OTR and COTA collaborated in developing treatment goals based on the information gathered through ongoing assessment. The long-range goals of acute care were to prevent soft tissue contracture and deformity that might affect later rehabilitation and to aid in psychological adjustment to the injury. The goals were to:

1 Reduce edema of the upper extremities.
2 Prevent contracture/deformity.
3 Prevent further tissue trauma.
4 Provide psychological support.

The goals during the wound closure stage, in addition to the ones previously stated, included (1) protection of grafts, (2) maintenance of range of motion and strength, (3) encouragement of functional independence as permitted, and (4) assistance in situational coping.

Techniques and Media

The OTR and COTA again collaborated in selecting techniques and media to achieve treatment goals and in sequencing the activities. The priority during resuscitation was edema reduction. This was accomplished through elevation using slings on intravenous (IV) poles for height adjustment and/or foam wedges to place the extremities higher than the level of the heart as shown in Figures 15-1 and 15-2. Active exercise was also encouraged for the pumping action.

Prevention of tissue trauma was accomplished through daily skin checks of pressure points. Since the patient had good bed mobility and was aware, no problems were noted.

Soft tissue contracture and deformities were prevented or managed through therapeutic positioning opposite the expected deformity, using a foam shoulder roll to extend the neck and slings to extend the elbows and abduct the shoulder. The following listing details these and other commonly used antideformity positioning techniques and assistive devices:

1 *Head*:
- Position of comfort: rotated to one side.
- Optimum position: neutral.
- Devices: foam head donut; ear donut if side lying.

2 *Anterior Neck*:
- Position of comfort: flexed when burn is symmetrical; add a rotational component when burn is asymmetrical.
- Optimum position: extension with head in midline and head of bed elevated.
- Devices: foam back wedge, shoulder roll, folded towels, thermoplastic or foam collar with/without conformer inserts.

3 *Shoulder*:
- Position of comfort: adduction often with a slight internal rotation.
- Optimum position: 90 degrees of abduction and 15 to 20 degrees of flexion.
- Devices: net arm slings on IV poles, arm troughs, foam axillary wedges, breakfast tables with foam wedges or pillows and airplane splints.

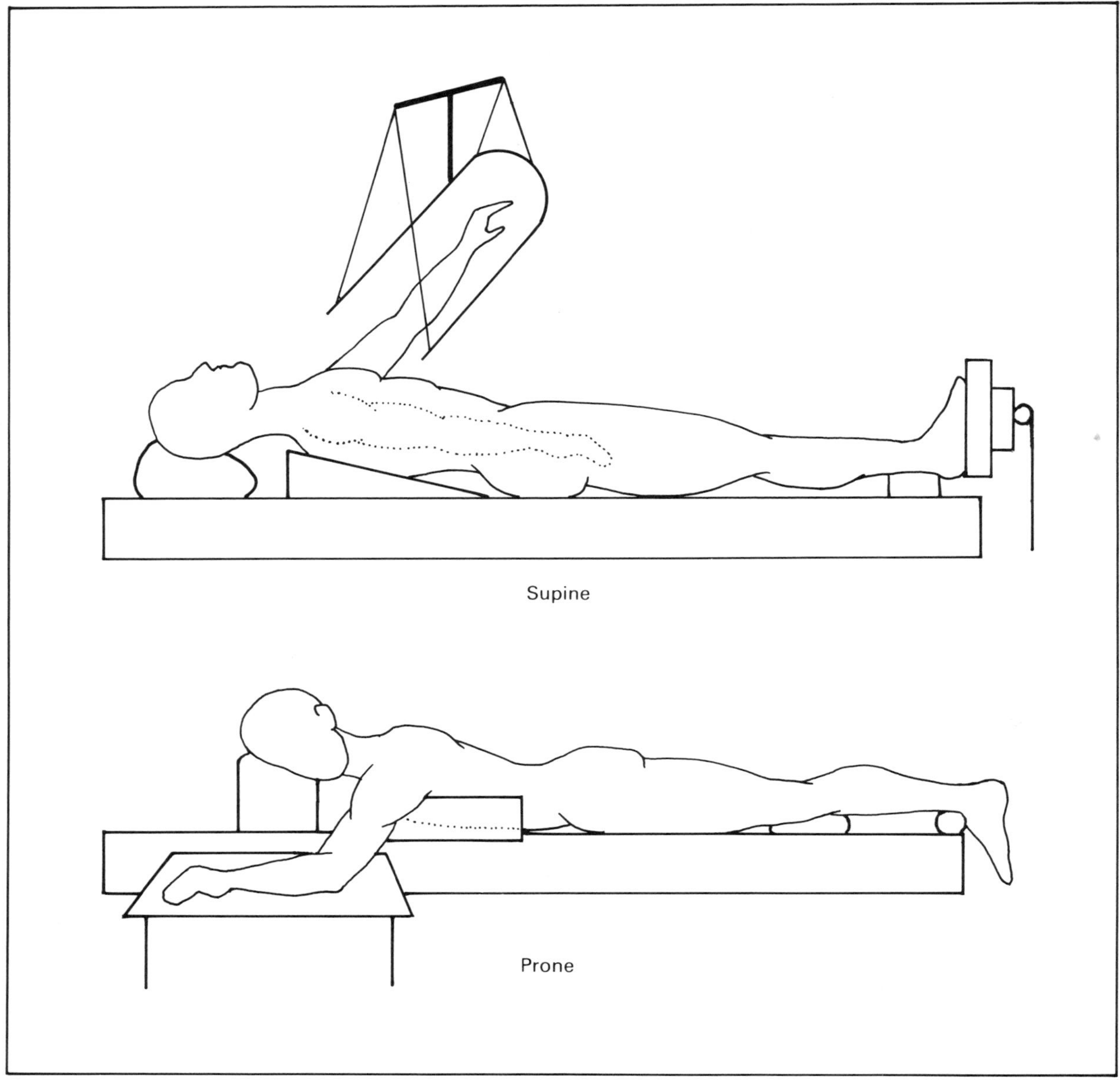

Figure 15-1

4 *Elbow*:
- Position of comfort: flexion and pronation.

Optimum position: anterior burn extension and supination; posterior burn—consider resting in about 10 to 20 degrees of flexion.

Devices: arm slings on IV poles, thermoplastic extension splints, tubigrip, conformers/inserts.

5 *Wrist*:

Position of comfort: flexion often with component deviation.
- Optimum position: 30 to 40 degrees of extension (exception is dorsal burns requiring a neutral wrist position).
- Devices: soft rolls, hard cones, thermoplastic cock-up splints.

6 *Hand*:
- Position of comfort: MPs flexed to 30

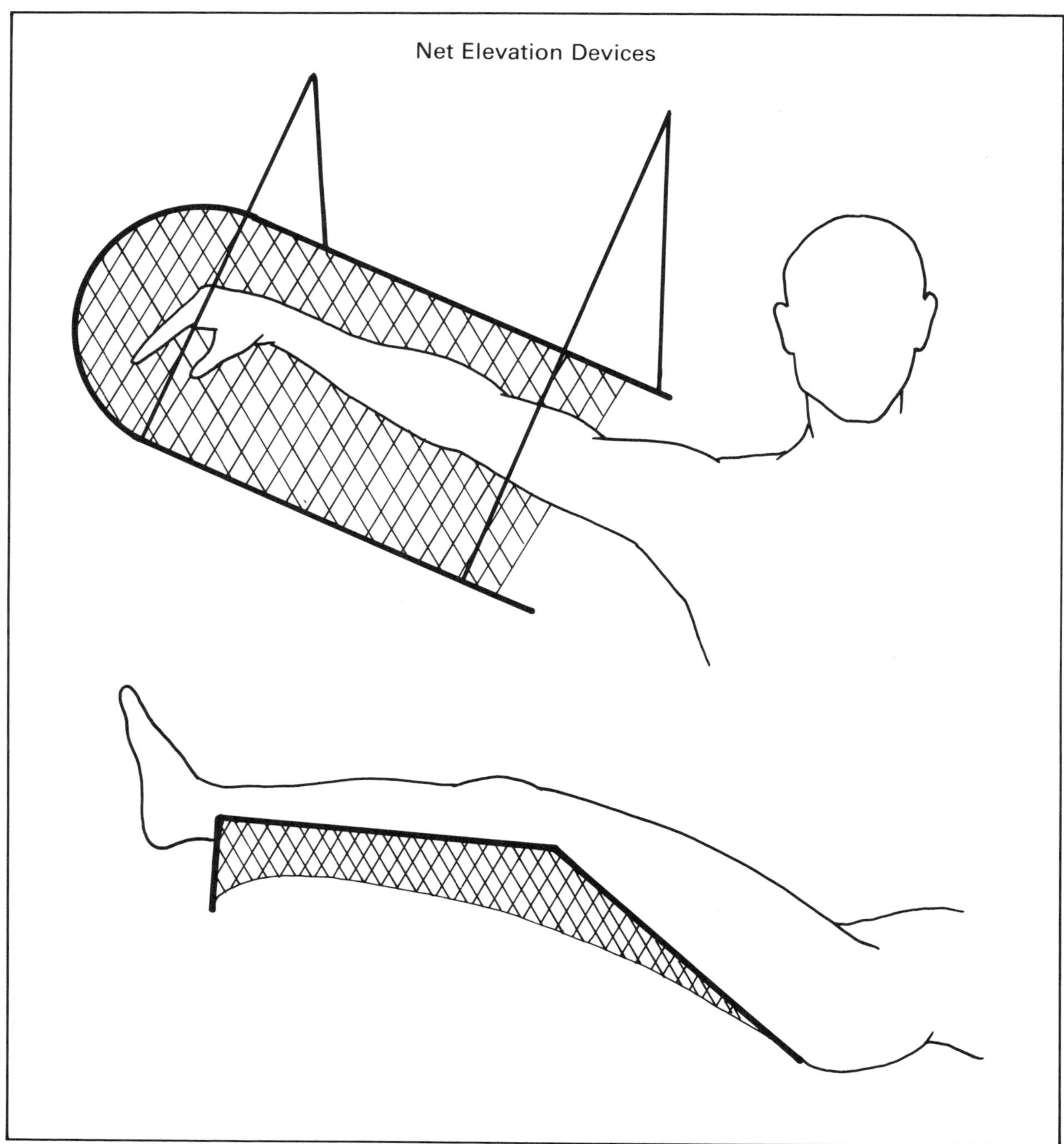

Figure 15-2

to 40 degrees; PIPs flexed to 45 degrees; DIPs flexed to 10 degrees.
- Optimum position: MPs in 90 degrees of flexion; PIPs and DIPs in full extension.
- Devices: thermoplastic splint in antideformity position (position of advantage), nail traction, web spacers (foam, elastomer), pressure garments.

7 *Thorax*:
- Position of comfort: flexion.
- Optimum position: prone with healed anterior burns but flat in supine position while still open.
- Devices: Prone—chest foam with diaphragm cut out, head donut, knee donuts; supine—flat or back wedge.

8 *Hip*:
- Position of comfort: flexion, abduction and external rotation.
- Optimal position: prone if possible; supine—completely flat with neutral rotation and slight abduction.
- Devices: As noted in No. 7 prone; foam separators as needed.

9 *Knee*:
- Position of comfort: flexion.
- Optimum position: extension.
- Devices: thermoplastic knee tabs, metal long leg splints; foam heel wedges.

10 *Ankle and Heel*:
- Position of comfort: inversion and plantar flexion.
- Optimal position: neutral in all planes.
- Devices: foot board, foot drop splint, heel wedges, pillows.

During the wound closure phase, the same techniques were used as during resuscitation/critical care but with several additions. Edema reduction was still a concern. The patient was allowed to be out of bed and encouraged to exercise. However, elevation was still used whenever the activity would permit and always when the patient was at rest. The same adjustable IV pole slings were used during the pregrafting phase of care. Foam wedges were used in the postgrafting stage.

Tissue trauma was of concern, particularly for splinted areas. The skin was checked every time the splint was removed.

Soft tissue contracture was managed through positioning and static night splinting during this phase. The hands were splinted with maximum flexion of the metacarpophalangeals (MP) and full interphalangeal (IP) extension. Elbows were extended in slings at night.

Grafts were protected through custom fitted static splints to maintain positions, as shown in Figure 15-3. The type of splint was determined by the OTR in collaboration with the physician. They were used continuously until grafts adhered (about five to eight days) and were used as night splints thereafter.

Strength and range of motion were maintained through combined occupational and physical therapy efforts. While the physical therapist provided ranging and exercise twice per day, the OTR and the COTA primarily used self-care and leisure activities to achieve range of motion. Particular media for such activities were chosen for ease of cleaning and freedom from irritating materials.

As healing occurred, hypersensitivity was reduced and skin was toughened through patient application of pressure and texture, beginning with lotion massage in the early stage. This progressed to having Bill rub various fabrics and use desensitization boxes containing different types of substances.

Independence in physical daily living skills was pursued through simulated work situations, such as skills necessary for school, such as writing drills, typing drills, calculator use, and drafting problems, applied over gradually increasing periods of time.

Psychological support was provided primarily through role playing, discussion, and stress management techniques to assist with situational coping.

Analysis and Adaptation of Activity

Bill was majoring in engineering at a local college. He was active on the debate team and enjoyed playing the guitar in his spare time. Whenever possible, activities were chosen by the OTR to involve these interests while meeting treatment goals. The COTA was instrumental in modifying and monitoring the use of the activity. Range of motion and strengthening activities included oversized games, which were positioned to require

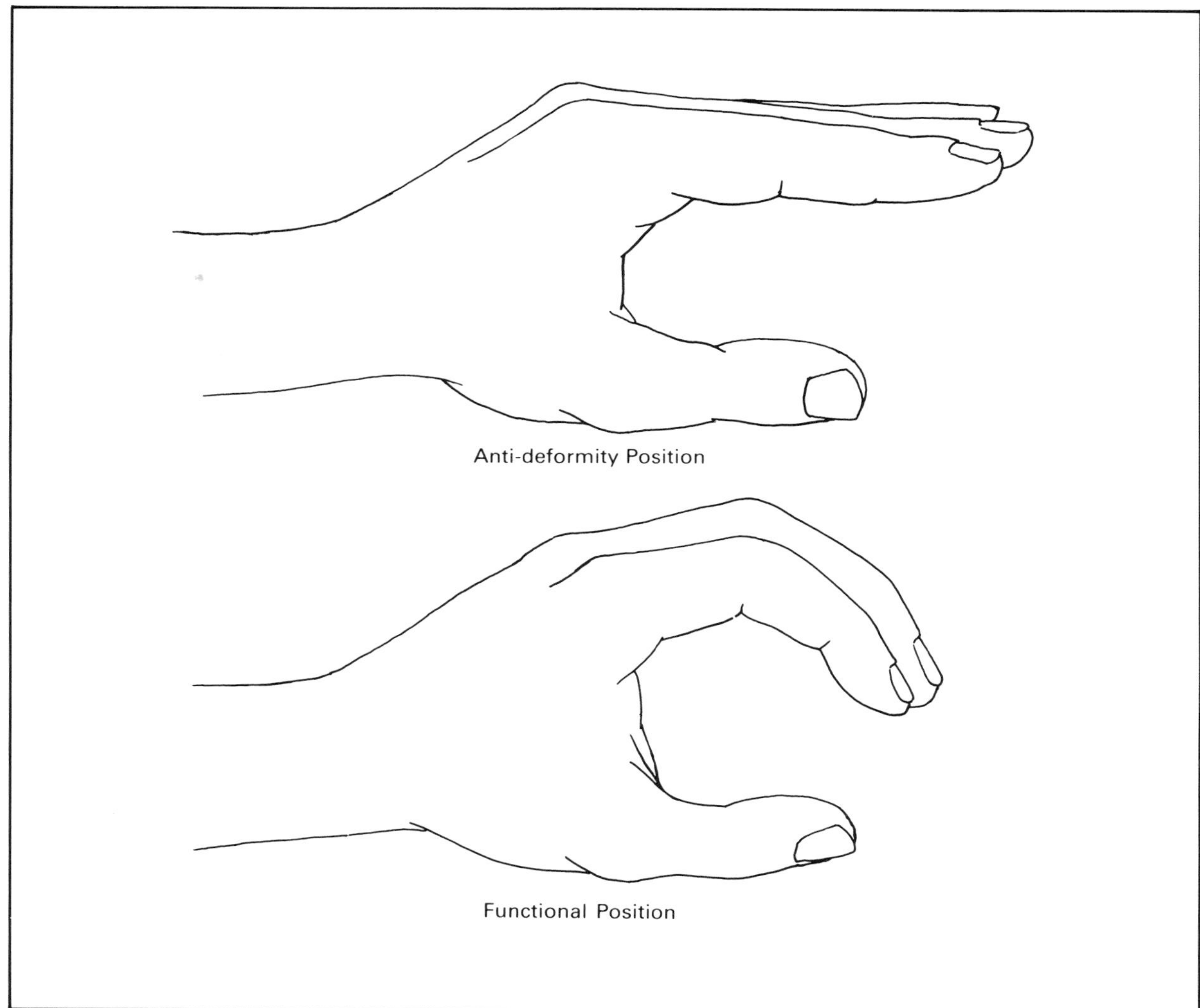

Figure 15-3

maximum stretch of the upper extremities. Hi-Q, checkers, and chess were among Bill's favorites. Pieces were graded from large to small to improve grasp. Strengthening was accomplished by adding velcro to board and pieces, using wrist weights, or both. A typewriter, calculator, and mazes were used for dexterity, and he was encouraged to practice his guitar when on pass. Just prior to discharge, when the wounds were well healed, he was given macramé and leather lacing, which had been modified with instructions for maximum stretch of shoulder abduction and graded with wrist weights.

Hand and elbow splints, as shown in Figure 15-4, were monitored daily for fit and were revised with decreased edema and increased motion until the optimal antideformity position was achieved. Foam positioning devices and neck collars were modified to achieve desired antideformity position. Conformers (Silastic elastomer inserts, custom molded to provide total contact with scar tissue) were worn under the collars to provide even pressure as hypertrophic scar began to form near the end of Bill's stay in the hospital.

Discussion of Goals and Methods

While Bill had some difficulty with concentration due to pain during the resuscitation period, he was able to comprehend most of the interaction

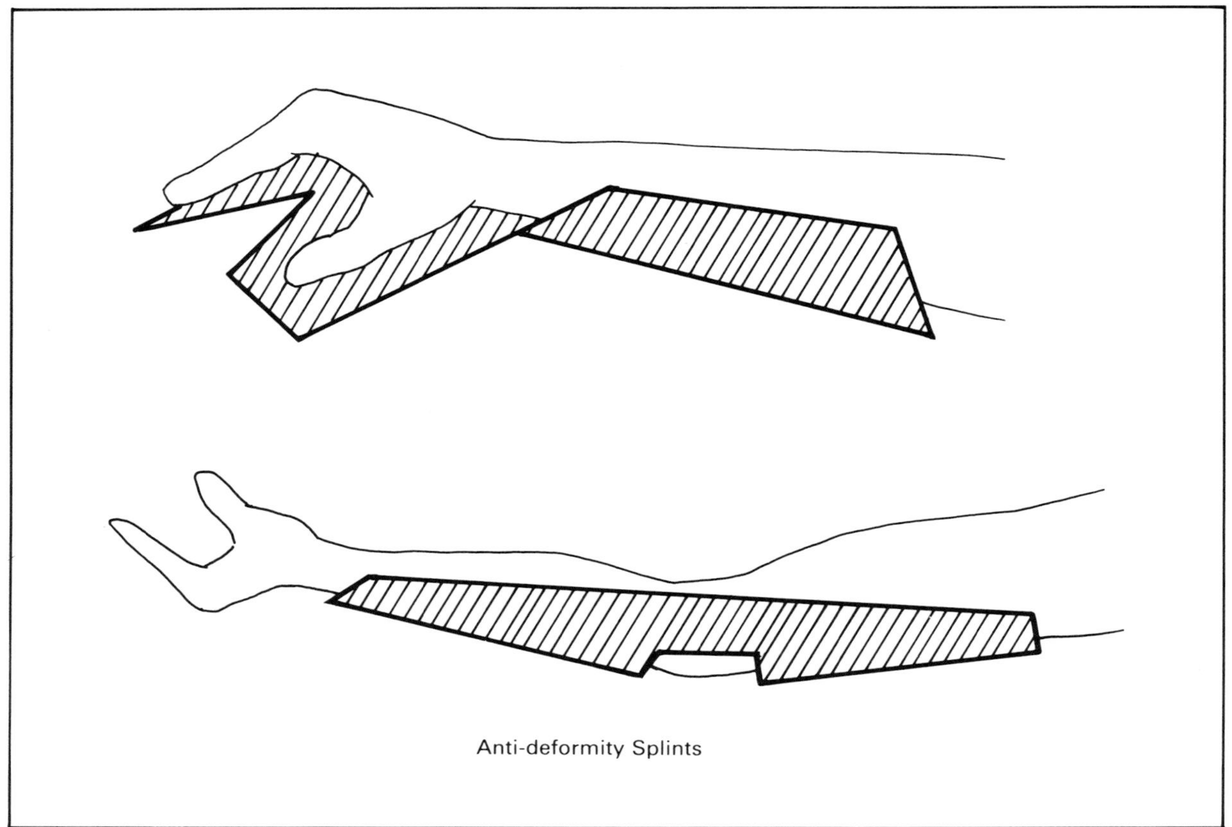

Figure 15-4

with the occupational therapy staff. As he improved, both the OTR and COTA reviewed the goals of treatment, the procedures and media to be used, and potential complications, such as edema, graft loss, soft tissue contracture, hypertrophic scarring, and deformity. The family was unavailable during the day, so the COTA interacted with them in the evenings to ensure their understanding and support during the treatment program.

The burn team made rounds every morning, and changes in Bill's program plan were discussed for each stage of recovery. The initial evaluation, assessment, and program plan were entered in the chart by the OTR. Progress notes and changes in the plan were documented by either the OTR or COTA after discussing observations with each other.

Occupational Therapy Treatment

Many aspects of the occupational therapy treatment have already been discussed. During resuscitation and wound closure, the patient's condition changed rapidly. Because of daily reassessment and modification of the treatment plan and modalities, the OTR and COTA worked together closely to ensure continuity and quality of care. During the rehabilitative phase, the COTA performed with more independence and less direction from the OTR.

Throughout treatment, the occupational therapist and the assistant both sought to maintain rapport with the patient to help with psychological adjustment. Bill was encouraged to interact with other individuals and to participate in the patient group, led by the clinical psychiatric nurse, as soon as he was allowed out of bed. He was taught relaxation techniques to aid in controlling pain. Both the OTR and the COTA always made it a point to explain procedures before beginning and to provide the patient with verbal reinforcement during his performance. Treatment was timed for about 30 minutes after pain medication, when possible, so as to decrease discomfort and increase compliance.

For the first three days after admission, the treatment consisted of patient education to ensure follow-through, elevation of his upper extremities to reduce edema, and therapeutic positioning of his arms in abduction and slight horizontal flexion to prevent soft tissue contraction/deformity. Net slings on adjustable IV poles were used. A shoulder roll was placed just below the base of the neck to facilitate neck extension. No pillow was allowed. Bill was checked at least three times per day to ensure proper elevation and positioning.

After diuresis began on the third day, Bill was evaluated for antideformity hand splints, as discussed and illustrated previously. On his right hand, he was able to demonstrate about 60 percent metacarpophalangeal (MP) flexion. Full proximal interphalangeal (PIP) extension of the right index and long fingers was achieved only when the occupational therapist blocked the metacarpophalangeal joints in flexion, indicating a need for night splinting to protect and position the proximal interphalangeal joints. The other splint was worn continuously except during supervised occupational therapy activities and when being exercised by the physical therapist or when bathing. The left hand required only night splinting since it was stiff but still had full active range of motion. To allow maximum functional use and exercises, the COTA did not apply the splint until bedtime each night. The OTR removed both of Bill's splints each morning before rounds to check for pressure areas and the need for adjustments. Therapeutic antideformity positioning of neck and arms was continued.

Bill was supervised 30 minutes in the morning and afternoon at board games such as oversized checkers, which were positioned vertically to achieve stretch of the upper extremities and to discourage neck flexion. Resistance was provided through the use of weights or velcro in the pieces. These activities were also supervised by the COTA and provided another opportunity to interact with the patient. Bill was encouraged to participate in these activities on his own throughout the day.

Fourteen days after admission, Bill underwent his first grafting procedure on his upper extremities and neck. A 1-inch foam ring was used to maintain neck extension and keep his head aligned. His arms and hands were immobilized with splints in the operating room at the end of the procedure, fabricated and applied by the OTR. On return to the ward, his arms were again elevated and abducted. The legs were also elevated with foam blocks placed under the calves to allow drying of donor sites on the posterior thighs. A foot board was provided for comfort and to assist in prevention of venous stasis. Bill was on bed rest for five days until the drying was accomplished. With arms immobilized and legs elevated, occupational therapy intervention consisted of verbal interaction. When daily dressing changes began, an OTR or COTA was on hand to reapply splints.

About eight days after surgery, when the grafts were judged adherent by the physician, all splints were changed to night-wear, and the regular program was resumed. The right hand was lacking enough flexion to grasp a fork, so a built-up handle was provided. As soon as motor function improved, the handle was discontinued, even though this made use of the fork less comfortable. Feeding was used to encourage increased active motion through functional activity. Pegs were used for game pieces to encourage making a fist and positioned to require reaching and neck extension.

During the second surgery, 32 days after the injury, the thighs and right arm were grafted. The right elbow was again immobilized by the OTR. Although Bill was on bed rest, his left arm and hand were free, and the COTA was able to provide treatment at the bedside. Since his left hand was nondominant, a plate guard was provided until he became more skilled at feeding. Space was not available for vertical positioning of games, so major emphasis was on forward reaching and strengthening. Pieces were either velcroed or weighted. No weight was used on the arm since the skin was still fragile. A foam neck collar was worn during activity to prevent flexion. Eight days after surgery, the right elbow splint was changed to night wear. Bill was allowed to walk short distances and be up in a wheelchair. At that point the regular occupational therapy treatment could be resumed.

About 45 days after injury, Bill's neck rotation had decreased, and the grafted area blanched with slight motion, both the result of scarring. The OTR fabricated a Silastic conformer and incorporated it into the neck collar to exert even pressure on the scar. This was worn continuously except for exercise sessions and bathing. Either the OTR or COTA performed skin checks twice a day to prevent maceration (softening). Elasticized stockinette was applied to both forearms, and web spacers were applied to the right hand to manage hypertrophic scars, which were beginning to form.

Fifty-three days after injury, Bill underwent his last surgical procedure for spots on his left thigh and right arm. No splints were needed for immobilization. Bed rest lasted for four days. Occupational therapy was similar to that provided after the second operation, but with some additional media since the wounds were now essentially closed. Graded activities included macramé, leather lacing, and woodworking for range of motion, strengthening, and endurance. Typing and writing drills were used to establish a data base and to provide treatment in preparation for his return to school. A right hand-based index and ring finger proximal interphalangeal extension splint was fabricated by the COTA and checked by the OTR. It was worn during the day. At night, static finger extension splints were worn. Self-desensitization of healed areas was continued under close supervision of the OTR. The therapist also measured the patient for pressure garments, even though he would be discharged to the outpatient occupational therapy facility by the time they arrived.

As discharge approached, the patient expressed more anxiety and concern regarding his appearance and the reaction of others. Bill was encouraged to talk, and the OTR and COTA worked with him in role-playing situations. Before discharge, the COTA assisted the OTR in completing a sensorimotor evaluation and reviewed proper care of the skin and the need to continue his therapeutic home program with Bill and his family.

Program Discontinuation

Inpatient treatment was discontinued with wound closure. While Bill had done well with treatment goals, rehabilitation was just beginning. Hypertrophic scarring was beginning to form and would not be mature for 12 to 18 months. He was referred to the outpatient clinic with an appointment in one week and a home program for range of motion, sensory re-education, and scar control until he could be assessed by the outpatient facility. A summary of inpatient treatment was provided to the facility by the OTR to ensure continuity of care.

Summary

This case study emphasizes the role of the OTR and COTA in the acute care of patients with major burns. Primary emphasis is on prevention of deformity, with techniques and media differing depending on the status of wound healing. Rehabilitation techniques are mentioned in brief.

The OTR is responsible for initial screening, evaluation, program coordination, and discharge planning. Of necessity, the entry-level COTA will need close supervision until he or she is thoroughly familiar with the antideformity positioning and splinting so essential to functional recovery. Once the COTA has attained a level of expertise with which both the OTR and the COTA feel comfortable, the COTA may function more independently in these areas. The COTA is also primarily responsible for patient involvement in therapeutic activity for range of motion and situational coping. However, because of the many physiological and psychological complications that the acutely burned patient is subject to during this period, the roles of the OTR and the COTA may not always be clearly differentiated, and may frequently overlap and complement each other. What is essential is that the COTA and the OTR work closely as a team to achieve maximal results in treating acutely burned patients.

Bibliography

Artz C, Moncrief J, Pruitt B: *Burns, A Team Approach*. Philadelphia: W.B. Saunders, 1979.

DiGregorio VR: *Rehabilitation of the Burn Patient*. New York: Churchill Livingstone, 1984.

Malick MH, Carr JA: *Manual on Management of the Burn Patient*. Pittsburgh: Harmarville Rehabilitation Center, 1982.

Salisbury RE, Newman NM, Dingeldein GP: *Manual of Burn Therapeutics*. Boston: Little, Brown, 1983.

CHAPTER 16

The Spinal Injury Patient

M. Laurita Fike, OTR
Melanie Wiener, OTR
with Sherise Darlak, COTA

Introduction

Nancy, was 25 years old when she sustained a C-6 fracture (incomplete) of the spinal cord after a 20-foot fall from a balcony. She was originally admitted to an acute care trauma center where she was placed in Gardner Wells tongs with traction for 27 days. Surgery was not indicated. Following traction, she was placed in a SOMI brace during the day and a Philadelphia collar at night. The patient's hospitalization at the acute care center was uncomplicated except for one instance of bradycardia, 5 days after admission, which resolved spontaneously. Her bladder was managed with intermittent catheterization every 4 hours. Oral laxatives and suppositories were used for bowel management. Nancy received occupational and physical therapy daily, consisting of range of motion and strengthening exercises for her arms, and limited training in activities of daily living. Two months after her accident, she was transferred from the acute care hospital to a rehabilitation facility which specializes in treatment of the spinal injured.

On the day of Nancy's admission to the rehabilitation facility, the occupational therapy department received the standard referral from the physician requesting occupational therapy evaluation and treatment; referral to occupational therapy is a routine order for all patients. The physician stated on the referral that the patient's neck was stable enough for the patient to sit, using only a soft collar as a brace for her neck and head. The OT unit supervisor assigned the patient to two staff members who worked as partners, one of whom was a registered occupational therapist and the other a certified occupational therapy assistant. After the OTR and the COTA jointly reviewed the referral, they decided which partner would conduct specified portions of the initial assessment to determine the patient's needs in occupational therapy.

Before meeting the patient for the first time, both partners read the patient's medical chart to obtain pertinent background information. The OTR and the COTA were able to coordinate their time so that they could introduce themselves to the patient together. They explained that they were from the OT department and briefly described their respective roles as partners. They informed Nancy that the COTA would begin the screening process later that day.

First, however, as is customary at the facility, the partners needed to start the patient on a "sitting program," so that she could come to the OT clinic for assessment in a wheelchair. The partners made the arrangements for the sitting program during this first visit to the patient's room.

In order for the patient to sit, the OTR had to complete a skin assessment to determine if there were any contraindications to sitting. These might have included red skin areas, skin breakdown, abrasions, bruises, or a rash. The OTR examined Nancy's skin on her lower back and buttocks, paying particular attention to the seating surface and bony prominences. The OTR then filled out the skin assessment form, noting any scars, pressure areas, or potential problem areas. Copies of the form were filed in both the medical chart and the occupational therapy chart. The patient was noted to have a mild rash due to incontinence, but this was not severe enough to prevent limited sitting.

The COTA then measured the patient's hip width to determine the size of the wheelchair and seat cushion needed by the patient. She consulted with her partner to choose the type of wheelchair and seat cushion most appropriate for Nancy. Because the patient had reported having dizziness and lightheadedness when sitting previously at the acute care hospital, the partners decided that a full reclining back wheelchair was indicated, and that the patient should initially sit at a 60° angle.

The patient also reported minimal sensation in the buttocks area, and a special seat cushion was recommended. This foam cushion had been tested during research at the facility, and was felt to provide adequate pressure distribution for most spinal injured patients.

The COTA obtained an appropriate wheelchair and cushion and arranged for the nursing staff to dress and help transfer the patient to the chair. Prior to transferring the patient to the wheelchair for the first time, the COTA took Nancy's blood pressure while she lay supine in bed, again immediately after the transfer, and then every 5 minutes until the pressure readings were stable. Significant drops in blood pressure can indicate orthostatic hypotension, a common problem for people with new spinal injuries, and the patient can suffer lightheadedness or even loss of consciousness. The patient's blood pressure was 120/80, a normal baseline. During the initial sitting session, it dropped to 105/70, but stabilized at 110/75; the COTA continued to monitor Nancy's blood pressure every 10 minutes during the first session.

Assessment

The occupational therapy initial assessment at the rehabilitation facility routinely consists of six parts:

1 Data base.
2 Areas of occupational performance affected.
3 Occupational performance components affected.
4 History/comments.
5 Patient's initial goals.
6 Occupational therapy intervention.

According to departmental policy, the COTA could be responsible for completing parts 1, 2, 4 and 5, while the OTR was required to complete parts 3 and 6.

Part 1, the data base, included the patient's name, age, sex, date of referral, date of onset, type of admission, hospital room number, diagnosis and/or medical involvement, and a description of life roles and occupations prior to onset. A separate section permitted initial grip and prehension strength readings to be recorded. The COTA obtained some of the information from the medical record, and interviewed the patient to gather other pertinent facts. Nancy was noted to have a cervical spinal injury, at the sixth vertebra, which resulted in involvement of all four extremities, and loss of bowel and bladder control. Her life roles and occupations prior to her injury had included being a daughter and sister, and an employee of a geophysical company, for whom she did computer-related work. She had no grip or prehension in her right (dominant) hand, while in her left hand she had one pound of gross grip strength and approximately one pound of prehension strength in lateral prehension, three-point prehension, and single-point prehension.

For Nancy, the areas of her occupational performance which were affected by her injury included self-care, work, education, and leisure. Through interview and observation, the COTA noted that the patient was unable to perform the following specific activities independently: eating, dressing, personal hygiene, functional mobility, homemaking, vocational, and avocational.

Pertinent history obtained through an interview noted that Nancy had attended college in New York and had graduated with a degree in mathematics. Her parents lived near New York City. Nancy had three brothers, one of whom was a hemophiliac, while another had Down's syndrome. She enjoyed traveling and skiing, and had also participated in team sports. Nancy had recently planned to return to work in New York; her accident occurred at her going-away party.

The COTA also discussed Nancy's initial goals with her, since these would suggest Nancy's level of understanding and acceptance of her condition as well as provide the COTA with direction to encourage the patient's active participation in rehabilitation. Nancy stated that her goals were "to walk out of the hospital" and to get back the use of her hands.

After these areas of the initial assessment were completed, the COTA showed Nancy a document entitled "Patient and Therapist Goals." These goals are based on the facility's many years of experience in working with spinal injured persons, and are considered "generic" goals; more individualized goals are developed as each patient proceeds through the rehabilitation process. By discussing these "generic" goals with Nancy, the COTA was helping Nancy to understand the role of occupational therapy as well as helping her to explore a broader range of goals. Columns are provided for both the staff member and the patient so each may place a check by those goals that, for example, the COTA felt applied to Nancy, and those that Nancy would like to accomplish. The COTA and Nancy jointly identified the following goals:

1 Increase sitting time.
2 Increase upper extremity muscle strength.
3 Increase upper extremity joint range of motion.
4 Improve trunk balance.
5 Increase endurance.
6 Improve independent living skill.
7 Evaluate and train in use of orthotic equipment, if needed.
8 Improve coordination and dexterity.
9 Order necessary equipment.
10 Explore avocational interests.
11 Pursue homemaking training.
12 Participate in adaptive driver's training.
13 Improve safety awareness.
14 Evaluate prevocational skills.
15 Take functional out-trips.
16 Follow a home program upon discharge.

At the end of the first session, the COTA's portion of the initial assessment was completed. She then explained the "sitting program" to Nancy, emphasizing the need to build up general sitting tolerance, but also skin tolerance by gradually increasing the amount of time spent sitting. The COTA also reinforced the need to change position frequently, by doing weight shifts which the patient would learn in physical therapy, and the importance of checking the skin for pressure areas. After returning Nancy to her room, the COTA waited 20 minutes and then checked Nancy's skin. She appeared to tolerate the session well.

The following day, the OTR transported Nancy to the clinic for parts 3 and 4 of the initial assessment. The occupational performance components which were affected by her spinal injury included: muscle strength, range of motion, muscle tone, coordination, pain, sensation, body image, self-esteem, family relationships, and ability or need for adaptive techniques and equipment. While interviewing and observing the patient, the OTR used the session to advance the sitting angle of the chair to 70°, which the patient tolerated well.

Program Planning

After the patient was returned to her room the OTR completed part 6 of the initial assessment, occupational therapy intervention, which consists of writing the formal plan for Nancy's OT program. The OTR reviewed the "Patient and Therapist Goals" completed by the patient and the COTA, as well as the information recorded by the COTA on the other parts of the assessment form. The OTR also discussed with the COTA her impressions and concerns about Nancy.

Although Nancy was always to be treated as a special individual, based on the occupational therapy initial assessment of her rehabilitation needs, she appeared able to benefit from a typical OT spinal injury program at this facility.

Short-Term Goals

The OTR specified the following as short-term goals which were expected to be completed within one week:

1 Complete manual muscle test (MMT).
2 Complete sensory evaluation.
3 Complete Evaluation of Personal Independence (EPI).
4 Begin hand skills assessment.
5 Increase progressive sitting to 1½ hours three times per day at 90 degrees.

Each week new short-term goals would be established, based on Nancy's progress.

Long-Term Goals

As long-term goals, expected to be completed by discharge, the OTR listed the following:

1 Patient will be independent in feeding, dressing, and personal hygiene.
2 Patient will sit 8 hours to 10 hours daily with no problems.
3 Patient will acquire basic homemaking skills.
4 Patient will acquire necessary equipment.
5 Patient will explore vocational and leisure interests.
6 Patient will receive home program prior to discharge.

These long-term goals are also typical for persons with spinal injuries at the facility, and experience over time has demonstrated that most patients like Nancy will be able to meet these goals during their hospitalization. The OTR and COTA discussed the goals and how the goals would be individualized for Nancy. Then both staff members signed and dated the initial assessment form.

Continued Evaluation

For the rest of the week, while beginning treatment to achieve her goals, Nancy also continued to receive specific tests of her functions. These evaluations provided the baseline information from which her progress could be measured. These same evaluations would be repeated periodically throughout her hospital stay, and immediately before discharge, and the results compared with these initial findings.

First, the OTR completed the MMT and the sensory evaluation, and found that the patient differed from the picture of a "complete" C-6 spinal injured person, because she retained voluntary bilateral elbow extension, wrist flexion, and left wrist and finger motion. Her left arm was significantly stronger than her right arm. Nancy's sensation was tested to the T-12 dermatome level for pain, light touch, pressure, temperature, and proprioception. In general, Nancy had intact sensation to the C-6 level, impaired sensation to the T-12 level, and no sensation below that level. Proprioception was intact throughout, except for her fingers on the right hand, which appeared to have no sensation. The OTR felt that sensation appeared better on the left side than on the right, since Nancy responded more quickly when touched on the left.

That same day the COTA completed the EPI (Evaluation of Personal Independence), which is a test of physical daily living skills that was standardized at the facility. The COTA observed while Nancy performed a variety of tasks that included communication, eating, hygiene, and dressing. Then she graded Nancy's performance from "1" to "4," with "4" being the most independent, on specific activities within each daily living skill area. In general Nancy was independent in most areas of communication, required minimal to moderate assistance in eating and sink hygiene, and required maximum assistance for all other areas. Her total

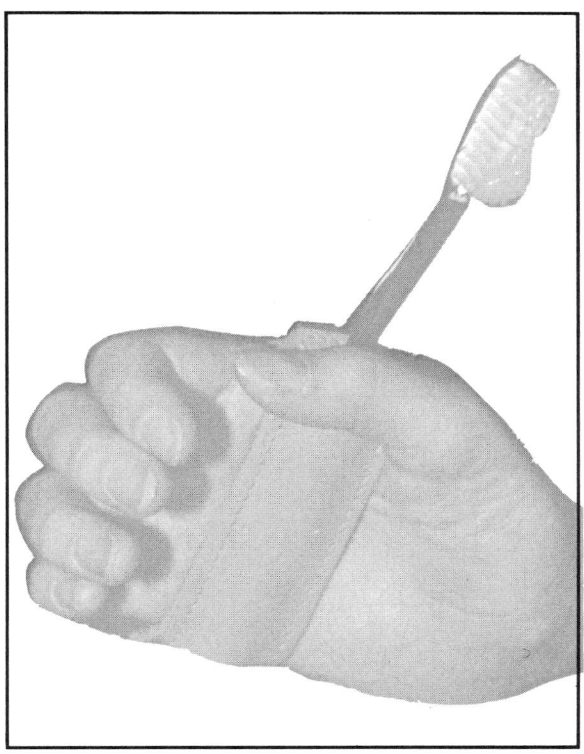

FIGURE 16-1. The Universal Cuff

score on the EPI was 520 of a possible 748.

The next day the COTA completed a hand skills assessment which had also been standardized at the facility. Nancy was unable to perform any bilateral hand skills subtests, and scored below 65 percent of the score for able-bodied persons on unilateral skills. The COTA also noted that on the unilateral tests Nancy stabilized herself by using one arm to hold onto the armrest of the wheelchair, which suggested that poor trunk balance might be interfering with Nancy's ability to use both hands together.

This completed the evaluation process for the patient. Baseline data had been obtained in the areas of personal independence, muscle strength, hand skills, coordination, and sensation. Goals had been established jointly with Nancy, and long-range goals for occupational therapy had been decided. Short-term goals would be updated weekly.

The partners decided that the COTA would take primary responsibility for Nancy's day-to-day occupational therapy program, with the OTR monitoring treatment by discussing the patient's progress with the COTA on a weekly basis, giving feedback and suggestions when appropriate, reading the COTA's progress notes prior to weekly interdisciplinary team rounds, and by treating Nancy on the COTA's days off.

Treatment Implementation

Week One

Although evaluation was the primary focus during Nancy's first week at the facility, treatment had also been in progress. The COTA ensured that the patient could continue the level of self-care she had attained in the acute care hospital by providing a universal cuff for different utensils. This cuff holds items to the palm of the hand and is useful when people have little or no grasping strength. Nancy used the cuff on her left hand initially, inserting her toothbrush, comb, and eating utensils. The COTA then made arrangements with other staff for these items to remain within Nancy's reach so she could maintain the highest possible level of independence. The universal cuff is shown in Figure 16-1.

The COTA also began passive range of motion to prevent joint stiffness in the right (nonmoving) hand and fingers. While some facilities use resting or static orthoses to prevent joint deformity and to facilitate development of functional hand positions, at this facility range of motion exercises and training with dynamic orthoses are used, unless the patient exhibits spasticity. This was not a problem for Nancy. The COTA instructed Nancy in the performance of short upper extremity exercises which she could do to prevent deconditioning, including the use of one-half pound and 1 pound wrist weights during simple active range of motion exercises.

In general, the patient tolerated her first week of treatment well, although she became lightheaded on several occasions when first transferred into her wheelchair. This was corrected easily by tilting the chair back for 1 minute at the beginning of each sitting session.

Week Two

By week two, the COTA felt that Nancy was ready to begin a more active therapy program. She asked her if she would like to try a ceramic project which could be set up in order to improve her strength, endurance, and coordination. Nancy agreed, and selected a small decorative ceramic box that had been previously poured using a mold. Nancy used a cleaning tool with a 1½ inch foam built-up handle to help increase the grip strength in her left hand. Moving the tool in a variety of planes to clean the seams of the box facilitated coordination. In addition, the COTA placed a 1-pound wrist weight on Nancy's right arm and 2-pounds on the left. Lifting her left arm to clean the seams and using her right to stabilize the ceramic project helped promote bilateral strength and endurance. She was able to work on this for 20 minutes, requiring several rest periods.

The COTA taught Nancy to perform self range of motion by using her more functional left hand to move her right wrist and fingers. She also cautioned her against hyperextending her fingers while her wrist was also extended, since this could excessively stretch the flexor tendons and prevent an effective tenodesis grasp.

Although her left hand was more functional, Nancy elected first to attempt writing by using her dominant right hand. Because Nancy had no functional pinch in her right hand, the COTA applied a wrist driven flexor hinge (reciprocal) orthosis from the department's supply of training equipment. Follow-up studies done by this facility indicate that early introduction to and training with such devices results in greater retention and usage after discharge. The greatest long-term use of reciprocal orthoses is by patients whose activities involve fine motor coordination, such as extensive writing and drawing. If a reciprocal orthosis proved practical for Nancy, a customized device could be made for her by the Orthotics Department; because such devices are quite expensive, the need for them must be carefully evaluated. By extending her wrist, Nancy could bring her fingers and thumb together to form a tripod pinch to hold a pencil. The COTA used simple connect-the-dot and tracing exercises to promote coordination, but Nancy had great difficulty with these, often overshooting the dots and drawing extremely crooked lines. Her attempt to write her name was barely legible.

The COTA worked with Nancy to establish adequate telephone skills since she received and made many calls; no special equipment was needed, because the COTA was able to suggest adaptive ways of lifting and holding the phone using both hands in place of single-handed palmar grasp. In self-feeding, Nancy continued to use her left, nondominant hand, but she progressed from a universal cuff to utensils with 1½ inch built-up handles. This change gave her more control, and she spilled less food. She was also pleased that she was eating more "normally." The COTA also worked with her on using a knife, and Nancy was able to cut soft foods, but still needed assistance with tougher items. Nancy began using the built-up handles for her personal hygiene as well.

Since Nancy was tolerating sitting at 90°, the COTA decided to procure an upright wheelchair with "quad pegs" (projections from the metal push-rim) on the wheels, so that Nancy could begin moving herself around the building. This would give her more independence, and the pushing would also increase her upper extremity strength and overall endurance. However, during the second week Nancy was able to push only 10 feet to 12 feet before tiring. At the same time her sitting time was advanced to 2½ hours, three times a day, with no skin problems.

Week Three

At the beginning of week three, the COTA used the dynamometer to re-evaluate Nancy's grip strength on the left. She found it had increased from 1 pound to 2½ pounds. There was still no measurable grip in the right hand. The patient continued to clean her ceramic piece, but the COTA cut the diameter of the built-up handles from 1½ inches to ½ inch. Wrist weight cuffs were continued, and the COTA used positioning of the ceramic project to force Nancy to reach higher and farther. Nancy was also able to increase the length of time she could work to 25 minutes.

Since the patient enjoyed playing cards and board games, the COTA suggested that these would be good activities to help promote right-hand dexterity and coordination. She demonstrated tenodesis grasp for Nancy, and had her use this technique to pick up game pieces and cards with her right hand. Nancy would alternate use of her hands since the right hand was not as functional as the left and tended to fatigue easily.

Nancy practiced propelling her wheelchair each day and was able to push herself approximately 20 feet. Her sitting time was advanced to 3½ hours, twice a day, with the additional option of 2 evening hours, which brought her total sitting time to an average of 8 hours per day. She continued to have no skin problems, and she took the responsibility for asking her nurse or therapist to assist her in performing weight shifts to reduce skin pressure.

Nancy expressed the desire to attempt writing with her left hand. With a ½ inch foam handle on a pencil she was able to write more quickly and legibly than with the reciprocal orthosis on her right hand shown in Figure 16-2. She decided she would like to practice with her left hand before deciding which hand she preferred to use for writing.

FIGURE 16-2. Reciprocal Orthosis

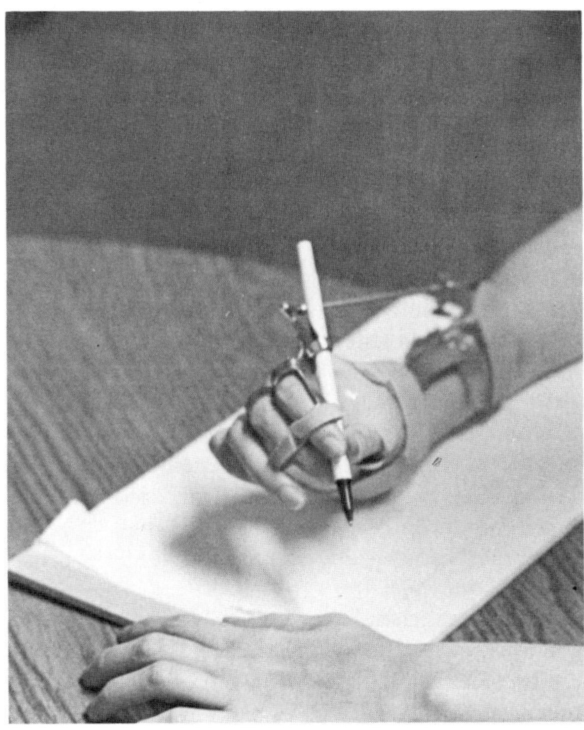

During this week, as she did every week, the COTA spent time discussing the physical and psychological value of each activity being used in therapy with Nancy. This appeared to help her continue to be motivated and to participate actively in her rehabilitation program.

As was done each week of the patient's stay, the COTA wrote a narrative progress note for the medical record. The OTR reveiwed this note and discussed the patient's progress with the COTA. The OTR then reported on Nancy's progress at interdisciplinary rounds.

Week Four

At the end of the first month of her hospitalization, Nancy appeared to have gained significant upper body strength and endurance. On the left, her lateral pinch had increased to 2 pounds and her grip strength to 3 pounds. The COTA and Nancy decided to remove the foam handles from her self-care equipment and her ceramic brush. Nancy expressed her pleasure that she no longer required such equipment.

The patient continued to paint her ceramic project, with wrist weights increased by 1 pound each, and positioning of her project was also increased. She was independent in moving her wheelchair around the clinic to get her ceramic materials and to set up her work area, as well as putting her supplies away at the end of therapy. Her handwriting improved gradually. Although awkward, she could write legibly within the lines of standard notebook paper using her left hand. She decided that she preferred to use her left hand to write, because she did not like how the orthosis looked on her right hand. At this point Nancy was using her left hand for most physical daily living skills, and in effect had switched dominance. This was supported by both the COTA and the OTR, since Nancy continued to have functional gains in her left hand, with very slow progress on the right.

Since her coordination and her endurance had improved, the COTA suggested she try typing with a typing stick in a universal cuff on her right hand. Nancy was able to use isolated finger movements to type with her left hand. She was familiar with the keyboard and had had a typing speed of 45 words per minute (wpm) prior to injury. On her initial typing trial she typed 9 wpm with 2 to 3 errors per line. By the end of the week she was able to type 12 wpm with very few errors.

The COTA provided Nancy with minimally resistive therapy putty and reviewed a hand exercise program with her. Nancy wished to do these exercises in her room during her free time, and since she was very motivated, the COTA permitted this. At the same time, the COTA cautioned the patient to exercise for only 10 minutes twice a day initially, so as not to overtire the muscles.

Because Nancy's trunk balance had improved, and she was maneuvering her wheelchair safely and with greater endurance, the COTA suggested that she try out a lightweight model, since many spinal injury patients, and younger people in particular, tend to prefer the sport-type wheelchairs for their permanent use. The chair selected did not have pegs on the wheel rims, so Nancy used push mitts to create friction and give her a stronger push. Using the lighter chair, she was able to push herself 60 feet with only two rest intervals.

Nancy's sitting time was increased to 4 hours twice daily, with an optional 2 hours in the evening. This sitting schedule continued for the duration of her hospitalization, and she continued to tolerate the schedule well, with no skin problems.

Week Five

It is customary at this facility for the interdisciplinary team to hold a discharge planning meeting with the patient and family members if possible. Nancy's mother came from New York to participate in the meeting and remained for 1 week to become familiar with her daughter's rehabilitation program. The COTA met with the OTR prior to the meeting to discuss the occupational therapy goals that should be accomplished before discharge. The COTA attended the meeting and reported that in addition to the activities Nancy had been doing, she could become independent in dressing, simple meal preparation, and in operating a personal computer. The COTA also said that Nancy would need to have a wheelchair ordered, since she was currently using one from the OT equipment pool. Nursing felt the patient should be independent in self-catheterization and turning and positioning in bed, and the physical therapist stated that Nancy should become independent in all transfers to and from her wheelchair.

Nancy agreed with all the goals except ordering the wheelchair. Although the physician had been explicit with her regarding her prognosis (since there had been no motor return in the legs), Nancy still believed she might walk, and did not want to buy a permanent wheelchair. She also said that although friends had invited her to live with them upon discharge she would prefer to get her own apartment. The team felt that her daily activities would take more time and energy than they had prior to her injury, and recommended that she consider having a roommate who could provide some assistance. The social worker planned to help Nancy work out suitable living arrangements prior to discharge.

Nancy's mother attended occupational therapy sessions with her daughter for the remainder of the week and participated in educational experiences, such as learning to assist her daughter with transfers in physical therapy and getting items set up for Nancy's self-care.

During this week, the COTA had to change Nancy's therapy time so that Nancy could work on self-catheterization on a very regular basis. The COTA was aware that at some facilities occupational therapy personnel also work with the patient on self-catheterization and bowel programs, particularly in the development of the necessary hand skills and acquisition of adaptive equipment. However, at this facility, the "Cath Team," a group of specially trained technicians supervised by the nursing department, was responsible for assisting Nancy in meeting this goal. Other team members, such as the COTA, primarily provided support, reinforcement, and schedule changes as needed.

The patient noticed movement in her right hand and discussed this with the COTA, who reported it to the OTR. The OTR re-evaluated Nancy's active range of motion and muscle strength on her right, and found that she had gained approximately 10° of active range in metacarpophalangeal flexion and extension. Nancy was extremely anxious to work toward strengthening the muscles of her right hand and had to be cautioned not to overwork her muscles. The OTR agreed to re-evaluate her range every day until discharge to detect any improvement.

Since Nancy's previous and future vocational interests had involved computers, she was interested in learning to operate the microcomputer in the OT department, and began the first of the three training tapes. She was able to insert and remove the disk from the disk drive, and to operate the tape recorder independently.

With the COTA's help, Nancy began working on upper body dressing and learned to put on a pullover shirt. She needed minimal assistance getting a front-buttoned shirt around her back while in her wheelchair, but could button it independently.

During this week the COTA obtained permission for Nancy to have a day-pass to begin community re-integration. She arranged for Nancy to go to the zoo and to a restaurant with her mother. Nancy reported that it was "very therapeutic" for her to be away from the hospital setting for the first time in 3 months. She pushed her wheelchair for a short period around the zoo and became very tired, but she was proud that she was able to feed herself at the restaurant, needing only to have her steak cut. She also said this day-pass helped her to realize how tired she would become if she did everything for herself when she was discharged. Nancy and the COTA discussed other out-trips she could take, either with an OT group, or with Therapeutic Recreation, and Nancy signed up for an outside activity the following week.

Week Six

Nancy continued to make steady gains. Her left hand grip increased to 6 pounds. She had nearly 20° of active range at the MCPs of her right hand. Her handwriting was more legible, and she was typing at 16 wpm. She was independent in wheelchair mobility throughout the day. In addition to the computer, she worked on a calculator and an adding machine. These were machines she had used on the job in the past and anticipated using in the future, so the COTA recommended working on hand function and vocational goals at the same time. Nancy finished her ceramic project and gave it to her mother as a going-away present. The COTA suggested copper tooling for a new activity, advising Nancy that it would be more difficult because of the resistance of the copper, but that it would help Nancy work toward greater strength and coordination. Nancy chose a mold of a skier, one of her favorite sports, and worked with a 3-pound weight on her right wrist and 4 pounds on her left.

With the COTA's help, Nancy practiced putting on her pants, using the elevating head of her bed to assist her to a sitting position and to maintain trunk stability. However, she was unable to roll side to side to pull the trousers over her hips. While rolling could be worked on in OT, since it was being worked on as a major exercise in physical therapy, the COTA and Nancy agreed to address other occupational therapy goals and to continue to work on dressing the following week.

Week Seven

This week Nancy was able to roll side to side, and learned to pull her pants over her hips. It took her 45 minutes to dress herself.

Nancy had finished the copper tooling, and was ready to sand the mounting board. The COTA set up the table so that sanding could be done on an inclined plane to work for increased strength and endurance. Because of the increased difficulty of this task, the wrist weights were removed.

During this week, Nancy worked on meal preparation, and was able to complete a simple meal of a salad and grilled cheese sandwich. She needed no special equipment, but did use adaptive techniques for holding and stabilizing cooking utensils. The COTA reviewed energy-saving techniques, such as placing frequently used items within easy reach. Modifying a regular kitchen to make it wheelchair accessible was discussed in detail. The COTA also talked with Nancy about safety precautions, especially the possibility of burns and cuts on the hands and arms due to diminished sensation.

Nancy's right hand active range had increased significantly, and she was now able to use utensils with a 2-inch foam handle. She was able to alternate hands for eating, and for other self-care activities, which seemed to reduce her fatigue as well as provide additional exercise to the right hand.

Nancy was still not psychologically ready to order a permanent wheelchair. In view of her impending discharge, the COTA arranged to order a rental wheelchair for Nancy's discharge.

Week Eight

During the final week of Nancy's hospitalization the focus was on refining her skills, completing discharge evaluations, and providing a home program.

Nancy was able to dress herself in 30 minutes, except for her shoes and socks, which she was still not strong enough to don. The COTA completed a final Evaluation of Personal Independence, and a discharge Hand Skills Assessment. Nancy had a score of 690 out of a possible 748 on the EPI, as compared with 520 at admission. Her hand skills scores increased by 20 percent in both hands.

The OTR completed a discharge evaluation of muscle strength and sensation. She found that Nancy had gained an average of ½ of a muscle grade in her upper extremities, in all but the thumb and IP movements of her right hand. Her sensation appeared to be intact to the C-7 level. All of her discharge evaluations indicated that Nancy had made significant progress during her admission.

Nancy completed her copper tooling project and the last of the computer training tapes. In addition, she had completed the goals set for her by nursing and physical therapy: she could transfer independently, turn in bed, and do self-catheterization.

Program Discontinuation

After discussing Nancy's progress and discharge status with the OTR, the COTA completed a written home program for Nancy. On Nancy's last day of treatment, the COTA reviewed the home program with her. The program included recommendations for progressive activities that Nancy could perform independently in her apartment to improve her strength, endurance, and coordination.

The COTA recommended that Nancy increase her sitting time of 4 hours by ½ hour per week. Since she only needed to return to bed for a few minutes to do self-catheterization, she could increase her tolerance to 8 hours to 10 hours at a time if she wished. The COTA stressed the importance of Nancy's monitoring her skin for red areas each day, and for decreasing her sitting time if red areas appeared. If actual skin breakdown occurred, Nancy was instructed to call her physician without delay.

The COTA also made sure that the rental wheelchair fit well and was adequate for Nancy's needs. The COTA reviewed wheelchair and cushion care, instructing Nancy to contact the rental agent if any problems occurred.

Realizing that Nancy had a very high level of motivation, with the potential for overexertion, the COTA again cautioned her to rest adequately and to exercise only as prescribed on the home programs from PT and OT. She also discussed with her the ways to ask for help when needed.

Finally, the COTA and Nancy discussed occupational therapy goals for her readmission, which was planned to occur in 2 months to 3 months. Nancy wished to continue working on the "Patient and Therapist Goals" which had been discussed at admission. In particular, she wanted to complete the adaptive driving program and learn to drive with hand controls, for which she would need more upper extremity strength than she currently had. The COTA also suggested that the second admission would be a good time to look at the need for a permanent chair, since the rental was a standard and not a lightweight, and Nancy agreed to discuss it at that time. Also, Nancy wanted to explore heavier homemaking skills, such as ironing, vacuuming, and additional meal preparation. Through her home program she could continue to work on building her strength and endurance as she had done during her hospitalization, and this would help her to be ready for more advanced work on the next admission.

Nancy was discharged to an apartment, with a roommate, 2 months after her admission to the rehabilitation center.

CHAPTER 17

The Schizophrenic Young Adult

Patty L. Barnett, COTA
Margaret Drake, OTR

Introduction

Owing to legislative reassignment of mental health funds, a state mental hospital was scheduled to close. Five hundred patients had to be located in new settings. The legislature had reappropriated funds from the hospital budget to be given to the home counties of each of the patients to set up a program for these relocations.

Jefferson County was the home of about 70 of those needing placement, so the county mental health association designed a program requiring registered occupational therapists, certified occupational therapy assistants, social workers, and a recreational coordinator. The program was located in a community-based center with an existing sheltered workshop. Adequate space was provided for additional offices and an occupational therapy clinic. There were 10 new group homes established in Jefferson County, with a capacity of six to eight patients each and having a 24-hour houseparent. Occupational therapy treatment took place in the center, where patients were brought by van for a six-hour program, five days per week. Occupational therapy personnel also provided treatment in the individual group homes whenever necessary (PRN basis).

Case Background

Gordon, a 23-year-old patient, was from an upper middle class suburban community. He was the middle child of three. His mother's career as a concert violinist had been stifled for a number of reasons, and she had started to mold Gordon into the musician she had always wanted to be. He had been considered a child prodigy. Gordon had willingly participated in this unstated plan by taking lessons and giving recitals until his schizophrenic break at age 16. Prior to his five-year stay in the state hospital, he had had numerous admissions at the local acute psychiatic unit of a major hospital and a private psychiatric hospital. At the time of the latter inpatient stay, the psychiatrist recommended that Gordon receive ongoing long-term care. It was felt that this action would also provide improvement for the entire family's mental health. Gordon had been diagnosed as schizophrenic from the onset, but the refined diagnosis for admission to the state hospital was schizophrenia undifferentiated.

The patient's childhood had been unremarkable, with the exception of a lack of peer interaction due to his mother's insistence on his violin practice. Teachers reported that Gordon was a good student, but expressed concern about his history of social isolation. No other unusual behaviors were noted until Gordon was in the eleventh grade. At this point, he became very strongly infatuated with his social studies teacher, who gently rebuffed his adolescent advances. His response to this apparent rejection ranged from abusive statements to auditory hallucinations. His "voices" had seemingly been telling him that the teacher was attracted to him and desired more than a student-teacher relationship. His increasingly disturbed behavior after this episode resulted in Gordon's first hospitalization. Subsequent exacerbations and rehospitalizations were related to hallucinations about a variety of slightly older females.

Gordon's older sister, like his mother, had been a nurturing, protective, and controlling influence. His relationship to her had been similar to that with his mother. His younger brother had had a close affiliation with his father, unlike Gordon, whose closest kinship was with his mother. His brother had been an athlete and a popular school leader. There had been almost no brotherly relationship between them.

The father was employed as a highly respected manager of a local television station. This job frequently required elaborate social gatherings at their home. Gordon's increasingly bizarre behavior had been an embarrassment at these events. The state hospital admission had removed him from the local scene, where his presence had been extremely disruptive to the family's life; however, the family remained supportive and genuinely interested in his receiving appropriate care.

Medication had controlled his worst symptoms but caused mild tardive dyskinesia, or late-appearing impairment of voluntary movement,[1] which had been controlled by other medication. Over the course of five years in the state hospital, a variety of antipsychotic (neuroleptic) medications were tried before an effective combination of antipsychotic and anticholinergic drugs, which serve to block the transmission of nerve impulses through the parasympathetic nerves,[1] was found. The latter drugs decrease parkinsonian symptoms, which occasionally occur with neuroleptic drugs.

Gordon's return to his home community was expected to cause adjustment problems for the family, since his parents, who were approaching retirement, remained in their home but were considering buying a condominium.

A discharge summary from the state hospital that preceded his placement in a group home indicated dysfunction in socialization, self-care skills, and absence of work skills and of some prevocational skills. Gordon had his violin in the hospital but was unable to use it often because of the medication's side-effects and also because the violin was locked up most of the time.

Assessment

One COTA and one OTR were assigned to work together as a team with a group of the recently relocated patients. The occupational therapy staff at the center established a plan to evaluate each patient upon arrival. Screening had been done by a multidisciplinary team before the patients were chosen for treatment at the center. Because of Gordon's past treatment and diagnosis, the following assessments were chosen: the Scorable Self-Care Evaluation (SSCE) and the Schroeder Block Campbell Adult Psychiatric Sensory Integration Evaluation (SBC). Evaluation of socialization skills was to be done on an informal basis by the occupational therapy team members. The outcomes of these evaluations were expected to be the basis of an individual program plan for the sheltered workshop as well as the occupational therapy treatment plan. The OTR/COTA team's goal was to complete the battery of Gordon's evaluations within a week after his first attendance at the center. They both met with the patient the first day to introduce themselves, briefly explain the purposes of the program, and verify their choice of assessments. Both team members had read the discharge summary and family history provided by the state hospital.

The most crucial aspect of re-entry into the community is self-care; therefore, the Scorable Self-Care Evaluation was initiated first. The SSCE, which is a structured test, was administered by the COTA under the supervision of the OTR. The results indicated the following information:

Initial Appearance

The first area evaluated was initial appearance. Gordon's clothing was mismatched. His dress slacks did not fit his 6'1" frame, and it was obvious he had been wearing his clothes for some time as they were speckled with spots and stains. His appearance was unkempt with a day's growth of whiskers and recently cut but uncombed hair. His fingernails were dirty, untrimmed, and tobacco stained. Gordon had the typical schizophrenic "S" posture with slumped shoulders and lordosis. His arms hung limp at their sides, confirming the occupational therapist's decision to also administer the Schroeder Block Campbell assessment.

Orientation

Gordon's orientation was appropriate, in that he knew where he was, could sign his name, and give his birth date. He was unable to accurately give his home address although he attempted to remember. Gordon's concept of time appeared to be almost absent. He did not wear a watch and stated that he hadn't since admission to the state hospital. Gordon reported that this had caused him numerous problems since he often had been late for or missed scheduled appointments. He also stated that when his parents had seen him the previous Friday, they had promised to buy him a new watch and some new clothes.

Hygiene

In the session of the SSCE addressing hygiene, Gordon was unable to say how often a person should shower, wash face and hair, shave, brush teeth, or comb hair. He said he had been told when to do these activities in the hospital but indicated he didn't know how often they were required for adequate hygiene.

Communication

When Gordon was given the telephone book and asked to look up emergency numbers, he exhibited unfamiliarity with the process of using the book.

First Aid

He could recall having had a first aid class in high school but could not remember any life saving and first aid procedures.

Food Selection

Gordon was presented with a blank menu sheet and asked to plan a balanced meal. He was unable to take the first step by naming a main dish he was accustomed to eating. However, he said he "loved barbequed pork rinds" and noted that "they almost never have them" in the snack machine at the hospital.

Household Chores

In organizing household chores such as dishwashing and laundry, Gordon was given cards with tasks to place in the proper sequence. He laid the cards in a row on the table and began to read them aloud, suddenly turning his head to the side to say, "No this is women's work. I'm not going to do this because she just wants me to do it with her so she can be my girlfriend. She is just like my social studies teacher in high school." He then turned to the COTA and said, "You want me to do this so you can touch me!" When the COTA asked who he had just been speaking to, he said the voice had told him not to do women's work and to be beware of women trying to seduce him. Since the patient did not appear excessively agitated, the COTA, speaking in a calm voice, assured Gordon that she did not wish to be his girlfriend and that her goal was to help him. Gordon's facial expression demonstrated that he accepted her statement. In a pleading tone of voice he said, "I really want help. Please help me." The evaluation was continued without disruptions.

Safety

In analyzing picture cards for dangerous situations, the patient seemed to be unaware of basic safety practices.

Leisure Pursuits

When asked about leisure pursuits, Gordon was unable to name any except playing the violin and smoking. He continued by discussing his desire to do more with his violin.

Transportation

Gordon was handed a city map and asked to find the street where his parent's home was located. He acted confused and overwhelmed with the task.

Financial Management

He appeared to have no problem with simple monetary transactions; however, he was unfamiliar with the basic check writing procedure, paying bills, and budgeting. Gordon knew that the group home operator would manage his money and provide him with an allowance for such items as cigarettes, snacks, and grooming supplies.

The Scorable Self-Care Evaluation scoring record form is shown in Figure 17-1.

The following day the OTR and COTA discussed the results of this evaluation. They went on with their planned administration of the Schroeder Block Campbell Adult Psychiatric Sensory Integration Evaluation, with the COTA administering two parts of the assessment: body image and self-reported childhood history. The OTR would be interpreting the results of these two sections.

In the body image section, Gordon was directed to draw a person. He took more than half an hour to draw the minute details of the female figure's clothing and hair. He appeared to be hallucinating during the drawing, turning his head to the side and "talking to the air." The COTA recognized that the picture was of her.

On the self-reported childhood history Gordon discussed his family environment. He felt that he could never achieve the perfection in music that his mother desired. When asked about other family members who might have had mental illness, Gordon recalled his mother's brother, who had been in a mental hospital in the West. He appeared to remember almost nothing about his own physical development milestones. He described his childhood as being "normal" with no particular scholastic difficulty. When asked about events related to his own birth, Gordon slumped over and seemed to be using his mother's words and tone of voice when he stated that the birth was painful and the pregnancy had not been planned. He also stated that he had always tried to please his mother to make up for the pain she had endured for him.

Figure 17-2 shows the Schroeder Block Campbell Psychiatric Sensory Integration Evaluation summary sheet.

The COTA and the OTR met and conferred about the results of this assessment. In reporting the part that she had administered, the OTR noted that Gordon appeared to have right-side dominance in eye, hand, and foot, which most likely contributed to his proficiency in playing the violin. Lordosis was present as were jerky neck movements (probably a result of the residual tardive dyskinesia). He exhibited a shuffling gait and had restricted arm movements. Fine motor strength and coordination of the hand and wrist seemed quite good, however. Gordon stated that he had done some hand exercises in the hospital which had been taught to him by his high school violin teacher. He did not appear to have any problem with visual pursuit except when his neck jerked, which occurred when he had intentional movement of the head but not when he was relaxed. This was further evidenced by his successful playing of the violin. Bilateral coordination and crossing the midline tasks were accomplished without difficulty. Gordon exhibited the classic Romberg sign, which is an inability to maintain balance with one's eyes closed while holding the arms out and feet together. His trunk and upper extremity strength was somewhat weak. He exhibited some overflow movements in his mouth and chin when exerting his whole body. His neck postures did not appear to have a reflexive basis. Gordon's protective extension was adequate, as was his equilibrium while sitting.

In discussing the body image drawing, the likeness of the COTA was immediately obvious to the OTR despite the primitive nature of the drawing. The COTA described the bizarre, hallucinatory behavior of Gordon during the drawing session. When questioned further, the COTA indicated that the patient seemed to have problems relating to women appropriately. She questioned whether he had ever had a normal heterosexual relationship. Recalling the family history, she noted that both the mother and older sister dominated Gordon. The COTA was aware of Gordon's interest in establishing a relationship with her.

Evaluation of socialization skills was informal. Part of this observation had occurred during the formal evaluations. The inappropriateness of his behavior toward females was the most obvious problem area. His hallucinations appeared to oc-

FIGURE 17-1. SSCE Scoring Record Form

SSCE Scoring Record

	Score			Maximum Possible Points
Personal care	_____	1.	Initial appearance	8
	_____	2.	Orientation	7
	_____	3.	Hygiene	6
	_____	4.	Communications	6
	_____	5.	First aid	24
	_____		SUBTOTAL	51
Housekeeping	_____	1.	Foods selection	26
	_____	2.	House chores	10
	_____	3.	Safety	6
	_____	4.	Laundry	15
	_____		SUBTOTAL	57
Work and leisure	_____	1.	Leisure activity	4
	_____	2.	Transportation	4
	_____	3.	Job seeking	4
	_____		SUBTOTAL	12
Financial management	_____	1.	Making correct change	4
	_____	2.	Checking	11
	_____	3.	Paying personal bills	5
	_____	4.	Budgeting	10
	_____	5.	Procurement of supplemental income	1
	_____	6.	Source of income	6
	_____		SUBTOTAL	37
Total score				157

Patient: ____

Date tested: ____________________

Reproduced Courtesy of Clark, EN, Peters, M: *The Scorable Self-Care Evaluation,* Thorofare, NJ: SLACK, Inc., 1984.

FIGURE 17-2. "SBC" Adult Psychiatric Sensory Integration Evaluation Summary Sheet

Client ______________________ Age ___ Sex ___ Subject No. ______________

Primary diagnosis ______________________ DSM III ___ ___ ___ . ___ ___ 1st Test Date ___ / ___ / ___

Secondary diagnosis ______________________ DSM III ___ ___ ___ . ___ ___ 2nd Test Date ___ / ___ / ___

Physical diagnosis ______________________ DSM III ___ ___ ___ . ___ ___ 3rd Test Date ___ / ___ / ___

Medication ______________ # ___ ___ , Dosage (24 hr. total) ___ ___ ___ ___ ___ mg.

Medication ______________ # ___ ___ , Dosage (24 hr. total) ___ ___ ___ ___ ___ mg.

Medication ______________ # ___ ___ , Dosage (24 hr. total) ___ ___ ___ ___ ___ mg.

(Key: 0 = no problem, 1 = slight, 2 = moderate, 3 = severe)

1. Dominance: ______ eye, ______ hand, ______ foot. (1 = Mixed dominance)
2. Posture .... ___
3. Neck rotation .... ___
4. Gait .... ___
5. Hand .... ___
6. Grip .... rt ___ lft ___
7. Fine motor control .... rt ___ lft ___
8. Diadochokinesis .... ___
9. Finger-thumb opposition .... ___
10. Visual pursuits .... ___
11. Bilateral coordination-UE .... ___
12. Crossing midline .... ___
13. Stability—UE .... ___
14. Stability—trunk .... ___
15. Classic Romberg .... ___
16. Sharpened Romberg, EO ___ EC .... ___
17. Overflow movements .... ___
18. Neck righting .... ___
19. Rolling .... ___
20. Asym. tonic neck reflex .... ___
21. Sym. tonic neck reflex .... ___
22. Tonic labyrinthine reflex .... ___
23. Protective extension .... ___
24. Seated equilibrium .... ___
25. Body image .... ___

Total score obtained
____
Divide by number of items tested and scored = Index score ☐

Reproduced Courtesy of C. Schroeder, OTR

FIGURE 17-2. "SBC" Adult Psychiatric Sensory Integration Evaluation Summary Sheet (continued)

SUMMARY

I. PHYSICAL ASSESSMENT:	☐	Norm	.50	Min	.90	Mod	1.30	Severe	3.00	
II. ABNORMAL MOVEMENTS:	☐	0	Norm	1	Min	3	Mod	5	Severe	14
III. CHILDHOOD HISTORY:	☐	0	Norm	2	Min	6	Mod	10	Severe	29

Therapist's signature ______________

Schroeder Block Campbell

cur only when in the presence of females. He seemed to have normal friendly relations with the other males in the group. Investigation by the social worker indicated that Gordon had been placed in an all male group home because of his inappropriate behavior with women.

On the basis of the assessment results, the following summary of Gordon's resources and problems was prepared:

Resources:

1 Concerned family.
2 Musical background.
3 Good level of cooperation.
4 Desire for help.
5 Ability to remember instructions.
6 Bilateral hand capabilities.

Limitations:

1 Relating to women.
2 General socialization.
3 Grooming and hygiene.
4 Prevocational skills.
5 Self-care.
6 Use of leisure time.
7 Decreased strength.
8 Positive Romberg sign.
9 Posture.
10 Tardive dyskinesia symptoms (neck jerk).

Treatment Planning

The COTA assisted the OTR in treatment planning in a session with Gordon. Basic objectives of the center's programs concerned self-care, readjustment to the community, familiarization with community resources, development of work and prevocational skills, and normalization. Gordon's problem areas fit into the guidelines of service provided by the center. With this in mind, the occupational therapy staff and Gordon considered which of his problems required habilitation and which required rehabilitation. Those that required habilitation could be approached in a developmental way, accepting Gordon at his current level of functioning and working with him to advance to the next level. Areas requiring habilitation were general socialization, relating to women, and physical strength. The other areas which required rehabilitation would be approached through re-education.

Long-Term Goals

The following long-term goals were set with Gordon:

1 Develop and demonstrate appropriate socialization behaviors.
2 Demonstrate independence in all self-care activities.
3 Attain long-term employment.
4 Develop improved sensory integration.
5 Utilize leisure time effectively.

The COTA and OTR talked with Gordon together during this session since both had administered parts of the evaluations. The team related Gordon's problem areas to things that had happened during portions of the evaluations. Gordon concurred with their observations and the goals they selected. These goals would be approached and achieved by working on short-term objectives. The short-term objectives were set to be accomplished in one week's time. Each week's progress was to be assessed and recorded, and the short-term objectives would be re-evaluated and updated if appropriate. The first set of short-term objectives for Gordon was chosen so that there was one specific goal related to each long-term goal.

Short-Term Goals

These were delineated as follows:

1 Participate in male and female group for 30 minutes without obviously hallucinating.
2 Arrive at center shaved, groomed, and appropriately dressed.
3 Utilize new watch to keep own schedule in the center.
4 Participate in at least 15 minutes of moderately strenuous group exercise.
5 Complete five page leisure check list.

Social Skills

This area would be worked on in a task group run by the COTA and held in the occupational therapy clinic. The format of the group required each participant to work on the same individual project. Through this activity, Gordon would have opportunities to share tools and supplies and also to discuss patterns and techniques. The COTA guided this interaction with the future objective of discussion of individual problems and solutions.

Appearance

In preparation for the "grand opening" of the center, the COTA and OTR had completed a checklist of grooming/hygiene requirements to aid participants in developing self-care skills. Gordon was given a copy, and the COTA reviewed each item with him. She answered his questions, such as how to use a fingernail brush and floss his teeth. His progress was to be checked by the COTA on a daily basis.

Punctuality

During the goal-setting conference, Gordon was provided with a written copy of the schedule the OTR/COTA team had developed. They stressed the necessity for punctuality with him, and Gordon earnestly agreed to observe the following schedule. Occupational therapy personnel responsibilities were also noted.

9:00 Grooming check by COTA
9:30 Task group—COTA
10:30 Refreshment break
10:45 Individual therapy/leisure counseling — OTR
11:30 Exercise group—shared by COTA and OTR
12:00 Lunch
1:00 Sheltered workshop employment
2:30 Refreshment break
2:45 Sheltered workshop employment
4:00 Time card check with workshop foreman

Exercise

Gordon's exercise program would take place within the context of a structured daily class of both men and women. His strength and balance were addressed here as well as providing opportunities for heterosexual socialization. The OTR and COTA conferred each day about which exercises would be emphasized, and how they would grade them to meet individual needs.

Leisure Checklist

Areas included in the leisure checklist were socialization, creative interests, exercises, spectator/audience events, and educational programs. He was instructed to find time at the group home to complete this form.

Treatment Implementation

At the end of the first week of his program, Gordon had successfully accomplished the first short-term objective, although he said it had been difficult not to answer the voice when it spoke to him. In the early part of the week, the COTA had to remind him when he started responding to the voice. She rewarded him with a large bag of pork rinds at the end of the fifth session. He held the bag and expressed surprise and gratitude appropriately, thanking her for both the gift and her interest. In the following weeks, the group was able to begin to identify individual problems and suggest solutions or possible alternatives. Gordon was an active participant. He had been able to use the grooming/hygiene checklist successfully. He had received praise and compliments from other staff at the center, which reinforced his efforts. As the weeks progressed, he seemed to develop a real pride in his appearance.

The occupational therapy team shared Gordon's short-term objective on punctuality with the other staff members, who agreed to report any deviations from his schedule to them. The sheltered workshop staff said that Gordon had been late from his break three days the first week. After adjustments were made in his paycheck, this behavior corrected itself, and he had not been late during the last two days of the week. The OTR discussed this with Gordon, and he agreed to continue working on this objective.

During the first week, there was no measurable change in strength or equilibrium. By the fourth week, Gordon demonstrated increased balance by walking back and forth on the balance beam to the cheers of his fellow exercise classmates. His strength increased very slowly, but the length of time he could endure exercise increased 50 percent by the fourth week.

Completion of the interest checklist indicated that playing the violin and socializing with others were most important. Successful interactions with the COTA and other female group participants appeared to influence this choice for him. He still had occasional lapses of inappropriate interaction, however. The OTR, working in collaboration with the night recreation coordinator for the group homes, developed a schedule of cultural events which included free concerts, museum visits, and plays. Gordon attended several concerts and participated in a museum outing.

Gordon's renewed involvement with his violin was a slow process. He tried to practice in the group home at night, much to the annoyance of the other residents. The recreation coordinator saw his potential and helped him to arrange a time and place that were less disruptive for others.

After observing Gordon's level of capability in the sheltered workshop, the OTR made an appointment for him with a vocational rehabilitation agency. After their assessment of his skills and potential, Gordon was assigned to an apprenticeship in which he learned the care and maintenance of stringed instruments.

Program Discontinuation

It is anticipated that Gordon will need a structured environment such as the group home and the mental health center indefinitely. Without close supervision, the staff members felt that he would revert to his previous level of dysfunction. He was discontinued from the occupational therapy program when all short- and long-term objectives had been accomplished. The coordinator of services at the center continued to follow Gordon's case and agreed to initiate a new occupational therapy referral if Gordon's behavior indicated that former problems were beginning to recur.

At the occupational therapy program discontinuation conference, the social worker noted that

Gordon, under the auspices of the vocational rehabilitation agency, was now employed at a part-time job in a local music store. The store allowed him to use a listening studio as a practice room, which eventually led to his involvement with other musicians and giving performances. Part of the process required that he learn to use the public transportation system. The vocational counselor also encouraged Gordon to take a class at the adult night school in order to complete his high school equivalency tests.

Gordon's interaction with his family increased and improved. His parents were proud of his efforts and accomplishments, both personally and with the violin. This led to their allowing Gordon to spend increasing amounts of time visiting them in their new condominium. He appeared happy and comfortable living in the structured environment of the group home.

Reference

1. Miller BF and Keane CB: *Encyclopedia and Dictionary of Medicine, Nursing and Allied Health*, 3rd Edition. Philadelphia: WB Saunders, 1983.

Bibliography

Mosey AC: *Activities Therapy*. New York: Raven Press, 1973.

Tiffany EG: Psychiatry and mental health. In: *Willard and Spackman's Occupational Therapy*, 6th Edition. Philadelphia: JB Lippincott, 1983.

CHAPTER 18

The Rheumatoid Arthritic Adult

Robin A. Jones, COTA/L
Sheryl R. Kantor, OTR/L

Introduction

Barbie, a 30-year old female, was diagnosed as having rheumatoid arthritis at age 25. She had bilateral involvement in the elbows, wrists, hands, knees, and metatarsophalangeal joints, her major complaints being pain and swelling of both hands and feet. Both hands were showing early signs of boutonniere deformities at the second, third, and fourth fingers. Mild volar wrist subluxations were present bilaterally; however, this did not interfere with her function. Crepitations at the shoulders and elbows were evident, more so on the right than on the left. A small subcutaneous nodule was noted on her right elbow, which was frequently irritated. There were no systemic manifestations; however, Barbie complained of mild dryness in her mouth. The patient's condition was persistent, and it progressively interfered with her daily lifestyle. She had decreased her activity and had difficulty caring for herself, her husband, and their active 3-year-old daughter. Barbie was forced to take a sick leave from her job.

The patient's rheumatologist started her on a bimonthly treatment with gold therapy. However, she eventually began using prednisone because of the persistence of the arthritis and lack of response to nonsteroidal anti-inflammatory agents.

Barbie continued to be followed by her rheumatologist; however, consultations with another rheumatology specialist were suggested since her health was deteriorating so rapidly. The laboratory data and x-ray reconfirmed the diagnosis of active rheumatoid arthritis with mild structural changes, but no extra-articular disease was clinically evident. The consulting rheumatologist's finding was: "The client was doing poorly and losing ground, despite a reasonable medical program." The physician recommended this as an optimal time for a thorough review of her disease process and a good multidisciplinary rehabilitation program. Active physical therapy and occupational therapy programs were strongly advised.

Barbie was seen in an outpatient arthritis clinic and was screened by a registered occupational therapist and a registered physical therapist (RPT).

It was determined that she could benefit from an inpatient stay at the rehabilitation facility. Owing to the location of the facility and her responsibilities for her young child, Barbie chose to have her therapy at home. A home interdisciplinary program was initiated which included nursing, occupational therapy, physical therapy, and social work. The treatment team felt that this was not the ideal course of treatment; however, because of the patient's concern for her family, it was agreed that therapy would continue in her home. (Homecare was covered under the patient's insurance policy.)

Assessment

In assessing management of this patient by the occupational therapist and the COTA in the home setting, it should be kept in mind that the OTR must be involved in the first visit and at least once a month thereafter, according to the American Occupational Therapy Association's publication, *AOTA Guidelines for Occupational Therapy Personnel*, which presents a format of recommended supervision.[1] The patient was to be seen for 1 hour, four times per week, for 6 weeks. All sessions were approximately 1 hour, except for the initial evaluation, which was nearly 2 hours. The OTR was involved on a weekly basis for supervision purposes, while the COTA visited daily.

Prior to scheduling the initial evaluation, the physician's orders were received by the OTR for the following services:

1. Range of motion evaluation and program.
2. Joint protection and teaching for all daily living skills: self-care, child care, homemaking, avocation, vocation, and community activities.
3. Work simplification evaluation.
4. Splinting evaluation.
5. Adaptive equipment/assistive devices evaluation.
6. Education regarding the diagnosis, management, and therapeutic process.

The precautions were to avoid sustained resistance since the joints were currently inflamed.

Together, the OTR and the COTA began the evaluation process through data collection, with each being responsible for specific areas of the evaluation. The OTR was responsible for selecting the evaluation process for assessment of the following skill areas and performance components: independent living/daily living, sensorimotor, cognitive, and psychological. The OTR evaluated passive range of motion (PROM), active range of motion (AROM), upper extremity function, and musculoskeletal status. The COTA completed a nine hole peg test, grasp and pinch test (one time only within limits of pain), sharp/dull, two point discrimination, and position sense tests. It should be noted that an entry-level COTA would need direct supervision until he or she displayed competence in the ability to complete these evaluation procedures independently. A joint OTR and COTA assessment for activities of daily living, home care, child care, community living skills and vocational/avocational needs was also completed as shown in Figure 18-1.

Barbie was interviewed using a structured format to gather information regarding her social history and personal goals. The OTR initiated the interview, while the COTA completed the assigned areas. Communication between the OTR and the COTA was ongoing, with data being jointly interpreted. Evaluation documentation was written by the OTR and discussed with the COTA, the therapy team, and the patient. A treatment plan outline, using the form shown in Figure 18-2, was developed by the occupational therapist and given to the assistant. The program planning outline, which is shown in Figure 18-3, presents the long- and short-term goals established for Barbie as well as the roles of the OTR and the COTA in relation to the goals.

Treatment Implementation

The COTA began occupational therapy treatment after the initial evaluation was completed and formally documented by the OTR. Under the direction of the OTR, the COTA started an upper extremity exercise program. The OTR wrote a specific routine designed to meet Barbie's range of motion needs, as shown in Figure 18-4. The COTA followed this program format, which took approximately 10 minutes to complete. It was recommended that Barbie perform this program two to three times a day in addition to her usual self-care routine. The Arthritis Foundation suggests

☐ BOWMAN HEALTH SERVICES, LTD.
☐ BOWMAN THERAPEUTIC ASSOCIATES, LTD.
OCCUPATIONAL THERAPY EVALUATION

Facility ______________________________ ☐ Home Visit

Type of Note: ☐ Initial ☐ Discharge # of Rx ________ Date ____________ to ____________

Type of Patient: ☐ Medicare A
☐ Private Pay
☐ Private Pay/Insurance

Occupational Therapy Plan of Treatment
Reviewed With: ☐ Patient ☐ Family ☐ Primary Caregiver ☐ Not Completed to Date ☐ Nursing Home Personnel

Patient Name ______ LAST ______ FIRST ______ MIDDLE ______ Patient Number ____________

Age ______ Sex ______ Diagnosis ______________________________

Orders ______________________________

______________________________ Date of Order ____________

Complications/Precautions ______________________________

______________________________ Physican ____________

PROBLEM II — PSYCHOSOCIAL

Observations:

Goal/Prognosis:

Plan:

PROBLEM III — SENSATION: N = Normal, I = Impaired, A = Absent

	L	R
Tactile (Sh/dull)		
2 pt. discrimination		
Proprioception: Sh		
Elbow		
Wrist		
Hand		

Observations:

Goal/Prognosis:

Plan:

PERCEPTION: (Observations interferring with function, ie. apraxia, R/L discrimination, visual field, attention, follow directions, safety, judgement, problem solving)

Goal/Prognosis ______________________ Plan ______________________

PROBLEM IV MOTOR SKILLS

CLINICAL STATUS			ROM L	ROM R	STRENGTH L	STRENGTH R
Shoulder	Flexion	0-180				
	Abduction	0-180				
	Extension	0-40				
	Int. Rotation	0-80				
	Ext. Rotation	0-60				
Elbow	Flexion	0-150				
	Supination	0-80				
	Pronation	0-80				
Wrist	Flexion	0-80				
	Extension	0-70				
	Ulnar Dev.	0-30				
	Radial Dev.	0-20				
Thumb	Flexion	MP 0-50				
		IP 0-80				
	Abduction	0-70				
	Opposition					
			MP | PIP | DIP	MP | PIP | DIP		
Finger	Flexion	2			S	
		3				
		4			P	
		5				
	Extension					
	Intrinsic					

Dominance: Premorbid:
Present:

Arm Placement: A = Able, P = Partial, N = Not Able

	L	R		L	R
Table Top			Grasp		
Top of Head			Lateral		
Side Reach			Palmar		
Overhead			Modified		
Lap			ABNORMAL TONE		
Feet			S = Spasticity		
Behind Head			C = Clonus		
Behind Back			R = Rigidity	L	R
Supination			Shoulder		
Pronation			Elbow		
Grasp			Wrist		
Release			Hand		

MOTOR CONTROL/COORDINATION:

ENDURANCE:

OTHER PERTINENT DATA:

Goal/Prognosis ______________________ Plan ______________________

Therapist ______________________ Date ____________

FORM 15 page 1

Figure 18-1 *continued*

OCCUPATIONAL THERAPY EVALUATION

Page 2

PROBLEM IV ACTIVITIES OF DAILY LIVING

METHOD OF GRADING:
- I = Independent
- I/S = Independent with Set-Up
- I/E = Independent with Equipment
- I/C = Independent with Cues
- S = Supervision
- A = Physical Assist Necessary
- D = Dependent

Note: NA = Not Applicable
NT = Not Tested

√ = Initial Status
X = Goal
Circle Discharge Status

FEEDING		I/S	I/E	I/C	S	A	D	EQUIPMENT/COMMENTS
Eat Entire Meal								
Utensil Feed								
Cut Food								
Finger Food								
Drink From Glass								
HYGIENE								
Brush Teeth								
Wash Hands/Face								
Shave/Make-up								
Comb Hair								
Toilet Hygiene								
UE Bathing								
LE Bathing								
DRESSING								
Cardigan On								
Off								
Slipover On								
Off								
Slack On								
Off								
Socks On								
Off								
Shoes On								
Off								
Underclothes								
Fastenings								
COMMUNICATION								
Write								
Type								
Phone								
Turn Pages								
MOBILITY								
Turn In Bed								
Bed Controls								
Toilet Transfer								
Bed Transfer								
Tub Transfer								
BALANCE								
Sitting								
Standing								
LEISURE								
Table Games								
Crafts								
TV								
Radio								
OTHER AREAS								
______								
______								
______								
______								
______								

ACTIVITIES OF DAILY LIVING OBSERVATIONS/ADDITIONAL COMMENTS:

ADDITIONAL PROBLEMS:

FAMILY INSTRUCTION/HOME PROGRAM:

COMMUNITY PLAN:

Goal/Prognosis:

Plan:

Physician ______________ Date ________ Therapist ______________ Date ________

FORM 15 page 2

Figure 18-1 *continued*

FIGURE 18-2. Treatment Plan Outline*

Please fill out and discuss with COTA prior to first treatment session.

PURPOSE: To aid in implementing treatment program.
To serve as a guide for writing progress and discharge notes.

INFORMATION ABOUT THE PATIENT:

Name: ______ Patient #: ______ Doctor: ______

Age: ______ Marital status: ______ Occupation: ______

Diagnosis: ______ Onset: ______

Authorized treatment duration: ______ Payment Source: ______

Complications/precautions:

Special approach:

Functional occupational therapy problems:

LONG TERM GOALS SHORT TERM GOALS

Date goals achieved: ______ Therapist: ______

*Printed with permission of Bowman Health Services, Ltd., Morton Grove, Illinois.

not replacing self-care completion by an exercise program.[2]

Training in principles of joint protection began immediately, since integration of these concepts is often difficult to incorporate into previously learned routines. The following principles of joint preservation were utilized:[3]

1 Avoid deforming postures.
2 Avoid deforming forces.
3 Maintain range of motion.
4 Maintain muscle strength.
5 Conserve energy.
6 Respect pain.

In teaching these principles, written tools were used along with demonstration and practice to assure compliance. All areas of self-care, home care, child care, job, and leisure were addressed.

Since Barbie was complaining of pain, due in part to structural changes, orthotic management was begun. The OTR saw Barbie during the second week of treatment intervention and fabricated bilateral resting orthoses and wrist gauntlet orthoses.[4] (A COTA with experience may demonstrate adequate skill to fabricate these orthoses independently.) The entry-level COTA assisted with adapting the straps so that Barbie could don and remove them independently. The COTA also monitored her use of the orthoses.

Following discussion of Barbie's progress over the past three treatment sessions with the COTA, the OTR suggested the following changes in the exercise program: 1) Review specific hand exercises, since the patient demonstrated a poor understanding of the method; 2) be more specific with joint preservation and identify instances when the patient does not follow identified techniques. For example, The COTA had observed that Barbie was starting to incorporate the joint preservation techniques in basic skills such as carrying her purse on her shoulder and lifting objects and closing and opening drawers with both hands. However, the COTA observed that Barbie was sitting in chairs that were too low, using poor body mechanics when picking up her daughter, and while she did plan ahead, she often tried to complete too many projects in too short a time. Both positive and negative feedback was required for Bar-

FIGURE 18-3. Program Planning Outline

Long-Term Goals	Short-Term Goals	Role Delineation* OTR	COTA
1. Independent use of bilateral orthosis at rest and for functional task completion and good application of joint protection.	1. • Fabricate bilateral resting orthoses.	X	X
	• Fabricate bilateral gauntlet orthoses.	X	X
	• Independent donning and doffing of orthoses.		X
	• Toleration of wearing orthoses when performing functional tasks.		X
2. Independent with and/or without equipment in all self-care, home/child care, and work tasks (individual modification of activities dependent upon stage of fluctuating disease process).	2. • Assess need for and provide necessary equipment.		X
	• Fabricate assistive devices.		X
	• Train in use of equipment and assistive devices.		X
	• Independent use of adapted techniques for performance.		X
3. Independent with daily exercise/graded activity program when active and inactive disease is present.	3. • Develop a home exercise/graded activity program that incorporates patient's needs and interests.	X	X
	• Incorporate performance of daily exercise /graded activity into patient's routine.		X
4. Application of joint protection, work simplification, and energy conservation techniques 75% of time with self-care, home/child care, vocational/avocational tasks, and community skills.	4. • Instruct patient in joint preservation techniques.		X
	• Monitor and facilitate patient application of joint preservation during daily routine (*i.e.,* ADLs, homemaking, child care, vocational/avocational, and leisure activities).		X

**Note:* This plan indicates task assignment for the purpose of this case study only.

bie to properly adapt her life-style to include joint preservation.

The COTA continued with the treatment program and adjusted it accordingly. Use of the resting and gauntlet orthoses was added to the patient's daily routine, as needed. When increased pain was present in the wrist and hands during the day or night, Barbie was encouraged to cease activity and put her resting splints on. If functional tasks were being completed, the wrist gauntlets were used to allow her hands to move freely, but still remind her to be careful and not to put too much stress on her painful joints. The COTA noted redness at the thenar eminence when using the gauntlets and reported this to the OTR, who directed the necessary modifications.

Activities of daily living became the major focus of Barbie's treatment program. Because of her young age and her family and work responsibilities, Barbie indicated to the COTA the importance of these skills in maintaining her current lifestyle. The patient's concern over longevity often interfered with her confidence and capacity to care for herself, her child, and her husband independently. The COTA voiced Barbie's concerns and anxieties in a discussion with the OTR. It was agreed that the focus for the next 2 weeks would be on daily living skills and home and child care issues, while continuing to incorporate joint preservation techniques. The patient's major complaints of pain during early morning and late evening hours indicated to the COTA that Barbie was overexerting herself in the morning from care for herself and her child and breakfast preparation for her husband and in the evening from dinner preparation, bathing herself and her child, and completing housework. (Housework tasks had accumulated since Barbie was working 5 days per week prior to her recent exacerbation.)

On days when Barbie experienced extreme pain,

FIGURE 18-4. Arthritis Home Program

When one has arthritis, it is important to carry out a regular program of exercise. The following is a program designed to put your joints through all necessary motions. Exercise should be performed twice a day, and each exercise should be repeated five to ten times. If pain lasts over 1 hour after exercise program is developed, discontinue. This is usually a good indication that you have done too much. Please do not hesitate to call if you have any questions. Good luck and keep up the good work.

1. Activities of Daily Living Warm-up: DO FIRST THING IN THE MORNING. Touch your hands to shoulders, mouth, nose, eyes, top of head, up and over head, behind neck, behind back, knees, ankles, and toes. You can do this while lying in bed if painful when sitting, and modify accordingly. Repeat before sleeping at night.
2. Bend elbows so hands are as close to shoulders as possible and straighten toward knees. Be sure to keep elbows at your side.
3. Keeping elbows at your side, hold a stick in your hand and turn it upward toward the ceiling, then down toward the floor.
4. Rest forearm on table top and lift wrist off table. HELP with other hand, if necessary, to keep forearm on table.
5. Place palm flat on table; raise each finger toward ceiling, one at a time, and hold each finger up for 5 seconds. Return finger to table before proceeding with next one; be sure palm is flat on table.
6. Place palm on table and bring fingers, one by one, toward thumb side. Make a fist; then open and begin again, bringing fingers, one by one, to thumb.
7. Make an "O" with your thumb and each successive finger.
8. Make large circles with thumb in both directions.
9. Hold pencil in hand and try to touch with fingertips. Remember: pencil should be at crease between fingers and palm.

DO THE FOLLOWING ONLY WHEN ACTIVE DISEASE IS NOT PRESENT

1. Heavy rubber band exercises of biceps and triceps for strengthening.
2. Bring arms to shoulder height; place 3-pound weight on upper arm and hold for 5 seconds. Take weight off, let arm down, and repeat.

Please contact us if you have any questions or problems.
R. Jones, COTA/L S. Kantor, OTR/L

she had difficulty with all self-care and child care activities; however, she forced herself to complete these chores, which resulted in increased pain. Following further discussion between the OTR and the COTA, it was decided that an activity analysis would be beneficial. The COTA gave Barbie an activity configuration form and assisted her in filling in her specific activities. Tasks that were often painful and difficult to complete were highlighted. A sample activity configuration is shown in Figure 18-5.

Tasks which were analyzed included buttoning, writing, carrying and bathing her child, and managing keys and the car door. It should be noted that there were other areas requiring analysis; however, the aforementioned tasks were chosen for the purpose of this case study. The task analysis consisted of the following steps:[5]

1 Identification of tasks by the COTA with the patient.
2 Description of task components, including activity characteristics.
3 Identification of solutions by the COTA, OTR, and patient.

The objective was to find less painful methods for task completion through the use of equipment, modification of the tasks, joint preservation techniques, and adaptation of clothing and environments. For example, buttoning was painful in the morning. Barbie tried a button hook and this resulted in fewer complaints of pain while completing the task. The COTA placed an elastic strap on the button hook which prevented her from using a tight grasp. A second area analyzed was bathing her daughter. This task had previously been done at night when Barbie took care of her own hygiene needs as well. It was recommended that Barbie bathe herself and her daughter in the morning since arthritis patients frequently report that this is beneficial in relieving morning stiffness.

FIGURE 18-5. Activity Configuration*

	Weekdays	Saturday	Sunday
Wake-up			
Early morning			
Late morning			
Early afternoon			
Late afternoon			
Early evening			
Late evening			
Bedtime			

*Printed with permission of the Rehabilitation Institute of Chicago, Chicago Illinois.

Barbie had always bathed her child while on her knees, leaning over the bathtub. The COTA suggested that she sit in a chair placed next to the tub instead, and that she obtain a light weight, hand-held shower for rinsing the child. Barbie's daughter enjoyed these changes in her bath routine and spoke of the experiences as "the new bath game." This made the task of bathing more enjoyable for both the mother and daughter. Further equipment needs were assessed and a long handled brush was suggested for cleaning the tub after use.

Lifting her daughter in and out of the tub caused Barbie a great deal of pain, so the COTA suggested that this be done by her husband. Since her husband was not always available, an alternate plan was also discussed with Barbie, which would be to allow her daughter to crawl over the edge of the tub with assistance.

Meal preparation was a third area analyzed, since Barbie needed to prepare two meals each day, five days a week, and three meals a day on weekends. The patient reported that cutting food, opening containers, and bending to get objects out of lower cabinets were her major areas of difficulty. The COTA suggested alternative methods for holding a knife and instructed Barbie in the best method for using an adapted container opener along with a rubber pad for added stabilization. The need to reorganize the kitchen cabinets was also discussed in conjunction with her joint preservation training.

While Barbie seemed to enjoy her role as a homemaker, she indicated that she hoped to return to active employment outside the home. An activity configuration for work related tasks was completed jointly by the COTA and Barbie. Following further discussion with the OTR, the decision was made for the COTA to visit the patient's work site. Barbie worked in a food processing plant, and components of her job included both carrying heavy objects to an oven and doing a great deal of writing. The COTA noted that the gauntlet orthoses would not be durable enough for her job and discussed the possibility of an alternate orthosis with the OTR. A more durable leather and elastic wrist orthosis was decided upon for use at work only, and was purchased by the patient.

Throughout the course of Barbie's treatment program, the OTR had been in daily communication with the COTA and continued to see the patient once a week to assess progress and coordinate any necessary adjustments in the program.

The OTR arranged a job site visit with Barbie's employer during the last week of occupational therapy treatment to suggest some modifications in Barbie's work routine, such as doing writing tasks at intervals rather than during a concentrated period of time.

Barbie progressed well in therapy and found it rewarding to involve her daughter in more of her own self-care. Notable changes in her attitude were evidenced by fewer complaints of pain when completing her daily self-care and child care tasks. Barbie's husband was very supportive and agreed to share in laundry, grocery shopping, and driving responsibilities.

Although Barbie was able to drive, securing her daughter in the special car seat, as required by state law, was both difficult and painful. The COTA and Barbie discussed the situation together and determined a solution that incorporated good body mechanics and joint preservation principles. Opening the car door was difficult for Barbie owing to pressure placed on the joints of her hand. It was decided that the use of a plastic-coated dowel rod to depress the door latch would be an effective solution. The COTA developed a light plastic built-up key holder, which was easier for Barbie to grasp and turn, thus enabling her to turn the key in the car door and the ignition.

Program Discontinuation

During the fifth visit the OTR made, she and the COTA discussed the degree of progress that had been achieved with Barbie and the need for further occupational therapy. It was mutually agreed that Barbie had made significant progress toward returning to a more active life style, and that occupational therapy treatment would be discontinued as planned. The follow-up program was discussed, and both Barbie and her husband reviewed the home exercise protocol, all literature provided, the use of equipment and adaptations, as well as resources for purchasing replacement equipment. The patient was encouraged to contact her physician if her disease and/or functional status changed. Further assessment for occupational therapy treatment would occur at that time.

The discharge evaluation was handled jointly by the OTR and the COTA. Evaluation of the musculoskeletal components was performed by the therapist with input from the assistant, while the functional skills assessment was completed by the COTA. Results indicated that the patient had achieved all goals determined in the initial evaluation. Both the OTR and the COTA recommended that Barbie become involved in the Arthritis Foundation because of the variety of beneficial programs and support groups it provides.

Agreement was reached between Barbie and her employer that she would return to work three days a week and increase to five days when she felt able. Her daily schedule would be adjusted to allow for her to do her writing at selected intervals rather than during long blocks of time.

Summary

The OTR and COTA roles in treatment intervention fluctuate with each patient served, depending upon specific needs. In looking at role delineation, an entry-level COTA requires additional supervision to perform various aspects of the evaluation and treatment program. Constant communication is necessary for a thorough treatment program to be developed and implemented. A continuing literature review to identify new approaches and treatment techniques is valuable in providing comprehensive care.

References

1. Guide for supervision of occupational therapy personnel. *Am J Occup Ther* 35:815-816, 1981.

2. Arthritis Teaching Slide Collection Manual. Arthritis Health Profession Section of Arthritis Foundation, Arthritis Foundation, 1980, p 5.

3. Watkins RA, Robinson D: *Joint Preservation Techniques for Patients with Rheumatoid Arthritis*. Chicago, IL: Rehabilitation Institute of Chicago, 1974, p 16.

4. Melvin J: *Rheumatic Disease: Occupational Therapy and Rehabilitation*, 2nd Edition. Philadelphia: FA Davis, 1982, p 329.

5. Hopkins HL, Smith HD, Tiffany EG: Therapeutic application of activity. In H Hopkins, H Smith Eds: *Willard and Spackman's Occupational Therapy*, 6th Edition. Philadelphia: JB Lippincott, 1983, p 226.

Bibliography

Entry-level OTR and COTA role delineation. *Occup Ther Newspaper* 35(July):8-16, 1981.

Feinberg J, Brandt KD: Allied health team management of rheumatoid arthritis patients. *Am J Occup Ther* 38:613-620, 1984.

Fries JF: *Arthritis: A Comprehensive Guide*. Reading, MA: Addison-Wesley Publishing, 1979.

Swezey R: *Arthritis Rational Therapy and Rehabilitation*. Philadelphia: W.B. Saunders, 1979.

The Role of the Occupational Therapist in Home Health Care. Rockville, MD: American Occupational Therapy Association, 1981.

Acknowledgments

The authors wish to express their gratitude to Sheri Intagliata, MS, MPA OTR/L, Patricia Conlon, OTR/L, Kathleen Burroughs, OTR/L, Mary Andre, OTR/L, and Jeffrey Blackman for their guidance and support in the development of this case study.

CHAPTER 19

The Adult Stroke Patient

Barbara A. Larson, COTA
Patricia M. Watson, OTR

Introduction

Recently, Mrs. H, a 68-year-old homemaker, became ill while preparing dinner. She experienced a severe headache and numbness of her left side. Her husband notified the paramedics, who transported her to a nearby hospital, where her vital signs were stabilized. Following examination and tests, Mrs. H was diagnosed as having a right cerebral vascular accident (CVA) with resulting left hemiplegia.

Mrs. H's physician referred her to occupational therapy for evaluation and treatment 6 days after the CVA. The occupational therapy staff consisted of two registered occupational therapists and one certified occupational therapy assistant. The department was responsible for providing services to both medical and surgical patients in this 300-bed hospital.

Assessment

Upon receipt of the referral, the occupational therapist initiated the data gathering process. The OTR began by reading the patient's chart to obtain information on her medical, social, and work history, vital signs, medications, and special precautions. She spoke with nurses providing care for Mrs. H, obtaining their observations of the patient, and also received an update on her medical status.

Mrs. H was then interviewed at bedside by the OTR. During this first contact, the therapist informed the patient of the occupational therapy referral and briefly described the therapy services. Thus, from the beginning, Mrs. H was included in the rehabilitation process. This visit also provided the therapist with an opportunity to make initial observations of the patient's mental status and attitude toward therapy.

The OTR learned from review of the patient's chart that Mrs. H had enjoyed good health prior to the stroke. The interview information indicated that she resided with her husband in a small, two-story home in the suburbs. While raising her four children, she had worked part-time as a department store clerk. Since her retirement 5 years ago, Mrs. H had enjoyed traveling with her husband and spending time with her children and grandchildren, who lived nearby. She also volunteered once a week at a senior citizen center, assisting in the congregate dining program.

Evaluation

Mrs. H was scheduled for an occupational therapy evaluation in the clinic. During the first 1-hour session, held in the morning, the occupational therapist began by outlining the process that was to be used for evaluation. Following this explanation, the OTR assessed Mrs. H's position in the wheelchair. The patient was in a slouched posture, leaning slightly to the left. The OTR placed a firm seat and back support in the wheelchair and issued a lapboard, providing the necessary stability for maintaining an improved posture. After the patient was placed in a more optimal position for performance, the evaluation continued. The OTR assessed upper extremity range of motion, muscle strength, sensation, coordination, muscle tone, and edema.

During the afternoon of the same day, the COTA saw Mrs. H for an additional half hour. The occupational therapy assistant used a functional coordination board that included buttons, zippers, snaps, and velcro closures to observe Mrs. H's skill in using the unaffected upper extremity. A leisure interest survey was also completed, allowing the COTA an additional opportunity to interview the patient.[1]

Early the following day, the OTR visited the patient's room and assessed upper extremity hygiene and dressing skills. When Mrs. H came to the clinic later that morning, the OTR continued administering other evaluation procedures. Perceptual motor, visual, and cognitive assessments were used to detect problems with body image, problem solving, sequencing, presence of field cut, and dyspraxia (the inability to motor plan). During the evaluation, Mrs. H was pleasant and cooperative, quickly completing tasks, unaware of her errors. A homemaking evaluation was completed that afternoon by the OTR. This assessment gave the therapist an opportunity to gain information on Mrs. H's judgment and reliability with more familiar activities.

On the following day, the OTR and the COTA met to discuss the evaluation results and to plan the treatment. The results were as follows.[2]

Positioning: Mrs. H displayed fair trunk balance. She was able to attain a vertical posture with minimal assistance, and remain in the midline with cuing. After the wheelchair insert was provided, the patient was able to maintain this position when reaching away from her body about 12 inches to 14 inches.

Upper Extremity Functioning: The patient's unaffected right side displayed strength and range of motion measurements within normal limits. Mrs. H was right-handed and results of coordination testing revealed speed of coordination to be within funtional limits. Her left affected extremity had minimal spasticity present in the biceps but this did not interfere significantly with function. Passive range of motion was within normal limits with no complaints of pain during movement. No shoulder subluxation (partial dislocation of the joint) was evident, but mild edema was present in the hand. Sensation was intact in the areas of proprioception (ability to identify the position of body parts in space) and stereognosis (ability to identify objects and forms through the sense of touch). Her responses to surface pain, light touch, and hot/cold stimuli indicated impairment in these areas.

Synergy Patterns: Mrs. H demonstrated a flexion synergy with the strongest components being elbow and shoulder flexion. She was able to flex and abduct her shoulder through one-third the full range of motion and to flex her elbow two-thirds of the way through the normal range. She was able to partially extend her elbow and wrist with gravity eliminated. Mrs. H demonstrated the ability to flex her fingers but had no functional grasp.

Mental Status: The patient was oriented to time, place, and person. She was talkative and had a bright affect. She exhibited moderate impulsivity, decreased insight into her problems, impaired problem solving, decreased attention span, and poor concentration.

Visual/Perceptual Motor: Mrs. H demonstrated left-sided unilateral neglect but did attend to the left, once cued. Mild problems with figure ground and spatial orientation were also evidenced. These appeared on more complex assessment tasks, which included locating a number in the telephone directory and completing a three-dimensional cube design.

Leisure Survey: The patient indicated that she liked to be with people. She expressed interest in handicrafts such as ceramics and needlework. She stated that she enjoyed cooking and entertaining as well as attending movies and sharing gardening chores with her husband.

Daily Living Skills (DLS): The DLS evaluation revealed that Mrs. H needed cues to complete thorough hygiene. She had attempted to use her left arm to assist with tasks after cuing. She demonstrated an ability to learn and follow through after cues and suggestions for dressing techniques were provided. Mrs. H required only minimal assistance with her upper extremity dressing. She was dependent in donning her brassiere. The patient needed moderate assistance with starting and pulling up lower extremity garments and was dependent with stockings and shoes. Upper extremity dressing and hygiene were done from a seated position, and lower extremity dressing was accomplished from a supine position.

Homemaking: The initial evaluation was completed with the patient working from a wheelchair. She demonstrated moderate impulsivity and poor planning when propelling the chair. Initially, she had difficulties with problem solving and displayed lapses in judgment and reliability but demonstrated an ability to learn from cues provided by the OTR.

Treatment Planning

Once the evaluation was completed and the OTR and the COTA had collaborated on the evaluation results,[1] the occupational therapist attended a team conference. This meeting involved the staff members providing care for the patient and included the physician, nurse, physical therapist, and social worker, as well as the OTR. It was determined that Mrs. H would be treated by physical and occupational therapy for a period of 2 weeks, with a team meeting held during the second week to discuss her progress. The rehabilitation goal was to return Mrs. H to her home environment with increased independence in functional living skills and provision of support services, if necessary.

Mrs. H was scheduled to receive occupational therapy services three times per day. She would be seen by the COTA for daily morning dressing sessions and one 30-minute to 60-minute afternoon period for group sessions or homemaking training. The OTR would treat the patient each morning during a 60-minute functional restoration session. The patient's long-term goals for occupational therapy were established as:

1 Independence in dressing and hygiene.
2 Independence in light meal preparation.
3 Accomplishment of household chores with minimal assistance.
4 Use of the left upper extremity in all activities that required active pushing, pulling, stabilizing, and grasp and release. (This is considered a maximal active assistive extremity.)
5 Return to former level of community involvement.

The patient's short-term goals were initially set as:

1 Patient will dress self with minimal assistance and cues after provision of an adapted brassiere.
2 Patient will demonstrate good judgment and problem solving in four sessions of homemaking training.
3 Patient will consistently use left upper extremity to assist with a single active motion in daily skills.
4 Patient will complete an adapted cutting board project, incorporating use of left upper extremity in this task.
5 Patient will demonstrate compensation for left neglect, requiring only one reminder during any treatment session.

The occupational therapist discussed the treatment goals and plans with both Mr. H and Mrs. H and incorporated their suggestions. Mrs. H's record, which included problems, evaluation results, and the treatment plan, was kept on file in the occupational therapy clinic. The OTR and the COTA updated the file three times per week. This proved to be the most effective means for providing consistency in treatment.

Treatment Implementation

Mrs. H was seen daily by the COTA for dressing training.[1] Initially, they worked on upper extremity hygiene and dressing. The patient sat in her wheelchair facing a mirror while at the sink and proceeded to brush her teeth, wash her face and upper torso, and apply deodorant. The occupational therapy assistant instructed Mrs. H to slow down and become more thorough with hygiene. The COTA demonstrated and provided written and illustrated step-by-step procedures for donning either a front button or a pullover blouse. After three sessions, Mrs. H was able to recall the correct sequence for dressing her affected left upper extremity first. She was able to don and doff her brassiere independently after the COTA adapted it with a front velcro closure. As the patient's balance improved, she progressed to lower extremity dressing. At that time, she was independent with light hygiene. During dressing training, the COTA attempted to enhance Mrs. H's awareness of her affected side while having her utilize the present function. The COTA assisted her in dealing with acceptance of the change in her body so that it could be re-integrated into the performance of tasks. As a result of this training, the patient progressed to complete dressing independence. She demonstrated an improved ability to problem solve and spent appropriate amounts of time in her performance of tasks, slowing down instead of accomplishing them hurriedly.

The OTR initiated a program to improve Mrs. H's left upper extremity function, maintain her right upper extremity strength, and remediate her visual perceptual motor problems, including left neglect, impulsivity, decreased attention span, concentration, and problem solving.[1] The therapist used an approach to treatment that incorporated bilateral upper extremity tasks. The COTA and the OTR collaborated so that during treatment sessions, all problems would be addressed by the use of various modalities. The therapist used clasped-hand activities such as large pegboard games, ball and bean bag toss, and a punching bag, incorporating trunk rotation into the movements. Left upper extremity weight bearing was used as Mrs. H worked on simple mathematics problems and progressed to check-writing, record-keeping, and use of a calculator. Visual perceptual motor needs were addressed as Mrs. H worked on paper and pencil activities. These included the use of the telephone directory, writing short pieces of information, and engaging in problem solving with hypothetical emergency situations.

The COTA conducted an afternoon CVA treatment group which met twice each week. The focus of the group was to aid integration of sensory, motor, and perceptual skills for improved performance in daily tasks. The peer support also enhanced social skills necessary for resuming former lifestyle patterns. The occupational therapy assistant instructed the patients in self range of motion for regaining specific body part movement and awareness. The group also engaged in card and board games to address visual and perceptual problems, while facilitating social interaction as well.[2] Mrs. H was an active participant in all of these activities.

During the one-to-one session, the COTA worked with Mrs. H on individual activities that addressed goals more specifically.[1] The patient sanded an adapted bread board using both hands and an adapted sander. Using the present arm movement, Mrs. H sanded at a downward angle with gravity eliminated. After working through the synergy pattern, she sanded on an inclined plane, thus providing resistance to shoulder flexion and elbow extension. The patient also worked on completing a rubber link doormat. This activity encouraged bilateral upper extremity use, increased perceptual skill, improved concentration, and maintained right arm strength when she worked with a weighted wrist cuff. To address Mrs. H's avocational interests, the COTA provided her with a short-term embroidery project on large mesh canvas. The patient worked on this evenings and weekends, placing the project on her bedside table and stabilizing the work with her left arm and hand.

Twice each week, during an afternoon session, Mrs. H participated in homemaking training with the COTA.[1] Initially working from the wheelchair, she progressed to performing tasks while standing at the counter. A narrow based "quad" cane was used for ambulation. As improvement occurred, the patient progressed from opening cans to using the stove top safely. Following the package instructions, the patient successfully baked a cake in the oven. The skills acquired during training enabled Mrs. H to compile a grocery list, sequence tasks properly, and independently prepare a light meal. Although fine motor skill was absent, she used the weight of her left hand to stabilize objects. A hoop apron with pockets and a utility cart on wheels were used to transport items.[3] The COTA incorporated work simplification and energy conservation techniques into the sessions. She specifically encouraged Mrs. H to follow these basic principles:[3]

1. Sit while working whenever possible.
2. Slide objects across the counter or table.
3. Keep frequently used items within easy reach.
4. Prepare one course meals.
5. Plan intermittent rest periods during daily routine.

The OTR and the COTA met daily for approximately 15 minutes to review Mrs. H's current status and to update her file when indicated. Both encouraged Mr. H to attend occupational therapy sessions so he could become more involved in his wife's recovery process. Mr. H, a retired salesman, appeared somewhat anxious about his wife's illness but was attentive and offered support whenever possible.

Following 2 weeks of intensive therapy, Mrs. H demonstrated much improvement. Her left upper extremity progressed through components of flexion and extension synergies and had gained relative independence from synergies. Upon reevaluation, she demonstrated antigravity movement of her affected upper extremity. She had developed voluntary movement, using her left arm to assist in single sequence activities during daily tasks. Mrs. H regained an active grasp which measured 2.5 pounds on the dynamometer. She developed some isolated finger movement, including partial opposition, yet she would need more therapy to strengthen and refine the motion. With returning hand function, the edema was diminished. The patient was not yet able to manipulate objects smaller than a tennis ball. Because of improvement in Mrs. H's balance and upper extremity function, the lapboard and wheelchair insert were no longer necessary.

Mrs. H was independent with light dressing and light hygiene but required minimal assistance with bathing. She needed a shower seat and a handheld shower head, minimal transfer assistance, and standby supervision during the shower.

Using an adapted bread board, a hoop apron with pockets, and a utility cart on wheels, Mrs. H had become more independent with light meal preparation. She required less cueing, had slowed down her performance, and was demonstrating improved problem solving ability. The patient was able to ambulate 20 feet using a narrow based "quad" cane but did require standby supervision. Mrs. H was independent in her bed mobility, requiring only standby assistance for bed to wheelchair transfer. The patient displayed self-cued awareness of the left side of her body, indicating that she had learned compensation for left neglect. Her attention span had improved greatly, allowing improved task performance.

The OTR and the COTA were responsible for daily documentation and recording of charges for their treatment sessions. Each recorded pertinent performance data and noted any changes seen during the treatment periods. Notes were written using a problem oriented approach to charting.

Discharge Planning

Prior to the final team meeting, the OTR and the COTA met to review Mrs. H's progress and to identify further needs. Mrs. H had expressed concern about her ability to function in her kitchen and bathroom at home. She was open to suggestions for improving the arrangement but was having difficulty describing the floor plan. With input from the COTA regarding other areas of progress and concerns, the OTR prepared a progress report to present at the team meeting.

In the team meeting, it was decided that the OTR would make a home visit during the additional week Mrs. H would be hospitalized. The OTR suggested that the patient accompany her. Following discussion of progress to date, the team decided that Mrs. H would be discharged to her home the ensuing week. It was recommended that the patient return for additional physical and occupational therapy treatment on an outpatient basis twice weekly following discharge. Both Mr. and Mrs. H agreed to this plan.

Mrs. H became very apprehensive at the prospect of returning home, even for a single visit. She expressed concern about her ability to manage in the home atmosphere and felt she would be a burden to her husband. With encouragement from the team members, however, Mrs. H and her husband participated in the home visit. Following the home assessment, the OTR made several suggestions on ways Mrs. H might manage her home more easily. The therapist also gained information that would assist her in focusing more specifically on what was required for Mrs. H to have increased independence once she returned home. The home visit also allowed the patient a brief opportunity to practice some of her hospital acquired skills. She was cooperative during the visit, secure in the knowledge she would return to the hospital for further treatment.

Following the home visit, the OTR and the COTA planned treatment for the final week. Dressing training was discontinued, since Mrs. H had become independent in this area.[1] Practicing one-handed techniques, organizing her work more specifically, and learning appropriate safety measures were the focus of her current homemaking training tasks. Her husband would assume responsibility for the laundry and heavy cleaning chores, with other family members assisting him as necessary.

Mr. H had observed his wife's occupational therapy sessions quite regularly. During the last week of inpatient treatment, he became an active participant in her program by assisting her with activities such as range of motion and providing cues for the proper energy conservation techniques. He encouraged his wife during the final homemaking sessions as she practiced one-handed techniques, such as pouring liquids and breaking an egg, using the function of her left upper extremity to assist her.[3]

The COTA and the OTR collaborated on the development of Mrs. H's home program. The therapist prepared a left upper extremity active range of motion guide with diagrams and written instructions. She also suggested activities which included washing and drying dishes, dusting furniture and objects, folding laundry, and getting dressed. These light resistive tasks incorporated grasp and release motions during daily functional activities, reinforcing compensation for left neglect. The COTA identified equipment that Mrs. H would need at home, which included adapted bathroom items previously mentioned, as well as an adapted jar opener, a hoop apron, and a long oven mitt. Mr. H agreed to purchase these. Diagrams and written information on work simplification and energy conservation techniques were also included in the program.

Home safety was discussed with Mrs. H. She was encouraged to remove scatter rugs, use nonglare floor wax, and store things within easy reach to eliminate unnecessary bending or reaching.[3]

During the final days of treatment, the OTR continued working with the patient, using activities to improve Mrs. H's left upper extremity function. The COTA engaged the patient in completing the rubber link doormat, with her left hand and arm more actively involved in the process.

Program Discontinuation

Prior to program discontinuation, both the OTR and the COTA encouraged Mr. and Mrs. H to gradually begin resuming their involvement in community activities. They discussed the possibility of Mrs. H visiting the senior citizen center to begin re-acquainting herself with friends and activities. Mrs. H was interested but appeared hesitant and expressed the desire to have more improved function of her left arm and hand before returning to the center. To reinforce what she had learned in the hospital and to gain confidence in her skills, Mrs. H was urged to visit family members and accompany her husband on short outings to the shopping mall.

By the time his wife was discharged, Mr. H demonstrated comprehension of the home program and was a willing participant in her ongoing rehabilitation. Having been provided with specific treatment suggestions and community resource information, the couple felt prepared to deal with situations they might encounter. The COTA and the OTR, as well as other members of the treatment team, looked forward to Mrs. H's continued progress. As her functional abilities improved, she would regain her self-confidence and experience an enhanced quality of life.

References

1. Entry-level OTR and COTA role delineation. *Occup Ther Newspaper* 35(July):8-16, 1981.

2. Hopkins H, Smith H, Eds: *Willard and Spackman's Occupational Therapy*, 6th Edition. Philadelphia: JB Lippincott, 1983.

3. Klinger JL: *Mealtime Manual for People with Disabilities and the Aging*, 2nd Edition, Camden, NJ: Campbell Soup Co., 1979.

CHAPTER 20

Parkinson's Disease: The Elderly Patient

Kathryn Melin-Eberhardt, COTA/L
Javan E. Walker Jr., OTR/L

Introduction

Parkinson's disease is a disabling and progressive condition which gradually results in the loss of physical mobility. Its onset is usually between 50 and 60 years of age, with an incidence of 20 per 100,000 people each year. It is a chronic disease of the nervous system which often produces rather remarkable clinical symptoms. These include rigidity, either "cogwheel" or "lead-pipe"; rhythmic tremor of the hands with a pill-rolling motion; stooped posture; and a mask-like face. The affected person demonstrates an involuntary tendency to take short accelerating steps when walking (festination); an abnormal slowness of movement (bradykinesia); and absence or poverty of movement (akinesia). A resting tremor occurs only when the patient is at rest and disappears when there is voluntary movement. Fine motor incoordination, contractures, fatigue, and weakness make activities of daily living difficult without assistance. There is poor standing balance in late stages of the disease which, along with a tendency toward rapid propulsion and difficulty in stopping, makes ambulation very dangerous. The gradual loss of joint range of motion, which affects the rest of the body, also inhibits oral articulation, causing the patient to demonstrate slurred speech (dysphagia), and drooling, due to excessive salivation.[1,2]

There is no cure for Parkinson's disease, although in some cases symptoms may be alleviated by surgery or medication. Rehabilitation management by a treatment team composed of the registered occupational therapist, certified occupational therapy assistant, physical therapist, and physician can do much to assist the patient faced with this disabling condition. As the disease progresses and breathing problems are encountered, a respiratory therapist often provides treatment as well.

Case Study Background

Willie, a 59-year-old widowed janitor, had had Parkinson's disease for five years. Although he was still able to ambulate safely, he was forced to retire from his job owing to the increasing physical difficulties related to his disease process. An active man who enjoyed athletic activities, he had begun to attend the George Washington Carver Older Adult Center in his neighborhood.

The center is staffed with a social worker, activity therapists, and counselors as well as a certified occupational therapy assistant. The local hospital provided the COTA with an OTR supervisor who spent one afternoon each week evaluating patients and developing treatment programs for the COTA to carry out on a day-to-day basis.

Willie's primary interest in coming to the center was to give him social contacts and allow him to remain active. At his last visit to his physician, however, he complained about increased problems when performing household chores around his apartment, and he reported difficulty with some self-care activities. The physician referred Willie to the occupational therapy department at the rehabilitation hospital, which also provided services to the Carver Center. When the OTR received the referral, she called the COTA and asked her to initiate the screening process that they had developed and to report her findings to the therapist the following day.

Screening

During the initial interview, the COTA explained the role of occupational therapy to Willie and began obtaining some information that was indicated on the standard evaluation form. She asked about the architecture of his home, emphasizing the stairs, kitchen and bathroom layout, as well as the characteristics of other rooms. Knowing that he lived alone, she inquired about the type of help he had or felt he needed in taking care of his apartment and doing his shopping and laundry. Other questions were asked about his goals, knowledge of his disability, and his awareness of his prognosis. Following the initial screening, the COTA organized all of her screening data, and reported it to the OTR.

On the following Monday, the OTR visited the center and analyzed the screening data which the COTA had submitted to her. She then decided on the evaluation tools that would be used and arranged a meeting with the assistant to discuss those parts of the evaluation that the COTA would complete.

Evaluation

The OTR felt that there were four areas of evaluation that they should conduct: independent living/daily living skills, sensorimotor components, cognitive components, and psychological components.

Since the COTA had received outstanding training, the therapist felt comfortable having her assist in assessing the patient in several areas, which included further data collection using a structured format, observation of the patient, and administration of structured testing in several areas.

Prior to her evaluation, the OTR discussed her concerns with the COTA and explained the other areas that she wanted the COTA to focus on, such as using her observational skills during the evaluation to further assess the patient's functional motor skills. She stressed the importance of the COTA assisting the OTR by reporting her observations to her following the evaluation. The areas indicated for COTA evaluation were daily living skills, upper and lower extremity status, fine motor and gross motor coordination, and strength and endurance during the daily living skills evaluation; cognitive skills and some sensory integration skills were to be observed and evaluated also.

COTA Evaluation

The COTA set up an appointment with Willie to complete her portion of the evaluation. She began by having him fill out a structured interview form which gathered additional data about his family history, self-care abilities, school and work history, and his leisure interests and experiences. The COTA performed her assessment in the following areas:

Daily Living Skills:

Head/neck and oral hygiene.

Grooming.

Feeding skills.

Upper and lower extremity dressing.
Bed mobility.
Transfer skills (bed, toilet and tub).
Balance and endurance while sitting and standing.
Functional communication, including writing skills.

Upper and Lower Extremity Status:
Observation of active/passive ROM in functional activities during the daily living skills evaluation.
Testing of gross and fine motor coordination with structured tests.
Observation of strength and endurance during functional activities.

Cognitive Skills
Orientation as to time, place and person.
Observation of comprehension/attention span.
Observation of cognitive integration.

Sensory Integration/Perceptual Skills
Observation of body integration during daily living skills evaluation.
Observation of perceptual functioning.

At the completion of her evaluation, the COTA summarized the evaluation data and reported the findings to the OTR. They both studied the data, and the COTA indicated her recommendations at that time, based on her own evaluation data. The OTR then set up an appointment with the patient to complete the evaluation.

OTR Evaluation

The OTR evaluated the patient's neuromuscular status, concentrating on active and passive range of motion and the presence or absence of tremors and rigidity. She performed a manual muscle test and made an assessment of his fine motor and gross motor capabilities. She also noted that the patient did not appear to experience any pain or discomfort while the evaluation procedures were being carried out.

As part of her assessment, the OTR queried the patient about his emotional status and further explored his leisure skills and interests following his retirement and the death of his wife.

Following the completion of all evaluations, the OTR made an analysis of the data collected, synthesized it, and documented her findings and recommendations in the patient's chart. It was determined that the patient was having decreased range of motion in upper and lower extremities, problems with gait and balance, tremor, and some problem with articulation. He did have a positive attitude and was willing to work on his problems. His leisure skills, which included attending local baseball games, playing cards and board games, and hiking, appeared appropriate for his age and situation. His daily living skills evaluation indicated beginning problems in maintenance of personal hygiene, dressing, feeding, home maintenance, shopping, and communication when writing. The therapist prepared a report and sent a copy of the evaluation findings to the referring physician.

Program Planning

The OTR, with the assistance of the COTA, began to develop long-term and short-term goals for a program of treatment to be carried out by the COTA. The three factors identified were: establishing a daily pattern of functional activities at the center and at home to maintain active range of motion, maintaining the present level of strength and endurance, and continuing a life of productivity.[2]

Goals were developed for independent living/daily living skills, sensorimotor skills, strength and endurance, and cognitive and psychosocial skills. Some of the long-term goals identified were:

1 Independence in functional activities to prevent further deterioration of independent/daily living skills.
2 Maintenance and/or increase of fine and gross motor coordination in functional activities.
3 Maintenance of cognitive and psychosocial skills.

Treatment Planning

Following the identification of long-term and short-term goals, the OTR and the COTA began to discuss how a treatment program could be developed to involve the patient in activities at the center and at home which would meet his therapeutic goals. It was significant that both the therapist and the assistant had perceived Willie as a highly motivated patient, who was capable of working independently in the treatment program. The OTR stressed that movements should be rhythmical and that adjuncts such as music, clapping, counting out loud, or a metronome might be useful during some aspects of treatment. After further discussion, both the COTA and the OTR agreed on the following program for the occupational therapy assistant to carry out:

Independent Living/Daily Living Skills

Grooming and hygiene: Work with the patient in a group activity; assist in personal grooming skills.

Feeding/eating: Assist the patient as needed during the noon meal and provide large-handled, weighted utensils for feeding at home and at the center to decrease tremors.

Assist the patient in developing fine motor skills in activities such as buttoning and zipping by using a button hook and zipper pulls.

Functional mobility: Even though bed mobility is still intact, standing balance has decreased.

Work on challenging activities such as ball catching in a group.

Patient may need further assistance with transfers to tub, toilet, or car. This area will be evaluated further.

Functional communication: Focus on ability to use telephone accurately in an emergency, and maintenance of a legible signature.

Psychological/Emotional Daily Living Skills

Self-concept/self-identity: Work with patient in small groups and one-to-one focusing on feelings about his disability including his facial features, tremors, and gait.

Recommend support group.

Community involvement: Involve patient with members of the community and agencies which that focus on safety measures and safety while living alone, such as a telephone reassurance program.

Play/leisure: Work with patient individually and in a group to discuss leisure skills and their role in his life.

Interest in hiking may not be possible owing to progression of disease; encourage daily strolls in the neighborhood.

Involve patient in group card and board games and encourage continued attendance at baseball games.

Sensorimotor Components

Range of motion: Involve patient in range of motion exercise that can be done at the center or at home.

Gross motor skills: Work with patient on cone stacking activities and games, sitting or standing, to improve gross motor skills. Involve in sports activities at the center, such as shuffle board, pitching horseshoes, and relay games.

Fine motor skills: Work with patient on craft activities that require fine motor skills, such as mosaic tile work, copper tooling, stenciling, or leather work.

Strength and Endurance

Work on progressive resistive exercise (PRE) program and grade his activities, which should include a woodworking project, using a hand saw to cut out pieces; project should require sanding.

Ensure that postural balance is incorporated in all the activities.

Therapeutic Adaptations

Assistive/adaptive devices may be needed for daily living skills activities. These could include a button hook, zipper pulls, adaptive silverware or plate guards, and equipment for tub and toilet transfers.

Prevention

Energy conservation, work simplification, and body mechanics should be stressed.

Home Program

In addition to a home treatment program including activities identified, the OTR and COTA will make a home visit to determine whether modifications need to be made to ensure that the program is effective in the patient's environment.

Treatment Implementation

Since the treatment program established for Willie was carried out over a long period of time, the following brief excerpt is provided to acquaint the reader with some of the specific treatment activities.

The treatment plan was implemented the next day by the COTA. Willie joined the craft group at the center and selected a mosaic trivet project constructed with 1-inch tile. While waiting for the glue to dry prior to applying grout, he started work on an oak book rack. Since he hadn't used a hand saw for a long time, the COTA suggested that he practice on a piece of pine first. This also served as a way to grade the activity, as pine offers less resistance than oak. Involvement in these activities addressed the treatment objectives in the areas of range of motion, fine and gross motor skills, and strength and endurance.

The COTA observed Willie while he was eating lunch and determined that a plate guard would be needed. She asked Willie to try eating with a 6-ounce wrist cuff on his right hand. He agreed and stated: "This really helps get rid of some of my shaking."

During the afternoon, Willie participated in a leisure skills discussion group and later joined some of the group members in walking around the neighborhood. The COTA gave Willie a copy of the recreational calendar of events sponsored by the center and encouraged him to attend the baseball outing and to participate in shuffleboard that week.[2] She also made an appointment with him so that she and the OTR could evaluate his apartment. Before he left the center for the day, the COTA instructed Willie in a home range of motion program that emphasized crossing the midline. The assistant recorded observation and progress notes, and called the OTR to report this information as well as to verify a date and time for the home visit.

The home visit was conducted the following Monday morning. The COTA observed Willie while he was washing his face, brushing his teeth, and shaving. The latter activity presented some new problems, not observed in the initial evaluation. Willie was using a small manual razor, and the COTA suggested that he try a heavier electric razor which she had brought along. Willie stated: "I'm going right out to buy one of these!" The COTA also observed Willie while he donned a long sleeved shirt with front buttons. Noting his frustration in fastening the buttons, she instructed him on how to use a button hook. With some embarrassment, Willie stated that the only other dressing problem he had was zipping up his pants. He was surprised to see how easily the problem was solved with the use of a zipper pull. The OTR had brought portable grab bars for the bathtub and the toilet, and after observing Willie's transfer techniques, she installed the equipment and had the COTA instruct him in using it correctly and safely. Because of trunk and lower extremity rigidity, the OTR also recommended that an elevated toilet seat be used.

Both the OTR and the COTA noted that Willie's general housekeeping was less than adequate so, with Willie's permission, arrangements were made with a neighborhood church to have a volunteer youth group come in to do heavy cleaning every two weeks for a nominal fee that was used to support church activities. The OTR recommended that Willie join a group at the center, which the COTA led, to learn work simplification and energy conservation techniques related to daily cooking and housekeeping tasks. Since Willie lived alone, he agreed to be enrolled in a telephone reassurance program sponsored by a local senior citizens group.

Program Discontinuation

Because of the nature of this progressively debilitating disease, no program discontinuation was anticipated. Instead, the OTR and COTA conducted frequent reassessments of the patient's progress and continually adapted the program to his gradual loss of independence. It was anticipated that they would contact a therapist in a nursing home if and when it became necessary for Willie to transfer to an intermediate care facility.

At the present time, however, Willie is doing quite well. His spirits have improved as a result of his continued ability to maintain an independent existence. Although he recognizes his present level of difficulty, he has expressed appreciation to the occupational therapy staff for their assistance in maintaining his sense of dignity by helping him to remain independent.

References

1. Okamoto G: *Physical Medicine and Rehabilitation*. Philadelphia: WB Saunders, 1984, pp 181-182.

2. Spencer EA: Functional restoration-specific diagnosis. In H Hopkins, H Smith Eds: *Willard and Spackman's Occupational Therapy*, Sixth Edition. Philadelphia: JB Lippincott, 1983, pp 405-407.

CHAPTER 21

Alzheimer's Disease: The Elderly Patient

Ilenna Brown, COTA
Cynthia F. Epstein, OTR

Introduction

Alzheimer's disease, first described by the German physician Alois Alzheimer in 1907, is a neurological brain disorder which causes both intellectual and physical decline and, eventually, death. Early stages of the disease are characterized by a gradual, and sometimes imperceptible, decline in many areas of intellectual function with accompanying physical decline. Initially, only memory may be noticeably affected. There may be difficulty in learning new skills or with tasks requiring abstract reasoning.

As the disease progresses, impairment in both language and motor ability is seen. Inability to find the right word or words to describe things and increasing difficulty in understanding explanations (expressive and receptive aphasia) become evident. Changes in personality and outbursts of anger may be seen. Late in the illness, such varying symptoms as incontinence, inability to walk, and inability to recognize people are characteristic. Alzheimer's disease usually leads to death in about seven to nine years.

An estimated 1.3 million to 1.8 million Americans over 65 years of age have this disease. Another 80,000 or more Americans in their 40's and 50's also contract it. To date, there is no cure for Alzheimer's disease, and death occurs probably not from brain deterioration itself, but from physical infirmities such as pneumonia and pulmonary embolism that can accompany the disease.

A final diagnosis of Alzheimer's disease rests on the presence of neurotic plaques and neurofibrillary tangles in the structure of the brain. A brain autopsy is the only way of making this determination, and these are not routinely done at present. Currently, clinical observation, the absence of any other causes for the condition, and a compatible CT (computerized tomography) scan are the basis on which a diagnosis of Alzheimer's disease is made.[1,2]

Case Study Background

Gertrude was born on April 6, 1910, in New York. She was the oldest of four children, two of whom are still living. Gertrude never married and lived by herself, employed as a secretary, until her retirement at age 65 in 1974. She then went to live with her sister and her husband, where she was a productive member of their household. In 1979, her sister noticed that Gertrude was becoming increasingly forgetful, often misplacing personal belongings or leaving pots unattended on the stove. Additionally, Gertrude could not concentrate on an activity, and she didn't seem to enjoy participating in family discussions the way she had in the past. Her sister attributed these problems to Gertrude's "getting older," not recognizing them as possible symptoms of early Alzheimer's disease.[1]

By 1983, the home situation had significantly worsened. The sister's husband became ill and was hospitalized. When he returned home, he required a great deal of time and care. Gertrude had become a serious management problem for her sister. She was withdrawn, spoke very little, and often had sudden outbursts of temper over seemingly inconsequential matters. She would frequently leave the house and then not be able to find her way home. One day Gertrude walked out of the house without putting on her shoes or stockings. It was at this point that her sister, recognizing the seriousness of the problem and feeling unable to cope any longer, took Gertrude to a geriatrician, a physician who specializes in working with older people.

The diagnosis was Alzheimer's disease. The physician referred the family to a community support group, which was sponsored by the local chapter of the Alzheimer's Disease and Related Disorders Association, to help them to cope with the situation. As the family realized the severity of the problem and the increasing demands Gertrude's illness would make upon them, they began to consider nursing home placement. They visited many facilities, seeking one which would be supportive of patients with this disease. Guidelines provided by the support group helped the family to identify important services, such as occupational therapy, which should be available in the nursing home.

The nursing home selected was well known in the community for its supportive care to such patients. They even had a special family council, where families met together with staff to plan special events for the patients. Because of its excellent reputation, the facility had a waiting list. The family decided that it was worth waiting and obtained homemaker assistance and the help of the sister's grown children and grandchildren. This allowed Gertrude's sister to manage her invalid husband and Gertrude at home until a bed became available in the nursing home.

During the month of waiting, Gertrude became progressively worse. At the time of her admission, presenting problems were: increased confusion and forgetfulness, rapid mood changes, and catastrophic reactions involving a refusal to participate in such daily living skills as bathing, dressing, and undressing.[2]

Assessment

A referral for occupational therapy evaluation was made by the physician upon the patient's admission. As part of the screening process, the registered occupational therapist assigned the certified occupational therapy assistant to perform the preliminary chart review. Using a structured reporting format, the COTA gathered information on the patient's educational and occupational history, her leisure interests, and her prior living situation. With this information on hand, the OTR then met with the family to obtain a more comprehensive picture of the patient's functional level prior to admission.

In assessing a patient with Alzheimer's disease, the care givers provide an important source of information, since the patient is not usually reliable. The family reported that the patient's increasing forgetfulness, unsteady gait, and increasing incontinence had made home management unfeasible. They indicated that she had never been very social, but was, at times, pleased to be involved in small homemaker chores such as folding linen and paring vegetables.

The evaluation procedure was carried out over a week and a half so that the patient would not become overly stressed or agitated. The procedure utilized formal evaluation by the OTR and observational assessments done by the COTA and OTR.

The evaluation covered performance of selected physical and psychological daily living skills as well as sensorimotor, cognitive, and psychosocial components. In daily living, it was found that the patient was incontinent of bowel and bladder, unable to perform self-care activities without physical assistance, unable to self-feed when presented with a meal tray, and had difficulty in transferring in and out of bed. The patient could verbally make her needs known, but at times would be unable to express herself coherently. She could not make appropriate decisions regarding performance of such daily living tasks as when to brush her teeth or hair, when to go to the bathroom, or when to go to sleep.

In the sensorimotor area, the patient's range of motion and muscle strength were essentially within normal limits for her age and status. She ambulated with an unsteady slow gait, stooped posture, and almost complete absence of arm swing. Visually, she was able to follow an object, but visuospatial deficits were noted in figure-ground discrimination and form constancy. There was an identified hearing loss, greater in the left ear, which had been fitted for a hearing aid. The patient refused to wear this. When engaged in purposeful tasks, Gertrude tired easily, sustaining only 3 to 4 minutes of activity. Difficulty was also noted in right/left discrimination and in such tasks as writing, buttoning, and cutting.

Selected cognitive assessment tools were used to help develop baseline data. The patient's short attention span and tendency toward agitation limited the testing. Since the COTA had begun visiting the patient daily and was establishing a supportive relationship, it was decided to incorporate selected aspects of the cognitive assessment into these visits. The COTA was able to assist in administering some of the structured test material and reported her findings to the OTR. It was also possible for the OTR to observe the COTA as she worked with the patient during the assessment process, thus providing additional important information.

The patient was given a 10-item test, called the Mental Status Questionnaire (MSQ), which is used to assess orientation and recent and remote memory. A rating of 6 to 8 errors indicates moderate-to-severe chronic brain syndrome. The patient made 8 errors, answering only two questions correctly.

Another test given was the FROMAJE.[3] This test covers seven areas: function, reasoning, orientation, memory, arithmetic, judgement, and emotional state. The test follows a structured interview format and utilizes information from family members, the patient, and current care givers such as nursing, social service, and occupational therapy staff. The COTA was able to perform portions of this assessment under the direction of the OTR. A rating of 13 or more on this test indicates severe dementia or depression. The patient scored 19. During this portion of the evaluation it was noted that the patient became highly agitated and at times physically abusive, when presented with problem solving tasks that were beyond her capabilities.

Psychosocially, the patient was noted to have signs of depression, including lethargy, withdrawal from social interactions, suspiciousness, and sudden mood swings. Gertrude would not participate in any group activities and was highly selective in her dyadic interactions, requiring maximum encouragement and support from care givers in order to obtain meaningful responses.

The evaluation results were summarized in a written report prepared by the OTR. This report, which was to form the basis for the treatment plan, identified the following problems which occupational therapy would address:

1 Incontinence.
2 Relocation in new environment.
3 Dependence in self-care daily living skills.
4 Lack of purposeful activity.
5 Poor physical endurance.
6 Depression.
7 Significant cognitive deficits.

The treatment plan would include the use of specific activities and therapeutic methods in the areas of daily living skills training as well as sensorimotor, cognitive and psychosocial treatment. In addition, the treatment plan incorporated specific training for other staff care-givers.

The occupational therapy treatment plan was one component in the overall plan of care for Gertrude. In order to develop a realistically comprehensive plan, the OTR and COTA met with the full team to develop the program plan.

Program Planning

A post-admission team conference was held with family, patient, and staff involved in the case. Owing to the patient's cognitive and behavioral problems, the conference was conducted in two stages. The initial part of the meeting took place without the patient's involvement. At this time, team members reviewed findings and presented their suggested goals for the team's information and consideration. After discussion, it was agreed that the long-term goals would be to:

1 Encourage the patient's optimal functioning within the nursing home environment
2 Establish a DLS maintenance program which could be periodically re-evaluated and adjusted.
3 Maintain the patient's functional physical capacity within the limits of the disease process.

The occupational therapy program plan and goals were presented and discussed with the team by the OTR. The COTA, designated as the person responsible for primary treatment of the patient, explained the initial occupational therapy treatment objectives in relation to the goals. These goals, in order of priority, were:

1 Re-establish continence in conjunction with nursing.
2 Adapt and stabilize physical environment to enhance cognitive performance.
3 Establish structured plan for performance of self-care activities.
4 Identify feasible work and leisure activities.
5 Involve patient in purposeful activities on a regular basis.
6 Provide inservice for nursing staff on unit to assure carryover of structure and environmental adaptations.
7 Integrate patient into small group exercise program in conjunction with activities department.

The team accepted the occupational therapy goals. Specific objectives for interdisciplinary goals were incorporated into the treatment plan for each respective discipline. It was agreed that the initial team focus would be the re-establishment of continence and independence in eating. The COTA would work with the nursing staff on the unit to provide inservice regarding the procedures and structure for guiding the patient.

Gertrude was present for the last part of the conference. Owing to her cognitive deficits, the goals established were discussed in very general terms, focusing on the team's desire to help her feel more comfortable and independent in her new home.

In accordance with the team plan, the initial

FIGURE 21-1. Action Plan

Staff:	Action Plan for Stabilizing and Adapting Environment:
OTR/COTA	1. Assess patient's room in light of her limited cognitive abilities and existing environmental barriers. Develop plan to modify room.
COTA	2. Draw up plan.
OTR/Nursing/ Housekeeping/ Maintenence	3. Meet with supervisors from nursing, housekeeping, and maintenance. Request assistance from their staff in modifying the patient's room, using the plan developed by the occupational therapy department.
OTR/COTA/Social Service/Family	4. Meet with social service and family to request help in bringing familiar objects and furnishings for the patient's room.
COTA	5. Analyze self-care activities, including toileting, so that the modified environment would facilitate patient's motor and cognitive daily living skills performance. Begin to implement plan.
COTA	6. Contact other departments for assistance as needed (*i.e.*, maintenance to make sign for toilet and housekeeping to move furniture).
OTR/COTA	7. Meet periodically to discuss and document progress. Modify plan as needed.
OTR/Team	8. Keep team supervisors informed of progress and ongoing needs.
OTR/COTA/Team	9. Meet with the team, including family, as needed, to assure continuity and continue stabilization of new environment.

occupational therapy treatment plan had a primary focus in the area of daily living skills. Techniques, media, and activity sequence were identified by the OTR. Input and discussion between the OTR and COTA helped to refine and formalize the initial plan. A primary key to facilitating the daily living skills for this patient was the stabilization and adaptation of the environment. In order to do this, it was important for the team to be involved in the occupational therapy treatment plan.

A similar action plan, developed for each of the short-term goals, is shown in Figure 21-1.

As the patient progressed, a daily living skills maintenance program was to be instituted. This would require that nursing aides understand and demonstrate the ability to provide Gertrude with needed structure and sequence so that she could perform daily living skills tasks under their supervision. In accordance with the guidelines developed by the occupational therapy department, a "care plan card" was to be made by the COTA for each general daily living skills area. These cards would contain environmental guidelines to assure stabilization; key phrases to use when guiding the patient in an activity; and special approaches which would help the patient to refocus if she became agitated or confused with the task at hand. The plan also required that the COTA provide inservice to the aide staff so that they would understand how to use the cards when working with the patient.

In conjunction with the activities department staff, headed by another COTA, a plan was developed to integrate the patient into a small exercise group. This was to be accomplished by having both COTAs co-lead the group while Gertrude became acclimated to the setting. The group leader would also reinforce the patient's work and leisure roles in this group structure. The initial plan was to have Gertrude hand out name tags to each group member when they met and collect them at the conclusion of the meeting.

It was hoped that this plan would allow the patient to become more independent and comfortable in her new environment, and the staff to be more capable of carrying over the specifically designed structure. The OTR and the COTA were then to develop a monitoring plan to be carried out after the patient was discharged from the occupational therapy treatment program

Treatment Implementation

After long-term and short-term goals had been established and the program plan developed, a treatment program based on these goals was initiated by the COTA. Gertrude was now familiar with the occupational therapy assistant by sight, although she could not remember the COTA's name. To establish structure for the patient, she was treated at the same time five days a week, and a routine was adhered to as strictly as possible. In addition, the physical environment was set up simply.

In light of the environmental problems presented, the COTA worked with the staff to make certain changes. The bathroom door in the patient's room looked very similar to other doors in the room, and Gertrude was unable to distinguish among them. To give the patient visual cues, a sign saying "Toilet," along with a picture of a woman of the type seen in many public rest rooms, was affixed to the bathroom door.

Gertrude shared a room with another woman, and she frequently confused her bed and closet with those of her roommate. The room was rearranged so that Gertrude's bed, with the bedspread from home, was nearest the door. Her dresser from home was brought in, as well as a small lamp and doily, which were placed on top. In order to help Gertrude remember where her clothes were in the dresser, the COTA made labels and affixed these, along with appropriate pictures, to each of the drawers.

The patient was seen daily in a corner of the day room that contained a table and two lounge chairs. Each day, after the COTA greeted Gertrude, she offered her a glass of juice, which she seemed to enjoy. During this initial part of the treatment session, the COTA attempted to engage the patient in conversation. It was difficult for Gertrude to respond to questions that required anything but a yes or no answer. She had problems finding words and would often make statements such as, "Well, of course, you know, don't you?" or "What day is it you want to know? Well, you know," rephrasing the question asked of her. The COTA would then respond, supplying the answer, "Yes, I know. Today is Wednesday." In this way, the patient was given the opportunity to answer herself, and was also given the correct information without being placed under stress.

After this initial period of several minutes, a plan to reinforce Gertrude's adapted environment was implemented. Each day, the patient was taken to her room. She was given a flower to place in a vase on her dresser, and she was complimented on how beautiful her room looked. She was then shown where her bathroom was and was made aware of the word "Toilet" on the door. After Gertrude used the bathroom, she was again reminded of how beautiful her room looked with the flower on her dresser, her bedspread, and the special lounge chair nearby. The COTA then escorted Gertrude back to the day room. At subsequent intervals during the day, nursing staff accompanied the patient to the bathroom; thus a team approach was used to meet the goal of reestablishing continence.

Mealtime for Gertrude was another problem. Meals were given to the patients on trays. Paper plates and cups were used as well as plastic utensils. The patient's response to receiving a tray full of food, plates, and cups was to just sit and look at it. She appeared unable to feed herself. When staff members urged her to eat, she would say, "I'm not food." The occupational therapy department worked in conjunction with the dietary department and nursing staff to normalize and simplify the patient's mealtime. Instead of paper goods and plastic utensils, Gertrude was provided with ceramic dishes and stainless steel utensils. Nursing aides no longer placed a full tray of food in front of the patient but, rather, gave her a small portion of food on a plate or in a bowl, and handed her the appropriate utensil. The rest of the meal was placed outside of the patient's visual field. Gertrude was able to eat when presented with one item at a time.

Because of previous discussion with Gertrude's sister, it was felt that the patient might agree to participate in concrete, meaningful tasks which took place in her immediate environment. The job of sorting mail was chosen as an appropriate one in which Gertrude could become involved. Since room numbers appeared on the envelopes as part of the patient's address, Gertrude was directed to sort the mail by these numbers. The patient responded positively to this activity, feeling that she was being helpful to others. She was very pleased to discover her own mail mixed in with the other envelopes, as the abstract concept that the nursing home was now her home was still not clear to her. Even after several weeks, Gertrude continued to be surprised when she discovered an envelope with her name on it.

Another activity in which Gertrude became involved was helping to serve juice to the other patients in the afternoon. The COTA structured the task so that all the juice was poured into cups that were set on a cart for Gertrude, who would then push the cart to each patient in the day room and say "Juice?" and hand the patient a cup. The activity proved satisfying to the patient, as it provided a concrete task for interaction with others in a nonthreatening way. In subsequent weeks, this activity was carried out in the morning in conjunction with nursing staff. An attempt was made to increase the complexity of the task by having Gertrude pour the juice, but the addition of another step interfered with the patient's ability to interact with others so it was discontinued.

During the treatment period, weekly meetings were held between the COTA and the OTR. The patient's progress was discussed and suggestions were made as to ways in which the treatment program could be modified or enhanced. The COTA reported observations related to the patient's ability to perform simple activities, make her needs known, and participate in daily living tasks.

The COTA worked closely with the nursing staff throughout Gertrude's treatment program to help them incorporate the structured and sequenced approach needed to effectively manage this patient. It was found that with the environmental adaptations in her room, and with supervision and verbal cuing, Gertrude was eventually able to dress herself. The patient responded well to verbal encouragement, so that the nursing staff was able to dress Gertrude's roommate, while at the same time offering Gertrude the supervision and positive feedback which she needed to be independent in morning care. Through the activities of serving juice and sorting mail, the patient began to feel useful and needed. Nursing staff began to see her as an asset rather than the difficult behavior and management problem she had been when she entered the nursing home.

Toward the end of the treatment program, the patient was seen by the COTA three times a week instead of five. The nursing staff worked with Gertrude on the other two days, using the care plan cards developed by the occupational therapy assistant. The COTA met with the members of the nursing department at the end of each week to discuss problems which had arisen, offer suggestions, and clarify areas on the care plans which were unclear.

In the activities area, the COTA worked cooperatively with the head of the department, also a COTA, to help integrate the patient into a small group exercise program. Gertrude was initially resistant to becoming involved with this group. During the first several days, she observed the other patients. By the end of the first week, with encouragement from both COTAs, the patient was performing some exercises. She much preferred the beginning and end of each session when she distributed and collected name tags with the assistance of the COTA, as this task made her feel special and important.

After several weeks of co-leadership, the activities director was able to work independently with the patient in the group. Gertrude had responded positively to the group setting and performed her assigned tasks with satisfaction.

By using this method, a smooth transition was established from the occupational therapy treatment program to a continuation of structured supervision by the nursing and activities staff. The patient became used to associating a structured, positive approach with nursing and activities tasks as well as with occupational therapy. Thus this patient was provided with the kind of supportive environment which would enhance her optimal functioning.

Program Discontinuation

The monitoring program, formulated jointly by the OTR and the COTA, was presented to the team as a part of the occupational therapy program discontinuation. This program provided for periodic review of the patient's performance in the areas where treatment had been provided. A structured checklist, completed by the COTA, was to be done every three months after discharge. Should there be regression, a re-evaluation would be performed by the OTR.

The occupational therapy department would also work cooperatively with the activities department regarding the patient's performance in work and leisure activities. If the COTA who was in charge of activities noted any changes, a request for re-evaluation would be made to the occupational therapist.

The care plan cards were reviewed as part of the team conference. The nursing department integrated the use of these cards into the daily plan of care for the patient. It was agreed that if the nursing staff noted any problems with the patient's performance, a request would be sent to the OTR for a re-evaluation.

A discharge summary was prepared by the occupational therapist with the assistance of the COTA. The summary documented the patient's progress, treatment outcomes, and the follow-up plan. The treatment program was then terminated, and the monitoring plan was implemented.

Summary

This case study of a patient with Alzheimer's disease, residing in a nursing home, illustrates the effectiveness of the team approach to patient care. The involvement of family and the social services, activities and nursing departments in the occupational therapy intervention program was the key component of its success. The development of a specific maintenance program for this patient allowed the OTR and the COTA to monitor the status after direct patient treatment services were discontinued. The relationship between the occupational therapist and the occupational therapy assistant, as demonstrated by this case, points up the importance of ongoing communication and interaction as the OTR and COTA work together to provide optimal patient treatment.

References

1. National Institutes of Health, Office of Scientific and Health Reports: *Alzheimer's Disease — A Scientific Guide for Health Practitioners*. Bethesda, MD: U.S. Department of Health and Human Services, 1984.

2. Mace NL and Rabens PV: *The 36 Hour Day — A Family Guide to Caring for Persons with Alzheimer's Disease*. Baltimore, MD: Johns Hopkins University Press, 1981, pp. 38, 71-108.

3. Snow, T: Assessing mental status. *AOTA Gerontology Special Interest Section Newsletter*, 1:1, 1983.

SECTION IV

Models of Practice

As evidenced by the preceding section, certified occupational therapy assistants work in a variety of settings providing services to individuals who have various abilities and disabilities. In contrast, this segment focuses on three different models of occupational therapy practice, presented as comprehensive examples of the many roles assumed and relationships established by COTAs.

Hospice care, work and productive occupation programs, and the activities director in a geriatric facility were selected as examples because they represent areas where the demand for health care and occupational therapy services is increasing. There are numerous descriptions and examples of practice within these settings and frameworks. Note the variety of different skills, tasks and responsibilities a COTA may be responsible for. The complimentary nature of the OTR/COTA team is also discussed as a model for the provision of occupational therapy services.

CHAPTER 22

The Role of the OTR and the COTA in Hospice Care

William Matthew Marcil, COTA
Kent Nelson Tigges, OTR

Introduction

Hospice is a medieval term for a place of safety; a place for travelers to stop, eat, sleep, and be refreshed on a long journey. The first hospices were used by the crusaders on their way to the Holy Land. The term hospice came into modern usage in the 1960s when Dame Cicely Saunders conceived and implemented a plan to provide a model of health care for people with advanced metastatic disease for whom there was no hope of a cure, whose life expectancy was 6 months or less. Saunders, who was a nurse, then a social worker, and subsequently a physician, recognized that the needs of the terminal patient could not always be appropriately assessed or met in traditional hospitals or nursing homes, as their model of care was either cure, rehabilitation, or long-term maintenance.

Saunders' model for hospice care did not emerge out of, or as, a medical speciality, but rather from a humanitarian model. Saunders opened the first modern hospice, St. Christopher's in England, in 1969. She continues to be the foremost authority on the subject, and most hospices in the United States and Canada are based on her model. The first hospice to open in the United States was the Connecticut Hospice in New Haven in 1971. The first Canadian hospice, at the Royal Victoria Hospital in Montreal, opened in 1973. In 1970 the National Hospice Organization was incorporated and provides guidelines for developing hospices and promoting the hospice model of care.

At the present time there are approximately 2,000 hospices in the United States offering varying levels of care. Regulations for certification of Medicare providers became effective in 1983, and presently 13 of the nation's health insurance carriers offer hospice coverage.

Tenets of Hospice Care

Medical Management of Pain and Symptoms

The single most significant reason why patients are referred to, or seek, hospice care is for the severe and unrelenting pain that frequently is associated with advanced cancer. In traditional medical situations pain alerts the physician that something is wrong and must be investigated. Once a medical work-up is completed, a course of treatment is undertaken to resolve the problem. When the problem is corrected, the pain ceases. If the pain does not cease, traditional physicians, not understanding the true nature of pain and being reluctant to use moderate or large dosages of narcotics, have patients that suffer unnecessarily.

In the case of advanced cancer, since the source of the pain cannot be removed or treated, it is the pain itself that becomes the major concern of medical treatment. During the past 15 years hospice physicians have studied and researched the pain experienced by the cancer patient and have developed successful chemotherapy protocols that will, in 98 percent of the cases treated, completely eliminate the pain. When appropriately medicated on either small, moderate, or high dosages of narcotics, hospice patients are free from pain, experience no addiction, and are sufficiently alert to be out of bed, bathe, dress, leave their homes, and in some cases return to work. The key to successful pain control is the physician's understanding of the disease, its associated pain, and the appropriate use of narcotics.

Diagnostic Honesty

All too frequently, when unfortunate, devastating, or life-threatening news is learned, both lay and professional people react in either one of two ways. *First*, not wanting to admit or accept that there is nothing that they can do to change the situation, the physicians proceed to bring about cure with all effort, or failing that, put their efforts into prolonging the patient's life. *Second*, as no one wants to be the bearer of bad news, with all the best intentions, people respond to the patient's inquires with a lie. Communications become strained when such situations occur. Eventually, when the patient learns the true diagnosis and prognosis and realizes that he has been deceived, communication may cease. With such deceptions, patients frequently experience the additional pain of isolation and abandonment.[1]

It is the hospice philosophy that patients not only have the right, but also the need to know the nature, course, and outcome of their diagnosis. It is felt that without such knowledge patients cannot make realistic plans for the remainder of their lives. Hospice staff members advocate an open and honest attitude. No matter what question a patient asks, an honest answer is given. In dealing with diagnostic honesty, great caution and sensitivity are always employed.

Quality of Life

There are advocates who believe that the two greatest deterrents to quality of life are physical pain and discomfort. If the pain is controlled and the patient's physical needs are met, it is felt that the patient will have an improved quality of life. Hospice philosophy recognizes that quality of living extends far beyond physical pain and discomfort. Quality of life is a concept which is relative rather than absolute. It is a concept that people define individually within the context of their social community. Factors that are inherent in determining a given quality of life include:

1 Excellence of character.
2 Achievement.
3 Accomplishment.
4 Personal/social status.
5 Sense of personal well-being.

When a terminal illness dashes all hopes for a future, it is not uncommon to see patients either relinquishing their desire to live, or struggling to maintain a desire to live. When individuals feel that they can no longer be independent, have a purpose, or be significantly contributing members of society, it is little wonder that they display an attitude of helplessness and hopelessness. In either situation it is of paramount importance for hospice professionals not only to be knowledgeable of the components necessary for quality of life, but also to take as much time as needed to help the patient work through the process of identifying what it is that he or she would like to accomplish before death. In the final analysis, hospice measures its success if patients die free from pain and adverse symptoms, and with feelings of excellence of character and personal well-being. To accomplish these tenets requires not only appropriate education, but also a composition of team members that are compatible with each other and have a close and respected appreciation for each other's contribution.

Training of the COTA for Hospice Care

As the treatment of the hospice patient is not an entry-level practice for either the registered occupational therapist or the certified occupational therapy assistant, more education and experience must be undertaken before entering hospice practice.[2] For the COTA, the education, training and selection should follow this protocol:

1 When a COTA shows an interest in working with the terminally ill, the OTR should hold an initial interview with the assistant. This interview is intended to specify the reasons why the COTA wishes to enter hospice practice. As the hospice movement is new, and gaining an increasing popularity with health professionals, many are eager to be associated with hospice care for a variety of reasons. The initial interview acts as a screening process to determine appropriate motives and suitability.

2 If the COTA is considered to be an appropriate candidate, the next step is to have the assistant complete a thorough review of the literature, summarize fundamental concepts and principles, and present the findings in an oral report.

3 The COTA is then given the charge to prepare for a series of four debates and role plays with the OTR. Topics to be covered are dying/death, spiritual/religious attitude, diagnostic honesty, and grief and bereavement. These topics are dealt with in two categories: first, personal beliefs and values; and second, professional attitudes and intervention.

4 Upon successful completion of these steps, the COTA begins a trial period of accompanying the OTR to team meetings and on assessments and treatments of patients.

5 The assistant then follows a minimum of two cases: one case with the OTR and the other under supervision. Both cases must include all aspects of intervention, e.g., assessment, treatment planning, treatment, and involvement during death, wake, funeral, burial, and/or shiva.

6 Upon completion of the training program, an exit interview is held to determine if the COTA is still committed to hospice care and if the OTR feels that the assistant is personally and professionally suited for hospice care.

Role and Supervision of the COTA

As the nature of the prognosis and the needs of the terminally ill patient are considerably different from patients with "traditional" diseases and problems, the role delineation between the OTR and the COTA does not follow the exact pattern established by the American Occupational Therapy Association.[3] The following is presented as a model for COTA involvement in hospice care.

Owning to the emotionally charged nature and personal vulnerability of patients and their families, it is essential that the OTR open every case. It is at the time of the first meeting with the patient and family members that the physical, emotional, and social status and needs of the patient are determined. Equally important, the personal, emotional, social, and interpersonal dynamics between the patient and the family members are also assessed. If appropriate future treatment planning is to occur, it is essential for the OTR to screen, make an initial evaluation, and establish short-term goals, and when possible, begin treatment at the first meeting with the patient.[4]

With all cases, it is not only advisable but also highly recommended that the COTA accompany the occupational therapist during screenings and evaluations. This is important for three reasons. *First*, the assistant is introduced to the patient and the family from the onset and conveys an impression of the close teamwork that will occur between the OTR and the COTA. *Second*, the assistant will be in a position to observe the interpersonal interactions and dynamics between the therapist and the family members. If the COTA should be assigned to the case, he or she will be in a substantially better position to follow through with the treatment. *Third*, the COTA can function in the capacity of separating the patient and the family member from one another. Although it is always advisable to include the family in the initial screening and assessment, there are times when it is either recommended or essential to speak to the patient alone and to the family member or members alone. Such situations occur under the following conditions:

1 The family member answers for the patient, and the patient cannot, or does not, participate in the screening or assessment.
2 The patient is apprehensive in being open and honest about personal needs, concerns, fears, or goals.
3 The goals or expections of either the patient or a family member are not compatible or agreed upon.

Depending on the nature and complexity of the case as determined by the OTR at the time of the first visit, the OTR will make one of the following determinations: 1) the OTR will follow the case exclusively; 2) the COTA will be assigned to the case; 3) the treatment requires that both the OTR and the COTA treat the patient simultaneously.

If the second decision is made, the assistant, under close supervision by the occupational therapist, will be responsible for carrying out all or part of the treatment plan, and continually assessing the patient's status. With advanced metastatic disease, it is not uncommon to observe either a situation where the patient has consistent fluctuations between loss of function and increase of function, or a steady physical deterioration. In both situations, it is the responsibility of the COTA to assess such changes and to report them to the OTR following each treatment. The occupational therapist will then make the appropriate modifications in the treatment plan.

The treatment and ongoing assessment of patients who experience temporary remission, accompanied by increased physical independence, pose quite a different set of problems for the OTR/COTA team. It is not uncommon for occupational therapy personnel to provide treatment to patients which results in a significant increase in physical independence. While one of the authors was visiting St. Luke's Hospice in Sheffield, England a conversation took place with noted writer E. Wilkes, who stated that following pain and symptom control, occupational therapy provides the single greatest contribution in maximizing patients' quality of life. This can only be accomplished if the occupational therapist and the assistant are practicing from an occupational behavior perspective (see Chapter 4 for more detailed information). Working from this point of view, the occupational therapy team focuses exclusively on maximizing the patient's roles in relation to self-care, work, and leisure.

There are cases when medical intervention affords patients a substantial remission in their disease process. With appropriate occupational therapy intervention, patients experience a significant "improvement" in physical function and independence. There have been situations where patients have been bedridden upon admission to hospice care, and subsequently have been able to return to work. In such "miracle" cases, it is extremely important for the OTR/COTA team to maintain an appropriate professional perspective and to keep foremost in mind that the increase in performance and independence is only temporary. If professional objectivity is lost, not only will the patient develop unrealistic hopes, but occupational therapy personnel may experience feelings of failure when the patient begins to deteriorate and dies. When professional objectivity is lost, treatment is jeopardized.

A second situation occurs when the patient perceives the increased improvement as "proof" of cure. This patient, regardless of what has been stated directly, is determined to believe that he or she will be a survivor. In such cases, the COTA responsible for treatment must be careful to not "feed" into the patient's false sense of reality. A fine line must be drawn: encouraging the patient to achieve, while at the same time not promoting false hope for survival.

Once the COTA has been assigned to a case, he or she must be constantly involved in assessing how the patient is perceiving new-found independence and must convey such information to the OTR so that appropriate clarification can be established between the patient and the therapist. In traditional clinical settings, diagnostic and prognostic communication with the patient has been the sole responsibility of the physician. In hospice care, it is the role and responsibility of all professional personnel. Occupational therapists and assistants, although they may be unfamiliar with such roles, must be prepared to talk to patients honestly and explain that increased function does not indicate that they will survive.

The third example involves the OTR determining that both the occupational therapist and the assistant should treat the patient simultaneously. This type of situation occurs when there are significant interpersonal stressors between the patient and family members. The following are examples of such situations:

1. The patient and/or a family member is excessively apprehensive regarding adjusting to any change in their established routine of living; they are immobilized by the situation and have few or no outside resources to support them.
2. The patient or family member is totally dependent or independent and goals cannot be agreed upon.
3. The family member, due to a sense of responsibility, becomes unnecessarily overprotective and renders the patient dependent.

No matter how independent the patient desires to become, he or she relinquishes this need out of fear of either upsetting or alienating the family member. With the OTR and the COTA treating the patient at the same time, appropriate strategies can be put into place to meet the individual and collective needs of the family.

An important consideration in treating the hospice patient, be it in a freestanding unit or in a home care setting, is seclusion. No matter how attractive or familiar the environment is, a sense of confinement and isolation can occur over an extended period of time. Occupational therapy treatment planning should always include the option and feasibility of setting goals that would allow the patient the opportunity to engage in familiar community activities or events.

Treatment Discontinuation

The discontinuation of treatment begins the day that the patient becomes confined to bed and is no longer able to cognitively or physically engage in any aspect of self-care, work, or leisure. In cases where the OTR/COTA had minimal involvement with the patient, treatment is discontinued with appropriate "goodbyes." When occupational therapy personnel have had a significant role and involvement, the patient should be followed to the end. This includes at least one member of the OTR/COTA team participating in the vigil and being with the patient at the time of death. If the occupational therapist is the only professional person present when death occurs, it is the therapist's responsibility to declare the patient dead and to carry out the routine procedures of caring for the body and giving support to the family until a nurse or physician arrives. Following the death of a patient, occupational therapy personnel assist in seeing the family through the wake, funeral, memorial service, burial, or shiva. It is only then that the case is officially closed.

The two following case studies illustrate the role of the COTA in hospice care.

Case Study — Bill

Bill, a 63-year-old, 6′ 4″, 240-pound man with a diagnosis of glioblastoma — a malignant tumor of the brain — was referred for occupational therapy services by his hospice physician. The OTR and the COTA made the initial visit to Bill's suburban home together.

After meeting with Bill and his wife to explain the hospice program and the services that could be provided by occupational therapy, the OTR obtained an occupational history from Bill. During this time, the COTA talked with his wife in another room in order to establish a relationship and to obtain information that might assist in Bill's treatment.

The occupational history revealed that Bill was a detective with the local police department — a job which he valued and to which he hoped to return. This was evidenced by statements such as "I'm only on sick leave." Bill continued to carry his badge. It was also determined that Bill was an active outdoors man who enjoyed camping and swimming.

A physical assessment indicated that the tumor had left Bill with a flaccid left-sided hemiplegia and a severe sensory loss. Bill was concerned that this condition had made it difficult for him to perform daily living activities such as bathing, dressing, and functional household ambulation. This, combined with his inability to work, interfered with his role as family provider. The increasing dependence on his wife led to feelings of anger, depression, and being "less of a man."

Bill asked the therapist what could be done to return function to his left side, and the therapist replied that nothing could be done for his hemiplegia. Bill then asked angrily what good could therapy do for him if this was the case. The therapist told him that although no function could be returned, he could help him use his time in a meaningful way regardless of his condition. Bill acquiesced to this response.

While the OTR worked with Bill in the living room, the COTA talked with Bill's wife in the kitchen. She stated that she was concerned with the amount of care that Bill required and feared that she might not be able to care for him much longer because of his size. She also told the assistant that due to the overall design of the house, it was difficult for Bill to move about in his wheelchair and impossible for him to go outside. She added that this was contributing to his depression and causing added friction between them.

Following the 2-hour assessment, the occupational therapy team departed. While driving back to the office, they compared notes from their separate interviews. Drawing from this information, with emphasis on Bill's occupational roles and interests, the following tentative treatment plan was formulated:

1 Increase Bill's independence in dressing.
2 Increase Bill's ability to assist with bathing and toileting, using adapted equipment as necessary.
3 Increase Bill's ability to assist in transferring from bed to wheelchair and wheelchair to chair.
4 Assist Bill in leaving the home a minimum of one afternoon a week for swimming and socializing.

The OTR and the COTA returned the following day and discussed the treatment plan with Bill and his wife. After explaining how the various activities would be accomplished, both Bill and his wife agreed to the goals, and the plan was implemented.

Work on the first three goals was initiated immediately. The OTR and the COTA had brought various pieces of adapted equipment which they had previously determined would help in Bill's self-care. Use of these items was discussed with Bill and his wife and they chose those which they thought would be most helpful. Decision-making opportunities such as these allowed Bill to take a more active role in his self-care and transfers and also gave him a sense of control over other events. The therapist and the assistant then demonstrated proper transfer techniques and body mechanics to both Bill and his wife. This assured safety and the prevention of back injuries for Bill's wife.

One-handed dressing techniques were demonstrated to Bill. It was agreed that the COTA would see Bill three mornings each week to reinforce the dressing program.

The final goal, assisting Bill to leave his home for short periods, presented the biggest problem. After inspecting the home and studying the design, construction of a traditional ramp was ruled out. To solve this problem, the OTR and the COTA designed a system of portable metal runner ramps and an electric winch which could be installed and removed in minutes. This made it possible to help Bill in and out of the house safely and easily.

Each Thursday afternoon, the occupational therapy team took Bill to a local health club and spa for a swim, steambath, and a shower. Bill looked forward to these weekly outings with great enthusiasm. His depression lifted and he would often state: "It's great to be alive." In addition to the psychological boost, the swimming session provided buoyancy to support Bill's left side. This also allowed an increase in passive range of motion which could not be achieved out of the water. Both the therapist and the assistant worked with Bill during these sessions in the pool.

Following the visit to the health club, Bill, the COTA, and the OTR would stop at Bill's favorite bar and grill for a meal and a drink. Bill would often meet old friends, many of whom he had not seen since becoming ill, and would spend time socializing. This time "out with the boys" would prove to be the best therapy for Bill.

Although he never denied that he would soon die, Bill began to believe that he would regain function of his left side. He convinced himself that the swimming, which allowed him to stand, as well as his increased independence in self-care, were sure signs of returning to normal. This situation is common among hospice patients and must be dealt with honestly by the therapist and the assistant.

One day, on the way to the health club, Bill asked when he could expect full return of use to his flaccid limbs. The COTA and the OTR had to deal with this one false hope by stating very frankly that there would be no return and that no amount of exercise would bring it about.

Bill cried heavily upon hearing this response — one that he did not want to hear. The treatment team parked the car and allowed Bill to continue crying. When he had composed himself, he said "I didn't want to hear that, but it's better than not knowing for sure. Thanks for being straight with me."

Three weeks later, when the OTR and the COTA came to pick Bill up for swimming, his wife, who was crying, met them at the door. Her husband at lapsed into a coma earlier in the day and the hospice physician told her that he would probably die within a few hours. The therapist and the assistant stayed with her to provide comfort and support. Two hours after they arrived, Bill died.

The OTR, after checking vital signs, pronounced Bill dead. The COTA called the hospice to notify them and stayed with Bill's wife offering continued support. Bill's wife was so upset that she was unable to call the funeral home to make the proper arrangements so the COTA took care of this matter for her. Both the OTR and the COTA assisted his wife in choosing the suit in which Bill would be buried.

At the wake, Bill's wife introduced the COTA and the OTR to family and friends, and, at her request, they both served as pallbearers at Bill's funeral.

Following the graveside services, a funeral breakfast was held which both the assistant and the therapist attended. It was here that the case was discontinued. By saying goodbye to both Bill and his family through ritual funeral attendance, the treatment could be considered to be finalized and closure complete.

Case Study — John

John, a 72-year-old retired grocer with a diagnosis of lung cancer with subsequent metastases to the brain and spine, was referred for occupational therapy evaluation by the hospice visting nurse.

The COTA and the OTR made an initial visit to meet with John and his wife. John was lying on the couch in the living room when the occupational therapy team arrived. The therapist obtained an occupational history and conducted a sensory motor evaluation while the COTA observed and assisted.

The occupational history indicated that John was a "homebody" who had few interests. He did, however, enjoy going for drives in the country or to an occasional movie. Since he had become ill, he had little desire to do anything but watch television because he was "too weak and tired to do anything." His wife stated that although he had generalized weakness of his right side, he was physically able to care for himself but he choose not to get dressed and received only an occasional sponge bath from his wife if she "nagged" him.

From the information obtained in this first meeting, the OTR and the COTA outlined the following program which would be carried out twice a week by the assistant with input and supervision by the therapist as needed.

Short-Term Goals:

- John will shower and dress daily.
- John will engage in a leisure/social activity of his choice two times a week at home.

Long-Term Goal:

- John will attend a movie or go for a ride with the COTA at least one time.

The following day the assistant arrived at John's home and found him watching television. He asked John if he might be more comfortable sitting in a reclining chair that was by a window. The patient agreed and was assisted in walking to the chair. The COTA then presented the treatment plan for John's approval.

John stated that he would like to shower and dress, but because he was so weak both tasks were difficult and he was also afraid that he might fall in the shower. He also stated that he had no leisure interests. In regard to the long-term goal, John stated that he did not want to be seen in public in his condition and was happy to stay indoors.

The COTA then explained to John that he could teach him alternate methods of dressing which would allow him to dress himself while expending as little energy as possible. In terms of the shower, the assistant explained that there were many assistive devices available to make the process easy and safe. John agreed to "give the plan a try."

It had been previously determined by the COTA and confirmed by the OTR that John could benefit from a long-handled bath brush and an adapted tub seat to aid in showering. The assistant removed these items from the car and carefully explained how the equipment could be used. The assistant then asked John if he would like to shower, to which he replied, "You mean right now?" The assistant nodded, and John carefully inspected the tub seat and asked the assistant if he was sure it was safe. When the COTA assured him that it would be, he agreed to try. It should be noted that it is important in hospice practice to engage the patient in activity as quickly as possible, because treatment time is at a premium and must be used effectively.

The COTA assisted John to the bathroom and asked his wife to accompany them. He demonstrated to both of them how to install and remove the tub seat, as well as the proper transfer techniques. John, who was initially skeptical about this activity, remained in the shower for 30 minutes and repeatedly commented on how "great" it felt and that he wanted to shower on a daily basis from then on.

Following the shower, the assistant demonstrated dressing techniques which John could perform while seated in an armchair and accomplish easily and independently. Once dressed, John looked in the mirror and told the assistant that he felt like "a human again."

The COTA assisted John with his self-care program for the next three days, and he became totally independent. While dressing on the third day, John told the COTA that he enjoyed playing poker but had not played since he had become ill — partly because his "poker buddies had stopped coming around," and also because he didn't want anyone to see him "like this." He stated that he would like to play again, and the assistant encouraged this activity, indicating that they would discuss it further on the next visit.

After each visit, the COTA recorded accurate notes on the patient's physical and psychological status and any progress achieved in relation to the established goals of the treatment plan. These notes were discussed with the OTR on a weekly basis and also signed by the therapist. Because the self-care goals had been met in a short period of time, the therapist encouraged the COTA to pursue the poker game as a leisure activity leading to social interaction.

At the next meeting with John, the assistant played a few hands of poker with him after he had showered and dressed. During the game, John talked constantly and expressed feelings of remorse about how he missed his weekly poker games with his friends, which allowed him to socialize, relax, and "get away from the little woman for a while." The COTA asked him if he would like to invite his friends over some night for a "real" game. John was apprehensive and hedged on the answer. The assistant, not wanting to press him and damage the rapport and trust that had been established, told John to think about it and changed the subject.

The following day, John told the COTA that he had thought about the game and decided he would like to do it. Together, he and the assistant made plans to schedule the game for the following week. The patient became more excited as the planning process continued and called to invite two of his friends that day. He also indicated that he would like the assistant to be present at the card party.

While John remained in the living room, the COTA explained the plan to his wife, who was in the den. He asked her if she could make plans to go out that evening. She readily agreed, since she had not been out of the house since her husband had become ill. She immediately went to the living room and informed her husband that he was doing the planning. John responded "good, that will give me a chance to visit with my friends." This particular interchange was significant because it gave John a feeling of control and a sense of having a "normal" poker game.

The night of the game, while John and the COTA were setting up, he asked the assistant if, now that he was able to function independently and was living a relatively normal life, he would be able to "beat" his cancer and resume life as it had been. The assistant, without benefit of another professional present, and knowing the tenet of diagnostic honesty, told him that his cancer was far too advanced to be treated. He also stressed the importance of the fact that it was still possible for John to make the most of the time he had left.

John was noticeably hurt by this response and said, "But I thought that I was getting better." The COTA responded, "You have gotten better in terms of what you can do, regardless of your disease, but you can't make your cancer go away." John began to weep and then said, "Well, this isn't going to ruin my night. Nobody is going to bring me down without a fight!"

The poker game was a success, and John had "the best night of my life." He was even able to tell his friends that although he wasn't going to live much longer, they were welcome to come by and play cards anytime.

The following week, when the COTA arrived at John's home, he found him on the couch, not feeling well. John told the assistant that he felt weak and didn't want to do anything. When asked if he would like the assistant to stay and talk, he agreed. They discussed the events which had taken place at the poker game, and John smiled at the memories. During the conversation, John had a seizure and lapsed in and out of consciousness. Sensing that John would die soon, the COTA went to inform his wife of the situation. John also sensed that he was dying and took this last opportunity to tell his wife that he loved her and to say goodbye.

While John and his wife were talking, the COTA recognized their need for privacy and left them alone for a brief period. He then called the hospice physician and the OTR to inform them of the turn of events. When he returned to the living room, John was dead. The assistant comforted John's wife and checked her husband's vital signs, determining that he had, in fact, died. The COTA then covered John's body and led his wife to the kitchen where he remained to console her until other hospice staff arrived.

Before he left, the COTA removed the bath bench and brush to spare John's wife any unnecessary memories.

Although John ultimately died, the COTA helped him to achieve a better quality of life in the time that was left to him. Without occupational therapy intervention, John would have remained immobile on his couch and would not have experienced some of life's pleasures.

Summary

The hospice philosophy has been considered to be the most innovative model of treatment developed in the 20th century. As the hospice model departs substantially from traditional medical and rehabilitative attitudes and values, a reconstruction of the roles of occupational therapy personnel, and particularly that of the COTA, have been outlined in depth. The tenets of hospice care highlight the important elements of medical management of pain and symptoms, the importance of diagnostic honesty, and the need to maintain quality of life for the terminally ill patient. The occupational therapy model of occupational behavior is used as a framework for the delivery of services. The occupational therapy process is modified to some degree, because the therapeutic intervention time is limited. Case study examples illustrate the many ways that the success of occupational therapy can be measured in helping the terminally ill *live* before they die.

References

1. Tigges K, Sherman L, Sherwin F: Perspectives on the pain of the hospice patient: The role of the occupational therapist and the physician. *Occup Ther in Health Care*, 4:55-68, 1984.
2. Tigges K: Occupational therapy in hospice. In: Corr CA and Corr DM, Eds: *Hospice Care: Principles and Practice*. New York: Springer Publishing, 1983, pp 160-176.
3. Entry-level role delineation for OTR's and COTA's. *Occup Ther Newspaper*, 35 (July):8-16, 1981.
4. Tigges K and Sherwin F: Implications of the pawn-origin theory for hospice care. *The American Journal of Hospice Care*, 2:29-32, 1984.

Bibliography

Flanigan K: The art of the possible — occupational therapy in terminal care. *British Journal of Occupational Therapy*, 45:274-276, 1982.

Picard H and Magno J: The role of occupational therapy in hospice care. *American Journal of Occupational Therapy*, 36:592-598.

Tigges K and Holland A: The hospice movement: A time for professional action and commitment. *British Journal of Occupational Therapy*, 44:373-376, 1981.

CHAPTER 23

The Role of the COTA in Work and Productive Occupation Programs

Kathlyn L. Reed, OTR/L

Introduction

Work is defined as the effort exerted to do or make something.[1] In American society, work usually is associated with employment at a job, vocation, profession, business, trade, or craft. However, not all work is for a paycheck. Thus the term "productive occupations" is used to identify such efforts as housework, volunteer activities, amateur pursuits, or student efforts.

Work includes an action and a purpose as illustrated in Figure 23-1. The action is the expenditure of physical or mental energy. There are three purposes for work according to sociologists: 1) to survive, 2) to preserve social institutions, and 3) to produce or distribute goods and services.[2,3] Occupational therapists have defined survival as daily living skills (DLS), or self-care, rather than as work. Nevertheless, there is a close relationship between daily living skills and work since most people must complete some daily living tasks each day before they can begin working. Furthermore, there is a relationship between DLS, work, and leisure. In an average day, some time is spent in all three areas. Achieving a balance among the three is an important task, according to occupational therapy theory. As Figure 23-2 suggests, there is a danger to health and well-being when the balance is not maintained. Therefore, although this chapter is primarily about work and productive occupations, references to daily living skills and leisure will be included where relevant.

A Word About Words

Americans are fascinated by words. They enjoy thinking up new words, changing terminology, and expanding the vocabulary. The "fun stops" when one must learn the variety of terms and synonyms associated with the same phenomenon. Alas, work programming is such a phenomenon. The terms *work*, *productive occupations*, and *work programming* will be used in this chapter because they are most recognizable. Other references may use a variety of different terms. Many of these have been organized in Figure 23-3.

FIGURE 23-1. Definition and Description of Work

Work =	Action	+	Purpose
	Expenditure of physical or mental energy		1. To survive 2. To preserve social institutions or 3. To produce and distribute goods and services

History of Work Programs in Occupational Therapy

Occupational therapy has been involved in work programs since the early 1900s. Work programs have included a wide variety of techniques and approaches to encourage work behavior and to develop work skills. These techniques are outlined in Figure 23-4. Early programs used arts and crafts as work situations, and workshops made and sold hand crafted items. The choice of handcrafts was deliberate. A popular view of health problems attributed illnesses such as tuberculosis, a lung disease, and neurasthenia, a mental stress disorder, to the industrial revolution, machine manufacturing, and the crowded conditions which resulted. A return to handcrafts was thought to promote more healthful living.

After World War I, the use of arts and crafts was changed. Art was rarely used, and crafts were analyzed according to the range of motion, muscle action, or physical strength the craft provided. During the 1930s, some work programs were not using any media or methods in occupational therapy. Rather, the occupational therapist assigned patients to other services in the hospital and monitored their work progress.

The 1940s saw a return to the occupational therapy clinic as a source of work programs. Understanding of work tasks and the skills needed to perform them had increased the emphasis on physical capacities. Analysis of jobs and assessment of individuals expanded rapidly during the 1950s. Job simulation and individual testing for job fitness became popular and led to the development of work samples.

During the 1960s, there was a growing awareness that there were people with special work problems. Some had multiple physical limitations, while others had emotional difficulties and intellectual deficiencies. Special work programs were developed to meet these special needs. Some of these programs, however, included work as only a minor part of the overall plan.

In the 1970s and 1980s, work programs developed and expanded to include other aspects of life such as daily living skills and leisure activities. There was a recognition that people do not live by work alone. Occupational therapists saw the concept of total rehabilitation as a core concept of occupational therapy and reasserted their interests in work programs. This interest has led to an increase in continuing education opportunities for therapists and assistants to develop their skills in providing work and work-related activities.

Effects of Federal Legislation on Work Programs

Federal legislation has had a significant effect on work programs in occupational therapy. Important legislative acts are summarized in Figure 23-5.

Prior to 1920, the profession of occupational therapy was unrestrained in its development of work programs since there were no federal or state guidelines for what constituted a work program. Also, few vocational training people existed.

After the 1920 Vocational Rehabilitation Act was passed, guidelines were developed which became procedures for determining eligibility for funds. Work programs which included medical services and rehabilitation were not eligible because there were no funds for medical services. The focus was on education and training only. Since occupational therapy was considered a medical service, it was not covered either. Thus outpatient workshops or free-standing workshops were difficult for occupational therapists to maintain financially and most closed. Only those in states that provided supplemental funds for medical services saw such growth in occupational therapy sponsored work programs. In the other states, work programs were run by vocational training personnel.

After 1943 the situation changed somewhat because medical services were covered. However, occupational therapy was viewed as a hospital ser-

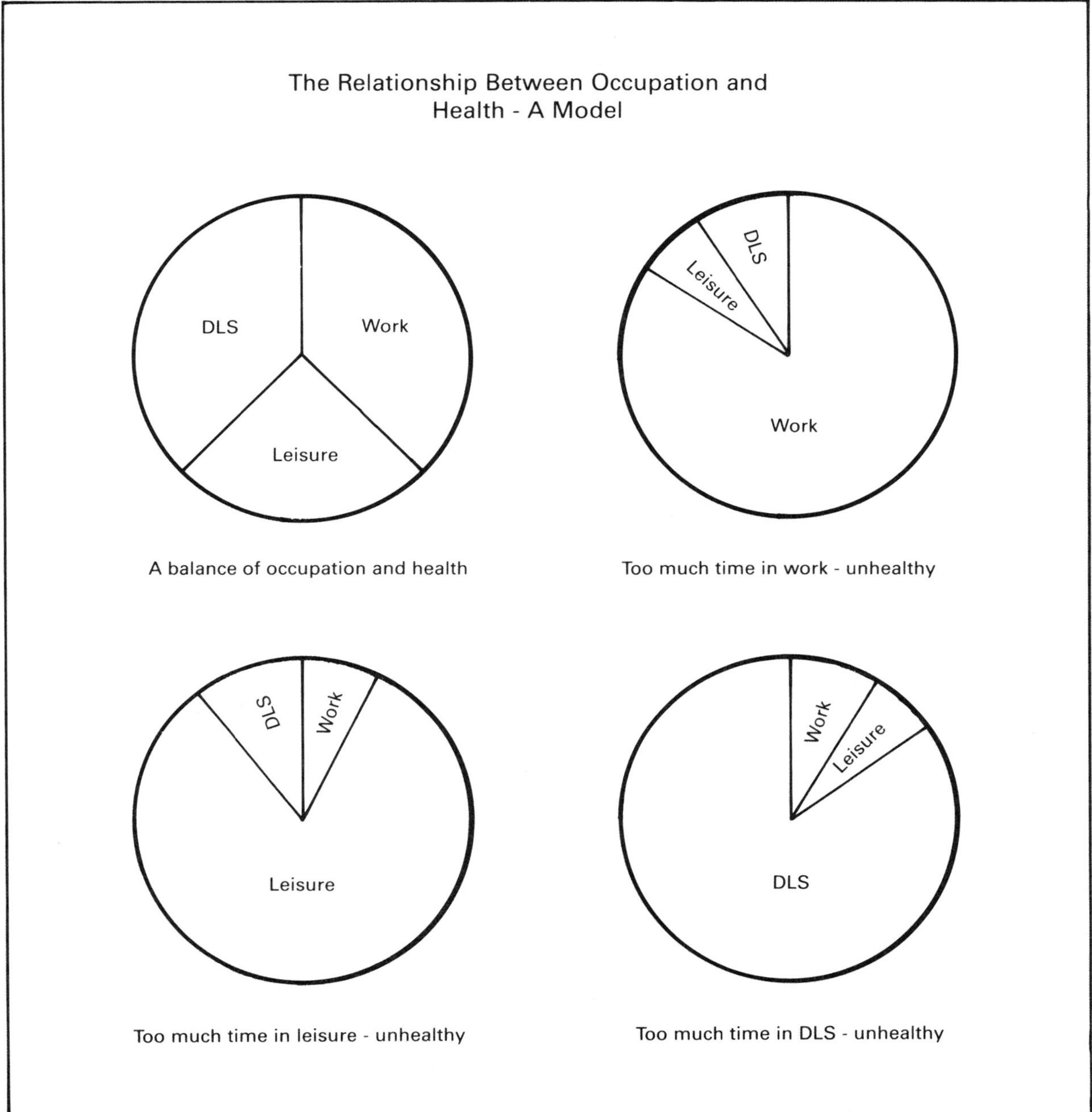
The Relationship Between Occupation and
Health - A Model
DLS
Work
Leisure
A balance of occupation and health
DLS
Leisure
Work
Too much time in work - unhealthy
DLS
Work
Leisure
Too much time in leisure - unhealthy
Work
Leisure
DLS
Too much time in DLS - unhealthy

Figure 23-2

FIGURE 23-3. Terminology in Work Programming

Meaning	Words Used
The nature of one's labor or toil	Work, occupation, vocation, trade, craft, job, business, profession
A program designed to teach work skills and prepare a person to work	Workshop, sheltered workshop, curative workshop, prevocational workshop, work program, work activity center, vocational workshop, work adjustment program
The teaching or training of people to work	Work therapy, industrial therapy, work readiness, vocational preparation, vocational readiness, career education, rehabilitation counseling, prevocational training, job training, work training, work adjustment therapy
The assessment of work skills and attributes	Work assessment, work evaluation, vocational evaluation, occupational assessment, prevocational evaluation, work sample, vocational guide, work capacity evaluation, work habits evaluation

vice during this time period, and rarely did occupational therapists get involved in work programs outside the hospital environment. The few therapists who were involved in work programs were employed by vocational training personnel.

The changes in the 1954 Vocational Rehabilitation Act had a profound influence on occupational therapy. Once again, occupational therapists were involved in nonhospital work programs, and there was an increase in hospital programs as well. Money for education and training supported the expansion.

By the 1960s, work programs became too expensive to operate in medically related settings and most closed. The separation between vocational training personnel and occupational therapy widened once again.

The 1970s and 1980s have witnessed an expanding role for occupational therapy. Career education, industrial insurance claims and training of special populations have contributed to the increase. Occupational therapists and vocational personnel are working together again to provide better work programs.

The Meaning of Work

Over the years Western man has attributed a number of viewpoints to the meaning of work.[3] The ancient Greeks saw work as drudgery and a curse. Work was to be avoided by everyone but the slaves. Hebrew tradition viewed work as man's lot because of original sin. Work was necessary but not fun. Early Christianity accepted the Hebrew point of view.

During the Protestant revolution, Martin Luther espoused the view that work was the key to life and would lead to salvation. Thus work became more than a daily "grind." Work well done could lead to eternal life. John Calvin augmented Luther's ideas, pronouncing that work was God's will. Therefore, work was good in and of itself. Idleness and leisure were the sins of the devil.

The Renaissance period viewed work as pleasurable. Artists, writers and craftsmen were seen as enjoying their work, as opposed to working out of necessity to gain God's favor.

Utopian, Socialist and Humanist views contain modifications of these themes. The Utopians felt that work could be pleasurable if the work was suited to the worker's character and was not done to excess. Socialists felt that people would work if the work was limited to what was needed with the remaining time spent in leisure. They viewed the demon of work to be the profit motive, which drove people to produce more than was needed in order to make more money. Finally, the Humanists viewed work as a fundamental human activity, which shaped a person's character and developed potential. Without work a man was not truly a man. Women's work was a separate issue. The various views on work are summarized in Figure 23-6.

The historical views of work have been organized by Bucholz into five belief systems expressed by workers today.[4] These belief systems can be useful in discussions of value clarification regard-

FIGURE 23-4. History of Work Programs in Occupational Therapy

Year/Program	Program Description	Reference
1904 Sanatorium workshop	Handcraft Shop in Marblehead, Massachusetts. Dr. Herbert J. Hall opened the shop to offer work instead of rest as a means of prevention and cure for psychiatric patients.	Luther J: Occupational treatment in nervous disorders. *Modern Hospital* 11:11–15, 1918.
1913 Hospital workshop	Outpatient Workshop, Massachusetts General Hospital, Boston, Massachusetts. Dr. Hall helped organize the workshop to help "sick and discarded" workers adapt to work that would be graded and controlled to meet any degree of handicap.	Hall HJ: Hospital and asylum workshops. *Journal of the American Medical Assn.* 61:1976–1977, 1913.
1914 Free-standing workshop	Consolution House, Clifton Springs, New York. George Barton, an architect, wanted a place where people could convalesce but also serving as a school, workshop, and vocational bureau.	Newton IG: Consolution House. *Trained Nurse and Hospital Review* 59:321–326, 1917.
1928 Curative workshop	Milwaukee Curative Workshop, Milwaukee, Wisconsin. The goal was to make a man functionally fit for work after an industrial accident or injury.	Goodman, HB: The Milwaukee Curative Workshop. *Rehabilitation Review* 3: December, 1929.
1936 Industrial therapy	Ypsilanti State Hospital, Ypsilanti, Michigan. Activities within the institution were used as sources of work for patients who produced articles and performed services useful to the institution.	Inch GF: Therapeutic placement of mental patients in state hospital industries. *Occupational Therapy and Rehabilitation* 15:241–248, 1936.
1946 Prevocational program	Lovell General Hospital, Fort Devens, Massachusetts. Occupational therapy clinic and hospital industries functioned as testing and learning situations to develop work habits and capacities.	Farwell MM: Occupational therapy in prevocational exploration. *Occupational Therapy and Rehabilitation* 25:198–199, 1946.
1950 Work evaluation	Rochester Rehabilitation Center, Rochester, New York. Actual job situations served to evaluate interests, skills, dexterity, coordination, rate of production, adjustment to routine and personnel, and general work habits.	Stevens AL: Work evaluation of rehabilitation. *Occupational Therapy and Rehabilitation* 29:157–161, 1950.
1957 Work therapy	May T. Morrison Center for Rehabilitation, San Francisco, California. Job simulation was used to assess and train people to develop work skills.	Wegg L: The role of the occupational therapist in vocational rehabilitation. *American Journal of Occupational Therapy* 11:252–254, 1957.
1964 Work adjustment	Work Adjustment Program, Lafayette Clinic, Detroit, Michigan. Goal of program was to evaluate patients with poor work histories to adjust to work conditions and to function on a job.	Llorens LA, Levy R, Rubin EZ: Work Adjustment Program. *American Journal of Occupational Therapy* 18:15–18, 1964.

FIGURE 23-5. Significant Legislation in Vocational Rehabilitation

Date	*Name and Purpose of Legislation*
1916	National Defense Act: Improved military efficiency and enabled soldiers to gain work skills for civilian life.
1917	Smith-Hughes Act: Created the Federal Board for Vocational Education (FBVE).
1918	Smith-Sears Act, or Soldiers Rehabilitation Act: Directed the FBVE to provide programs for disabled veterans who were unable to work.
1920	Smith-Fess Act, or Civilian Rehabilitation Act: Extended services to nonmilitary people. Emphasis was on basic education, vocational training, and placement. No medical services were provided. This act encouraged states to start vocational rehabilitation programs.
1943	Vocational Rehabilitation Act: Included coverage for medical services for the first time.
1954	Vocational Rehabilitation Act: Included money for training and education of health professionals such as occupational therapists.
1965	Vocational Rehabilitation Act Amendments: Increased services for severely disabled and socially handicapped individuals.
1973 – 1978	Vocational Rehabilitation Act Amendments: Emphasized total rehabilitation rather than just vocational rehabilitation, began independent living programs, and included section on moving architectural barriers.

ing the meaning of work. They are listed in Figure 23-7.

Another way to explore the meaning of work is to ask people why they work and what they achieve from working. Analysis of studies suggest that there are three major areas of meaning: economic, sociocultural, and psychological.[3]

Economic reasons include making money or having an income which can be used to purchase goods and services. In other words, a job provides a paycheck, which in turn pays the rent, buys groceries, and permits the purchase of a television, an audio system, or a vacation. Occasionally, someone comments that work is good for the economy. If no one in America worked, it would be difficult to buy American-made products.

Sociocultural reasons for working are that the work setting allows people with common interests to meet, get to know one another, and arrange social activities. Most people count coworkers among their friends. Another sociocultural reason for work is that it provides an identity and establishes a level of status in society. People are frequently known by what they do. A person may be a lawyer, a farmer, a salesman, a policeman, or business executive, for example. Each job title provides information about what the individual does or does not do. In addition, a job title can be translated into a level of status which society has attributed to the job. Most people can identify the level of status or occupational prestige of a physician, a teacher, and a used car dealer. A third sociocultural reason for working is to make a contribution to society. The value of the contribution may be measured in terms of years of work, occupational prestige, or level of income. Contributing to society is a positive value as opposed to being a "free loader" or "a lazy, no good bum."

Psychological reasons for working are quite varied. Some people mention that work permits them to be independent of family or welfare. Working allows you to stand "on your own two feet." Other people mention the satisfaction they get from working; they like to see the results of their work or to know that the job has been done well. Satisfaction often is coupled with the sense of self-respect. The individual feels that working demonstrates self-worth. A person who works hard deserves to feel good about himself or herself. Psychological reasons for working are often a reflection of the occupational status of the worker. Professional and white collar workers are more likely to provide psychological reasons for working. For blue collar workers or unskilled workers, work may have little psychological significance. They work because they have to work to get money and keep society "off their back."

For many people, however, the economic, sociocultural, and psychological reasons for working are interwoven and interrelated. Figure 23-8 illustrates the overlapping reasons people give for working.

Patients Suited to Work, or Productive Occupations Programs

There are five major groups of individuals who can benefit from work programs. These are people who 1) have never worked, 2) are underemployed, 3) are overemployed, 4) must regain old work skills or 5) must plan for a productive occupation.

Among those who have never worked are persons who are mentally retarded and people who are injured or become chronically ill during the teenage years. Persons who are mentally retarded must be assessed to determine whether individual abilities to function will permit employment in competitve situations or whether a sheltered workshop will be more appropiate. In addition, persons who are retarded may need programs to gain or increase their skills in performing daily activities and potential for independent living. Leisure skills need to be considered also.

Teenagers present a challenge to providing work programs. Their primary occupation is that of a student. At the same time, however, they need opportunities to explore the world of work as a volunteer, an amateur, or a part-time worker. Teenagers may have a well-developed interest profile or they may change their interests frequently. Those who have been handicapped for many years may not have had much opportunity to test their abilities in the real world. They do not know themselves or the world around them. Providing them with opportunities constitutes a major part of their work program.

Examples of people who may be underemployed are those with chronic mental illness, those who are blind or deaf, and those who are undereducated. People with chronic mental illness may have skill levels in educational achievement, job training, and aptitudes above the jobs in which they are actually employed. Therapy personnel may be tempted to encourage such individuals to seek jobs more in their skill level. Caution is needed because temperament and emotional behavior patterns may show such encouragement to be unwise, especially if the person cannot tolerate job stress.

People with sensory deficits may be viewed by potential employers as though they are mentally retarded. Sometimes behaviorisms of the blind or deaf person may contribute to the impression of

FIGURE 23-6. Historical Views on Work

Work regarded as drudgery and a curse, especially physical labor, and as a product of original sin.	Ancient Greeks
All work regarded as the key to life and the path to salvation.	Protestant (Luther)
All work regarded as the will of God and thus everyone should work for the sake of work. Idleness and pleasure were sinful.	Protestant (Calvin)
Creative work regarded as a joy.	Renaissance
Work can be pleasurable if it suits the person's character and is done a few hours a day.	Utopian
All work should be done for social use and not for profit. Then workers would have the zeal to work because there would be more leisure time.	Socialist
Work is regarded as an indispensable human activity. Work must be designed to help individuals discover their potential as human beings.	Humanist

FIGURE 23-7. Current Beliefs About Work*

Belief System	Work Attributes
Work ethic (also called the Protestant work ethic)	Work is inherently good in itself. It offers dignity to a person, and success is a result of personal effort. Anyone can succeed who tries hard enough.
Socialistic	Work is good for man if it fulfills man's needs. Work for profit is bad. Work that exploits man causes alienation.
Organizational	Work is good only if it contributes to a person's position in an organization. Work is bad if it does not contribute to an organized goal.
Humanistic	Work provides individual growth and development. The job is more important than the output.
Leisure ethic	Work is good if it is a means to personal fulfillment and the pursuit of leisure activities.

*Adapted from Bucchotz, RA: Measurement of beliefs. *Human Relations* 29:1177–1188, 1976.

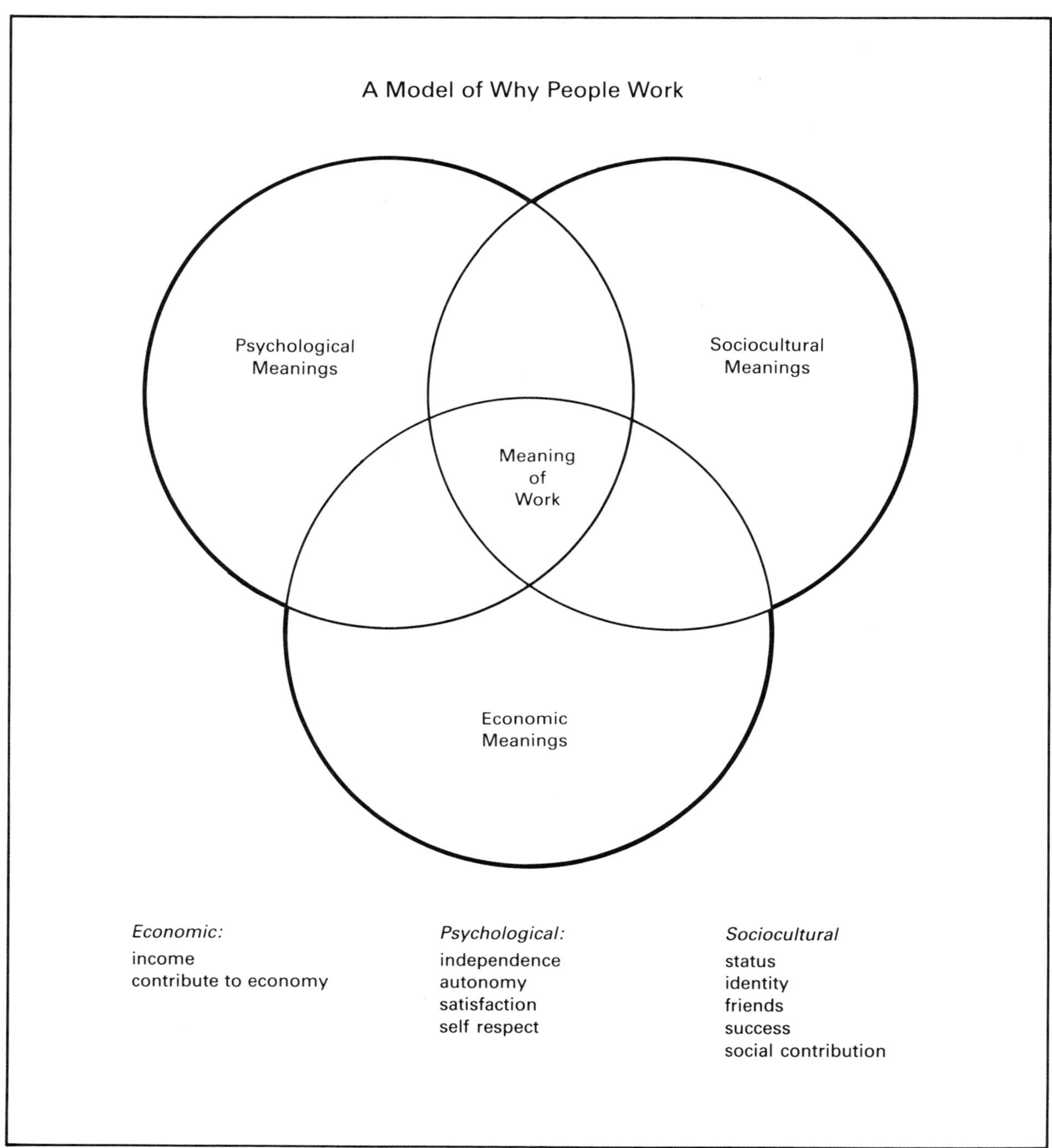
A Model of Why People Work
Psychological Meanings
Sociocultural Meanings
Meaning of Work
Economic Meanings
Economic:
income
contribute to economy
Psychological:
independence
autonomy
satisfaction
self respect
Sociocultural
status
identity
friends
success
social contribution

Figure 23-8

mental retardation. "Blindisms" include tilting the head down instead of toward the speaker's voice, swaying while standing in one spot, or shuffling the feet as opposed to walking with a heel-toe gait. "Deafisms" include cocking the head to one side and unclear pronunciation of words even though no structural problems exist in the mouth or tongue.

The undereducated may include underprivileged, social minorities, chronically ill, and institutionalized persons. Lack of education may be due to neglect or a learning disability. Whatever the cause, lack of education often equals lack of job opportunity. Work programs can help to narrow the gap between aptitude and ability by helping to identify the types of learning methods the individual responds to best.

The most common reason for overemployment is a head or brain injury which has caused changes in perceptual and cognitive skills. Such changes may not be obvious in performing daily living tasks that are routine and well learned. The deficits appear mostly when the person tries to perform a new task. Careful assessment is needed to identify the existence of a deficit and to determine the degree of the problem in performing work activities. Should the deficits in performance require a change of vocation, psychosocial problems usually arise also. Loss of status in the work setting is a problem often overlooked when a person must accept employment at a job with lower prestige than that before the injury.

Patients who worked in jobs requiring extensive physical abilities may need to change their line of work if their physical capacities change. Examples of such patients are those with spinal cord injuries, arthritis, amputation, heart disease, some forms of cancer, and ear disorders that affect balance. Muscle paralysis, joint range limitations, loss of vital capacity, irregular heart beat, loss of a body part, dizziness, and pain are common problems. Some people may be able to suggest their own change of career, but for others the loss of a career may be a serious problem. The loss of the job itself may not be as important as the loss of friends and related social activities. A new job and new friends will be important goals of the work program.

For some patients, the problem is to regain the old work skills. The injury, illness, or condition has not permanently changed the person's skill potential but has produced temporary changes that must be reversed. Common problems are muscle weakness, decreased range of motion, shortness of breath, lack of energy, and pain. The work program must be concentrated on increasing physical endurance, speed, accuracy, and quality control.

Finally, there are patients who are not candidates for paid employment but who need to participate in a productive occupation to keep their life in balance. The role of the student may become more meaningful if the person understands the need for academic skills in relation to expressed job interest.

The amateur may need to know how such skills could be used in performing work which benefits the community. For example, ham radio operators can be very useful in helping to track storms or tornadoes when "land lines" or telephones are not available or out of order because of a disaster.

Housework is a vital part of many people's lives but is often undervalued. If the work were done for pay, many families could not afford the cost. Housewives or housepersons perform as domestics, chefs, chauffeurs, handymen, babysitters, child care workers, teacher's aides, nurse's aides, financial managers, home decorators, telephone receptionists, executive secretaries, hostesses, and many other roles. Temporary role reversals often help other family members to understand the importance and complexity of being a housewife or houseperson.

Volunteer work can be a satisfying way of continuing to contribute to society for a retired person. For nonretired people, volunteering may provide a means of satisfying interests not met in the regular job. For those who do not need to work for pay or who are too young to work, volunteering becomes a means of seeing the world of work in action. Many social institutions such as churches, hospitals, and agencies could not operate without volunteers. Learning to be a good volunteer can be a useful and productive occupation.

The Work Program Team

The work program team may be only two or three people or may include a variety of individuals and professions. Other professionals who may serve as team members include career or vocational education teachers, special education teachers, vocational guidance counselors, clinical psychologists, work evaluators, rehabilitation counselors, physicians who specialize in occupational medicine, physical therapists, social workers, and industrial sociologists.

Each professional will be able to add certain information and contribute specific skills to the work program. It is important to get to know each team member and his or her skills. The team should discuss who is going to do what, because duplication of effort wastes time and lack of information may decrease the potential for good individual program planning.

Obviously the role of occupational therapy and the COTA will vary according to the size of the team, who is on the team, and the special skills each member possesses. Some general skills are useful, however. These will be discussed in the next section.

Specialized Knowledge and Skills Needed by the COTA

A COTA who is interested in work programs needs to become familar with the *Dictionary of Occupation Titles* (4th Edition) and its companion volume, *Selected Characteristics of Occupations Defined in the Dictionary of Occupational Titles*.[5,6] These two volumes describe the jobs available in the United States, organize the jobs into major categories, and indicate the level of education and training needed, as well as the general working conditions and physical demands at the job site. They also state many of the characteristics a person needs to perform a particular job. Job analysis and job assessment will be discussed in later sections.

A third useful reference is the *Classification of Jobs* (Revised Edition).[7] This book lists the aptitudes, interests, and temperaments needed for each job. It also cross references information given in other sources.

Use of these three documents will permit a person to understand the kinds of jobs available and skills needed to do the job. They can enable a person to become familiar with any job without ever seeing the job performed.

Another special knowledge and skill required by the COTA is familiarity with tests for aptitude, achievement, interests and values, and work sampling. Many of these tests are standardized and norm referenced. The directions must be followed carefully, and the evaluator must determine whether the test norms can be applied to the patient being tested. Scoring criteria must be observed and followed. A stop watch is used frequently as a means of measuring speed of performance. Practice in test administration is a must. A good method of learning to administer such tests is to have someone administer them to the therapist or assistant or to administer the tests to other professionals. Courses in tests and measurements can be taken at local colleges or universities.

A third area of knowledge is familiarity with the kinds of jobs found in the city or state which are suitable for the types of patients seen frequently in the work program. The state employment service should be able to provide a list of jobs, but the therapist will have to determine the suitability of the jobs for the participants in the work program. If there is a work team, all members should participate in identifying suitable jobs.

Finally, interviewing and observing skills are critical areas in work program planning. A good interview may identify important information about the interests and talents of a person that have not been identified by anyone else. Observing how a person performs a work task may be more important than what is done. For example, accidents frequently happen in setting up or preparing to do a task. Carelessness, failure to follow directions, or sloppy work habits are often the causes. How a person plans a task is as important as doing it.

Using the Dictionary of Occupational Titles and Related References

The DOT or "big orange book" is the primary reference on jobs in the United States. Each job is classified into an occupational category, but all jobs are listed in alphabetical order in the index at the back of the book. A few jobs are listed in the *Supplements*.[5]

To find a job, begin by looking in the index to locate the occupational code. For example, to look up information on the certified occupational therapy assistant, one begins by removing certification and licensure titles. The DOT uses generic titles only. Thus the job is listed as "occupational therapy assistant" in the index. The occupational code number is 076.364.010. Numbers beginning with "0" appear in the front of the book because the jobs are organized in numerical order. Next look for "076" and so forth.

The significance of the numbers will be discussed later. Other information is more useful. Figure 23-9 provides the information on "occupational therapy assistant," and each item contained in the definition is identified. The lead statement and task element statements are the most useful items in planning work programs. A worker should be able to do all task elements stated in the definition.

The next reference to consult is the *Selected Characteristics of Occupations Defined in the Dictionary of Occupational Titles,* commonly called the "little orange book" or "Selected Characteristics."[6] It is divided into two parts: Part A and Part B. Start with Part B because it is organized using the DOT numbers. Find 076.364.010. Reading from left to right, the next number is 10.02.02. This is the number for the occupational therapy assistant in the *Guide for Occupational Exploration*.[8] The GOE code is used to organize information in Part A.

Part A lists important worker characteristics, which are outlined and explained in Figure 23-10. Full explanation for all subcategories is given in the Appendix.

The worker characteristics identified in Part A are physical demands, environmental conditions, mathematics and language development, specific vocational preparation, and aptitudes. Other information has been compiled in the 3rd Edition of the DOT, which is out of print; therefore, one must use an alternate reference called *The Classification of Jobs*, Revised Edition, or COJ.[7] It lists all the information from the "Selected Characteristics" plus information from other sources. The DOT code number will identify the information on interests and temperaments as well as additional codes used to identify the occupational therapy assistant in other federal documents.

Code numbers abound in federal information; however, only two will be discussed — the DOT code number and the GOE code number. In the DOT code, the first digit designates one of ten occupational categories. The categories are professional, technical and managerial; clerical; sales; service; agricultural, fishery, forestry; machine trades; bench work; structural work; and miscellaneous. The second digit refers to a division within the occupational category. The third digit refers to an occupational group within the division.

Digits 4, 5, and 6 refer to skill levels within three characteristics of jobs. These job characteristics are called worker functions and are divided into data, people, and things. Digit 4 refers to the skill level needed in handling data; digit 5 represents the skill level needed for handling people; and digit 6 refers to the skill needed in handling things.

Digits 7, 8, and 9 are used to provide each occupational title with a unique number. The dig-

FIGURE 23-9. Parts of the DOT Definition

	1. Occupational Code	2. Occupational Title	3. Industry Designation
	076.364.010	OCCUPATIONAL THERAPY ASSISTANT	(medical ser.)

4. Alternate titles, if any
5a. Lead statement
5b. Task element statements
5c. "May" items
6. Undefined related titles, if any

Assists occupational therapist (medical ser.) in administering occupational therapy program in hospital, related facility, or community setting for physically, developmentally, or emotionally handicapped clients: Assists in evaluation of clients' daily living skills and capacities to determine extent of abilities and limitations. Assists in planning and implementing programs utilizing activities selected to restore, reinforce, and enhance task performances, diminish or correct pathology, and promote and maintain health. Designs and adapts equipment and working-living environment. Fabricates splints. Reports information and observations to supervisor. Carries out general activity program for individuals or groups. Assists in instructing patient and family in home programs as well as in care and use of adaptive equipment. Prepares work materials, assists in maintenance of equipment, and orders supplies. May be responsible for maintaining observed information in client's records.

FIGURE 23-10. Sample Translation of Worker Trait Codes for the COTA

Worker Trait Category and Code	Translation	
Physical Demands M 3 4 5 6 See Selected Characteristics . . . Appendix F(1)	M	= Medium work strength usually required, which is defined as "lifting 50 lb maximum with frequent lifting and/or carrying of objects weighing up to 25 lb"
	3	= Indicates job usually requires stooping, kneeling, crouching, and/or crawling
	4	= Indicates job usually requires reaching, handling, fingering, and/or feeling
	5	= Indicates job usually requires talking and hearing
	6	= Indicates job usually requires seeing functions, including near and far acuity, depth perception, normal field of vision, accommodation, and color vision
Environmental Conditions I 6 7 See Selected Characteristics . . . Appendix F(2)	I	= Indicates job is performed inside at least 75% of the time
	6	= Indicates there are hazards on the job "in which the individual is exposed to the definite risk of body injury"
	7	= Indicates there may be conditions in which fumes, odors, toxic conditions, dust, or poor ventilation is present in the work environment
Mathematic and Language Development M 3 L 4 See Selected Characteristics . . . Appendix F(3)	M3	= Mathematical skills should include all levels up to and including algebra and geometry
	L4	= Language skills should include ability to read and understand novels, newspapers, journals, manuals, etc., to write business letters, summaries, and reports using prescribed format etc., and speak at panel discussions or extemporaneously, etc.
Specific Vocational Preparation 6 See Selected Characteristics . . . Appendix F(4)	6	= Indicates that the job training time is over one year up to and including two years in duration
OAP 50 See Selected Characteristics . . . Appendix F(5)	Means the occupational aptitude pattern number. Includes the COTA job aptitudes as measured on the Specialized Aptitude Test Battery, which is drawn from the GATB	

FIGURE 23-10. Sample Translation of Worker Trait Codes for the COTA (continued)

Aptitudes 22333322234 See Selected Characteristics . . . Appendix F(5)		G2,V2,N3,S3,P3,Q3,K2,F2,M2,E3,C4
	G	= General learning ability or intelligence
	V	= Verbal understanding of words and ideas
	N	= Numerical ability to perform arithmetic operations
	S	= Spatial ability to comprehend forms in space
	P	= Form perception ability to perceive details in objects, pictures, or graphs
	Q	= Clerical perception ability to perceive details in verbal or tabular materials
	K	= Motor coordination ability to coordinate eyes, hands, or fingers with speed and accuracy
	F	= Finger dexterity ability to manipulate small objects
	M	= Eye, hand, and foot coordination (not a GATB score)
	C	= Color discrimination (not a GATB score)
	2	= Person should score in the highest third, exclusive of the top 10 percent of the population
	3	= Person should score in the middle third of the population
	4	= Person should score in the lowest third, exclusive of the bottom 10 percent of the population on that subtest
Interests 3B 4A Appendix F(6)	3B	= Person should have a preference for activities of an abstract and creative nature
	4A	= Person should have a preference for working for the presumed good of people
Temperaments J P T V Appendix F(7)	J	= Person should be able to make generalization, evaluation, or decision based on measurable or verifiable criteria
	P	= Person should be able to deal with people beyond giving and receiving instruction
	T	= Person should be able to deal with situations requiring the precise attainment of set limits, tolerances, or standards
	V	= Person should be able to perform a variety of duties, often changing from one task to another of a different nature without loss of efficiency or composure

FIGURE 23-11. Translation of Occupational Codes

Occupational Code 076.364.010 from the *Dictionary of Occupational Titles*

0 Designates a professional occupation.

7 Designates an occupation in medicine and health.

6 Designates a therapist.

3 Designates the level of skill with data the person should have: should be able to gather, collate, or classify information about data, people, or things and should be able to report and/or carry out a prescribed action in response to the information.

6 Designates the level of skill with people the person should have: should be able to talk with and/or signal people to convey or exchange information.

4 Designates the level of skill with things the person should have: should be able to use body parts, tools, or special devices to work, move, guide, or place objects or materials.

Occupational Code 10.02.02 from the *Guide for Occupational Exploration*

10 Indicates that the job is based on humanitarian interest, defined as "helping individuals with their mental, spiritual, social, physical, or vocational concerns."

10.02 Indicates a subclassification of humanitarian jobs called "Nursing, Therapy, and Specialized Teaching Services."

10.02.02 Indicates a further subclassification called "Therapy and Rehabilitation."

FIGURE 23-12. Comparison of Individual Assessment and Job Analysis

Individual Assessment:	Job Analysis:
Work history	Historical demand for specific job
Health conditions	Work or environmental conditions
Educational aptitude and achievement	Educational development
Job training completed or needed	Specific vocational preparation
Aptitudes available	Aptitudes required
Interests and temperaments expressed	Interests and temperaments needed
Worker skills	Work functions

Goal: To make a best fit between the individual abilities and the job demands.

its themselves have no significance.

The GOE code uses a similar system of grouping by occupational similarity. The first two digits represent an occupational category; the GOE uses 12 categories instead of 10 because recent studies have identified 12 interest areas rather than the 10 used to organize the DOT.

Digits 3 and 4 represent divisions with the occupational categories. Digits 5 and 6 refer to specific occupational groups. Analysis of the codes is summarized in Figure 23-11.

Assessment of Work Potential

This section is based on the categories outlined by the United States Department of Labor in analyzing jobs. The parallel categories for the assessment of individuals are listed in Figure 23-12. The job analysis categories are included in Appendix F.

The first category of assessment is the collection of data on the individual, including work history, personal and social history, education and training level, daily living skills, and leisure interests. Structured forms for self-reporting or interviewing usually are developed by each facility. Some sample questions on work history are presented in Figure 23-13.

Physical capacities constitute the second category (see Appendix F). This category includes many movements and positions which occupational and physical therapy personnel are used to assessing. However, the items must be assessed according to the terminology used by the government if communication between the treatment facility and the employment setting is to be maintained. Therefore, occupational therapy personnel need to be able to translate terms to those learned in school. For example, reaching is basically the same as upper extremity range of motion of the shoulder. If an individual scores in the normal range on a range of motion test, he or she has normal reaching skills. Handling and fingering include the items assessed in a hand function test such as cylindrical grasp, finger tip prehension, three jaw chuck (thumb, index, and middle fingers) prehension, and hook grasp. Feeling is the same as stereognosis, or the ability to identify objects by touch with vision occluded.

When testing for physical capacities, the evaluator must remember that the physical activities such as standing, walking, carrying, and climbing are done within a job task. In other words, the goal is not to stand but to stand in order to reach for a tool or put something on a shelf. Walking is done for the purpose of getting somewhere to do a task, not for the purpose of seeing whether someone can walk *per se*. The difference is important because the brain must be able to monitor the physical skill at the same time it is cognitively attending to a task. Walking while talking is a good example. A person who is relearning how to walk and maintain balance cannot talk easily. All attention is needed to keep from falling. In the work situation, walking must be more automatic.

Two of the better tests of physical capacities are the *Smith Physical Capacities Evaluation*, originally developed at Woodrow Wilson Rehabilitation Center in Fisherville, Virginia, and the *GULHEMP* developed by Leon F. Koyl, MD, at the de Havilland Aircraft Corporation in Canada.[9,10] Both cover the strength factors, climbing and balancing, and stooping, kneeling, crouching, and crawling categories. Both, however, are weak in the areas of reaching, handling, fingering, and feeling.

Other tests can be useful as well. The best test for reaching is the *Valpar Whole Body Range of Motion Test*.[11] This test requires the individual to unscrew and rescrew three plastic geometric forms while assuming four different body positions: reaching over the head, reaching in front of the body, reaching while crouching with vision occluded, and returning to standing. Another useful Valpar test is the *Upper Extremity Range of Motion Test*.[11] It requires the person to screw on two sizes of nuts while reaching through a hole in a

FIGURE 23-13. Work History Questionnaire Sample Questions

1. What was your first (second, third, etc.) job? (Note: include part-time work such as babysitting, newscarrier, yard work.)
2. How did you get that job? (Important for assessing job seeking skills.)
3. For whom did you work? (Try to determine whether the person has worked for people who are not relatives, neighbors, or friends who may overlook skill deficiencies.)
4. How long did you do that job, and why did you quit? (Look for a pattern of failure to perform any job for more than few days or weeks.)
5. Why did you start working at that job? (Look for motivation.)
6. Describe your job duties. (Be alert to unusual skills or interests that might not be obvious from the job title or typical description of that job.)
7. What did you like about the job? (Look for interests.)
8. What did you dislike about the job? (Look for dislikes that could interfere with future job performance.)
9. What was the hardest part of the job, or took the most skill, energy, or time? (Try to get additional information not given in item 8.)
10. What was the easiest part of the job? (Again, try to get additional information.)
11. What skills did you learn on the job? (Include such items as being on time, being courteous, and sticking to the job, as well as items such as learning how to take inventory, or learning to operate equipment.)

Go back to item 1 and repeat questions for the second job and then the third until all jobs have been discussed.

FIGURE 23-14. Hand Function Tests for Handling and Fingering Assessment

1. Box and Block Test[13]
   - Unilateral activity, but both hands are tested
   - Finger pad prehension
   - Uses 1-inch square blocks
   - Assesses shoulder function
2. Crawford Small Parts Dexterity Test[14]
   - Uses small tools: tweezers and 3½-inch screwdriver
   - Unilateral and bilateral activity
   - Small diameter pegs
   - Finger pad prehension
3. Hand Tool Dexterity Test (Bennett)[15]
   - Uses large hand tools: wrenches and screwdriver
   - Bilateral activity
   - Palmar grasp
   - Tests organization skills in laying nuts, bolts, and washers down for ease in pick-up for reassembly
4. Groove Pegboard[16]
   - Not standardized
   - Unilateral, but both hands can be tested
   - Finger tip prehension
   - Form perception
5. Minnesota Rate of Manipulation Test[17]
   - Bilateral activity
   - Finger pad prehension
   - Turning and placing large diameter pegs
6. Minnesota Spatial Relations Test—Revised[18]
   - Unilateral activity
   - Tests ability to develop a strategy for organizing the task
7. Pennsylvania Bimanual Worksample[19]
   - Bilateral activity
   - Finger pad prehension
   - Requires screwing motion of fingers
   - Can be done by blind person
8. Purdue Pegboard[20]
   - Finger tip prehension
   - Unilateral and bilateral activities
   - Small diameter pegs
9. Stromberg Dexterity Test[21]
   - Placing task in space
   - Finger pad prehension
   - Large diameter pegs
   - Following directions

box. Inside the box are bolts located on top, side, and bottom. The left hand screws on the nuts on the right side of the box, and the right hand does the reverse.

Handling and fingering can be tested together using the *Jepson Taylor Hand Function Test*.[12] This test must be constructed according to instructions, as it is not available commercially.

There are several good commercial tests which assess various aspects of hand function. These tests are summarized in Figure 23-14. It should be noted that they can be used in a variety of combinations. For example, the *Purdue Pegboard* tests finger tip prehension, while the *Minnesota Rate of Manipulation* tests finger pad. Both the *Purdue Pegboard* and the *Crawford Small Parts and Hand Tool Dexterity Test* use small diameter pegs, but the *Crawford* test requires the use of small tools which permits observation of manual dexterity of the fingers (Purdue) as opposed to the use of tools (Crawford). The *Crawford* test permits a comparison of small tool with large tool use. Thus there are many opportunities to cross check and validate test information.

Feeling (stereognosis) can be tested using a group of common objects of various sizes, textures, and shapes which are placed in the hand for identification. Vision must be occluded. Common items used are a key, paper clip, ball of yarn, rubber band, and bottle cap. Other objects such as a short pencil, ¾-inch diameter button, or eraser can be included to increase the list. Stereognosis testing is quick and gives useful information about tactile discrimination.

Talking (speech) and hearing may be assessed by a speech pathologist and audiologist, if consultants are available. If the occupational therapy personnel must do the testing, the *Wepman Auditory Discrimination Test* is a good basic test.[22]

Seeing (sight) may be evaluated by an optometrist or an ophthalmologist. If these professionals are not available, a *Snellen Eye Chart* (visual acuity), the *Titmus Stereo Test* (depth perception), and the *Dvorine Color Vision Test* (color blindness) will give a quick overview of seeing abilities.[23,24,25]

The third area of work assessment is aptitude testing. The state employment service uses the *General Aptitude Test Battery* (GATB).[26] It measures nine aptitudes, which are summarized in Figure 23-15. The GATB requires special training to administer, and information about training sessions may be obtained from the state employment service.

A test which is similar to the *GATB* is the *Occupational Aptitude Survey,* which is part of the *OASIS* system or *Occupational Aptitude Survey and Interest Schedule.* It measures six aptitudes, including intelligence, vocabulary, computation, spatial relations, work comparison, and making marks (motor coordination). The test is easy to administer and score. Other sources of information on aptitudes are summarized in Figure 23-16. Note that many of the manual and finger dexterity tests have been included.

Interest and temperament assessment is a fourth area of testing. The *Strong-Campbell Interest Inventory* and the *Kudor Preference Interest Survey* are used by most work evaluators, but these tests must be scored by computer.[28,29] There are, however, many other tests which can be hand scored. The list is not comprehensive, but includes the following:[27,30-35]

1 *Jackson Vocational Interest Survey.*
2 *Kuder Preference Record-C* (vocational interest survey).

FIGURE 23-15. The Nine Aptitudes Measured by the Twelve Tests in the General Aptitude Test Battery

Aptitudes and Codes:		Test Items:
Intelligence	G	Vocabulary Arithmetic reasoning Three-dimension space
Verbal	V	Vocabulary
Numerical	N	Arithmetic reasoning Computation
Spatial	S	Three-dimension space
Form perception	P	Tool matching Form matching
Clerical perception	Q	Name comparison
Motor coordination	K	Mark making
Finger dexterity	F	Assembling and disassembling pins and collars
Manual dexterity	M	Placing and turning pegs

FIGURE 23-16. Other Tests of Aptitudes

Category:	Name of Test:
Intelligence	Weschler Adult Intelligence Test-R[44] Stanford-Binet Intelligence Scale[45]
Verbal	Shipley Institute of Living Scale[46] Peabody Picture Vocabulary Test[47]
Numerical	Wide Range Achievement Test-R[42] Numerical Section Differential Aptitude Test[48] Numerical Section
Spatial perception	Minnesota Spatial Relations Test[18] Valpar Size Discrimination[11]
Form perception	Minnesota Paper Form Board Test[49] Valpar Problem Solving[11]
Clerical perception	TOWER Clerical Items[50] Differential Aptitude Test[48] Clerical Section
Motor coordination	Stromberg Dexterity Test[21] Box and Block Text[13]
Finger dexterity	Crawford Small Parts Dexterity Test[14] Purdue Pegboard[20]
Manual dexterity	Hand Tool Dexterity Test (Bennett)[15] Minnesota Rate of Manipulation Test[17]

3 *Kuder Preference Record-D* (occupational).
4 *Occupational Interest Schedule* (OASIS).
5 *Ohio Vocational Interest Survey* (OVIS).
6 *Self-Directed Search and Vocational Preference Inventory*.

For people who cannot read or who have dyslexia, there are tests that use pictures. These include the following:[36-39]

1 *Wide Range Interest and Opinion Test* (WRIOT).
2 *Reading-Free Vocational Interest Inventory*.
3 *Giest Picture Interest Inventory*.
4 *Picture Interest Inventory*.

Several of the tests listed previously also include information about temperament. These tests include:

1 *Geist Picture Interest Inventory*.
2 *Jackson Vocational Interest Survey*.
3 *Self-Directed Search*.
4 *Strong-Campbell Interest Inventory*.

Other tests which may be useful are the *Leisure Activities Blank*, which tests both past and present interests, and the *Work Values Inventory*, which tests the intrinsic and extrinsic values a person holds about work.[40,41] Special tests for specific occupational interests such as artistic aptitude, mechanical ability, clerical skills, and musical talent are also available. These specialized tests should be considered only if there are several patients who can benefit from such testing. Keeping track of so many tests can be a logistical problem.

Educational aptitude and achievement is the fifth area of testing. If a clinical or school psychologist is available, a referral to that person is preferable because a psychologist has had experience in giving and interpreting intelligence tests. Generally, occupational therapy personnel should not be administering intelligence tests unless they have had education and training as a psychologist.

Achievement testing, however, can be done by occupational therapy personnel if no psychologist is available. The easiest and best instrument to use is the *Wide Range Achievement Test* (WRAT).[42] This test has separate forms for children and adults and measures reading, spelling, and mathematics. The *Peabody Individual Achievement Test* (PIAT) is a good alternative choice.[43] Both of these are rapid screening tests. If more detailed information is needed, a referral should be made to a psychologist or psychometrist.

The final two areas of assessment are job training needs and determination of health conditions. The level of job training is given for each occupation in the *Selected Characteristics of Occupations Defined in the Dictionary of Occupational Titles*.[6] Usually the therapist's role is to determine the feasibility of the person's being able to attend the classes or training sessions if the educational program is offered in the community. Architectural barriers are a common problem as is the attitude of instructors toward special populations and handicapped individuals. A third problem concerns the obtaining of special equipment which may be needed such as a Braille typewriter or an optical reading machine. Finances may be an issue if the person is not eligible for vocational rehabilitation. Finally, the likelihood of getting a job if the education and training are completed must be considered.

Health conditions may play a role in the selection of an educational program as well as the selection of a job. Learning and working conditions must be examined. A person with pulmonary or lung disease must consider whether fumes, dust, and other toxic conditions exist. A person with a high level spinal cord injury should work in an environmentally controlled area since the body is unable to adapt quickly to temperature changes. A person who is easily distracted probably should not work in an area that is noisy. Hazardous conditions are undesirable for everyone but may be especially dangerous for someone with sensory loss of vision, hearing, or touch.

In summary, there are seven areas of individual work assessment in which the COTA can participate. These are work history, physical capacities, aptitudes, interests and temperaments, educational achievement, job training, and health conditions.

Work Programs

There are several types of work programs. The following descriptions of selected work programs are general and represent an average rather than a specific program. Each situation requires modification of the details, but the overall format provides a general guide.

FIGURE 23-17. Work Fields*

Alphabetical Listing of Work Fields

Code	Work Field
051	Abrading
291	Accommodating
232	Accounting-Recording
295	Administering
211	Appraising
141	Baking-Drying
005	Blasting
071	Bolting-Screwing
053	Boring
153	Brushing-Spraying
034	Butchering
094	Calking
132	Casting
052	Chipping
031	Cleaning
161	Combing-Napping
263	Composing
146	Cooking-Food Preparing
003	Cropping
142	Crushing
135	Die Sizing
202	Developing-Printing
144	Distilling
242	Drafting
111	Electrical Fabricating-Installing-Repairing
112	Electronic Fabricating-Installing-Repairing
122	Electro-Mechanical Fabricating-Installing-Repairing
154	Electroplating
244	Engineering
183	Engraving
297	Entertaining
181	Eroding
182	Etching
041	Filling
145	Filtering-Straining-Separating
061	Fitting-Placing
082	Flame Cutting-Arc Cutting
062	Folding-Fastening
006	Gardening
063	Gluing
294	Healing-Caring
133	Heat Conditioning
012	Hoisting-Conveying
001	Hunting-Fishing
151	Immersing-Coating
192	Imprinting
282	Information Giving
271	Investigating
032	Ironing
165	Knitting
092	Laying
241	Laying Out
272	Litigating
011	Loading-Moving
002	Logging
033	Lubricating
057	Machining
091	Masoning
121	Mechanical Fabricating-Installing-Repairing
131	Melting
292	Merchandising
055	Milling-Turning-Planing
004	Mining-Quarrying-Earth Boring
	Mixing
143	Molding
136	
	Nailing
072	
042	Packing
262	Painting
201	Photographing
134	Pressing-Forging
191	Printing
147	Processing-Compounding
293	Protecting
014	Pumping
231	Recording
251	Researching
073	Riveting
152	Saturating
056	Sawing
171	Sewing-Tailoring
054	Shearing-Shaving
083	Soldering
162	Spinning
021	Stationary Engineering
221	Stock Checking
101	Structural Fabricating-Installing-Repairing
264	Styling
243	Surveying
281	System Communicating
296	Teaching
013	Transporting
093	Troweling
298	Undertaking
102	Upholstering
164	Weaving
212	Weighing
081	Welding
163	Winding
043	Wrapping
261	Writing

*U.S. Department of Labor, Manpower Administration. *Handbook for Analyzing Jobs.* Washington, D.C.: Government Printing Office, 1972, p. 84.

Work Hardening Program

Work hardening programs are designed to increase or improve a person's endurance, physical tolerance or stamina, and to increase or improve the quality, quantity and complexity of the work performed. The goals of a work hardening program are as follows:

1 Increase the length of time a person can work without undue fatigue.
2 Increase physical strength.
3 Improve posture and use of body mechanics during performance of work activities.
4 Increase speed and accuracy of work performed.
5 Improve quality of product output.
6 Increase the worker's ability to handle the complex demands of the job.

Immobilization is known to reduce a person's physical capacity. A few days of bed rest or relative inactivity decreases vital capacity, cardiac reserve, and muscle strength. Fatigue occurs more quickly. Posture becomes more flexed or hyperextended. The mental processes seem to slow down, also. Speed and accuracy decrease, and simple tasks become complex. In short, the worker becomes unfit to work regardless of how well the injury may have healed or whether the illness has been cured. If disability is present, it adds to the need for work hardening because the feasibility of work must be reassessed.

Work hardening programs are designed around work simulation tasks. Therefore, the therapist must know what work has been performed, or would be performed, if the worker changed jobs. The U.S. Department of Labor lists 100 work fields which describe work tasks (Figure 23-17). For example, to move materials from one place to another there are four possible work tasks: to load, to hoist or convey, to transport, or to pump. Jobs may require a number of combinations. The worker may do the task by hand or by machine. A person may load a truck and drive (transport) it somewhere. Another person may use a crane to hoist a crate onto a flat car. A third person may transport gas and pump the gas into the holding tank of a filling station

Increasing the length of time a person can work needs to be done gradually. The gradual approach is important particularly if disability has been prolonged or muscle tendon injuries are involved. Units of 15-minute increases are used commonly, but physicians may recommend other time units. A basic work hardening schedule is started with 15 minutes of work and 15 minutes of rest. If no adverse effects are noted after 3 days, the work time can be increased another 15 minutes after the rest period.

Adverse reactions can include rapid increases in pulse, breathing, or blood pressure. The person may feel faint. The skin may become flushed or cold and clammy. The injured part may become sore and the skin reddened, swollen and tender to touch — all are signs of too much activity. Rest and relaxation are the best remedy.

The same schedule and precautions apply to increasing physical strength. The primary difference is that physical strengthening must be done using increased amounts of weight. The starting weight should be an amount which is easy to lift, carry, push, or pull. Then 5-pound units can be added every two to three days. Additional signs to observe for overexertion are changes in posture or mechanics from correct to incorrect, too much time moving the weight, and facial grimacing.

If the hand or hands are to be strengthened, start with a weight that is easy to pick up, hold, and place. Increase the units by 2 pounds to 3 pounds rather than 5-pound units. For finger strengthening, 1-pound units usually are enough to be noticeable.

An important concept to remember is that weights can be added to the extremities in addition to those external to the body. Therefore, if a cement block weighs 15 pounds and the person is ready for 20 pounds, continue to use the cement block but add 2.5-pound weights to the forearms.

Improving body mechanics and posture usually requires a demonstration and lots of practice. A mirror is useful, but the therapist must continue to observe. Changing body movement patterns is easy if conscious attention is maintained. The goal, however, is to have the improved body mechanics and posture become an automatic part of work habits. Changes in habits seem to take 7 days to 10 days to become "permanent" behavior. Therefore, a program of less than 7 days will be ineffective.

Increasing speed and accuracy requires attention to detail. Problems in speed and accuracy can be caused by poor set-up of the task, inefficient use of the body, and lack of practice. Occasionally, visual perception disorders may reduce speed and accuracy.

Tasks should be set up to require the minimum amount of movement possible and still get the job done. Usually the work space should be organized at the midline of the worker's body. Reaching should kept to a minimum, and reaching overhead should be eliminated if possible. The individual should practice error-free performance. If errors increase, slow down and increase speed more slowly.

Visual perceptual disorders do occur with the aging process. More commonly, visual changes occur after an injury to the brain. If the brain cannot control the eye muscles of both eyes simultaneously, double vision, loss of depth perception, and visual ground problems may occur. Specific testing for visual disturbance may be indicated before speed and accuracy can be improved further.

Improving the quality of output also requires attention to detail. First, the problems of quality must be identified. Then the person must be observed doing the process that results in that part of the product. Errors or poor workmanship must be noted and corrected. Sometimes quality control is a matter of helping the worker to understand why quality is important in the particular product. Demonstrating how the product is used may clarify the reason a standard of quality is important.

Finally, work hardening may be needed to increase the worker's ability to handle complex job situations. Usually the program begins with a simple activity and later the complexity of that activity is increased or other activities added. Another approach is to begin with the activity that is repeated most often on the job. Then add the next most frequent task, and so on. This approach may enable the worker to return to the job sooner because the three tasks the person is able to do constitute 85 percent of the work performed. The other 15 percent of the work may be reassigned or backlogged for a time.

Work Experience Program

The goals of a work experience program are the following:

1. To try out different work tasks.
2. To practice performing specific work tasks.
3. To develop or to improve work habits and skills.
4. To develop or to improve personal appearance and social skills in the work settings.

Trying out work tasks may be accomplished by assigning patients to actual stations as apprentices for one to two weeks. More commonly, work samples are used. There are several types, which must be considered in relation to the persons seen. There are work samples for people who are mentally retarded, deaf, physically disabled, high-school age, or adults. Some work samples take up floor space; others can be put away in cabinets. Also, some work samples are useful only for assessment, while others can be used for both. In a work experience program, the work sample should permit the worker to make a product which can be evaluated.

Another approach to trying out jobs is to subcontract with local industry or agencies to do selected tasks, such as stuffing and stamping envelopes, packaging nuts and bolts, or tying ribbons into bows. The limitation of this approach is that the work is highly repetitive. For some patients (such as those who are retarded) the sub-contract approach may be useful, but for others the work may be too simple or boring. Once the tryout period is completed, the person can be assigned specific work tasks to do. The amount of time, number of tasks, or amount of work may be graded to permit continued assessment of progress.

At the same time, work habits and skills can be observed. Work habits include punctuality and punching the time card, going to one's assigned work station, following directions, asking for clarification if needed, maintaining good posture, using good body mechanics, working without reminders, paying attention to work quality, maintaining a work output schedule (units of work per time period), and cleaning up. Skills may include any of the previously shown fields and activities listed in Figure 23-17. Personal appearance includes proper work dress and grooming. Social skills include greeting others and talking about subjects of interest at breaks or lunch.

Job Seeking Program

The goals of a job seeking program are as follows:

1. Clarify values and goals an individual holds about work.
2. Identify individual strengths and limitations in the job market.
3. Develop skills in locating sources of jobs and setting up interview appointments.
4. Practice interviewing skills and preparing a résumé.
5. Evaluate job offers in terms of benefits and work expectations.
6. Review importance of daily living skills in relation to work, especially appropriate dress and grooming.

Clarification of work values and goals may be done through self-assessment checklists, tests of work values, one-on-one discussions, or group discussion. The focus is on identifying the existing values and goals in relation to the job market.

Attempts to change values or goals should be done in individual sessions by experienced practitioners. The same techniques and cautions apply to identifying individual strengths, preferences, and limitations. Some people overstate their strengths and underestimate their limitations. Others understate their strengths and and overestimate their limitations.

Skills in locating jobs may require teaching a person to read the classified ads in the newspaper or professional trade publications. Another activity may be scheduling a field trip to the state or local employment service. A third activity could be inviting an employment service representative to speak to the members of the job seeking program. A fourth activity might be to use the yellow pages of the telephone book to locate names and telephone numbers of potential employers. Finally, role playing could be used to help prospective employees call for an appointment to interview. If a résumé is needed, there are several good publications which can be used as a guide. Also, employment service people can provide guidelines based on their knowledge of industries in the area.

Evaluation of one or more job offers is an important step in the program. Many young people do not know how to weigh the value of fringe benefits in relation to their total earnings. Some young adults may not understand payroll deductions, which reduce the amount of their take home pay. Listing fringe benefits and figuring gross versus net pay are useful learning tasks.

Discussions about grooming and dressing for work may be important for groups who have never worked or who have been out of the work force for many years. Illustrations about how work clothes may differ from everyday dress may help clarify the ways in which working is different from everyday routines.

Time management may also need review. Determining when to get up may be important. Allowing enough time for dressing, grooming, eating breakfast, and getting to work may be a new experience. It may also require a cultural adjustment if the individual is from a cultural group that does not view time in 60-minute hours, but rather as simply morning, noon, afternoon, and evening.

Independent Living Program

The skills included in an independent living program are much more comprehensive than those usually listed in a daily living skills program. Otherwise the goals are similar, including the following:

1. Identifying the skills the individual needs to function as an autonomous person in the community.
2. Teaching those skills which the individual does not possess.
3. Identifying and obtaining any adapted or assistive devices and aids which the person needs.
4. Providing opportunities to practice the skills in the real world, when possible.

Some skills that should be considered are: how to locate and rent an apartment, how to buy a new or used car, how to get a chauffeur's license, how to buy a bus or airline ticket, how to make a motel or hotel reservation, and how to buy automobile insurance. These are not the most commonly needed skills in daily life, but they could decide whether a person is employable.

Career Exploration

The goals of career exploration programs are as follows:

1. To learn about work as a life task.
2. To learn about different kinds of work and the skills required.
3. To define individual career goals.
4. To compare interests and aptitudes with the job market.
5. To explore the jobs that most closely fit the individual's personality and abilities.

Work as a life task needs to be explored from several points of view. As already discussed, work has sociocultural, psychological, and economic dimensions. Workers and potential workers hold various beliefs about work. In addition, work is only one aspect of a balanced life and must be integrated with self-care and leisure. Discussions, role playing, and self-assessment techniques are some methods for meeting this goal.

There have been two major approaches to exploring different kinds of work. One is based on the theory of John Holland.[51] Holland organized jobs into six occupational categories: artistic, investigative, realistic, conventional, enterprising, and social. The categories are based on Holland's analysis of personality types. In other words, a

FIGURE 23-18. Comparison of Holland Occupational Categories to USES Interest Areas of Work†

The relationship of the Holland Occupational Categories to the USES Interest Areas of Work is as follows:

Holland Occupational Categories	USES Occupational Interest Areas
Artistic	01 Artistic
Investigative	02 Scientific
Realistic	03 Plants and Animals 04 Protective 05 Mechanical 06 Industrial
Conventional	07 Business Detail
Enterprising	08 Selling
Social	09 Accommodating* 10 Humanitarian 11 Leading-Influencing** 12 Physical Performing

*A relatively narrow area, but it includes a few occupations covered by Holland's Enterprising and Realistic Categories in addition to those covered by the Social Category.

**A broad area including, in addition to occupations covered by the Holland Social Category, business management and law/politics occupations covered by the Enterprising Category, and social science occupations covered by the Investigating Category.

†U.S. Department of Labor, Employment and Training Administration. *Occupational Exploration.* Washington, D.C.: Government Printing Office, 1979.

person with an artistic type of personality is most likely to enjoy working in a job that requires artistic skills such as art, music, drama, or writing. Few people, however, are exclusively artistic in personality. Most people are combinations with varying degrees of several personality types. Therefore, Holland suggests that the assessment based on his theory consider the three personality traits with the highest scores as most reflective of an individual's total personality.

The U.S. Employment Service (USES) uses Holland's approach in organizing jobs but expands the six categories to 12 by subdividing the realistic and social categories. Figure 23-18 shows a comparison of the two approaches. The publication entitled *Guide for Occupational Exploration and Exploring Careers* provides a wealth of information and ideas for discussing and learning about different careers.[8,52]

FIGURE 23-19. Definitions of Interest Factors

1. **ARTISTIC:**
   Interest in creative expression of feelings or ideas.
2. **SCIENTIFIC:**
   Interest in discovering, collecting, and analyzing information about the natural world and in applying scientific research findings to problems in medicine, life sciences, and natural sciences.
3. **PLANTS AND ANIMALS:**
   Interest in activities involving plants and animals, usually in an outdoor setting.
4. **PROTECTIVE:**
   Interest in the use of authority to protect people and property.
5. **MECHANICAL:**
   Interest in applying mechanical principles to practical situations, using machines, handtools, or techniques.
6. **INDUSTRIAL:**
   Interest in repetitive, concrete, organized activities in a factory setting.
7. **BUSINESS DETAIL:**
   Interest in organized, clearly defined activities requiring accuracy and attention to detail, primarily in an office setting.
8. **SELLING:**
   Interest in bringing others to a point of view through personal persuasion, using sales and promotion techniques.
9. **ACCOMMODATING:**
   Interest in catering to the wishes of others, usually on a one-to-one basis.
10. **HUMANITARIAN:**
    Interest in helping others with their mental, spiritual, social, physical, or vocational needs.
11. **LEADING-INFLUENCING:**
    Interest in leading and influencing others through activities involving high-level verbal or numerical abilities.
12. **PHYSICAL PERFORMING:**
    Interest in physical activities performed before an audience.

*U.S. Department of Labor, Employment and Training Administration. *Guide for Occupational Exploration.* Washington, D.C.: Government Printing Office, 1979.

Defining career goals usually requires some self-assessment questionnaires. Examples of questions are: (1) If you could be anyone you wanted to be, who would you be and why? (2) If you had just won a million dollars and would never have to work, how would you spend your time? (3) Date your paper 5 years ahead of today's date. Write what you would be doing on that day. These questions and statements may be repeated several times before the person is able to give answers which reflect realistic self-assessment.

In order to compare interests and aptitudes, some tests must be given to each individual. If test scores are available already, job comparison and matching can begin. If assessment must be done, those tests which can be self-scored or scored by hand provide a starting point. Begin by comparing the interest scores against the twelve interest areas used in the *Guide for Occupational Exploration* rather than the five bipolar interest areas listed in the handbook for analyzing jobs (Figure 23-19).[8,53] The bipolar interests have proven to be unreliable and are no longer used. Temperament likewise has been dropped as a separate item of assessment.

Exploration of jobs which best match the individual is aided greatly by the use of the *Guide for Occupational Exploration* and the *Job Selection Workbook*, which is designed to be used with the *Guide*.[8,54] The *Workbook* can be used as a self-paced learning packet or with groups. It contains six steps:

1 Think about your interests.
2 Select one of the work groups to explore.
3 Explore the work groups you selected.
4 Explore subgroups and specific occupations.
5 Put it all together.
6 Plan your next steps.

These steps parallel the goals stated at the beginning of this section on career exploration.

Industrial Consultation Program

Industrial consultation requires experience with work programs and knowledge of the industries in the area. Goals for an industrial consultation program will vary according to the needs of the industry that contracts. Selection is usually made from the following list:

1 Eliminate barriers and reduce hazards for employees and consumers entering, moving about and exiting from the building.
2 Make the work station(s) and tools more compatible with human form and function.
3 Improve the safety and efficiency of work areas.
4 Improve the communication methods used to identify places and things in the work environment.
5 Analyze jobs to better understand job requirements and train workers needed to do the jobs.
6 Organize a recreational or leisure development program.
7 Plan a preretirement program.

Knowledge of barrier-free design is essential to a program to eliminate barriers and reduce hazards. Architectural or structural barriers are only part of the problem. Knowledge of common visual and auditory perception problems is important also. For example, some architects design outside stairs with small risers (height of back of step) to make stair climbing easier. What the architect fails to appreciate is that the small riser does not cast an observable shadow to alert many older people that the stair exists at all. Thus, an elderly person may fall down a 2-inch riser but would have stepped down a 5-inch riser with no difficulty.

Another common problem is the choice of floor surface in the lobby area. Architects, in an attempt to create unique decors, create floor surfaces which are visually pleasing but are often hazardous to anyone on foot. Some floors, such as cobble, brick, or poured floors, are uneven. Others are so slick that ice skates would be appropriate. The challenge is to find a floor surface that allows people to move about easily and safely but at the same time is visually appealing.

A third problem is the information desk, which is often located where sounds reverberate from other activities in the building. The person asking directions cannot always hear the answers clearly and may get lost for 25 minutes in the maze of hallways.

Making work stations more compatible with human form and function requires the knowledge of ergonomics or human engineering. Furthermore, the information must include the changes in function that occur with certain disabilities. For example, a person with arthritis or a spinal cord injury may have a reduced range of motion and hand function. Objects in the work environment need to be located more centrally to the body. Some objects may need enlarged handles to decrease problems of grasp.

Safety can be improved by using color to identify dangerous and safe areas. Red is used for the most hazardous, orange designates less hazardous areas, and green identifies safe areas. Marking the floor space where doors swing open is a simple but effective safety procedure. Another is to use mirrors at the point where two hallways intersect. Mirrors allow each person to see who is coming and prevent collisions.

Efficiency can be improved by organizing hand tools on a pegboard. Each tool has a place which is marked by a silhouette on the board. Anyone can tell at a glance whether a tool is missing. Larger tools may be put in a box that has a label identifying the tool by name. When several people use the same work station, such as at jobs done in shifts, each worker can quickly check to determine whether all tools are in place. An efficient check system such as this saves time looking for a tool during work activities.

Other efficiency ideas include organizing the work tasks in a sequence which reduces or avoids "back tracking." Work activities move in one direction. The same idea applies to stock rooms. If supply requests and stock piles are organized by the same numbering system, supplies can be taken from the shelves or bins in one continuous trip.

Communication often is a problem in industrial settings. The common solution is printed signs and written memos. For persons with educational problems, the message may be missed. People who are mentally retarded or learning disabled, or who have terminated their formal education in the elementary grades, often have reading difficulties. If signs are in picture form or commonly understood symbols, the message may be clearer. Signs and memos may also use cartoons since they rely more on action than on words to convey a message.

Analysis of jobs can be done from two frames of reference: the manager's and the worker's. Management usually knows what the job is designed to do. The problem is getting the worker to do the job. Highly repetitious jobs are boring to people with average or higher intelligence. When a person is bored, he or she may be prone to carelessness or "slacking off." The right worker for the job is an important concept. If the work is repetitious, perhaps a person who is retarded could adapt to it as well as or better than someone with normal ability. If the work requires sitting all day, perhaps a person with a spinal cord injury would be a better choice than an able-bodied person.

Planning a recreation or leisure program can be a real challenge. The objective has to be broader than organizing a few team sports. Activities need to be available for people with "two left feet" as well as for older workers. Quick activities must be alternated with activities that require more time. Cultural differences must be considered, and location of commercially available forms of recreation such as bowling alleys is important as well. Transportation almost always is a major consideration. For industries located away from towns and cities, such as logging camps, a recreational and leisure program can increase work output by keeping the workers active and interested during nonworking hours as well as working hours.

Another challenge is planning a preretirement program. Retirement is not a single phenomenon. There are as many kinds of retirement as there are retirees. The goal is to help each person plan for his or her retirement by thinking ahead and gathering the resources and information together. If the person sees himself or herself as being in charge of the planning, a major step has been made. The individual should view retirement as an opportunity rather than a liability of old age.

This section on intervention programs has covered only a few program ideas. Other ideas, innovations, and combinations are possible. Good programs start with creative ideas and individuals who have a willingness to seek advice, try things out, learn from experience, and try, try, again.

Case Study

David was 16 years old when he misjudged the depth of the pool and dove into water only 5 feet deep, while visiting friends at an apartment complex after a party. His head hit the cement bottom of the pool and instantly he felt something "snap" in his neck. He remembers feeling himself sink to the bottom but was powerless to stop himself. He thought he would drown, but fortunately a man living near the pool had wondered who could be using it at 1:30 a.m. The man reached his window in time to see the dive and realized something was wrong when Dave did not surface. The man and one of Dave's friends pulled him out.

After 10 weeks of hospitalization, Dave was referred for a work assessment. His rehabilitation had been slow primarily because Dave could see little point in living. His world had revolved around sports, and he had been sure he could get a sports scholarship if he decided to go to college, although he was not particularly interested in education. Sports were more exciting and the pay was good. He found football, baseball, and basketball attractive, but suddenly they were all out of reach. His legs were useless and his arms weren't much better. He stated that his "life was over before it really got going." Who would want a cripple on a professional sports team, he wondered?

Dave viewed work assessment as another ploy on the physician's part to get him out of his room, which resembled a sports museum more than a hospital room. He could not understand why he should be evaluated for work when he could not even pick up a pencil without the help of his hand splint. Employers do not want cripples either, he reasoned.

Nevertheless, he was on his way to the work assessment room. The orderly transporting him was a big man with strong arms and legs who told Dave to "quit complaining and get with the program!" Dave could not think of a snappy comeback and he certainly couldn't run away.

The COTA in the work evaluation program introduced herself to Dave and told him about the objectives of the program. She asked him some questions about his work experience, schooling, family relations, and leisure interests. Dave said that he had had a paper route when he was 14 years old but quit after two months because he did not like getting up early in the morning and did not like trying to collect from people who were never home. He did not feel that he had learned anything useful from the experience.

Dave indicated that he did not like any school subjects. His hobbies were sports and sports related activities, such as collecting baseball cards. Although he did not like reading, he would read the sports section of the newspaper and the comics; *Sports Illustrated* was his favorite magazine.

When the COTA asked what he thought his parents would like to see him do with his life, he was not sure. He thought his father had supported his interest in becoming a professional sportsman but he did not think his mother did. He remembered her commenting about how dangerous sports could be and that most players did not last more than 10 years. However, she did seem to think coaching or managing a team was all right.

The occupational therapy assistant knew that she should assess Dave's physical capabilities, but a standard test was not possible. Dave had no functional use of his lower extremities; therefore items such as standing, walking, and lifting were not scorable. The COTA decided to to use the form as a guide, not using the items as stated. This decision would be recorded in the summary of the evaluation results.

Dave was able to sit, but only in a chair with arms. Using his electric wheelchair, he could carry objects in his lap for "quick trips" or on his lapboard for longer time periods. For example, using his lapboard, he could carry a lunch tray, notebook, or calculator. He could push and pull objects on the lapboard, but friction had to be minimal and the distance a few inches. Climbing, balancing, stooping, kneeling, crouching, and crawling were activities that were clearly not feasible. Reaching was limited to the space directly in front of him and up to his head. With his tenodesis splint, he could handle objects weighing up to 6 ounces. He was learning how to pick up a pencil, but objects smaller than 3/8 inch were impossible. Stereognosis was poor. Speech, hearing, and sight were normal.

Aptitudes were assessed using OASIS. Again, the instructions had to be modified because Dave could not mark the form himself. Therefore, the scores achieved would be estimates. The marking section was omitted because of his disability. His scores were G5, V4, N6, S4, and P5, or about average.

To further explore his interests, the COTA administered the *Wide Range Interest and Opinion Test*. This instrument was selected because Dave told her that he had trouble reading. She also hoped that the picture format would hold his interest better and therefore give a more accurate assessment. Dave thought that some of the pictures were "weird" but he finished the test.

Dave's educational achievement was assessed using the *Wide Range Achievement Test — Re-*

vised, Level 2. Again, the instructions had to be disregarded and the COTA had to mark Dave's answers, except for the oral reading section. Scores were: reading 78, spelling 90, and arithmetic 109. Since the normal scores are 100 with a standard deviation of 15, it was apparent that the reading score was low.

The COTA also assessed Dave's medical condition in relation to environmental conditions found in work settings. Dave's quadriplegia would require him to work inside where temperature and humidity could be controlled. All extremes of temperature and humidity needed to be avoided because his body could not sweat from the chest down, his breathing capacity was reduced, and his sensation was poor except for the face, neck, and upper chest. The reduced sensation also required that hazardous situations be avoided.

A team meeting to discuss Dave's work assessment information was attended by Dave's physician, his hospital teacher, the psychometrist, vocational rehabilitation counselor, the COTA's supervisor, an OTR, and the COTA.

The work history and physical capacities data were reviewed. The vocational counselor verified the COTA's findings regarding Dave's aptitudes. Numerical computation scores were good, and other aptitudes were average or below except for manual coordination and dexterity items which were not tested. Results of the *Strong-Campbell Interest Inventory* suggested that Dave would like jobs which had social, enterprising, and conventional aspects to them.

Both the teacher and the psychometrist had found results similar to the COTA's on academic performance in class and data from the *Metropolitan Achievement Tests.* Dave's school records indicated that the *Weschler Intelligence Scale for Children — Revised* had been administered the previous year. His full intelligence quotient was 111, suggesting that Dave's ability was higher than his daily performance would indicate. His low reading scores may have reflected lack of interest or practice rather than limited ability. The teacher's observations supported the concept of average ability but low interest. She had noticed that Dave seemed to be able to read the sports news but not the class assignment.

In discussing Dave's interests, it was noted that he had scored high in sports, numbers, and sales. His literature and social science scores were above average. The OTR suggested that Dave seemed to like group sports, could work with numbers, and could persuade or influence people. He communicated with words and was interested in the actions of people and groups. These were his strengths. His limitations included reduced physical capacity, lack of work skills, low reading rate, and low interest rate in general.

The vocational counselor did not feel that Dave was a good candidate for vocational training at that time. He needed more therapy to maximize his physical capacities in the upper extremities, more education, and, hopefully, more realistic goals.

Members of the team concurred, however, that the next question was, what should be done in the meantime? The COTA asked whether there was some way to capitalize on his interest in sports. The vocational counselor suggested "nonplaying" jobs connected with sports such as sports writer, sports announcer, sports statistician, sports manager, or sports promoter. It was recommended by the teacher that Dave be asked to read a sports story each day and summarize it for the class. He could also write a short story each week on a sport or a sports figure. The physician suggested that the story could be posted for everyone to read. The OTR added that Dave could post the daily sports scores for those too busy to read them. Thus, the COTA's original question sparked a series of ideas which could improve Dave's educational skills, develop his work habits, and provide direction for future goals.

Dave was invited to come into the meeting at this point, and the physician reviewed the discussion with him including the suggested activities. Dave was sure that he could read a sports story but was hesitant about writing. The teacher proposed that he might begin by first taping his story and then writing or typing it. He was reminded by the OTR that this would also give him an opportunity to practice typing with his typing sticks and writing with his tenodesis splint. His stories could meet several goals at the same time and Dave was pleased with the idea. He also agreed to compile daily sports scores, which would require him to write more. He noted that he might need a computer to keep track of the scores over several days or weeks. The vocational counselor said that developing computer skills could be useful in later career planning. The team meeting ended with each person taking responsibility for following up on the ideas generated.

Summary

Work programs require special knowledge and skill. Whether a COTA or an OTR is able to conduct a successful work program depends on the willingness of the individual practitioner to learn the details. The details exist in the following questions: What is the meaning and value of work in this area? What specific jobs are common in the area? What special skills do those jobs require? What strengths and weaknesses do the patients being seen have in meeting those requirements? How can their strengths be increased and their weaknesses minimized? What resources are needed? Who is available to provide help? What methods can the OTR and COTA use to gain the knowledge and skills needed to be effective in carrying out a work program?

References

1. Guralnik DB: *Webster's New World Dictionary*, 2nd College Edition. New York: Simon and Schuster, 1982.
2. Braude L: *Work and Workers: A Sociological Analysis*. Malabar, FL: Robert E. Kreiger Publishing, 1983, p 14.
3. Parker S: The work-leisure relationship under changing economic conditions and societal values. In B Gardell, G Johansson, Eds: *Working Life: A Social Science Contribution to Work Reform*. Chichester, England: John Wiley and Sons, 1981, pp 115-132.
4. Bucholz RA: Measurement of belief. *Human Relations* 29:1177-1188, 1976.
5. United States Department of Labor, Employment and Training Administration: *Dictionary of Occupational Titles*, 4th Edition. Washington, DC: U.S. Government Printing Office, 1977, Supplement, 1982.
6. United States Department of Labor, Employment and Training Administration: *Selected Characteristics of Occupations Defined in the Dictionary of Occupational Titles*. Washington, DC: U.S. Government Printing Office, 1981.
7. Field TF, Field JE: *The Classification of Jobs*, Revised Edition. Athens, GA: VDARE Service Bureau, 1984.
8. United States Department of Labor, Employment and Training Administration: *Guide for Occupational Exploration*. Washington, DC: U.S. Government Printing Office, 1979.
9. Baxter PL: A focus on work, therapy and vocational direction. In JM Hunter, et al, Eds: *Rehabilitation of the Hand*. St. Louis, MO: CV Mosby, 1978.
10. Matheson LN: *Work Capacity Evaluation*. Trabuco Canyon, CA: Employment and Rehabilitation Institute of California, 1984.
11. *Valpar Component Work Sample Series*. Tuscon, AZ: Valpar International, 1974.
12. Jebsen RJ, et al: An objective and standardized test of hand function. *Archives of Physical Medicine and Rehabilitation* 50:311-319, 1969.
13. Mathiowetz V, et al: Adult norms for the Box and Block Test of manual dexterity. *Am J Occup Ther* 39:386-391, 1985.
14. Crawford JE, Crawford DM: *Crawford Small Part Dexterity Test*. New York: Psychological Corporation, 1956.
15. Bennett GK: *Hand-Tool Dexterity Test*. New York: Psychological Corporation, 1965.
16. *Grooved Pegboard*. Lafayette, IN: Lafayette Instrument Co.
17. *Minnesota Rate of Manipulation Tests*. Circle Pines, MN: American Guidance Service, 1969.
18. *Minnesota Spatial Relations Test*, Revised Edition. Circle Pines, MN: American Guidance Service, 1979.
19. Roberts JR: *Pennsylvania Bi-Manual Worksample*. Circle Pines, MN: American Guidance Service, 1945.
20. Tiffin J: *Purdue Pegboard*. Chicago: Science Research Associates, 1968.
21. Stromberg EL: *Stromberg Dexterity Test*. New York: Psychological Corporation, 1951.
22. Wepman JM: *Auditory Discrimination Test*. Los Angeles, CA: Western Psychological Services, 1973.
23. *Snellen Eye Chart*. Tucker, GA: WCO Ophthalmic Instrument Division.
24. *Titmus Stereo Test*. Tucker, GA: WCO Ophthalmic Instrument Division.
25. *Dvorine Color Vision Test*. Cleveland, OH: Psychological Corporation.
26. United States Department of Labor Manpower Administration: *Manual for the USES General Aptitude Test Battery*. Section III, Development. Washington, DC: U.S. Government Printing Office, 1970.
27. Parker RM: *Occupational Aptitude Survey and Interest Schedule*. Austin, TX: PRO-ED, 1983.
28. Campbell DP, Hansen JC: *Strong Campbell Interest Inventory*, 3rd Edition. Stanford, CA: Stanford University Press, 1981.
29. Kuder BF, Diamon EE: *Occupational Interest Survey — Kuder DD*. Chicago: Science Reasearch Associates, 1979.
30. Jackson DN: *Jackson Vocational Interest Survey*. Port Huron, MI: Research Psychologists Press, 1977.
31. Kuder GE: *Kuder Preference Record — C*. Chicago: Science Research Associates, 1960.
32. Kuder GE: *Kuder Preference Record — D*. Chicago: Science Reserach Associates, 1961.
33. Ayres GDC, et al: *Ohio Vocational Interest Survey*. New York: Harcourt Brace Jovanovich, 1969.
34. Holland JL: *The Self-Directed Search*. Palo Alto, CA: Consulting Psychologists Press, 1979.
35. Holland JL: *Vocational Preference Inventory*. Palo Alto, CA: Consulting Psychologists Press, 1978.
36. Jastak JF, Jastak S: *Wide Range Interest-Opinion Test*. Wilmington, DE: Jastak Associates, 1979.
37. Becker RL: *Reading-Free Vocational Interest Inventory*. Circle Pines, MN: American Guidance Service, 1981.
38. Geist H: *The Geist Picture Interest Inventory*. Los Angeles, CA: Western Psychological Services, 1968.
39. Weingarten KP: *Picture Interest Inventory*. Monterey. CA: Test Bureau, 1958.
40. McKechnie GE: *Leisure Activities Blank*. Palo Alto, CA: Consulting Psychologists Press, 1975.
41. Super D: *Work Values Inventory*. Atlanta, GA: Houghton Mifflin, 1970.
42. Jastak S, Wilkinson GS: *The Wide Range Achievement Test — Revised*. Wilmington, DE: Jastak Associates, 1984.
43. Dunn LM, Markwardt FC: *Peabody Individual Achievement Test*. Circle Pines, MN: American Guidance Service, 1970.
44. Wechsler D: *Manual for the Wechsler Adult Intelligence Scale — Revised*. New York: Psychological Corporation, 1981.

45. *Stanford-Binet Intelligence Scale*. Boston: Houghton Mifflin, 1960.

46. *Shipley Institute of Living Scale*. Los Angeles, CA: Western Psychological Services, 1967.

47. Dunn LM, Dunn LM: *Readbody Picture Vocabulary Test — Revised*. Circle Pines, MN: American Guidance Service, 1981.

48. Bennett GK, Seashore HG, Wesman AG: *Differential Aptitude Tests*. New York: Psychological Corporation, 1947.

49. *Revised Minnesota Paper Form Board*. New York: Psychological Corporation, 1970.

50. *Testing Orientation and Work Evaluation in Rehabilitation (TOWER)*. New York: Institute for the Crippled and Disabled, 1967.

51. Holland JL: *Making Vocational Choices: A Theory of Vocational Personalities and Work Environments*, 2nd Edition. Englewood Cliffs, NJ: Prentice-Hall, 1985.

52. United States Department of Labor, Bureau of Labor Statistics: *Exploring Careers*. Washington, DC: U.S. Government Printing Office, 1979.

53. United States Department of Labor, Manpower Administration: *Handbook for Analyzing Jobs*. Washington, DC: U.S. Government Printing Office, 1972.

54. United States Department of Labor, Employment and Training Administration: *Job Selection Workbook for Use with Guide for Occupational Exploration*. Washington, DC: U.S. Government Printing Office, 1979.

CHAPTER **24**

The Role of the COTA as an Activities Director

Sally E. Ryan, COTA

Introduction

The position of activities director, coordinator, or supervisor is one for which the certified occupational therapy assistant is well qualified. The COTA's educational background in human development throughout the life span and understanding of disabling conditions, group dynamics, and activity analysis, as well as an understanding of every individual's need for purposeful, meaningful activity, allows him or her to carry out activities programs of exceptional quality.

Activities directors are employed in a variety of settings, including community centers, large apartment and condominium complexes for the well and the disabled, group homes and institutions for the mentally retarded and the chronic mentally ill, and long-term care settings for the elderly. Since a large number of COTAs are employed as activities directors in geriatric, long-term care facilities, this chapter focuses on principles and applications for those settings. Definitions, regulations, and job descriptions are discussed, and detailed information is presented about developing activities plans and implementing programs. Recording and reporting aspects are outlined, as well as information about basic program management tasks and the use of consultation.

Definitions and Regulations

An activities program may be defined as an ongoing plan for providing meaningful activities which are determined in relation to the individual needs and interests of the patients. Such programs are designed to include a variety of opportunities for patients to participate in activities, the goal being to promote their physical, mental, and social well-being.[1] The term "patient" is used in keeping with the terminology adopted in the 1974 Medicare and Medicaid standards for skilled nursing facilities, as well as to provide consistent use of terminology within this text. The reader, however, should recognize that the term "resident" may be used in a number of settings, particularly board and care facilities.

An activities director is an individual who is employed by the facility and is directly responsible for planning, scheduling, implementing, and documenting an activities program. The program is designed with the overall goal of meeting the individual patient's needs for healthy activity that will assist in maintaining optimal levels of functioning.[2]

An activities consultant is a qualified individual who is employed by the facility to provide guidance to the activities director concerning all aspects of the activities program. This person may also consult for other staff members and departments, as requested by administration. Occupational therapists, experienced occupational therapy assistants, therapeutic recreation specialists, and social workers, among others, are often called upon to provide consultative services.

In 1974, the Department of Health, Education and Welfare (DHEW) published the following *Standards for Certification and Participation in Medicare and Medicaid for Skilled Nursing Facilities* (SNFs):[1]

> 405.1131 *Condition of Participation—Patient Activities*
> "The skilled nursing facility provides for an activities program, appropriate to the needs and interests of each patient to encourage self-care, resumption of normal activities, and maintenance of an optimal level of psychosocial functioning."
> (a) *Standard: Responsibility for Patient Activities.*
> "A member of the facility's staff is designated as responsible for the patient activities program. If he is not a qualified patient activities coordinator, he functions with frequent, regularly scheduled consultation from a person so qualified."
> (b) *Standard: Patient Activities Program.*
> "Provision is made for an ongoing program of meaningful activities appropriate to the needs and interests of the patients, designed to promote opportunities for engaging in normal pursuits including religious activities of their choice, if any. Each patient's activities program is approved by the patient's attending physician so as not to be in conflict with the treatment plan. The activities are designed to promote the physical, social and mental well-being of the patients. The facility makes available adequate space and a variety of supplies and equipment to satisfy the individual interests of patients."
>
> 405.1134 *Condition of Participation—Physical Environment.*
> "The skilled nursing facility is constructed, equipped and maintained to protect the health and safety of patients, personnel and the public."
> (g) *Standard: Dining and Patient Activities Rooms.*
> "The facility provides one or more clean, orderly, and appropriately furnished rooms of adequate size designated for patient dining and patient activities. These areas are well-lighted and well-ventilated. If a multi-purpose room is used for dining and patient activities, there is sufficient space to accommodate all activities and prevent their interference with each other."

In addition to these federal regulations for skilled nursing care facilities, others exist for intermediate care facilities (ICFs). Most state health departments and licensing agencies have specific regulations for activities programs as well. The activities director must have a complete understanding of all of these regulations before initiating an activities program.

The director must also have a job description that specifically outlines all responsibilities and expectations. The following items should be included:[2]

1. Job title, supervisor, and supervisees.
2. Qualifications, including formal education and training and any specialized training that might be required such as remotivation, reality orientation and reminiscence techniques, cardiopulmonary resuscitation, and first aid.
3. Licensure and/or certification requirements.
4. Other skills such as effective written and verbal communication and related public relations activities.
5. Required participation in continuing education and professional activities.
6. Specific activities responsibilities such as assessing individual patient activities needs; planning, scheduling, implementing, documenting, and evaluating the activities program. Definitive time lines should be included, e.g., weekly, monthly, or quarterly.
7. Participation in the care planning process, including specific requirements for attending meetings and frequency.
8. Staff and volunteer recruitment, training, supervision, evaluation, and termination.
9. In-service education training responsibilities for staff and volunteers.

10 Reports to be prepared and frequency.
11 Procurement of supplies and equipment.
12 Orientation activities for new employees in the facility.
13 Other responsibilities such as coordinating barber and beautician appointments and making arrangements for voting.
14 Methods and frequency of evaluation; conditions of probationary employment.

Job descriptions should be reviewed and modified as necessary, at least on an annual basis. Sample job descriptions for activities directors are often available from state health departments.

Developing an Activities Plan

The first step in developing an activities plan is to collect data about the patients. The medical record and the patient care plan will provide information regarding the primary and secondary diagnosis, precautions and limitations, physician's approval for activities participation, the patient's birth date, nationality, and social history, and the name of a family contact.[2]

Interest Questionnaire (see Appendix N)

Another step in the data collection process is to determine the interests of the patients. A structured questionnaire or checklist should be developed that seeks information in the areas of social, creative, productive (work substitute), educational, leisure, and spiritual activities.

Social Activities

Activities in this category include parties, picnics, meals at community restaurants and "tea time"; the primary goal is to provide an opportunity for patients to interact socially. Family members should also be invited to some of these events.

Creative Activities

Crafts, calligraphy, creative writing, and oil and watercolor painting are examples of creative activities. Such endeavors provide an outlet for creative expression, and while they often are presented in a group setting, socialization is not required.

Productive (Work Substitute) Activities

Many elderly people have a need to be engaged in a productive activity. Work on community service projects such as filling fund raising packets for the American Cancer Society or stuffing envelopes for a local charity should be provided. Other work-related activities include writing and producing a facility newspaper, rolling bandages for the Red Cross, and baking items for a bazaar. Productive endeavors such as these allow the elderly to continue to make a meaningful contribution to society.

Educational Activities

The opportunities for life-long learning are virtually endless. Photography clubs, music appreciation groups, and book review and discussion groups are a few examples. Individual activities such as learning to speak a foreign language or to operate a microcomputer should also be included. Reality orientation sessions should be scheduled for confused patients as a means of re-educating them as to person, place, time, season and so forth.

Leisure Activities

Most everyone needs time set aside to read a good book, write letters, listen to the radio, or view a favorite television program. Strolling in the park or just sitting on the patio observing and enjoying nature can be meaningful, refreshing pastimes.

Spiritual Activities

Spiritual needs can be met in a variety of ways such as participation in Bible study groups, a choir, or regularly scheduled religious services in the facility as well as the community. A missionary group often assists in fulfilling spiritual needs.

Interviews should be arranged with each of the patients to obtain the needed activity information. Volunteers may assist in this task. If patients are reluctant to discuss items on a questionnaire, a more generalized approach may be used by asking open-ended questions: "What activities did you enjoy doing before coming to the nursing home?"

"What are some of the things you did during your spare time this week?" "If you were the activities director, what do you think would be an important activity to provide?" The interviewer should provide added cues as necessary to keep the responses to questions on target. Speaking with family members and other staff is also recommended to gain as much additional input as possible. Once the data are gathered, they must be tabulated, categorized, and prioritized in terms of available staff, volunteers, space, existing supplies and equipment, community resources, and operating budget.

If, for example, the category of creative activities indicates that a large number of patients are interested in arts and crafts, a general session should be scheduled daily. Perhaps a small number are interested in knitting. While they could participate in the general group, they may also enjoy forming a knitting club that meets once a week to work on a special project such as knitting hats and mittens for a children's home.

Initial activity planning can best be done by setting up a "mock" weekly calendar with dates on the left, including Saturday and Sunday, and the six major categories of activities listed across the top. Enter the large group activities first—those which patients indicated the greatest interest in, such as crafts, movies, concerts, games. Next, enter the small group activities, such as baking, gardening, oil painting and the like. Determine which of these activities existing staff and volunteers can supervise and identify additional needs. Be sure that required space, supplies, and equipment are available. Look for gaps in the plan and be creative about introducing new activities. It is also important to determine whether activities are primarily active or passive in terms of degree of participation. Every effort should be made to schedule activities such as picnics, shopping tours, and visits to museums and zoos so that patients maintain contact with the community. Some patients will not wish to join groups, and therefore time must be set aside for individual activities participation.

Individual activities needs cannot be totally met by a program that only schedules events Monday through Friday during the usual daytime working hours. Flexibility is necessary, and every effort should be made to provide some activities in the evenings and on weekends. Arrangements can usually be made for the staff members assigned to take compensatory time off during the regular work week. The proposed activities plan should also be evaluated to assure that at least some of the activities are held at a time when family members can participate.

Once the mock plan is developed and staffing patterns are established, it is important to look at the timing of events. Consideration must be given to "set" activities such as meals, doctors' rounds, occupational and physical therapy schedules, and visiting hours.

When the final monthly plan is developed, it must be communicated as widely as possible. Copies should be provided to administration and all departments in the facility. Large weekly posters should be made and posted in prominent locations throughout the building; individual posters should also be made to advertise special events such as a concert or bazaar. If a public address system is in place, utilize it to make daily announcements of forthcoming events. Flyers can be mailed to family members when events are scheduled in which they can participate. The community should also be informed through providing local newspapers with press releases of activities of interest, such as a patient's 100th birthday, or an announcement of the patients who received "ribbons" for their entries in the county fair.

Activities planning must always be done at least one month in advance. Failure to do so will result in undue stress for the director, staff, and volunteers and unmet patient activities needs. Even the most thorough planning will not be flawless. The activities director must have alternatives to draw upon when the high school band fails to show up for a concert or a torrential rainstorm ruins picnic plans. Flexibility, adaptability, and resourcefulness are important attributes of the successful activities director.

Individual activities plans should be developed for every patient and be included in the total patient care plan. Problems and needs are identified and specific objectives are established along with methods for accomplishing the goals. State regulations should be obtained to be sure that all required information is included. Figure 24-1 represents a sample activities plan:[2]

A card system should be developed for each patient's individual activity plan. The patient card should also have information on the primary and secondary diagnosis, limitations and precautions,

FIGURE 24-1. Sample Activities Plan

NAME:	Mary Smith
LONG-TERM GOAL:	To reduce boredom by participation in leisure and social activities.
DATE:	9/18/85
PROBLEM:	Spends much time sitting alone in day room.
APPROACH:	Invite to attend social activities and assign a "volunteer" friend to accompany her.
OUTCOME:	Is participating in weekly bridge group and attends musical programs. Has joined in afternoon walking group 3 to 4 days per week. S. Jones 9/25/85
DATE:	10/8/85
PROBLEM:	Appears to be depressed owing to recent death of roommate; had been ill with flu and unable to attend the funeral.
APPROACH:	Arrange for minister to visit to help work through the grieving process; provide transportation to visit the grave site.
OUTCOME:	Speaks openly about roommate's death and seems to have reached a stage of acceptance; planted a rose bush in her memory and has resumed participation in activities as noted 9/18/85. S. Jones 10/15/85

physician's permission to participate in activities, birth date, and other pertinent social history facts. Locating the card system in a central place, such as the activities department office, will allow all staff members convenient access to it. Additional information on patient care planning and specific activities plans appears in the section on records and reports.

Implementing the Activities Program

Once initial planning has been completed, the activities program is implemented, often on a gradual basis over several weeks. As activities take place, the activities director must carefully monitor all aspects to ensure that the programming is effective in helping to meet patient goals. The following items are of particular importance:

1 General attendance and degree of participation.
2 Adequacy of staff and volunteer coverage.
3 Adequacy of space, furnishings, equipment, and supplies.
4 Adequacy of lighting, ventilation, and temperature control devices and general safety.
5 Effectiveness of communication with other departments.
6 Timing of events in relation to other activities taking place in the facility.
7 Specific ways to improve the activity the next time it is presented.

Keeping a clipboard close at hand is a good idea so that observations on these points may be recorded immediately. It is also important to seek critiques from participants as well as staff members and volunteers. An activities planning committee could be established to review past events and make recommendations for future activities.

Another helpful method is to break activities down into very specific components, particularly if they tend to take too much time or participation is less than expected. An example would be the weekly songfest. This activity is made up of at least 12 distinct parts, which include:

1 Furniture arrangement.
2 Transportation for nonambulatory participants.
3 Introduction of song leader and pianist.

4 Distribution of song sheets.
5 Use of an overhead projector with enlarged words to songs.
6 Use of clapping and marching activities.
7 Distribution and use of rhythm instruments.
8 Playing "name that tune" game.
9 Collecting and storing supplies and equipment.
10 Returning nonambulatory patients to their units.
11 Rearranging furniture.
12 Documenting participation.

Patient Motivation

A successful activities program involves much more than planning and carrying out a variety of activities. It must also include the creation of an atmosphere that is warm, friendly, and caring and is as nonthreatening as possible; an atmosphere that offers decision making opportunities and promotes independence; an atmosphere in which patients are offered encouragement and support but are never coerced or forced to participate. These are important motivational factors.

The main activities room should serve as a central gathering spot for those who just want to get away from their rooms for a while. Space should be provided for people to observe the activities taking place, particularly new patients. Serving coffee and tea is way to include observers in the activities group in a comfortable way. It encourages socialization and may increase motivation to become directly involved in the activity at hand.

Motivation comes from within, but it can be enhanced by showing a genuine interest in the patients. Sometimes writing a short personal note to invite a patient to participate will be a motivating factor. Others will be motivated or drawn to activities because they can be assured of some degree of success or of feeling "needed" by the other group members. For example, a patient who isn't the least bit interested in working on the mosaic mural in the dining room may be willing to spend hours sorting tile so that the others can work more efficiently.

Records and Reports

A system of regular documentation must be established in keeping with the requirements of federal, state, and facility regulations. The general categories of documentation include patient care plans, activities plans, progress notes, activities schedules, and participation records. Confidentiality must be maintained for all patient reports. Records should also be maintained for all staff members and volunteers indicating hours worked and major responsibilities. Budget reports must be prepared regularly, and the administration of the facility may require monthly summary reports of the activities program as well as an annual report. The activities director will also be responsible for developing and maintaining an activities policies and procedures manual. It is advisable to keep records of supply needs and an inventory of equipment and furnishings as well.

Patient Care Plans

One of the main purposes of patient care planning is to assess needs and problems in a systematic way. Specific goals are established and methods are identified for accomplishing them. Comprehensive patient care plans promote a coordinated effort in providing medical as well as multidisciplinary services for the patient. Effective patient care planning must include the patient, the family, and significant others as well as all of the health care providers in the facility. Patient care plans must be reviewed and revised on a regular basis.

Activity Plans

Activity plans are developed, evaluated, and updated on a regular basis, usually monthly. They are a part of the patient's clinical record. The activities director must allocate specific blocks of time each week for this task to ensure that all plans are always up to date. To assist in this process, a system should be developed for staff and volunteers to record their observations of individual patients on a daily basis, if possible. A notebook with a page for each patient is a simple way of collecting the information. Observations might be written in this way:

12/5/85-Mr. Jones began a mosaic flower pot project and worked one hour.

S. Smith, Volunteer

12/7/85-Patient finished mosaic project and said he didn't like it; expressed interest in making a wooden jig saw puzzle for his granddaughter.

M. Jones, Act. Aide

12/8/85-Patient worked on puzzle and stated he was a little "nervous" about being the discussion leader for the current events group.

S. Smith, Volunteer

In addition to contributing to the activities plan, observation notes such as these will also assist the activity director in evaluating the patient's degree of progress in attaining goals.

Progress Notes

Progress notes are included in the patient's clinical record and should be written whenever change is noted or at least once a month. A good activities progress note should include a summary of the kinds of activities the patient has been participating in, the frequency of participation, and the time involved. Quotations may be used. All notes must be dated, written legibly in ink, and signed. Use of abbreviations should be avoided unless the facility has an approved list of abbreviations for use in records. Progress notes must be objective, accurate, and complete. They should relate directly to the activity plan and the total patient care plan.[2]

Progress Notes—Sample

3/21/86 Mr. Johnson is actively participating in woodworking activities every weekday morning for one or two hours. He frequently takes a nap after lunch and participates in the weekly photography club and the current events group in the afternoons. He has served as discussion leader of the current events group on three occasions. He also visits the library frequently and stated that "Reading is one of my greatest pleasures."

Jane Doe, COTA, Activities Director

Participation Records and Activities Schedules

Participation records should be maintained on a daily basis to provide an overall view of activity trends and fluctuations. Such records will reflect individual patient inactivity as well as overactivity,[3] and serve as a barometer of interest in specific activities. These records may also be used as justification for hiring additional staff members. Graph paper may be used to develop a simple participation recording form. The names of all patients are listed on the left-hand side, and the different activities are listed across the top. To save space, use a coding system such as "C" = Crafts, "B" = Baking, "G" = Gardening. It is important to keep in mind that if a person comes to the activity area and falls asleep, he or she has not participated!

Activities schedules are generally the monthly calendar of events. These should be filed, as they provide specific information about the variety of activities offered and when. The schedules may also be coded to indicate whether activities require active or passive participation and the number of staff members and volunteers that are needed for each activity. A review of past schedules is a great help in planning for future events.

Activities Reports

Summary reports of the activities program are written on a regular basis as required by the administration and at least annually. A typical report might include information on the number of patients participating in the six major activity areas (social, creative, productive, educational, diversional, and spiritual) with a breakdown of individual and group activities. New or unique events may be highlighted. Budget information should be included in the categories of income, expenditures, and cash on hand. The number of staff and volunteers should be noted as well as consultation services received. Inservice training programs for staff and volunteers should be briefly described.

Policy and Procedure Manual

The activities director is responsible for developing, reviewing, and revising the departmental policy and procedure manual. A policy may be defined as a statement that describes how basic objectives can be met. Policies are not subject to frequent change. Procedures are methods for carrying out the policy and are subject to modification as need arises. For example, the policy and procedures for conducting a birthday party might be written in the following manner:[2]

SUBJECT: Birthday parties

POLICY: A monthly birthday party shall be held in the facility.

PURPOSE: To honor all patients who are celebrating a birthday during that month.

RESPONSIBILITY: The activity director shall be responsible for planning and carrying out the party.

PROCEDURES:

1 Written invitations will be sent to all patients celebrating a birthday during a given month. Invitations may also be sent to family members.
2 The date, time, and location of the party will be advertised at least two weeks in advance. All patients and staff are invited.
3 Corsages and boutonnieres will be provided for those being honored.
4 Cake, ice cream, and beverages must be ordered from the dietary department at least one week in advance of the event.
5 Prizes may be awarded to the youngest and the oldest birthday people.
6 Musical entertainment will be provided.

Staffing Needs

The literature yields little information on this topic. This author believes that the employment of one full-time activities director for every 50 to 60 patients should be an absolute minimum in skilled and intermediate care facilities. Individual state regulations and licensing agencies may specify other minimums for activities personnel. It should be kept in mind that providing a minimum number of activities personnel may not allow maximal services to be provided in meeting the patients' individual activity needs.

As more patients become actively involved in the activities program and increased needs are identified, it may be necessary to increase the staff size. Prior to hiring additional personnel, a specific job description must be developed which includes many of the items described in the beginning of this chapter. Administration must approve all new staff positions. Plans and procedures must also be developed for orienting and evaluating new employees and making provision for their continuing education. While volunteers are a most important asset to any activities program, it is this author's belief that volunteers should never take the place of paid staff under any circumstances.

Before a volunteer program is initiated, legal and insurance issues must be considered to assure that adequate liability safeguards are provided. Volunteers should be recruited, screened, and trained as needs arise to enhance the program. They can often provide some of the extra services that help to personalize the program, particularly in relation to individual needs. Volunteers can carry out a variety of tasks, including letter writing, personal patient and departmental shopping, leading songfests, teaching creative activities, and typing. The recruiting of volunteers may be accomplished in many ways, such as facility posters, more formal advertising in church bulletins, high school and college newspapers, and general announcements at neighborhood events. All volunteers must have specific job descriptions and hours and should participate in an orientation and training program. All volunteers should be formally recognized for their contributions on at least an annual basis; certificates or pins should be presented at a special gathering in their honor.

Program Management

As a departmental manager, the activities director must develop systems and approaches that will provide for the most effective and efficient delivery of activities services to meet the goals of the department and the health care facility. Failure to do so may result in decreased motivation and interest on the part of workers.

It is the responsibility of the supervisor to develop and utilize objective tools such as job descriptions and evaluation forms to measure performance. The supervisor should also encourage the staff to participate in self-evaluation activities on a regular basis. Individual job performance goal setting should be a collaborative process between the supervisor and the supervisee. When specific deficits in performance are noted, the supervisor should be constructive in the criticism given by providing guidance, resources, and opportunities that will assist the worker in skill improvement.

Above all, an effective supervisor must be caring, honest, objective, and open in his or her relationships and willing to carry "a fair share" of the work load. A supervisor who provides a strong role model for everyone he or she supervises and demonstrates a sincere interest in their well-being is indeed effective.

Financial Planning Role

The activities director is responsible for financial planning for the department and must have skills in developing and managing a budget. The main categories that must be considered in budgeting are salaries, nonexpendable equipment, expendable equipment and supplies, maintenance and repair, travel, and professional development. Projected income and cash-on-hand figures should also be included.

Salaries

Salaries are generally the largest budget item. In planning, consideration must be given to actual salary amounts as well as post-probationary raises, merit and cost of living increases, overtime costs, and annual bonuses. Social security contributions, costs related to health and retirement plans, and life insurance benefits must also be calculated.

Nonexpendable Equipment

Purchase of major items such as phonographs, tables, and desks, are included in this category. Before requesting purchase of new equipment, it is wise to check with other departments such as housekeeping to see whether the needed items are in storage or available from another area of the facility.

Expendable Equipment and Supplies

This is a category of budget planning in which most mistakes take place owing to false assumptions or inaccurate information. The big problem lies in determining just exactly what is "expendable." The "Ryan Rule," developed by the author, states that: "Anything smaller than a large bread box that is not bolted down or kept under lock and key or constant surveillance is eventually expendable." Table looms, radios, coffee pots, and hand tools are among the items which frequently disappear.

Another aspect that makes budget planning difficult is "who pays for what" when several departments participate in an activity. For example, when a picnic is held in the park, is the cost of food charged to the dietary department or the activities department? If a nurse's aide is designated to assist with the activity, are the hours she works charged against the nursing budget or the activities budget? Matters such as these must be resolved with administration. Once these questions have been answered, more accurate planning can be done. One method is to keep track of actual expenses for a period of 3 months, multiply that amount by 4, and add 20 percent to cover inflation and margin of error.

Maintenance and Repair

Routine maintenance is required for sewing machines, powered woodworking tools, and all audiovisual equipment. Departmental painting and redecorating may also be included in this category.

Travel

Expenses incurred for bus rentals for patient outings are generally the largest item. If the facility has a vehicle for patient use, determine whether any charges are made to your department. Reimbursement of employee and volunteer mileage for such tasks as errands and shopping should also be covered in this budget category.

Professional Development

Continuing education courses and workshops, conventions, meetings, books, journals, and mileage are items that should be covered.

Income Sources

Cash donations, bazaar receipts, and bake sale proceeds are examples of income sources. It is of the utmost importance that the activities director have a clear understanding of exactly what the administration's expectations are for income-producing activities. While some activities may be self-supporting in terms of revenue generated, it is unrealistic to expect an activities program to generate enough income to cover expenses. Activities programs should never be forced to exploit patient endeavors to raise money.

Continuing Education Role

We live in an age when change is occurring very rapidly, particularly in our health care delivery systems. The activities director in collaboration with administration, staff, and volunteers, and with necessary outside consultation, must identify continuing education needs and develop a plan to meet these needs. Such a plan must include the required financial support. For example, many facilities require all staff members and volunteers to take a first aid course, and some require specialized training in cardiopulmonary resuscitation (CPR). As patients' needs change, staff members may also need to be trained in the techniques of reality orientation, remotivation, and reminiscence therapy. The activities director and everyone involved in the delivery of activities services must be given opportunities to participate in continuing education courses and workshops to ensure that the existing skills are maintained and new ones are acquired. Continuing education is important to provide necessary activities services, to enhance those services, and to be responsive to the changing needs of the patients.

Interdisciplinary Role

Most health care facilities view the activities director as a department head and an integral member of the health care team. The activities director should participate in all department head meetings and patient care planning conferences, as the delivery of effective activities services is dependent upon cooperation from and coordination with a number of other departments. Efforts should be made to develop both structured and informal communication channels that will assure quality patient care and the attainment of goals.

Consultation

A consultant is a person who is employed by a facility on a contractual basis to provide indirect service. Consultants may be utilized to give information, assist in strategy development and problem resolution, clarify issues, and advise.[5] Typically, a consultant is employed by administration to provide services to a department or several departments in relation to specific concerns. Consultative services may be as short as a one-time visit or may extend over several months or years depending on the nature of the consultation required. It is important to understand that a consultant works "outside" the facility and brings expertise and an objective viewpoint to the facility.

The activities director might utilize a consultant to assist in providing information about and interpretation of federal and state regulations regarding activities programming. Other areas in which a consultant might offer assistance include continuing education and general community resources, activity suggestions for nonparticipating patients, establishing patient care planning goals, and ways of improving departmental management procedures. A consultant can also be a valuable resource for developing strategies for improved communication with another department or individual.

It is very important to note that when an occupational therapist is employed as a consultant, it does not mean that occupational therapy services are being provided. Further clarification of this point is found in the official position paper of the American Occupational Therapy Association entitled "Roles and Functions of Occupational Therapy in Long-Term Care: Occupational Therapy and Activity Programs," which has been reprinted in full in Appendix I.

Summary

The role of the COTA as an activities director offers many challenges and opportunities. Skills in assessing activities needs and in planning, implementing, documenting, and evaluating programs are essential. The activities director must also have strong leadership and management abilities. The need for qualified activities personnel in long-term care facilities for the elderly is increasing, and the educational background of occupational therapy assistants provides them with excellent preparation for such positions.

Employment of a certified occupational therapy assistant or a registered occupational therapist consultant does not mean that occupational therapy direct services are being provided.

References

1. Skilled nursing facilities—Standards for certification and participation in Medicare and Medicaid programs. *Federal Register*, 39:12, 405.1131, Jan.17, 1974.
2. *Functional Model for an Activity Program*, Minneapolis, MN: Minnesota Department of Health, 1978.
3. Bachner J and Cornelius E: *Activities Coordinator's Guide*. Washington, D.C.: U.S. Government Printing Office, 1978.
4. Tso ML and Catherine D: *Activity Programs In Long-Term Care Facilities*, Hyattsville, MD: Carroll Manor, 1974.
5. Pochert L: Our new role challenge: Occupational therapy consultation. *Am J Occup Ther*, 2:1-2, 1970.

SECTION V

Concepts of Practice

As a profession we have entered an age of rapid technological advances which affect on the delivery of occupational therapy services. The invention of the microcomputer is but one example of the influence of a machine on human performance. It has allowed people with a variety of problems to achieve many goals both in occupational therapy treatment and in their personal lives. It has in many cases revolutionized our society. Simple, inexpensive microswitches allow individuals to actively interact with their human and mechanized environments in ways never thought possible. The use of video recording is also making new inroads as a tool for evaluation, treatment, patient education, record keeping, and leisure enjoyment. All of this new technology also affects on the management of occupational therapy service programs; thus, topics on organization and administration are included in this section.

The reader should focus on the specific technologies in terms of skills and application and also consider the greater implications for basic management and system development in health care. It is also important to heed the words of Dunford, who states, "Traditional occupational therapy skills must be the basis for a practical approach to using technical aids."

CHAPTER 25

Contemporary Media: Video Recording

Azela Gohl-Giese, OTR

Introduction

Recent advances in technology have allowed video equipment manufacturers to market systems that are highly automated and simplified in operation to the extent that practically anyone can produce a video product of reasonable quality. This has resulted in the involvement of occupational therapists and assistants, who are creating ways of adapting the media for individual patients and groups.

This chapter focuses first on the video recorder as a machine. A simplified explanation of the mechanical aspects is presented, and diagrams illustrate the relationships between input and output devices. Next, the use of video recording to provide a historical library is presented. Historically referenced tapes can be of great value to the educator, the researcher, and the writer, as well as occupational therapy personnel involved in day-to-day treatment activities. Some recordings may "sit on the shelf" for years, while others which present education topics to the patient, parent, or family may be used daily. Standard treatment procedures that are used frequently can be taped for use with patients as well as new staff members as a part of the orientation process. A video tape library will be commonplace in every occupational therapy clinic in the future.

The use of video recording as a mirror which reflects an objective view of the subject on camera is then considered. The intent is to provide immediate feedback to an individual or a group on how they performed or reacted in a particular situation during a specific time interval. Replay of the video tape can assist in recalling the actions that took place as well as the feelings that may be associated with these actions. In a group situation, the replay will assist in focusing the group so that the critique will be based on input from everyone. These recording are generally not catalogued and stored.

Occupational therapy staff members seeking specific, objective feedback on such skills as interviewing or supervising can replay a videotape at their convenience, in privacy if desired. This can be an effective way to improve skills. Camera shy people may have difficulty in using video for this purpose; however, the fact that the tape can be erased instantly may give them added comfort in using this medium of self-evaluation. It need not be an embarrassing experience.

The fourth part of this chapter describes the use of video recording as a projective tool. Segments of commercial television such as "soap operas" and news broadcasts may be used as a part of the treatment milieu. Psychodrama techniques may be added to tailor the roles of particular characters in the television program to the patient's real life situation. The psychodrama skit may also be taped for later viewing and discussion. Finally, video recording is presented as a tool for creating. The intent is to emphasize the human quality of creativity and encourage the patient to use video for this purpose. Future trends in the creative use of video recording are explored along with the importance of keeping abreast of new technological advancements.

The Machine

Over the last 20 or more years, video recording has evolved from an amateur's nightmare to a fairly common leisure time activity. In the past, it seemed that only a person with a degree in electrical engineering could possibly cope with the technical maze of connecting a video camera, recorder, monitor, and microphone system. Today, because of the tremendous advances made in automating video recording equipment, a person who is familiar with a 35 mm still camera and with making adjustments on a commercial television set may feel fairly comfortable using a video camera and recorder after minimal instruction. There is a standard electrical connection system for operating video equipment. Once this basic system is understood, extra enhancements, such as use of a character generator for titles and dubbing in background music on a second audio channel, can be tried when more professional recordings are required.

The following neurological analogy provides a basic understanding of the video recording system. Consider the camera as the eye and the microphone as the ear picking up environmental sounds and actions that become *input* and travel via cables, which are the nerves of the system. The cables connect directly to the video tape recorder and store the information on tape just as the brain stores information in memory. When *output* is needed, the "play" button on the video tape recorder is depressed, and the recorded information is sent to the television monitor via an *output* cable. Three basic principles must always be followed when using video recording equipment:

1 The camera and microphone must be connected to the input terminals of the recording unit.
2 Output cables are connected to the output terminal of the recorder and the input terminal of the monitor.
3 When taping a commercial television program, the monitor is providing input; therefore, it is connected to the input terminal of the recorder.

The diagrams in Figure 25-1 show specific connecting patterns for four different uses of video equipment. Either commercial power outlets or batteries may be used.

It should be noted that the camera and the microphones provide input only. When one or both of these pieces of equipment are being used, the "record" switch on the video tape recorder must be turned on in order to record the information on tape and view it on the monitor. Newer camera models have built-in microphones with a fairly long range, and thus the camera cable contains both the audio and video connections. When connecting the various components of the system, it is important to apply firm pressure, but never force. If force seems to be necessary, it is likely that an improper connection is being attempted. Consult the operation manual for possible errors in the procedure.

The quality of the video recording is determined when it is being produced. There is little that can be done to improve a flawed or inferior recording while it is being viewed on the monitor, no matter how sophisticated the monitor's tuning system may be. Therefore, at the time of recording it is very important to check and recheck the functioning of the camera, recorder, and monitor. By making a short "trial" tape and viewing it on the monitor, the following areas in which video problems frequently occur can be avoided:

1 Poor color or black and white contrast.
2 Improper focus.
3 Inadequate lighting.
4 Inaudible or unclear sound.

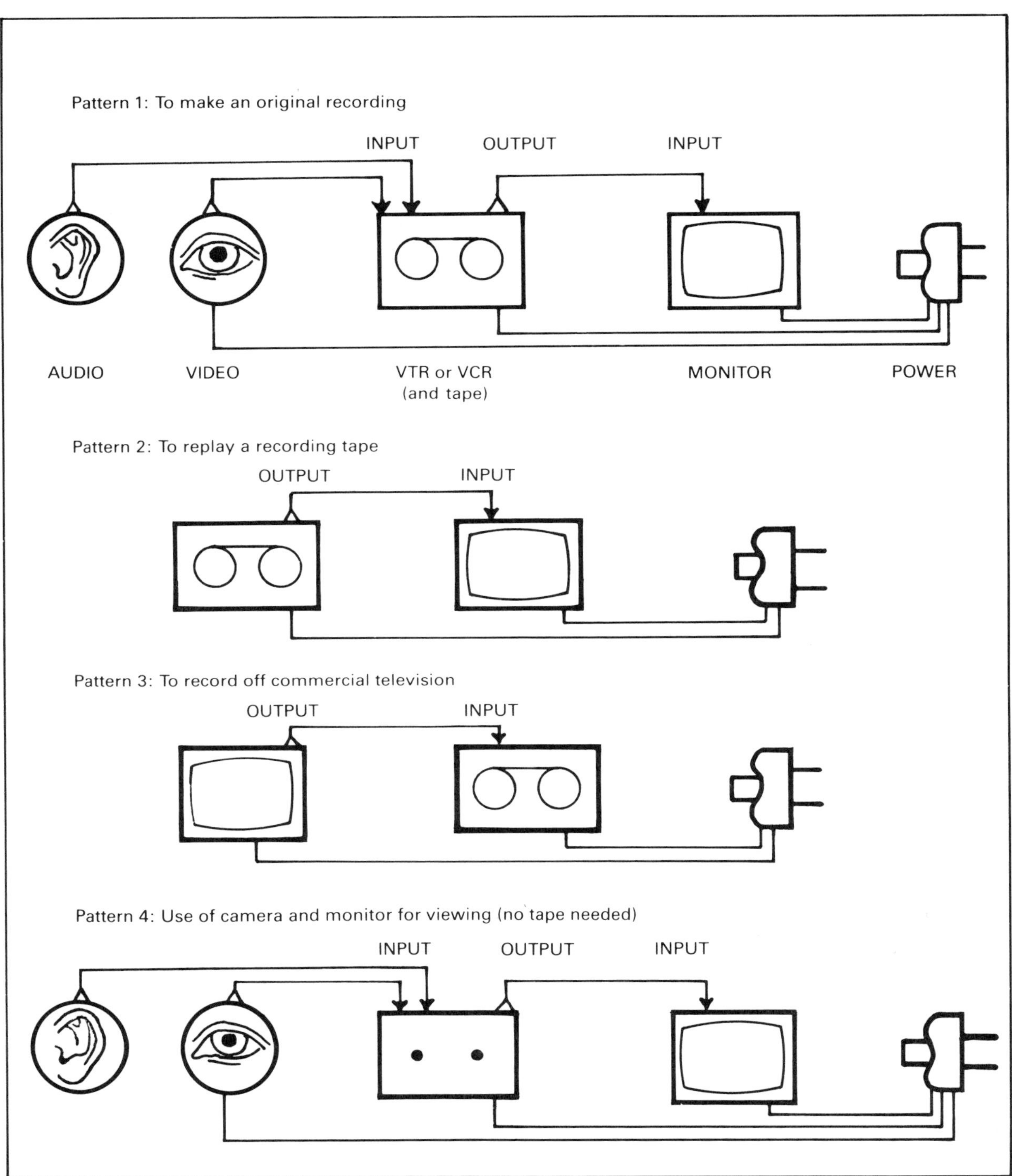
Pattern 1: To make an original recording
INPUT
OUTPUT
INPUT
AUDIO
VIDEO
VTR or VCR
(and tape)
MONITOR
POWER
Pattern 2: To replay a recording tape
OUTPUT
INPUT
Pattern 3: To record off commercial television
OUTPUT
INPUT
Pattern 4: Use of camera and monitor for viewing (no tape needed)
INPUT
OUTPUT
INPUT

Figure 25-1

By checking the monitor for proper contrast and sharpness of images, the camera can be adjusted for both focus and level of light. In some environments it may be necessary to use auxiliary lighting. Sound problems can generally be solved through the use of extra microphones and the elimination of background noise such as traffic, air conditioning, and fans. It takes several practice sessions to successfully accomplish all of these tasks and develop the skills necessary to produce a quality tape.

Video equipment in current use is designed for either a VHS or Beta cassette tape format used on a video cassette recorder (VCR), with the VHS type being the most popular; a reel-to-reel tape used on a video tape recorder (VTR) which is rapidly becoming obsolete; or the newer disk mode which is similar to a phonograph record in shape. Care must be taken to use the proper size and mode of recording material that fits the specific video recorder available, as the various formats are not interchangeable. For example, a ¾ inch video cassette tape cannot be used on a video recorder that is designed for ½ inch tape. Once the correct tape is selected, it is fairly simple to insert the cassette or to wind the tape from reel to reel in the machine. When the tape is in place and the camera is connected to the recorder, the recording process may begin.

Lighting

It is important to evaluate the lighting in the room where the video tape is to be produced. Before recording a trial tape the following steps should be taken to assure adequate lighting. The subjects should be positioned so that their faces are not in a shadow. If there is bright sunlight, the camera should be positioned with the light coming from behind. Never point the camera lens into the sun or other bright light, as this can cause damage. Most clinical settings that have fluorescent lighting provide adequate illumination for video taping. If other lighting is needed, it may be necessary to use auxiliary lamps to "bounce" light off a wall or the ceiling. Place these lights so that the stands or shades do not appear on camera. Producing a video tape out of doors can be particularly difficult owing to the wide range of light and shadows present. Camera lens filters may provide a partial solution in this situation. Seek advice from a factory representative or a local audiovisual consultant as to which style filter works best on the particular camera you are using.

Other Environmental Considerations

The more isolated the area selected for making a video tape, the less likely that background noise and interruptions will interfere with the production. It is advisable to close windows to help eliminate noise from traffic and aircraft, unplug telephones, and turn off fans and air conditioning units. Post a sign on the door or doors that states "Video Taping in Progress — Do Not Disturb!" Interruptions of any kind can mean that the work must be retaped. When a highly professional tape is required, it is best to use a soundproof video studio.

Arrange all furniture and equipment that will be needed in the production to assure that the camera can be moved about the area with ease. Consider the location of electrical outlets to be used for the camera and other video equipment. If the placement of electrical cables is likely to interfere with the tape production, battery power should be used.

Focusing and Timing

The key to good video tape production is focus and timing. Most video cameras have "zooming" power. This literally means that the lens is capable of quickly moving very close to the subject for a close-up view. Many new users of a video camera will overuse this technique, which tends to distract or tire the viewing audience. It is better to try to provide a mixture of varying distances and angles, using the zoom technique occasionally for emphasis or a detailed close-up picture, to help keep the viewer interested in the subject. Record what is being communicated by the subjects both orally and physically, for the person may be saying one thing while body posture or action may be conveying a different or conflicting message. It is important for patients to see such incongruence in order to develop self-knowledge and to improve communication.

Timing is also essential for keeping the viewer's attention. It is important to maintain a balance; moving the camera too fast will result in the viewer's missing the action; moving the camera too slowly may cause the viewer to become bored and some important action may be missed. As you move the camera, keep the motion as smooth as possible. Avoid sudden stops and starts as the videotape will appear jerky when it is shown.

There are definite advantages to having the camera securely supported on a tripod. This allows the camera operator to have both hands free to focus and move the camera smoothly about the room. There is also less danger of the camera's falling or being bumped. The one great advantage of having a small, portable camera is the flexibility of moving quickly into a narrow space or at a specific angle to the subject for a special shot. A tripod does not allow that motion in most cases. The trade-off is safety and smoothness for accuracy and immediacy.

If written material, such as titles, is included in the tape production, focus the camera on each line of print from 4 seconds to 5 seconds to give the audience sufficient time to comprehend the message. When in doubt, add an additional second or two. The chances of maintaining the viewers' attention are better with too much time than with not enough. Above all, try to maintain a professional approach and avoid giving the impression that the producer was a clever person with a brand new camera.

Portability

The elements of videotaping described up to this point differ little from one brand name to another. However, there is a great deal of difference in the degree of portability among the various models of videotape production equipment. Heavy-duty systems tend not to be moved about too much except on carts made especially for that purpose. Portable video recorder units weighing as little as 25 pounds to 30 pounds come in packs that have harness-type straps that secure them to the waist and shoulders in much the same manner as a backpack. The lightweight cameras have various types of hand grips and shoulder rests, which provide some added stability. Their disadvantage is that they tend to be easily dropped, bumped, or shaken beyond the normal limits. For these reasons, mechanical adjusting needs to be made on a regular basis in order to assure proper functioning. Care must be taken to evaluate the amount of use the equipment is to withstand before investing in new equipment.

Maintenance and Problem Solving

Like any precision tool, a video camera and recorder require a certain amount of maintenance in order to operate properly. Use of dust covers and storage in a clean area make it unnecessary to clean the vital parts of the equipment before each use. Excess dust can scratch video tape. The operation manual gives precise instructions on specific areas to be cleaned and the frequency of cleaning to ensure long-term service. For example, if you notice that the picture on the monitor seems "grainy" or distorted, it may be caused by an accumulation of dust and dirt on the recording heads of the video recorder. Follow the operator's manual instructions carefully when cleaning. If this does not solve the problem, the distortion could be caused by using a tape that was recorded in a different timing format. For example, if the video recorder being used is designed for two-hour tapes, it will not play a tape recorded in a four-hour format. Another tape recorder will have to be used that has this capability.

Careful handling of tape will prevent many maintenance problems. While cassette tapes have plastic cases for built-in protection, reel-to-reel types do not. Avoid touching the surface of the tape when threading as body oil left on the tape will attract dust quickly that will be deposited later on the contact points of the tape pathway of the recorder. This may cause a poor replay picture.

It is advisable to keep a record of each time the equipment is cleaned, as well as when it is sent out for professional repair or maintenance. Information on the replacement of parts and other adjustments should be noted together with costs and may well serve as justification for replacement when necessary.

Video tapes last longer if they are stored in closed cabinets in an area where the temperature is moderate and the humidity is low. It is best to set the tapes on edge rather than flat so that the tape does not become distorted by binding to the edge of the container, particularly in the case of cassette tape.

FIGURE 25-2. Production Title: "Activity Analysis of Knitting"

CAMERA CUES:	DIALOGUE:	
4 feet from teacher	Teacher:	"Knitting is frequently used as a treatment modality in occupational therapy. What are the major therapeutic strengths of this activity?"
Move to student A	Student A:	"I think knitting is relaxing now that I've learned how to do it. It might be a good activity for an anxious patient."
Move to student B	Student B:	"I agree, but my field work supervisor said that knitting could only be used in the clinic, where the patients are closely supervised. This surprised me—it looks pretty harmless."
Move to teacher Zoom in on yarn and needles	Teacher:	"While yarn does indeed appear harmless, a depressed, suicidal patient might use it to braid a noose. Knitting needles can be used to inflict personal injury."

Developing Scripts

Once the user has made several short video recordings, preferably in varying environmental settings with both group and individual subjects, it becomes essential to develop a taping "layout" or a script explaining exactly how the equipment will be used in order to maximize its unique qualities in the production. Initially, one must determine what the objectives are for using videotape recording: Why is it essential to have a visual record of the situation? Would an audiotape and still photographs or slides be just as effective? If not, then lay out a general plan to determine what equipment is to be used, where it is to be placed, and when it should be moved. Try to anticipate how the events will unfold and generate ideas about possible events so that the camera operator knows what is important and what might occur. The latter is a particularly important aspect in the recording of group interactions. Realistically, all group actions cannot be recorded; however, fewer surprises will occur if careful planning takes place prior to the actual videotaping. The following is an example of a segment of a production script for a video tape on the topic of learning to knit:

Production Title: "Learning to Knit"

Initial Camera Location: Five feet from table and title easel.

1 Zoom in on title for 5 seconds.
2 Film presenter from waist up during introduction.
3 Zoom in on specific pieces of equipment as they are described, then back to presenter.
4 Move camera to the left and behind the presenter for demonstration of "casting on stitches."
5 Maintain this position throughout this segment, using zoom initially.
6 Change camera angle to show one or two students practicing the technique.
7 Move from presenter to students as dialogue occurs.

A video tape on this or other craft techniques can be a valuable aid in student learning. The tape can be viewed at the student's convenience, perhaps in a media center. The program can be designed to allow the student to look at one or two segments and then stop the tape to practice the required skills before moving to the next step. The student may watch the tape again, prior to a test, to review the material.

It is important to note that the script for the camera operator is different from a dialogue script. The latter reads in much the same way as the script for a play and is used for productions in which factual interchange is the primary objective rather than spontaneous conversation. This script should also be prepared in advance and rehearsed with the participants. Once the script is decided upon, the camera cues can be added directly to the dialogue pages, the goal being to give the camera operator as much information as possible to ensure a quality production. Figure 25-2 presents an example of how a dialogue script may be written.

Since activity analysis is such an important aspect of occupational therapy, a student who is absent when this information is discussed can view the tape at a later time, thus gaining necessary knowledge that may not have been recorded in notes borrowed from a classmate.

Editing, Tape Re-use, and Tape Transfer

While it is fairly simple to do "add on" editing at the end of a tape, most individuals who need more sophisticated editing take their tapes to a professional studio because most health care facilities do not have the necessary equipment to do a professional job. If reel-to-reel tape is used, it is possible to erase a segment of tape and splice the remaining program together; however, even with the use of special adhesives and tools, such splices often appear jagged and are noticeable to the audience.

Video tape can be re-used by simply rerecording over it. As the new material is recorded, the recorder automatically erases the material that was on the tape before. The number of times this can be done successfully is dependent upon several factors, including the original quality of the tape, the age of the tape, and the number of times the tape has been used.

Both occupational therapists and occupational therapy assistants can be involved in making video tapes, dependent on their individual interests and skills as well as the particular needs of the department. Two helpful resources for information on both the mechanical and production aspects of video recording are *The Video Guide* by Charles Bensinger and *Video the Better Way* by R.J. Kerr.

As technological advances continue to improve the video recording process, new formats will be marketed. Fortunately, as part of this development, techniques are available to transfer existing tapes to these new formats. When replacing video equipment, it is important to retain the old recorder until all tapes that are to be retained can be transferred from the old format to the new.

Other General Considerations

Policies for honoring the patient's rights of freedom and confidentiality apply to video recording. Each occupational therapy department should have a written policy and necessary consent and release forms on file and available to patients. The policy should outline the specific instances in which video taping will be used as a therapeutic technique, as well as the conditions under which the tapes will be used for other purposes, such as student education. Some facilities require that all patients sign a consent and release form prior to participating in any video projects, whether used internally or externally by the facility. The right of the patient not to be videotaped must always be respected.

The Historical Library

One of the most common uses of video recording is to make a permanent audiovisual record of the treatment of a patient over a period of time. Owing to the complexities of some treatment regimens, a visual record is essential in recording the patient's progress or lack of progress. It is a way of objectively documenting the changes and improvements that have been gained and those that have not. In some pediatric programs, a video tape record is made at regular intervals over several months or in some cases several years. Thus all pertinent details of work with the child are documented. If the therapist's memory fades, the recording maintains a firm image. A written record usually accompanies the tape and serves as a sequential index of the recorded content. The tapes are then catalogued using a convenient library system for efficient retrieval.

The key to the effective use of a video tape library is the accuracy of the index. A good index includes not only the title, producer, and date but a detailed listing of the location of specific categories and events on the tape as well as what are referred to as "time locations." The critical measure in determining accurate time locations is to check that the timing gauge is on zero at the beginning of the recording session. Once the tape is running, begin a recorded log of the general categories and significant events. Such information will allow the user to quickly locate a particular segment when needed. When viewing the tape again, return the time gauge to zero before beginning. If there is a frequent need to use tapes in this way, an automatic time gauge can be purchased.

Occupational therapy personnel are also using

video tapes to record evaluation procedures. If the same person is repeating the evaluation, there is an opportunity to review the previous assessment in order to duplicate the procedures accurately. If a different person is doing the procedure, viewing the tape will help ensure consistency in administering the evaluation.

This video recording technique was used to establish rater reliability while using a checklist of behaviors designed for a research project.[1] A number of video taped sessions were produced showing an occupational therapist testing children on an individual basis. The tapes were then viewed at a later time by occupational therapists who were asked to observe the children being tested and to record their observations on the checklist. The advantage of using the videotaped programs as part of this research was that a number of participants in the research project were able to contribute over a period of time at different locations. They did not have to be present at the actual time or place of the testing. More important, all viewers were observing the same testing situation, thus assuring a more valid research procedure.

Holm describes another use of video recording in which information is taped to be used at a specific time in a treatment program when the patient is ready for it.[2] She cites the situation in which a patient can view a tape of another patient engaged in an activity. By viewing another patient engaged in the activity, instead of watching a nondisabled therapist demonstrating it, the patient may show less resistence to attempting an unfamiliar or difficult task. A number of different tapes can be kept available in the clinic for this use. If new tapes are made of different patients on a regular basis, the library will be current and aid in a variety of patient informational and motivational needs. Holm also describes the use of video in providing an orientation for patients who will be having a new experience or who feel uncomfortable with attempting an activity. The therapist filmed the environment in which the activity was to take place and then showed it to the patient as a means of "rehearsing" prior to the actual experience. This allowed the patient to visualize where and how to approach the unfamiliar, thus reducing anxiety and even enhancing some of the enjoyable aspects of the activity.

Another common reason for developing video tapes is for staff inservice or continuing education. The Minnesota Occupational Therapy Association Continuing Education Committee has begun building a library collection of video tapes for this purpose. The project was given impetus when the public service department of a local television company agreed to provide free use of their equipment and recording studio. The committee had to furnish the video tape, script, and actors. Several video tapes on such topics as feeding techniques and wheelchair adaptations have been completed and are available to therapists and facilities for a modest fee to cover postage and handling. This education method is particularly helpful for occupational therapy personnel residing outside metropolitan areas where continuing education opportunities may be less available.

This educational service demonstrates one of the advantages of using video recording rather than 16 mm film production. A video product may be produced at less cost and more quickly because the processing time is shorter, requiring only the time necessary to record the tape. The advantage of 16 mm film over video tape is that the film provides sharper color distinction. Owing to the structure of film, it may also provide a better slow-motion mechanism because it can be moved forward one frame at a time, a feature which videotape does not have.

The educator in the classroom or the clinic has many tape libraries to draw from across the country. Often these libraries are found at larger universities, which may furnish catalogs of their current holdings upon request. Usually the tapes are available in more than one format, and the exact type required must be specified when ordering.

A Mirror of Behavior

The video camera is often compared to an eye focusing in on the action. Just as a famous individual, because of his or her degree of notoriety, can detract the viewer from the content of a television interview the person is participating in, the presence of a video camera in an occupational therapy clinic can detract from what otherwise would be spontaneous action. Until the subjects being taped have become comfortable with the camera and less aware of its focus on them, the viewing of their actions must be tempered somewhat when interpreting what is on the monitor.

Add to this predisposition the historical situation for most people in middle-class society; they have watched television for many hours during their lifetimes. The content viewed and the normal viewing environment will surely have an impact on how seriously they view the monitor in a therapeutic situation. If they have maintained a regular schedule of watching certain quiz shows and situation comedies, their participation in a videotaped psychodrama as a part of psychiatric occupational therapy treatment may not make a lasting impression. This could be because they may view television primarily as fantasy that can be turned on and off. Such individuals may also "turn off" a display of their anguish or hostility as they view the playback of the psychodrama. For the most part, television is passive in nature. Nothing is required of the viewer except to select the channel and make slight tuning adjustments from time to time. This passive viewing pattern is difficult to alter because of long-term conditioning and the fact that most individuals see television as a form of entertainment.

Cater speaks of this conditioning and suggests an additional conflict that may be present for the television viewer who happens to be left-brain dominant in mental development. Such individuals show resistance to taking the television media seriously, as it is a type of medium that appeals more to the right hemisphere of the brain. It does not fit into the intellectual analytical thinking of the left-brained viewer. Thus from a therapeutic standpoint, the right-brained individual may be more adept at using video feedback than the one who is left-brain dominant. If the video feedback can be structured in a sequentially analytical manner using propositional thought, perhaps the left-brained person will also become engaged in using video feedback therapeutically.[4]

A simple measure that helps patients reach a comfort level with this medium is to demonstrate how easy it is to erase the tape used in the treatment session. Knowledge of this fact can aid the patient in relaxing and being spontaneous during the videotaping. While few patients request erasure of a tape, the fact that the possibility exists provides continuing reassurance. Once the patients recognize the value of the feedback, their anxiety over the recording is reduced. Engaging the patient in the mechanical control of the video equipment provides him or her with a sense of control over what is going to take place in the therapeutic session. If the patient feels in control, he or she is likely to make a greater investment in and commitment to changing behavior or risking new behavior. With the availability of instant replay, the patient is able to receive immediate feedback on what effect his or her behavior has in relation to the human and nonhuman environment. He also gains a perspective of how his behavior was seen by others viewing the tape.

Engaging the Viewer in the Results

Though the recording process is basically the same, the reasons for making the video recording and the manner in which the tape is viewed may differ considerably. The following are six situations that offer methods for actively engaging the viewer in the results shown on the tape.

Example 1

The video recording of a staff member or a student who wants to improve a skill, such as interviewing a patient or administering a patient evaluation, may be set up at his or her convenience. Once the tape has been made, the individual can review it at a later time either privately or with a colleague who has agreed to review the performance. By allowing these two options, the individual is able to choose the one with which he or she is most comfortable. The tape does not make any judgements; the person being taped is in control of how the tape will be used. Once the person has viewed the first taped experience, some confidence will be gained, and the next taping is much easier to accomplish.

Example 2

The complex situation of using video feedback in a group therapy session can be invaluable to the group. The technical aspects of filming should be accomplished with ease and in the most unobtrusive manner possible. The use of two cameras and two operators is ideal, as the amount of camera movement can be reduced significantly. If a second camera cannot be used or operators are not available, consider having group members take turns being the group observer and operating the camera. This alternating of tasks allows the individuals to continue in their roles as group members while also contributing to the collection of objective feedback that will be shared with the group at the appropriate time. Using a system of this type frees the group leader to address the immediate needs of the members as they occur. It should be noted, however, that it is best to have a non-group member operate the equipment. An occupational therapist or an occupational therapy assistant is an ideal person to run the camera because he or she possesses knowledge of group process and dynamics.

Placement of the camera or cameras should minimize distraction. The type of action to be focused on should also be discussed. Usually there are clues provided by the group's action that may suggest what should be emphasized. Because of the size of some therapeutic groups, all activity and dialogue may not be able to be taped. Larger groups generate more background noise that may affect the clarity of the sound track. Adding extra auxiliary microphones and a second group observer may assist in providing accurate feedback.

Example 3

One form of video feedback that has been found invaluable to parents is viewing taped therapy sessions of their children. Often parents find it difficult to believe that their child acts differently in an environment away from home. With the help of tapes that are made over a period of weeks or months, insight may be gained as to how the child is behaving and the degree of progress that is being made to improve inappropriate behaviors. The tapes may also show the parents how specific reinforcement techniques can be used with the child at home. Since progress may be slow, or very minimal at times, a tape may provide contrast if viewed again at a later time. Occupational therapy personnel have noted that the use of video tape can be an effective way of obtaining support from parents during the treatment of their child.

Example 4

Video feedback may also be used to motivate patients to make behavioral changes on their own behalf. Patients who experience seizures or have behavior disorders may be appropriate candidates for this approach as they are unable to control themselves and are unaware of what is happening during an episode. By viewing the specific event on video tape with a staff member present for support, the patient can gain insight into what is happening. Patients may be more willing to cooperate with the staff in taking the prescribed medication or attending the group therapy sessions that often are so uncomfortable for them.

Example 5

The use of the video camera and monitor without tape can be of great assistance in presenting information to a group of people, particularly when the content being emphasized requires close-up viewing for comprehension, and a permanent record of the material is not necessary. When demonstrating how to correctly use small tools such as needles, be sure to focus the camera on the detail so that each member of the audience can see an enlarged view of the proper technique. This is a very effective method for teaching students the detailed steps in beginning or ending double cordovan leather lacing, for instance. It could also be used to show a group of stroke patients how dressing techniques can be adapted to the use of one hand or the best methods for paring vegetables unilaterally. Recording on tape may occur at the same time as the viewing, but, as stated earlier, it is not essential unless a permanent record is needed.

If the room being used is too small to accommodate both the audience and the subject and equipment, the camera and subject can be placed in a smaller room, and extension cables can be connected to the monitor or monitors in the larger room.

Example 6

While some people are camera-shy, other individuals enjoy being filmed, finding it stimulating and energy generating. This increased patient energy can be used to advantage by filming the patient when he or she is exhibiting appropriate behaviors. Occupational therapy personnel must structure the experience so that the patient does not become overstimulated and lose self-control.[5] Later viewing can serve as a reinforcement and, in many cases, can enable the patient to gain greater confidence and self-esteem in attempting the unfamiliar. Use of such a reinforcement technique can help many to live more enriched lives.

A Projective Tool

In contrast with other aspects of video taping, when emphasis is placed on more subjective aspects of the medium, the tool may become an effective projective technique. As in finger painting and clay modeling, videotaping is pliable, leaving room for personal interpretation. There are at least three facets of video recording that may be a part of a projective technique.

The first and one of the most common video projective tools is the commercial television "soap opera" serial. This can be viewed on a daily basis, or prerecorded and shown at a time that is more therapeutically appropriate. It is essential to structure the viewing and discussion so as to involve the patients in an active manner. The highly defensive person may assume an attitude of being passively entertained and be unwilling to become involved in the projective exercise.

The viewing of the program can be structured by providing the group members with carefully constructed questions in advance. Such questions may focus on a particular role being portrayed or the patient's reactions to a particular event or situation. One of the advantages of prerecording the television program is that a specific segment can quickly be replayed. This technique aids in uncovering emotional material that some patients may not wish to acknowledge by insisting that they do not remember what was being depicted or said. Once the discussion has covered the specific content, the next segment of the program can be viewed. The primary objectives in using this method are to explore the roles and situations the patient identifies with, support any insights gained, and enable the patient to risk a change in behavior.

The plot of the "soap opera" may play as important a function in the projective process as the identification of a particular role by the patient. When the patient views the program on a regular basis, the questions used to structure the experience may direct the focus to how a situation developed and what actions were being taken to alter the results, which may be healthier for the people involved. The patients may be willing to describe attempts that they have made in similar situations and discuss the degree of personal satisfaction gained from this action. In other instances, the patients will take this new information or approach and apply it to similar situations in their own lives.

By having the entire group watch the same video action, much can be learned by noting the varying perceptions of the individual group members. The leader needs to assure all members that all perceptions are acceptable and that no moral judgements will be made as to the "rightness" or "wrongness" of their perceptions. It is helpful to the group to see how differently a given action can be perceived. Gaining an appreciation of this fact may allow viewers to expand their knowledge, their communication skills, and their sense of self-worth.

The use of video as a projective technique relies heavily on the cognitive ability of the viewer. However, the technique may be adapted to various levels of maturation and functioning by the questions formulated by the OTR and COTA, who may serve as co-leaders. This adaptation begins with the careful selection of the program to be viewed, the questions to be addressed, and the methods for processing the patients' projective reactions throughout the discussion. There is no substitute for effective group facilitation on the part of the therapist and the assistant. Neither the viewing of the video nor the questions asked can, in and of themselves, bring about a therapeutic experience.

Psychodrama has proven to be an effective adjunct to "soap opera" viewing. Patients who have just viewed a particular scene may wish to adapt that scene to their personal situation, using fellow group members to play needed roles. The psychodrama is also videotaped and replayed for discussion. When this method is used, patients are often more attentive and curious about viewing themselves and their personal vulnerability, rather than watching a professional actor or actress on the monitor. This curiosity is a part of assessing body image and self-image as well as congruency and incongruence. It provides another example of how video can serve as an effective projective tool.

A second format produced by commercial television and useful to occupational therapy personnel is the news or documentary broadcast. While the technique used is similar to the one used with a "soap opera," the content of the news is more conducive to helping the patient relate to the world at large instead of being solely occupied with the inner self. It is advisable to create a degree of structure to assist the patient in meeting the main objective of relating to the societal realities presented through discussion of current events. The use of predetermined questions or a viewing guide outline encourages involvement in both viewing and discussion. Observing the patient's responses to the news program can provide information relative to cognitive and affective levels as well as values. Such observations of responses, together with other information, may serve as measures of appropriate adapted behavior. It also may be a way of determining whether a patient is approaching the time for hospital or facility discharge.

A Tool for Creating

A vital part of most occupational therapy programs is facilitating the patient's needed behavioral changes. The key to making these changes in behavior is the internal motivation of the individual. Creativity is individual and requires a certain freedom of space and time. When the elements of change and creativity are combined in treatment planning, the patient is able to be involved in the therapeutic process. Through such involvement in a creative endeavor, verbal and nonverbal communication takes place between the patient, the activity, and the therapist.

Occupational therapy personnel are often challenged to introduce activities that will motivate the patient to become actively involved. Creative activities are attractive to many because they offer the creator total control over the materials used as well as a tangible product. If external limits are imposed, the creativity can be stifled or lost.

Using the activity of making a videotape as a medium for creative expression may communicate information about how the patient sees the world. The impressions of a paraplegic individual who will be in a wheelchair for the rest of his or her life can be very different from those of a neurotic patient who has many unresolved societal and environmental fears. The simplicity of operating many types of video equipment makes this activity feasible for most age groups, except the very young. While staff instruction and supervision are generally required, once initial learning has taken place, the individual can often proceed with a fairly high degree of independence, focusing energy on the creative process and product rather than on the equipment. When the videotape is completed, it may reveal significant information about the patient, which can be used as a communication tool to effect the behavioral changes needed in order to achieve a more productive and meaningful life.

Goldstein describes the use of video production by individuals and groups.[6] Staff members served as consultants in the use of the equipment and provided structure in the activity process as need arose. The communication that resulted during the production of the video recordings provided important information for therapeutic intervention. Each patient was experiencing a different level of self-confidence; some were intimidated by the equipment, while others wanted to control the camera. Several of the adolescents in this group were able to use the taping experience to better adapt to the treatment institution and eventually to make some behavioral changes. The staff also gained insight into some hospital procedures that were improved upon as a result of this treatment project.

An elderly population that may not have "grown up" with television increasingly depends on it to meet social needs. The Mount Sinai Medical Center received grant funding to assist in addressing the problem of isolation felt by the elderly, such as those living in an apartment complex in East Harlem.[7] By means of a cable television system, each resident's television set was connected to a service which utilizes an unused channel exclusively for the tenants in the 20 story high-rise apartment building.

The grant program provides a number of television services, one of which is resident-produced programs. Residents were involved in the overall program early in its development by video taping group discussions about the living conditions and social activities of the apartment complex. The initial shyness of some participants was soon overcome, and in a short time about 100 residents had appeared on camera. It should be recognized that it often takes a longer period of time for the elderly to become comfortable with handling the equipment, because they did not have exposure to this technology at a young age.

One group project featured several residents demonstrating their favorite recipes, and another focused on discussion of growing up in early America. As involvement increased, so did the number of residents viewing the special channel. By becoming regular viewers, many also participated in the health care program offered under the grant sponsorship. This program was designed to reduce the health care costs of the elderly through televised and other mass media health care education.

During the next stage, resident involvement was on an individual basis. Since video tapes featuring the elderly were not that readily available for rent or purchase, the taped programs were designed to show individual residents engaged in interviews, leisure time activity demonstrations, tenant news broadcasts, and a health tips program. Once the recording was made, the resident could watch it in the privacy of his or her own apartment. Provision was also made for individual residents to visit the studio during the recording sessions.

The elderly have many life-time experiences to share, and this sharing enhances the quality of their life within their environments. Video recording provides a vehicle that the elderly can use to communicate to others the social riches and skills that they have gleaned throughout their lives.

The use of video recording for creative purposes need not be restricted to patient or client populations. This medium has great potential for the student in the classroom. Many educators who previously required that all assignments be prepared in either oral or written form are recognizing the value of making a videotape. Since increasing numbers of curricula have access to video recording equipment, students may be given the option of making a videotaped presentation as a creative approach to completing assignments such as case studies or research projects.

Case study video productions may dramatically contrast normal and abnormal behavior and conditions. Role plays may be used if actual patients are not available to participate. The effective production and use of a short, 10-minute video presentation can often convey a stronger and more accurate message than a 10- or 15-page paper.

Researchers are finding that video tape is a valuable method for documenting their findings. This medium has helped to demonstrate specific research methods and has assisted those conducting research in duplicating previously completed studies. Information that may have been overlooked in studying the written research report is often found when the video recording is viewed.

Future Trends

As the communication industry continues its rapid advances, videodisk technology is beginning to make an impact. This format employs a combination of videotape and computer disks, which currently are not readily compatible with existing video cassette recorders. While videodisk players are not in the mass production phase currently, what is known of this technology shows great potential for occupational therapy education and practice. The fact that disk players can be controlled with a joystick instead of a keyboard is a particular advantage for the physically handicapped population. This format also allows the individual to participate actively in the program by answering questions and making decisions. Once production costs decrease and more competition occurs in the marketplace, the possibility of investing in this format should be considered.[8,9] While not directly related, it has been noted that as this format emerges, the Beta videotape format appears to be receding somewhat.

Another type of equipment which may become more commonly used in the future is the camcorder. This system has both a camera and a recorder housed in one lightweight unit. It is packaged in a manner that allows it to take the place of the 8 mm movie camera, and it can use battery power, which makes it extremely portable.

In the not too distant future, the increased development and expansion of video technology will provide the general population with many new services that are now in their early stages of development. For example, communication systems for every household may include video telephones connected directly to frequently used services such as the bank, supermarket, department store, and primary health care provider. When considering the latter, it is feasible to predict that the annual physical examination by a physician may be conducted in the privacy of one's home by means of a combination of video, telephone, and a microcomputer system connected to a health center. Medical history, current symptoms if any, and other pertinent data can be entered into the computer. Simple electronic devices will automatically record temperature, heart rate, and blood pressure, and interactive video will enable the individual to talk with the physician. If additional diagnostic tests or services are required, the monitor will display these along with times they can be scheduled, thus automatically making appointments and printing a list of them for the individual.

The home health care delivery system may be dramatically different in the future. For example, occupational therapy personnel could gather some screening and evaluation data through a computerized questionnaire and an interactive video system that would allow discussion of work, play, and self-care skills and problems. The individual could move a small video camera about the house that would assist the occupational therapist in making an initial evaluation of the environment. Other health professionals will also be using video techniques and will utilize "video visits" as a supplement to actual home visits. Such measures ultimately could result in reduced health care costs and increased efficiency in service delivery.

As more and more families find that economic pressures require both parents to be employed, the responsibility for day-to-day child care is placed in the hands of people other than the parents. As this trend increases, there appears to be a growing concern on the part of young parents that they are not able to have the desired influence on their children during their formative years. Occupational therapists and assistants may become much more involved in the well community in the areas of normal child development and child care. Their services could include the use of video tape and computer programs which address such topics as the roles of parents and ways to develop "quality time" activities with their children. Programming may enable the parents to view the current relationships they have with their children and contrast them with other approaches and options. This might provide one method to individualize the child-parent relationship and offer resources to draw upon when problems occur.

Another aspect of child development that could be addressed is the lack of quality commercial television programming for the toddler and preschool child. There is a good market for occupational therapy personnel to apply their knowledge of child development and related developmental life tasks and activities to create new programs. Programming that engages the child in active viewing and learning, somewhat like that presented on public television, is needed. Adding a parent education and interactive video discussion segment to each presentation would allow both the parents and the child to gain from the viewing experience.

The development of sophisticated satellite relay systems for video signal transmission has aided in the advancements of space science. It has made a particular impact on mass media coverage of events world-wide which are presented to the public on a regular basis. Of equal importance is the way this technology can improve the quality of life for the handicapped. Resourceful individuals asking the question "how" will continue to find new applications when assessing individual patient needs.

Summary

Each of the functions of video recording described can play an important role in the delivery of occupational therapy services. Assessing the patient's situation, treatment planning and implementation, re-evaluation, and discharge planning provide numerous opportunities to use this medium. The ways that video recordings can be used — as an historical reference, a spontaneous feedback mechanism, a projective instrument, or a creative experience — all address the components of the occupational therapy process. The examples of specific uses of video recording are intended to challenge OTRs and COTAs to adapt the techniques to fit the needs of the populations they are serving.

The future of video recording applications for occupational therapy is virtually unlimited. As technological advances are made, it is imperative that members of the profession seek this new knowledge and develop the skills necessary to help the physically and emotionally handicapped to maximize their potential and improve their quality of life.

References

1. Bauer BA: Tactile sensitivity. *Am J Occup Ther*, 31:357-361, 1977.
2. Holm MB: Video as a medium in occupational therapy. *Am J Occup Ther*, 37:531-534, 1983.
3. Bensinger C: *The Video Guide*. Santa Barbara, CA: Video-Info Publications, 1977.
4. Cater D: The intellectual in videoland. *Saturday Review* 12:12-16, 1975.

5. Heilveil I: *Video in Mental Health Practice*. New York: Springer, 1983.

6. Goldstein N: Making videotapes: An activity for hospitalized adolescents. *Am J Occup Ther*, 36:530-533, 1982.

7. Wallerstein E: Television for the elderly. A new approach to health. *Educational and Industrial Television*, April:28-31, 1975.

8. Meyer R: Borrow this new military technology, and help win the war for kids' minds. *Am School Board J*, June:23-28, 1984.

9. Kehrberg KT: Videodiscs in the classroom: An interactive economics course. *Creative Computing*, 8:99-102, 1982.

Bibliography

Kerr RJ: *Video The Better Way: A New Art for a New Age*. Yokohama: Victor Company of Japan, 1980.

CHAPTER 26

Contemporary Media: Small Electronic Devices and Techniques

*Mary Ellen Lange Dunford, OTR/L**

with contributions by Sally E. Ryan, COTA

Introduction

Patients with severe physical handicaps and multiple disabilities are often limited in the amount of interaction they have with others and with their environment. Modern technology and advanced technical aids have revolutionized many areas once restricted for handicapped individuals. Powered wheelchairs and adapted automobiles provide independent mobility. Communication aids allow independent oral and written communication. Environmental control units offer access to the operation of lights, radios, coffee makers, and other electrical appliances. There are now sophisticated instructional devices for teaching educational skills to the severely physically and cognitively disabled.

Technological advances have provided versatile opportunities for the disabled to exercise control within their environment, to live and work semi-independently, to communicate, to learn, and to be constructive, contributing members of the community. Technology has created new avenues of therapeutic intervention for health professionals and educators who work with the handicapped. The use of electronic aids is a new phenomenon in occupational therapy. It presents a challenging treatment modality as well as a valuable evaluation tool.

One of the electronic components being used to adapt devices for the handicapped is the microswitch. A microswitch is a small on/off lever switch. When combined with the appropriate circuitry, it can be used to replace common on/off switches found on battery operated devices such as toys and tape recorders. Instructions for the construction and therapeutic use of a Plexiglas pressure switch operated by a microswitch are described later in this chapter.

The Evaluation Process

Traditional occupational therapy skills must be the basis for a practical approach to using technical aids in treatment sessions. An assessment of each patient and his or her individual needs is essential, and the first step toward incorporating electronic devices into the practice of occupational therapy.

A patient's needs can first be assessed through a brief and informal interview with the patient and his or her family. An interview will identify the needs and establish objectives to be accomplished with microswitch technology. For instance, a patient with a spinal cord injury may want a switch fabricated to operate a microcomputer or an environmental control unit, whereas the parents of a handicapped child may want to have their child use switches to play with toys that he or she is not able to operate with conventional switches.

The patient evaluation also includes an assessment of physical limitations and functional abilities such as mobility, communication, and object manipulation skills. Sensorimotor components, which include range of motion, muscle tone, reflex integration, gross and fine motor coordination, developmental skills, strength, endurance, and sensory awareness, are also assessed. Other aspects of the evaluation include the cognitive and psychological areas of intelligence, cognitive development, motivation, and attitude.

Positioning and seating considerations for the patient are important in the evaluation process. Secure and stable positioning is necessary to enhance learning and skill development.

Patient evaluations should be a team effort. Input from other health and educational professionals working with the patient can provide valuable information and insight. Ideally, a team should include an electrical engineer or a rehabilitation engineer to provide consultation about electronic aids, devices, and systems. While this may be considered a rarity in most occupational therapy work settings today, engineers will play a major part in the therapeutic application of electronic technology in health care professions in the immediate future. Currently, in occupational therapy practice, it is recommended that the registered occupational therapist be responsible for the overall evaluation procedures, whereas either the therapist or the certified occupational therapy assistant could be responsible for the fabrication and use of electronic devices in treatment sessions.

Control Site

When the evaluation of the patient is completed and it has been determined that a microswitch adaptation is an appropriate measure, a control site for switch activation must be determined. A control site is defined as an anatomic site with which the person demonstrates purposeful movement.[1] The location of control sites can be divided into three general anatomical areas: the head and neck, the trunk and shoulders, and the extremities.

Individual control sites from the head and neck include the head, chin, lips, tongue, mouth, eyes, and isolated facial muscles. The trunk and shoulders, when used as control sites, offer gross movements such as rolling, lateral tilting, and shoulder elevation, depression, retraction, and protraction. Specific control sites for the extremities include elbows, arms, hands, fingers, legs, feet, and toes.

Each site being considered for switch activation is assessed for range of motion, strength and ease, and amount of control. Once the site has been chosen, the method of activation is determined. The method of activation is defined as the movement or the means by which a control site will activate a switch.[1] For instance, elbow extension, lateral head movement, or some type of external device such as a headstick or a mouthstick may be used.

Selection of a Switch Control

Commercial as well as hand-made switches can be made to be extremely simple or highly complex. Switches vary greatly in their versatility. The following are some of the general characteristics to consider when choosing a switch: feedback, weight, size, shape, safety, mounting and positioning, stability, durability, adaptability, portability, reliability, appearance, simplicity, warranties, and availability and ease of part replacement.

There are three types of feedback provided from a control switch:[1]

1 *Auditory feedback*, which is the noise the switch makes when it is activated.
2 *Visual feedback*, which is the movement of the switch when it is activated.
3 *Somatosensory feedback*, which includes the texture of the surface of the switch, the force required to activate the switch, and the position of the patient's body when the switch is operated.

The feedback provided can enhance training and the patient's successful use of the specific switch.

The weight and size of a control may also need to be considered. Small, lightweight controls are easier to mount and to transport from place to place. Large and heavy controls can be awkward but they also offer the advantages of having more surface area and thus requiring less motor precision for activation. These larger switches might be used by children with cerebral palsy.

Safety is a critical factor in the use of switches. They must be both physically and electrically safe to operate. Physical safety refers to the materials used to make the switch. Sharp edges and rough materials that irritate the skin must be avoided. Electrical safety is not a significant concern when the switches are connected to low voltage, battery operated toys and devices, but it is a concern when they are connected to commercial electrical outlets, such as those found in the home or treatment facility. When using hand-made switches with electrical outlets, it is important to be sure that they are properly grounded. An electrical or rehabilitation engineer should check the switch, the mounting, and the grounding before it is used by a patient. If the patient frequently drools, and this is a common problem with children, be sure to keep the switches well covered or mounted in a position that will prevent them from becoming wet.

Mounting and positioning of the switch are as important as the positioning of the patient for the most effective use. Frequent documentation of positions and mounting techniques used during the assessment can be useful during later training sessions. Specific patient responses such as spastic movements should also be recorded, as they may interfere with the switch placement.

Stability and durability are also important characteristics to consider. A switch must be sturdy and able to withstand reasonable use. In some instances, modifications will need to be made to protect the switch. A switch that is adaptable can be modified as the patient's needs change. This is especially important when working with children as they grow and change.

The degree of portability of the switch is another important consideration. If a patient operates several devices or uses the switch in different seating arrangements, the switch may need to be moved from one place to another or multiple switches may need to be constructed.

A switch must work when the patient needs it. To help ensure reliability of the switch, standard and easily replaceable components should be used in constructing hand-made controls. It is a good idea to make a second switch for use as a "back up" in emergencies.

The physical appearance of a switch is an important element for many patients. It should be cosmetically pleasing and not overly noticeable. Hand-made switches should be as simple as possible and not "overdesigned." Consider warranties and the availability of repair services for commercial switches used.

Evaluation of Switch Effectiveness

Technical research documents the necessity for evaluating the effectiveness and efficiency of a switch.[1] Evaluative measures include the speed of response, accuracy of response, fatigue, and repeatability.

Speed of response can be assessed in relation to two performance components: tracking time and selection time. *Tracking time* is the amount of time needed for a patient to move from a resting position to activation of the switch; *selection time* is the time needed to operate two switches or two functions of a switch. An example of selection time would be the amount of time required to activate a dual switch system for a Morse code communication device. Special computer software programs that come with an "adaptive firmware card" are available that assist in keeping track of progress.

Accuracy of response is measured from the percentage of errors and the percentage of correct responses recorded during the tracking and selection times. These percentages and the speed of response provide a crude estimation of the degree of accuracy. Poor speed or accuracy responses are generally related to one or more of the following factors:

1 Switch feedback.
2 The weight and size of the switch.
3 Positioning of the individual.
4 Mounting and positioning of the switch.
5 Inability of the individual to respond and manipulate the switch.

Re-evaluation, making the appropriate modifications, and monitoring are necessary to improve the patient's performance.

Fatigue is assessed by making comparisons between the speed of responses and the accuracy percentages recorded at the beginning of a training session and at the end of the session. Repeatability refers to the ability of the patient to repeat the performance over a specific period of time. It can be assessed by making comparisons between the speed of responses and the accuracy percentages documented at different training sessions over a designated time period.

Case Study

Evaluative measures for the selection of a switch are exemplified for a male child with cerebral palsy, a spastic quadriplegic. An initial interview with his parents identified the child's need for a microswitch. The parents wanted a means for their child to communicate, to play with toys, and to have some control over his environment.

Since the child attended a public school, various evaluations were administered by speech, psychology, education, and physical and occupational therapy personnel. The child was nonverbal with normal intelligence. An occupational therapy assessment indicated severe physical limitations. Increased muscle tone and neurological impairment delayed motor development significantly. The patient lacked functional use of his extremities, and trunk and head control was limited.

The child was positioned in a customized seating system built by a local carpenter. His head was chosen as the control site for the switch. The patient had minimal side-to-side head movement, and thus head turning to either side was determined as the method of switch activation.

Two commercial microswitches (round pressure type, Du-It Control Systems Group) were chosen as the most desirable. They were lightweight, small in size, easy to mount, and durable and provided a "click" for auditory feedback. Mounting was accomplished by gluing pieces of velcro to the back of the switches and attaching strips of counter velcro to the headrest of the child's wheelchair. The switches were positioned in such a way that as the child turned his head to either side, his cheek bone brushed against a switch and activated it.

The switches were interfaced with two battery operated toys, and tracking time trials were taken for each switch. The first four trials required 30 seconds to 35 seconds for each switch activation. Selection time, the time needed to operate both switches, was approximately 95 seconds. Accuracy of response (the correct number of switch activations) was 60 percent (six activations in 10 trials) for the switch mounted on the right side. The switch mounted on the left had an 80 percent accuracy of response.

Speed of response increased and accuracy of response decreased after the first four trials. This indicated that fatigue interfered with performance.

On the basis of this information, adjustments were made in the position of the headrest angle, and the position of each switch was changed slightly. Records of speed of response and accuracy percentages were compiled during the next six treatment sessions. Speed of response decreased and accuracy increased. This indicated that the switches appeared to be working efficiently for the child.

Repeatability was seen as the patient was able to improve and repeat his best performance level over several weeks. Eventually, the child was able to use the two switches to operate a computer, an environmental control unit, and a Morse code system for written communication.

Selection of Interfaces and Assistive Devices

Completion of the evaluation process should result in a recommendation for a switch that can be operated efficiently by the patient. Assistive devices and switch interfaces are determined after the switch has been selected and the patient has been trained to use the switch.

The operation of electronic assistive devices requires the use of switch interfaces. Interfaces are electrical circuits that connect switches to the assistive devices. With the appropriate interface, switches can be used to operate microcomputers, environmental control units, communication systems, and battery controlled devices.

Various interfaces may be purchased through manufacturers or hand-made interfaces can be fabricated. Purchasing controls for assessment and training can be very expensive as there are numerous products available, and it is difficult to know exactly what to buy to get started. When doubt exists about purchasing a particular switch, it may be beneficial to make one first for experimentation. A resource list of supplies, equipment, and related information appears at the conclusion of this chapter.

Basic Principles of Electricity

Electricity needs a pathway of circuits to conduct energy. The pathway of circuits for the operation of battery-operated devices consists of a power source (the batteries), an on/off microswitch, and the toy, light, tape recorder, or other device.[2]

When the microswitch is closed or turned on, it completes the electrical pathway and allows the electricity to flow from the battery to the device, thus turning it on, as illustrated in Figure 26-1. When the microswitch is open or off, the electricity is not allowed to flow from the battery and thus the device is not turned on, as shown in Figure 26-2.

In order to construct a Plexiglas pressure switch, there are three basic electrical components that must be purchased: the subminiature microswitch, the subminiature jack, and the subminiature plug. The subminiature microswitch is the on/off lever switch, and the subminiature jack and plug are the two counterparts that make up the electrical connection between the switch and the interface. Either subminiature or miniature jacks and plugs can be used; however, the different sizes are not interchangeable and must match in size to fit together correctly. Subminiature components are not as readily available as miniature parts. It should be noted that when using a tape recorder, the subminiature plug will fit directly into the remote control jack on the recorder, and an interface is not necessary. Detailed instructions for making a switch will be provided later in this chapter.

Technical Procedures

The technical procedures necessary to construct switches include splitting a wire, stripping a wire, and soldering.

Splitting a Wire

To split a wire means to separate the two strands of the wire. Each strand is coated in plastic. With either wire cutters or scissors, cut and separate the two strands, as shown in Figure 26-3. Care must be taken to avoid penetrating each plastic strand so as to not to expose the wires.

Stripping a Wire

To strip a wire means to remove the plastic coating from a segment of the wire. If wire gauges are marked on the wire stripper, place both strands of the wire in the 22-gauge hole, which is the size recommended for projects described in this chapter. Place the jaws of the stripper about 3 inches down from the end of the wire. Gently squeeze the wire stripper handles together and quickly pull up to remove the plastic coating. Care must be taken, because if the wire stripper is squeezed with too much force, the wires may be cut off. If this should happen, try the procedure again.

There are several varieties of wire strippers that may operate differently from the one just described. The wire gauge is not marked on some, and it is necessary to adjust a bolt and set the cutter for the size of the wire. Once the plastic coating has been cut, place the wire in a separate hole marked on the stripper to pull off the plastic coating.

Soldering

Soldering is the process of fusing two pieces of metal together to facilitate the passage of electricity between them. The following procedure should be followed:

1. Some wires, plugs, jacks, and other electrical terminals may need to be cleaned with steel wool.

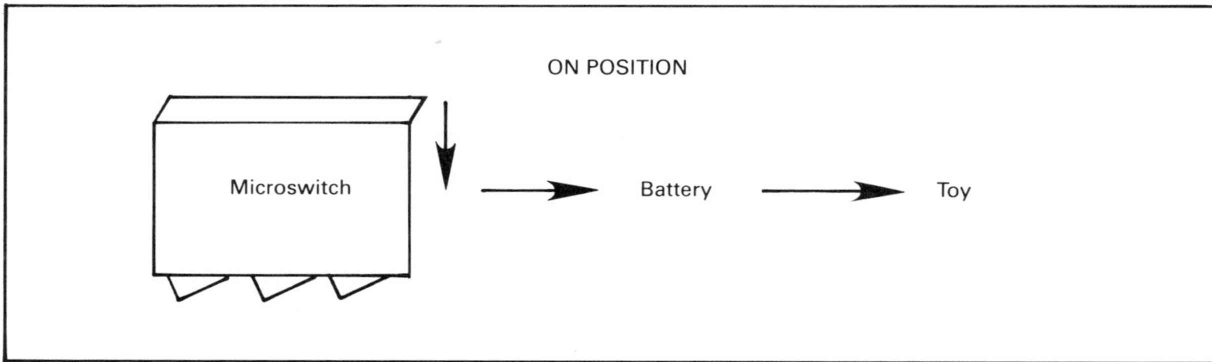

Figure 26-1

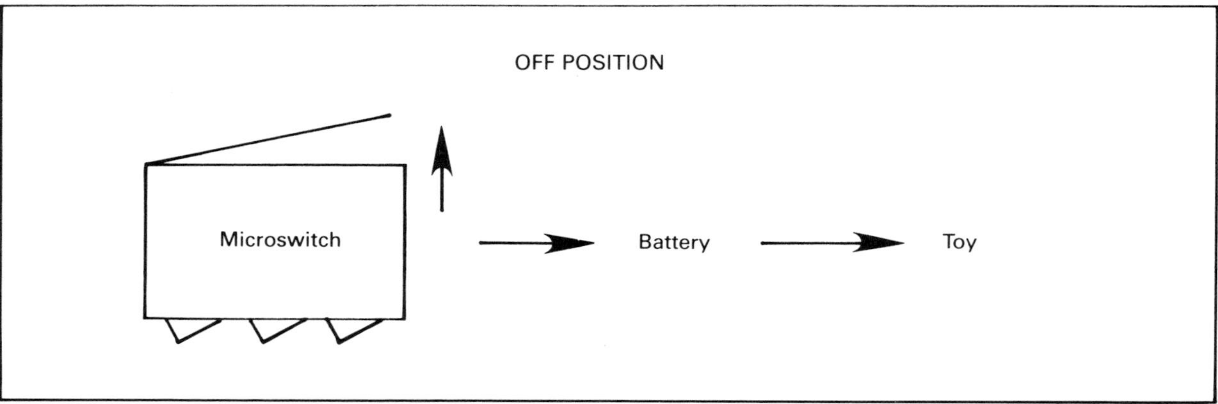

Figure 26-2

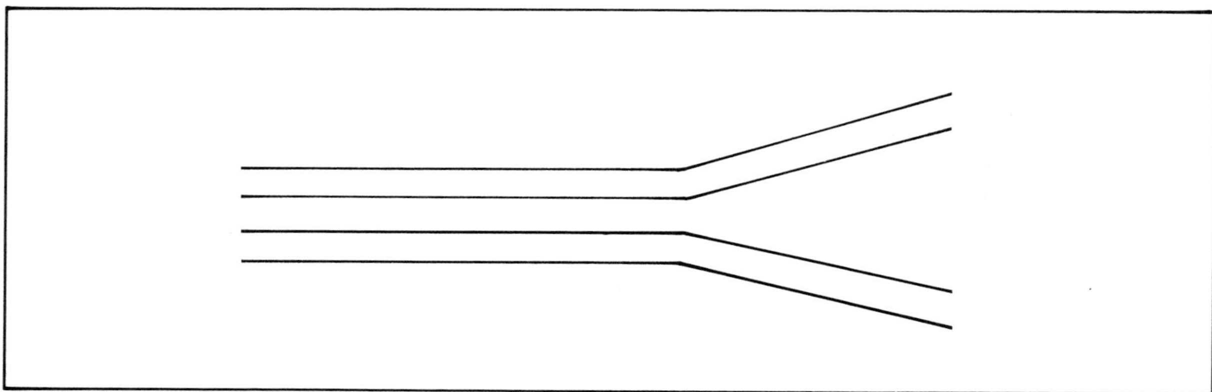

Figure 26-3

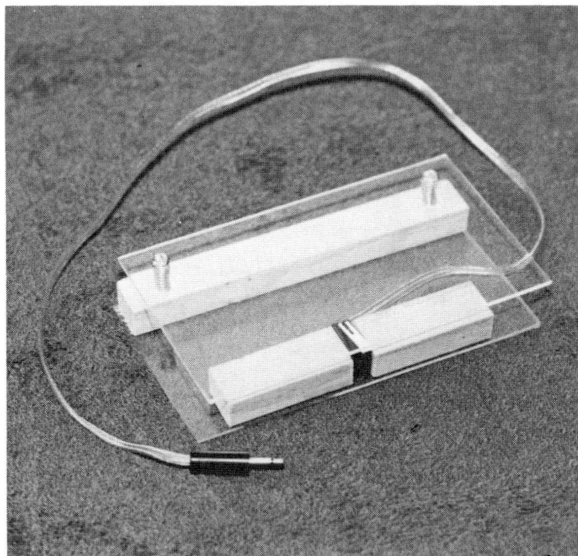

Figure 26-4. Plexiglas Pressure Switch

2 After the wire is threaded to the terminal, hold the parts with a pliers or tape them to the table. A small table vise may also be used. This is necessary, as the components become very hot and it is difficult to hold them while soldering.

3 To solder, first heat the wire and terminal parts at the same time by holding the soldering iron tip firmly against them. (Be patient and wait until both the wire and terminal are hot.) When both parts are hot, touch the rosin core or electrical solder to the connection. The solder should melt and flow evenly to coat the surfaces. Hold the soldered parts in a stable position until cool. If the parts have not been heated enough, the joint will lump. This is known as a cold solder joint and will make a poor electrical connection. If this occurs, simply reheat.

4 *Use Caution*. The soldering iron must be used carefully. It becomes extremely hot and can cause severe burns and ignite fires. Avoid overheating the switch itself as high temperatures can damage internal parts.

Instructions for a Plexiglas Pressure Switch (Using Subminiature Components)*

Basic Materials:

2 pieces of Plexiglas, each cut to 5½ inches by 3 inches.

2 sheet metal screws, No. 6 diameter and ¾ inch in length.

3 wooden strips cut from ½-inch thick pine stock: 1 piece cut to 5½ inches in length by ½ inch width and 2 pieces cut to 2 inches in length by ½ inch in width.

1 spring that will fit under the screw head and is 1 inch in length; the tension of the spring is the individual's choice depending upon the amount of strength the user can exert. (It's a good idea to have a variety of springs on hand.)

1 lever type on/off microswitch.

1 subminiature plug (miniature can be used).

1 22-inch piece of 22-gauge speaker wire.

Other Supplies and Equipment:

Rosin core or electrical solder, soldering iron, super glue, masking tape, electrical tape, hand drill, screwdriver, wire stripper/wire cutter, knife or taped, single edge razor blade, needle nose pliers, awl, needle file, varnish, and sandpaper. (The assembled switch is shown in Figure 26-4).

Instructions:

1. Sand the edges and corners of the Plexiglas until smooth.
2. Sand all surfaces of the wood strips until smooth.
3. Varnish the wooden strips and allow to dry overnight.
4. Glue the 5½-inch strip of wood along the 5½ inch edge of one of the pieces of Plexiglas with super glue.
5. Split 2 inches from both ends of the 22-gauge speaker wire with a knife or a taped, single edge razor blade.

**Note:* The author is not responsible for any damage or harm that may be caused by the use of any devices for which instructions are given.

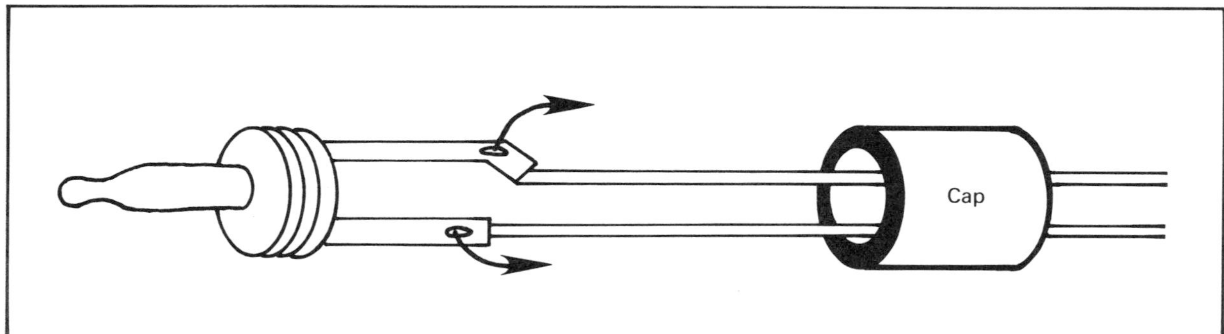

Figure 26-5

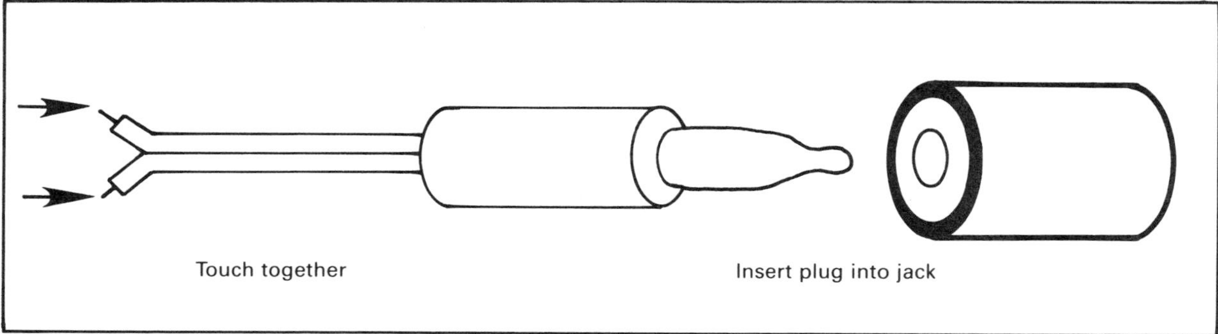

Figure 26-6

6. Strip about ½ to ¾ inch of plastic coating off each strand on both ends of the wire.

7. Unscrew the cap from the subminiature plug.

8. Thread the wires through the metal holes of the plug. Thread from the inside through the holes to the outside. Bend the wires back and trim to ⅛ inch. Be sure to pull through so that the plastic coating touches the inside of the metal hole (see Figure 26-5).

9. Solder the wires to the plug. Use only a small amount of solder so the cap will screw back on. If too much solder is used, the excess can be removed with a needle file.

10. Using needle nose pliers, bend the two metal prongs at the end of the plug around the plastic coating of the wire passing through that hole. This helps hold the wire securely.

11. Screw the cap back on.

12. Test the plug by plugging it into a subminiature jack adapted to a battery-operated toy or plug it into the remote jack of a tape recorder. The toy or tape recorder needs to have the existing switch mechanism turned to "on." Touch the two wires at the opposite ends together; if the toy or tape recorder turns on, the plug is working properly (see Figure 26-6). If the plug does not work, unscrew the cap and check to see whether the wires soldered are touching each other. If this is the case, put electrical tape around one wire and a metal prong to keep them separated.

14. Solder the wires to the switch and trim off any excess wire.

15. Test the circuitry again with a battery-operated toy or a tape recorder.

16. Glue the 2-inch strips of wood, one on each side of the switch lever and placed on the opposite edge from the 5½-inch strip glued earlier. It is best to glue one piece, let it dry 30 seconds, place the lever switch snugly against the glued piece, and glue the second 2-inch strip next to the switch. It is important to note that the microswitch is placed

with the "C" terminal facing the inside of the switch, as illustrated in Figure 26-8.

17. Drill two 5/32-inch holes in the second piece of Plexiglas, ½ inch from each edge of the 3-inch side, and 3/8 inch from the 5½-inch edge, as shown in Figure 26-9.

18. Place the Plexiglas with the holes over the glued 5½-inch strip of wood. Use an awl or a nail to mark the screw holes on the wood.

19. Cut the spring in half with a wire cutter.

20. Put the screws through the holes in the Plexiglas, slip one piece of spring on each screw (springs under Plexiglas), and screw them into the wood. Tighten the screws so the tension of the springs keeps the top piece of Plexiglas above and not touching the microswitch.

21. Retest the microswitch for operation.

This switch can be made either larger or smaller than the specifications given.

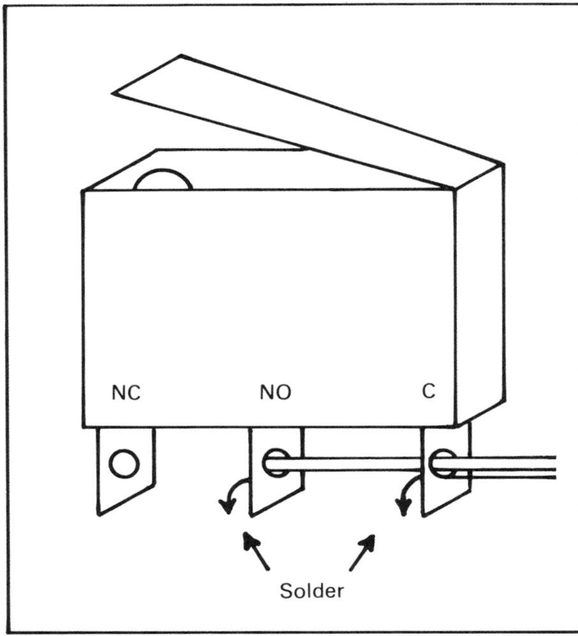

Figure 26-7

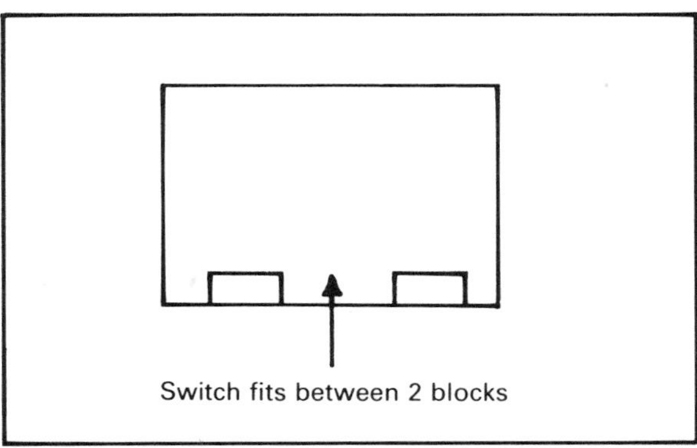

Figure 26-8

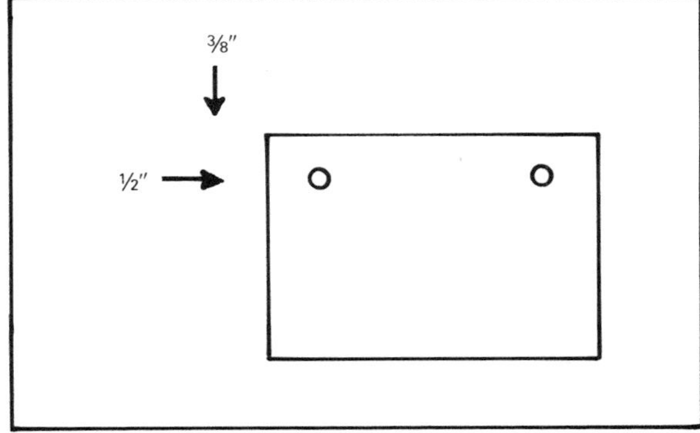

Figure 26-9

Instructions for an Interface for a Battery Operated Device Using Subminiature Components*

Basic Materials:

1 12-inch piece of 22-gauge speaker wire.

1 subminiature jack.

1 small piece of double stick tape, ½ inch by ¼ inch.

2 small pieces of copper tooling foil, cut slightly smaller than the double stick tape.

Other Supplies and Equipment:

Wire stripper/cutter, knife or taped single edge razor blade, soldering iron, rosin core solder or electrical solder, scissors, and ruler. (An interface for a battery operated device is shown in Figure 26-10.)

Instructions:

1. Using a knife or a taped single edge razor blade, split 2 inches from one end of the 22-gauge wire and split ½ inch from the other end.

**Note*: The Author is not responsible for any damage or harm that may be caused by the use of any devices for which instructions are given.

2. Strip about ½ to ¾ inch of the plastic coating off each strand on both ends of the wire. Twist the strands of each separate split piece of wire.

3. Unscrew the cap from the subminiature jack.

4. Thread one end of the split and stripped wire through the metal holes in the jack. Thread from the inside through the holes to the outside. Bend the wires back and trim to ⅛ inch. Be sure to pull the wires through the holes so that the plastic coating touches the inside of each hole, as illustrated in Figure 26-11.

5. Solder the wires to the jack; file off excess solder if necessary.

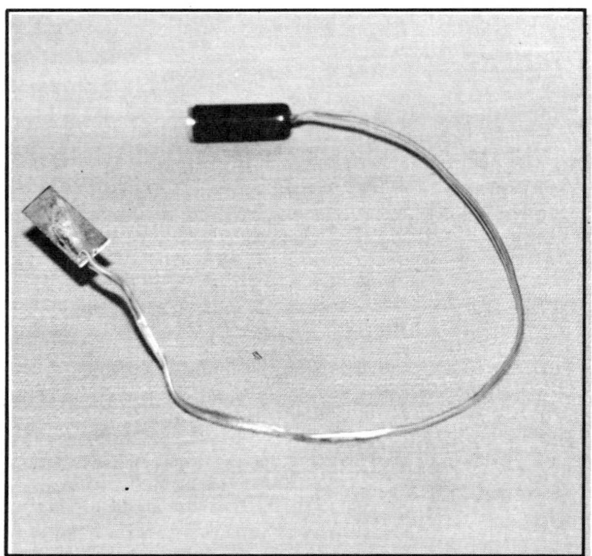

FIGURE 26-10. Interface for a Battery Operated Device.

6. Using a needle nose pliers, bend the two metal prongs at the end of the jack around the plastic coating of the wire passing through the hole. This helps to hold the wire securely.

7. Thread the wire through the cap and screw the cap on.

8. Cut a small ½ by ¼ inch piece of double stick tape.

9. Cut two pieces of copper tooling foil slightly smaller than the ½ by ¼ inch piece of double stick tape.

10. Place the copper tooling foil pieces on either side of the double stick tape. The tape acts as insulation and is necessary because the two pieces of copper must not come into contact with each other.

11. Place the ½ inch split and stripped wires, one on each side of the copper chip, and solder each wire to it. Be sure that the plastic coating on each touches the end of the copper chip. This keeps the wires from touching each other, as shown in Figure 26-12.

12. Test the interface by using a battery-operated device in this manner: Remove the cover from the battery compartment and place the copper chip between the two batteries or between a battery and its contact. Turn the device on. It should not run. Connect a microswitch with a subminiature plug to the subminiature jack. Activate the microswitch and the device should work.

Variation:

An insulated copper circuit board, cut to the same specifications, can be used to replace the

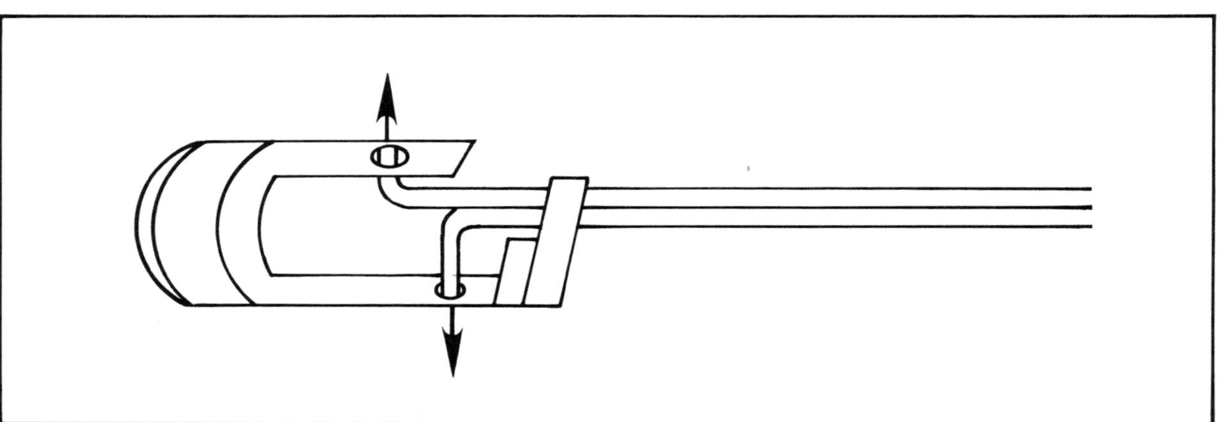

Figure 26-11

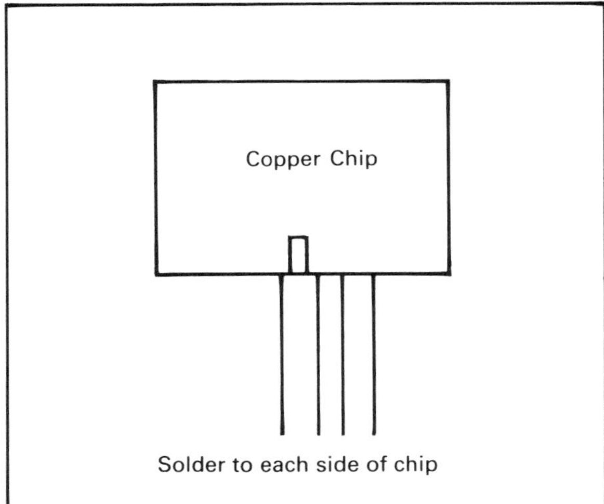

Figure 26-12

copper foil and double stick tape. If this option is selected, the wires are soldered to each side of the circuit board. It should be noted that chips made from circuit board are thicker and often more difficult to fit into a battery compartment. Foil constructed chips are more flexible and fit compartments more easily. The disadvantage of using them is that they often break and will wear out faster.

Selection of Toys and Battery Operated Devices

Toys provide valuable learning and growing experiences for children. Switches combined with toys encourage and motivate handicapped children and provide opportunities for them to play alone or with peers, and actively participate in learning situations.

When purchasing battery-operated toys, it is important to select the ones with on/off switches. Check the battery box to be sure there is room for insertion of the copper chip from the interface. Some battery boxes are so small that once the batteries are inserted, there is not enough room for a small copper chip.

Toys that provide movement are very stimulating for children. Some action toys have a "bump and go" movement; they accelerate forward until they bump into a boundary or object and then reverse direction. Toys that are safe, durable, and colorful, make noises, and have lights are good choices for handicapped children. Some favorites include small trains or engines, police cars with sirens, and animal characters that play musical instruments.

In addition to toys, small battery-operated fans and vibrators can provide sensory stimulation. Flashlights and other battery powered light devices can be used for visual tracking and visual stimulation activities.

Tape recorders are also useful. Favorite songs and tunes, voices, and noises can be recorded and used as a play activity or as a reinforcement for correct performance. For example, a handicapped child who correctly moves an electronic car through a simple maze might be rewarded with a short taped segment of his or her favorite song, which is activated when the car reaches the final point. When using a tape recorder with a switch that has a subminiature plug, an interface is not necessary. The subminiature plug fits directly into the remote control jack on the tape recorder.

Toys that have more than one control switch and radio-controlled toys are difficult to adapt and require sophisticated wiring. An excellent resource that provides detailed information about complex toy adaptations is *More Homemade Battery Devices for Severely Handicapped Children with Suggested Activities* by Linda J. Burkhart. Toys that perform stunts or require a track to run on are not recommended for use with switches because the wires become twisted and break.

Safety Precautions

When using microswitches and battery devices, it is important to consider the patient's responses and needs. Watch for seizures and signs of boredom, fear, or annoyance. Change or stop the activity in response to the patient's behavior.

Low voltage battery-operated devices will not cause an electric shock. They do, however, contain battery acid, so care must be taken that patients do not put them in or near their mouths.

The type of solder commonly used to join electrical connections contains lead; therefore, never let patients put these soldered parts in their mouths. Exposed soldered areas can be easily covered with electrical tape, or electrical solder that is 100 percent tin can be used.

The switches discussed in this chapter are to be used with battery-operated devices only. When using a tape recorder, run it on the batteries, *not* plugged into an electrical socket.

When in doubt, always consult with an electrician or someone with electrical expertise before using a device with a patient.

Treatment Applications

The successful use of microswitch controls and other technical devices as treatment activities depends upon the abilities and ingenuity of the occupational therapist and the assistant. Hundreds of controls are available, and not all are operated by a microswitch. Joysticks and mercury, toggle, grasp, breath control, and voice-activated switches are examples of controls that are not operated by a microswitch. Treatment activities vary depending on the type of switch being used. A joystick can be used to assess a quadriplegic patient for operation of a powered wheelchair. A mercury switch attached to a patient's head can be used to facilitate head control. The following discussion provides treatment suggestions for the Plexiglas pressure switch.

Tactile stimulation can be provided by placing different textures over the Plexiglas switch. Sandpaper, terry cloth, burlap, lambs' wool, felt, and carpet pieces provide an assortment of textures for both stimulation and discrimination.

Battery-operated fans and vibrators provide sensory stimulation. When a pinwheel is placed in front of the fan, it spins and provides a stimulating visual activity. Brightly colored toys and lights can be used to encourage visual localization, tracking, and discrimination. Auditory stimulation can be provided by toys that make noise, such as radios and tape recorders.

By combining switches with therapeutic handling techniques, positioning of a patient can be maintained or inhibited. To encourage sitting, "on all fours," kneeling, or standing, a patient may be placed in the position and required to weight-bear on the switch. The activity provided through activating the switch diverts attention and motivates the patient to maintain the position. To inhibit excessive or abnormal movement, the switch can be placed so that it turns on when the patient is positioned correctly and turns off with the undesirable movement, thus reinforcing the proper motor response.

Stacking blocks or various objects on the surface of the switch encourages prehension patterns. Squeezing the switch with the fingers to turn it on and off facilitates pincer grasp patterns. Switches can be used to train patients in developing headstick and mouthstick skills. Target areas can be placed on the surface of the Plexiglas and graded in size as skill develops.

Combined with specific interfaces, switches can be used with microcomputers. Computer software programs written to use the technique of scanning must be used with microswitches. Scanning is a technique that bypasses use of the keyboard and provides input directly to a cursor or an arrow which appears on the computer monitor. The user activates the microswitch to select specific characters. Microswitches combined with scanning techniques allow computer access for severely handicapped patients.

The use of switches can also provide leisure and entertainment. Adapted computer software games and modified toys are both enjoyable and educational. These activities offer the opportunity for patients to entertain themselves as well as a means to interact and socialize with others.

In many educational systems, the use of switches is included in the curriculum to teach cognitive skills. Concepts like cause and effect, object permanence, and other early learning skills can be taught to handicapped children. For example, a child learns cause and effect by understanding that if a switch is touched, the toy will be turned on. Shape discrimination can be taught by placing a switch in a formboard. If the child places the shape in the correct spot, the switch is turned on, activating a reinforcement for the right answer, such as a bell ringing.

Goals and Objectives

Switches combined with various devices offer enjoyable, motivating, and rewarding activities. As with all therapeutic activities, the use of switches must be included in the treatment goals and objectives. They must be used with a therapeutic purpose. The following are four examples of goals and behavioral objectives that incorporate switches and devices into treatment sessions for severely handicapped children.[3]

1. *Goal: Patient will improve gross motor skills.*

Behavioral Objective: Patient will bear weight on extended arms for at least 30 seconds.

Procedure: Assist patient into a prone position over a large bolster or ball. Rock slowly forward and place arms and hands on floor. Encourage weight bearing on arms by having patient push pressure switch with both hands. Record length of time for weight bearing on switch.

2. *Goal: Patient will increase fine motor skills.*

Behavioral Objective: Patient will reach for and activate a pressure microswitch without assistance at least three times in five trials given.

Procedure: Position patient in a prone position over a body wedge. Place a toy and switch in front of patient. Encourage activation of the switch.

3. *Goal: Patient will improve gross motor skills.*

Behavioral Objective: Patient will walk up one step with the assistance of a handrail in three of five trials given.

Procedure: Place patient's hand on railing. Stand close but offer no physical assistance.

Alternate Activity: Place large flat microswitch on a step. Encourage patient to step on step and switch using railing and wall for support. The switch should be attached to a toy and be activated by stepping up.

4. *Goal: Patient will increase fine motor skills.*

Behavioral Objective: Patient will place four objects into a container on request on four of five consecutive days.

Procedure: Place a switch in the bottom of a container (dishpan, can, basket, etc.) and attach the switch to a toy, computer, or tape recorder. Give the patient a weighted object to place in the container which is heavy enough to activate the switch. After the patient places one object accurately, offer objects of less weight so that two, three, or four objects are needed to activate the switch.

Summary

The application of small technical devices in the evaluation and treatment of severely handicapped individuals is becoming a significant aspect of health care. Combined with the traditonal skills of assessment, use of functional, meaningful activities, and the ability to evaluate performance through the achievement of goals and objectives, this new array of therapeutic intervention techniques offers challenging opportunities for the profession of occupational therapy. There appears to be an increasing need for this technology in many segments of the treatment population. Since the role of occupational therapy personnel is not well defined in this area, it is open for expansion and exploration of new ideas and applications.

References

1. Williams J, Csongradi J, LeBlanc M: *A Guide to Controls, Selection and Mounting Applications*. Palo Alto, CA: Rehabilitation Engineering Center, Children's Hospital at Stanford, 1982, pp 5-7.

2. Wethred C: *Toy Adaptations*. Toronto, Ontario, Canada: Association of Toy Libraries, June, 1979, p 1.

3. Bengtson-Grimm M, Snyder S: *Daily Goals and Objectives Written for Severely Handicapped Using Microswitches*. Clinton, IA: Kirkwood School, 1984.

Resource Guide

Sources of Supplies for Handmade Switches and Battery Operated Devices

Active Electronic Sales Corporation
P.O. Box 401247
Framingham, MA 01701

Barbey Electronics
333 North 4th Street
Reading, PA 19603

BNF Enterprises
119 Foster Street
P.O. Box 3357
Peabody, MA 01960

Chaney Electronics, Inc.
P.O. Box 27038
Denver, CO 80227

Digi-Key Corp.
P.O. Box 677
Thief River Falls, MN 56701

Digital Research Parts
P.O. Box 401247
Garland, TX 75040

Edlie Electronics
2700 Hemstead Turnpike
Levittown, NY 11756

Electronic Handicapped Equipment
1299 Portland Avenue
Rochester, NY 14621

GMI Electronics
715 Armour Road
North Kansas City, MO 64116

Godbout Electronics
Building 725
Oakland Airport, CA 94614

Jameco Electronics
1355 Shoreway Road
Belmont, CA 94002

Micro Switch: A Division of Honeywell
Freeport, IL 61032

Mouser Electronics
11433 Woodside Avenue
Santee, CA 92071

Local Radio Shack Stores

Sources for Commercial Microswitches, Controls and Interfaces

Adaptive Peripherals
4529 Begley Avenue North
Seattle, WA 98103

DU-IT Control Systems Group, Inc.
8765 Township Road 513
Shreve, OH 44676

Handicapped Children's Technology Services
RFD 2, Box 60B
Foster, RI 02825

Mary Ellen Dunford, OTR/L
733 West Donahue
Eldridge, IA 52748

Prentke Romich
R. D. 2, Box 191
Shreve, OH 44676

Rehabilitation Engineering Center
University of Tennessee
682 Court Street
Memphis, TN 38110

Rocky Mountain Software, Inc.
1038 Hamilton Street
Vancouver B.C.
Canada, V6B 2R9

Southern California Research Group
P.O. Box 2231-S
Goleta, CA 93118

Technical Aids for the Severely Handicapped

2075 Bayview Avenue
Toronto, Ontario, Canada, M4N 3MS

Terry Pouliot Schlabach, OTR/L
Box 22
New Liberty, IA 52765

Touch Toys, Inc.
303 Ritchie Highway
Rockville, MD 20852

Washington Research Foundation
Suite 322, U District Building
1107 Northeast 45th Street
Seattle, WA 98105

Zygo Industries
P.O. Box 1008 Portland, OR 92707

Publications

Computer Technology for the Handicapped: 1984 Conference Proceedings.

Computer Technology for the Handicapped: 1985 Conference Proceedings.

Closing the Gap, P.O. Box 68, Henderson, MN 56044.

Computer Technology for the Handicapped in Rehabilitation and Special Education: A Resource Guide. International Council for Computers in Education, 135 Education, University of Oregon, Eugene, OR 97403.

Control Battery Operated Toys: Instructions for Constructing a Large Area Flap Switch (LAFS) to Allow Disabled Children to Control Battery Operated Toys. G. Fraser Shein, Biofeedback Research Project, Rehabilitation Engineering Department, Ontario Crippled Children's Centre, 350 Ramsey Road, Toronto, Ontario, Canada M4G 1R8.

Guide to Controls, Selection and Mounting Applications. Rehabilitation Engineering Center, Children's Hospital at Stanford, 520 Willow Road, Palo Alto, CA 94304.

Home Computers for Home Health Care. JA Preston Corporation, 60 Page Road, Clifton, NJ 07012.

Homemade Battery Powered Toys and Educational Devices for Severely Handicapped Children, second edition. Linda J. Burkhart, 8315 Potomac Avenue, College Park, NJ 20740.

Information on Communication, Writing Systems, and Access to Computers for Severely Physically Handicapped Individuals. Trace Research and Development Center on Communication, Control and Computer Access for Handicapped Individuals, University of Wisconsin — Madison, 314 Waisman Center, 1500 Highland Avenue, Madison, WI 53706.

International Software/Hardware Registry. GC Vanderheiden, LM Walsted, Editors. Trace Research and Development Center for the Severely Communicatively Handicapped, University of Wisconsin — Madison, 314 Waisman Center, 1500 Highland Avenue, Madison, WI 53706.

Proceedings of the Johns Hopkins First National Search for Applications of Personal Computing to Aid the Handicapped. IEEE Computer Society, P.O. Box 80452, Worldway Postal Center, Los Angeles, CA 90080.

Wobble Switch Toy Control Switch: A Do It Yourself Guide. B Brown. Trace Research and Development Center for the Handicapped, University of Wisconsin — Madison, 314 Waisman Center, 1500 Highland Avenue, Madison, WI 53706.

CHAPTER 27

Contemporary Media: Computers

Sally E. Ryan, COTA
with Brian J. Ryan, BSEE, and
Javan E. Walker Jr., OTR/L

Introduction

The purpose of this chapter is to provide a basic understanding of computers. Large, central computers are discussed; however, emphasis has been placed on the microcomputer because of its many uses in occupational therapy evaluation and treatment. These small machines have been described as enhancers or amplifiers of human ability.[1] They can assist disabled individuals in many areas, such as increasing attention span, developing communication skills, mastering eye-hand coordination tasks, improving sequencing and memory abilities, performing auditory and visual discrimination tasks, problem solving, and controlling their environment. The computer also provides creative outlets through the use of word processing and graphics programs. Both cognitive and creative abilities are utilized when patients learn to develop their own programs. In many instances, handicapped adults are finding that their computer skills are creating many new job opportunities and careers that were previously unavailable to them. These are just a few of the many applications possible.

Occupational therapy departments are increasing their use of computers for performing such tasks as maintenance of patient records, and generation of reports, budgets and other word processing and data management projects. Use of the computer also allows access to vast quantities of health care information worldwide.

Microcomputers are small machines that are relatively inexpensive, serve a variety of general purposes, and are easy to learn to use.[2] They don't require a controlled environment or highly specialized installation, and the space requirements are minimal. Many are capable of interfacing with large central computers. Battery-powered, portable microcomputer units are also available which allow work to be done in practically any location.

Central computers, also called mainframes, are

used primarily in large corporations, educational institutions, and government facilities that must process great amounts of data and information. These computer systems can handle hundreds of input/output terminals at the same time. For example, a corporation might install a terminal at the desk of all supervisors and managers and provide several for the secretarial group in each division. All of these people could be using a terminal at the same time, a system which is called time sharing. Engineers doing research and statistical analysis at home or at another location would also have terminals connected to the same system by telephone lines.[3]

Computer Terminology

In order to develop an understanding of how a computer works, it is necessary to know the meaning of the following basic terms:

Hardware

This is a term that refers to the computer and all of its electronic parts. It includes the keyboard, the wires, and the electronic components inside the computer case. Hardware is the "brain" of the computer.[1] It includes the *Central Processing Unit* (CPU).[2]

Firmware

The flat electronic cards that occupy slots inside the computer are called firmware or boards.[4] They perform such functions as connecting the disk drive to the computer, expanding the computer's memory capacity, and increasing the number of characters that can be displayed across the screen. For example, a computer might come from the manufacturer with a 40 column standard display. By adding an 80 column board, the display potential is increased to 80 characters across the screen, which is a great advantage in using word processing programs.

Software

Programs that send messages to the computer telling it to perform specific functions are known as software. Software is stored in the computer's memory on both a permanent and nonpermanent basis. Software program operations are described using the acronyms RAM meaning *random access memory* and ROM which stands for *read only memory*.

RAM refers to the part of the computer's memory that receives information and data. The greater the RAM capacity, the greater the amount of information and data that can be stored. When someone describes a computer as "64K" they are talking about RAM. The literal message is that the computer has a random access memory of 64 kilobytes or thousands of bytes of RAM. Byte is a term which is used to measure units of computer memory storage capacity. Another way to think about software is that it gives ideas to the brain in the hardware, the computer.[4] When the computer is turned off, all RAM memory is lost. It is regained by reloading information from a software program (see disk drive).

ROM, or read only memory, is a permanent part of the computer. Examples of ROM include mathematical computations and programming language such as BASIC, *Beginner's All-purpose Symbolic Instruction Code*,[2] which are built into the computer. When the computer is turned off, ROM always remains.[4]

Disk Drives

The disk drive is a piece of peripheral equipment. It may be mounted directly above the computer in the computer case or it may be a separate box connected to the computer with an electrical cord. The disk drive is also referred to as the DOS, or *disk operating system*. One of its main purposes is to send messages from a software program to the microcomputer's RAM memory. Some software programs may require the use of two disk drives. A tape recorder may be used in place of a disk drive; however, it is a much slower process and increasingly fewer software programs are available in this format.

Disks or Diskettes

Microcomputers use "floppy" disks or diskettes for software programs. These are made of plastic with a special magnetic coating that allows information to be recorded. The disk is placed in the disk drive and is activated to send information to the computer memory. This process is called *booting*. If the computer is turned off, the disk must be re-booted to continue the program. Disks must be handled very carefully, never bend them or touch the "oval window." Be sure that they are not exposed to excessive sunlight, heat, or magnetic sources.[5] Always make an extra copy (backup) of all program disks and store them in their protective envelopes in a secure place away from the computer work area.

Monitors

A monitor is another piece of peripheral equipment that is needed to see a display of computer information. The three main types are green screen, black and white, and color. The green shows green characters on a black background and is frequently used for word processing as well as other programs that do not require color. The black and white monitor is used in the same way. Color monitors are the most expensive but are very usefull for graphics, games, and a variety of educational programs. A monitor is often referred to as a CRT, or *cathode ray tube*. It is possible to use a television set in place of a monitor provided it is compatible with the computer. If a television set is used it should be noted that the display will not be as clear as that provided by a monitor. In technical terms, a monitor has higher resolution,[4] which means it displays more lines per inch on the screen. Display peripherals are referred to as terminals or video display terminals, rather than monitors, when they are a part of a large mainframe computer system.

Printers

Printers are available in three basic types: dot matrix, letter quality, and thermal, with dot matrix currently being the most popular.[4] A dot matrix printer will produce text in a variety of fonts or letter sizes. Many also produce graphics. The quality of the printed material is dependent upon the density of the dots. Printers with high density dot systems can produce printed material that is almost the same quality as that made by a typewriter.[1]

Letter quality printers are most frequently used by people who do extensive word processing and must produce written work of a professional quality. Most of these printers have a "daisy wheel" that produces characters, similar to a typewriter.[4] Some models also present excellent graphics.[1] Letter quality printers are more expensive than the dot matrix type and are considerably slower.

Thermal printers are the least expensive and are more portable than the others.[1] They produce both text and graphics using a heat process to reproduce characters on a special paper. They make less noise than other printers. The main disadvantages of this type of printer are the cost of the heat sensitive paper and the quality of the print when compared with the dot matrix.[4]

Modems

A modem is a device that allows computer signals to be sent over telephone wires to other computers and information to be received. The term modem is derived from *modulator/demodulator*. It converts electronic signals received from a computer so that they can be sent through a personal telephone.[1] It also converts information sent from another computer so that it can be received by the initiator. Use of a modem requires a special firmware card in the computer.[4]

Joysticks

A joystick is another peripheral that allows the user to interact with the computer. It basically sends six messages: on, off, up, down, right, and left, which are often used with games and elementary education programs. It operates in the same manner as the computer's arrow keys and can easily be adapted for patients who are unable to control the handle. Methods used include increasing the size of the handle with foam rubber, placing a rubber ball over the handle, or constructing a specialized adaptation with plastic splinting material or plastic pipe fittings available at most hardware stores.

Paddles

A paddle or a set of two paddles may be used in place of a joystick. The paddle uses rotational movements that the computer recognizes and has an on/off switch. Paddles may be adapted in many of the ways described for joysticks.

Microcomputer Input and Output Equipment

Operation of a microcomputer system requires correct electrical connections and a power source, most commonly regular commercial current of 110 volts. Follow the directions in the manual *exactly* as they are described when setting up a computer. Figure 27-1 shows a typical work station and the

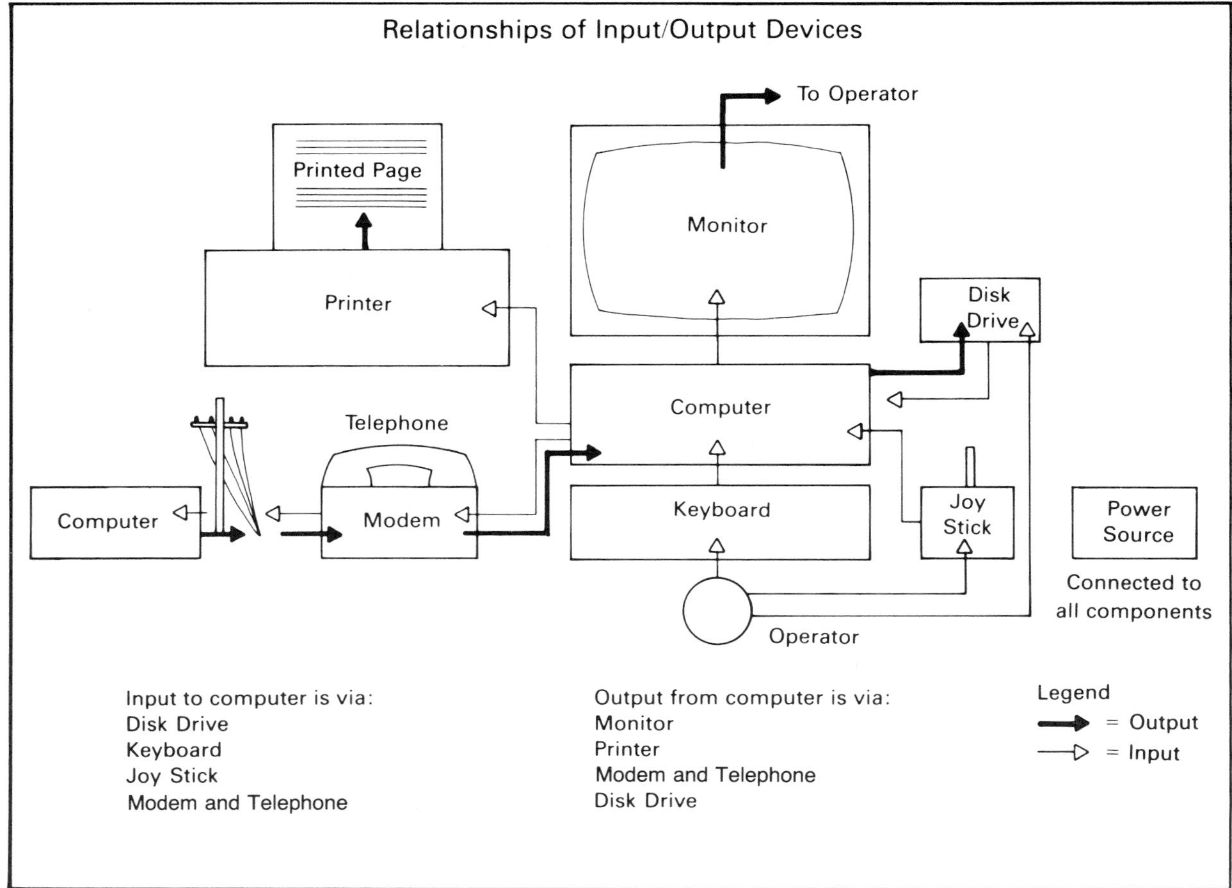

Figure 27-1

relationship of input and output equipment. Input is a term which means the ways the computer can receive information, or how information can be "put in." Output refers to the information that is sent from the computer, or "put out."

Input on a microcomputer can be accomplished in a number of ways which include the activation of the disk drive to load a software program, and use of a keyboard, joystick, or a modem.

In addition to being stored on a diskette in the disk drive, output can also be produced by the monitor, the printer, and the modem.

How Computers Work

A complete description of the many aspects of how computers work would require several chapters; therefore, only very basic information on this subject will be discussed as it applies to microcomputers. Computers are versatile machines that perform a variety of functions when they are instructed to do so by a software program. These functions include playing games as well as operating file, spreadsheet, database, and word processing systems. The electronic mechanisms within the computer respond to input from a number of sources and translate the information received into a binary system comprised of "zeros" and "ones." For example, if the user types "MARY" on the keyboard, small electronic components, referred to as microchips, will convert the letter "M" into a binary code of zeros and ones and store it, together with the other input information, in the RAM or random access memory of the computer. The computer's memory might be compared to a block of post office boxes, where "slots" exist to save and categorize information.

To more clearly illustrate some of the computer's functions, the use of a word processing program written in BASIC in a diskette format will be used as an example. The first step is to put the word processing program into the disk drive and turn on, or boot up, the computer and monitor. The program is then "LOADED" into the computer's RAM memory. Next, the user removes the word processing diskette from the disk drive and places an initialized "FILE" diskette in the drive. At that point, information can be entered via the keyboard or another type of input device.

Once all of the information has been put in, the user can "SAVE" it on the diskette by inputing the correct "SAVE" command and entering a short title so that the information can be easily retrieved if needed. In the event that the computer is turned off before the "SAVE" command is entered, all of the information will be lost. If the user also needs a printed copy or "printout" of the material then the "PRINT" command is used.

If it is necessary to add to the information at a later time, the user simply reloads the word processing program by placing the disk in the disk drive, turns on the computer, replaces the word processing disk with the file disk and enters the "LOAD" command. Once the information is loaded, additions, deletions and other modifications can be made. When the user is finished working on the document, the "SAVE" command must be entered so that all of the revisions are saved on the diskette.

Word Processors, Databases, Spreadsheets, and Terminal Programs

Certified occupational therapy assistants who are prepared to practice for the balance of this century and into the 21st will find using a computer no more a chore than dialing a telephone or driving an automobile. The "mystery and awe" which currently surround use of the microcomputer will gradually disappear, and it will be a tool as common as a video cassette recorder or a microwave oven.

Much of the mystery has revolved around the differences between the concepts of the computer programmer and the computer operator. In the early days of computing, one had to be a programmer because of the relative complexity of computers, and because there was a lack of "user friendly" software programs available. With the advent of more powerful microcomputers and the increase in available software, most occupational therapy assistants will be computer operators, rather than computer programmers. This opens up a wide variety of opportunities.

As a computer operator, the COTA may have access by terminal to either a large mainframe computer, such as one used by a hospital, or a microcomputer at a desk or departmental work station. Both can be linked to other computers for information sharing.

Information management is one of the most important factors which the computer offers to occupational therapy service programs. With access to an electronic bulletin board or database, occupational therapy personnel will have instant access to information about a variety of health care subjects.

Currently, occupational therapy departments use computers primarily for administrative purposes; however, use as a therapeutic tool in patient evaluation and treatment is becoming more widespread. The following four basic computer software programs are in the repertoire of the COTA who is a literate computer user:

1 A Word Processing Program.
2 A Database Manager (DBM).
3 A Spreadsheet Program.
4 A Terminal Program.

Word Processing

A word processor is software that allows a computer to function somewhat like a typewriter. It permits one to compose and edit text; move, duplicate or delete entire blocks of text; check for proper spelling; identify some specific elements of poor writing style; print the document with data inserted from the keyboard, from files, and from a database manager or a spreadsheet.[6]

The word processing program has become one of the most utilized programs for occupational therapy personnel. Many of the routine forms which are necessary for evaluations, progress notes, and discharge summaries can be placed on a computer to avoid unnecessary repetition. Through the use of either a terminal program to access a mainframe computer or a microcomputer and a printer, the therapist and the assistant can more efficiently manage the information which must be completed for every patient receiving their services.

In addition to patient information, there are letters, reports, patient education documents, public affairs information, and other routine pieces of frequently used printed material which can be stored on diskette in the computer's main core, and quickly called up for easy revision and printing.

Many word processing packages offer added features which may be helpful such as a spelling checker for the poor speller or typist; a way to link parts of different documents together, or reproduction of forms and mailing labels that are frequently used.

One of the authers worked on a psychiatric ward at Walter Reed Army Medical Center, during the 1970s, which allowed all pertinent staff members to record patient chart data on a computer utilizing a word processing program. The individual patient charts were literally maintained on the mainframe computer and hard copies were printed only when necessary. The occupational therapy staff wrote their weekly progress notes at the terminal and were able to have instant access to all data relevant to the patient. Although this was an experimental program at the time, it is becoming the norm in many hospitals, nursing homes, and other treatment facilities.

The advantages of utilizing a word processing program over pen and paper or a typewriter become obvious when the use of the program becomes routine. One of the problems with writing a note for a chart is that many therapists and assistants are not gifted writers and they would like to revise their notes from time to time. Using a pen and a blank progress reporting sheet, the result can sometimes be a sloppy note with error markings, or a recopied note. With the typewriter, revisions either require the judicious use of "white out" or the retyping of the entire note. In contrast, the word processing program allows instant revision. By merely moving the cursor, a visual electronic position indicator symbol, back a letter, a word, a line, or a paragraph, revisions can be easily made. In addition, entire paragraphs or blocks of information can be moved, edited or deleted before the final note is saved for later storage or retrieval.

Editor's Note: A large portion of this textbook was written on a microcomputer utilizing a word processing program. Once final editing was completed, the entire book was sent to the publisher on disks and to the printer via a modem.

Database Manager

Database managers (DBMs) maintain a file or a group of items that are related. A recipe file on small index cards is an example of a noncomputerized database management system.[7] The DBM is another software tool that is finding increased utilization in occupational therapy settings. It was created in response to the demand for a system to manage efficiently the volume of information created on the computer. A DBM allows access to that information in a predetermined way.

The easiest way to conceptualize a database management system is to think of a personal address and telephone directory. When there is a need to recall the telephone number of an individual named Schwann, one goes to the book and looks under the "S." Assuming there are not hundreds of Schwanns, the individual is quickly able to gain access to the correct number.

A DBM allows the same type of access, but with considerably more power and speed because of the computer. Perhaps there is a time when a therapist wants to identify all of the patients in the hospital records who had a diagnosis of myocardial infarction and have received occupational therapy services during the last six-month period. Using the more traditional file card or file drawer system, the therapist would review all of the occupational therapy records for that period, and select or note those patients who met the criteria. Obviously, this could be a long and tedious task in a large hospital. On the other hand, if the departmental records are a part of the hospital's mainframe computer system, or if the department has computerized its own files and maintained that information in a DBM program, access to the needed data is relatively simple.

A COTA who is seeking this specific information merely enters in the required "search parameters":

1 Hospitalization during last 6 months.
2 Treatment given by occupational therapy.
3 Diagnosis of myocardial infarction.

Depending on the program, such a computer search could take a matter of seconds but no more than several minutes. The information could then be printed out on paper to provide a "hard copy." If a need existed to contact the individual patients for information on a post-treatment questionnaire, the computer program would print the mailing labels. If a form letter were being sent, the computer could integrate the names and addresses of each individual in the selected group and repeat the patient's name in the body of the letter, thus making each one personal.

The DBM can be used to maintain inventories, patient information files, mailing lists, bibliographies, routine treatment techniques, and other collections of data which may be too large to maintain in a simple office filing system. It should be noted, however, that there are times when a basic, old-fashioned file card system may be more efficient. For example, if the database contains less than 20 or 30 files, with minimal information in each file, it is much easier to open an address book and get the needed information rather than boot up the computer, load the program, call for the data, and read the CRT or wait for a printout.

Spreadsheet Programs

A spreadsheet is a software program that manipulates numbers just as a word processor manipulates words. Electronic spreadsheets organize data in a matrix of rows and columns. Each intersection of a row and column forms a cell that holds one piece of information. The cells are linked together by formulas. When the user enters data to change one cell, the spreadsheet uses the power of the computer to automatically recalculate and alter every other cell linked to the original cell.[8] With the increased emphasis on accountability in health care service delivery, particularly in hospitals, a spreadsheet program can be an invaluable tool for handling the day-to-day maintenance and analysis of numerical data.

The spreadsheet allows the computer operator to perform "what if" scenarios. The program makes it quite easy to project the budgetary effect of adding or eliminating an item or a category of items. Using traditional methods, this information could only be obtained after the time consuming task of recalculating all of the budgetary figures had been completed.

Information typically needed in occupational therapy departments, such as daily treatment count, staff time sheets, budget, inventory, and other numerically based records, can all be easily maintained on a spreadsheet program. Once the initial format, or template, is established, it can be saved to disk and used over and over again for subsequent calculations.

Terminal Programs

A terminal program is a communications program which allows the computer to "talk" with the outside world. It is responsible for instructing the computer to send the characters that are typed through the telephone line to another computer; for establishing and maintaining the connection between the two systems; for making certain that incoming information is displayed correctly on the screen; and for performing other functions to enhance communications.[9] The capability for occupational therapy personnel to communicate with others through a computer system is perhaps the most promising aspect of computing. One of the problems in a profession such as occupational therapy is that there is an ever increasing volume of information. Maintaining access to this data through traditional methods can often be a cumbersome and time-consuming task. The combination of a computer, terminal program, and a modem, however, can open up the "whole world" of information on such topics as rehabilitation medicine to anyone who needs to have access to it. The modem, as described earlier, modulates and demodulates the computer's digital signals. Modulation occurs when the modem converts the information coming from the computer into audible sound signals that can be sent over a telephone line. Demodulation occurs when the modem takes the sound signals coming in from a correspondent's modem, converts them into digital pulses, and sends the pulses to the host computer.[9]

Bulletin Boards

Computers are frequently being used for information access. The information can be contained on an electronic bulletin board. Much like the cork board in the office, computerized bulletin boards are established for the relaying of information or sending and receiving electronic mail between computers. They exist as both private and commercial operations.

These two fundamental uses — gaining or exchanging information — are the primary reasons for using a terminal program. The former is frequently accomplished by contacting commercial networks such as COMPUSERVE, DIALOG, or the SOURCE. Each of these boards allows one access to a variety of separate electronic databases. Most offer an on-line encyclopedia, the ability to track stocks, access various news wire services, select flights, and order airline tickets or shop and do one's banking electronically. Researchers and consultants have compiled a large database of literature available on scientific, medical, and engineering subjects. More detailed information on bulletin boards may be obtained through most local libraries or computer centers at colleges and universities.

Networking

The second use of a terminal program involves networking, or electronic interfacing of individuals through their computers to share information, seek answers to specific questions, or just talk with someone electronically. This is accomplished either by sending an electronic message to someone (electronic mail) or by simultaneously exchanging information from keyboard to keyboard. There are many free "public domain" programs which can be downloaded and saved to disk for later use.

COMPUSERVE, for example, has an on-line interest section for professionals and consumers interested in medicine. One can send a message to individuals or the general public, which will be answered by anyone accessing the special interest section. On many bulletin boards, there are conferences established to deal with specific subjects. Individuals who happen to be on-line at the pre-established time are able to comment and exchange ideas.

There are several bulletin boards that have been specifically established for health professionals. Some of these are operated by universities and medical schools and are quite costly, while others are being developed by professional associations or private groups and have very reasonable rates.

With access to a commercial or private board, much information is obtained. The sharing of information among individuals is helping to limit the isolation which occupational therapists and assistants often feel when working in small communities, or within highly specialized treatment areas. There is no reason, for example, that a board could not be developed to address the needs of the occupational therapy assistants and be available to focus on their specific interests. Many of the professional journals which are now in print form, such as the *American Journal of Occupational Therapy* (AJOT), may soon have electronic copies placed on a bulletin board. Authors will check their electronic mailboxes and respond to questions about their article, or link up with others who have similar interests.

In those instances where a consultant or a supervising therapist is not on site on a daily basis, a combination of the word processor and a terminal package offers some unique options, as illustrated in the following case:

Case Study

Jim Smith, OTR is an occupational therapy consultant and direct service supervisor at the R and R Nursing Home in Paducah, Kentucky. Because he travels to several communities to evaluate patients, communication with Anita Brown, the COTA he supervises at this home, is difficult at times. The OTR and the COTA have found that using computers makes communication much more efficient. Jim and Anita utilize electronic mail to send each other messages and other information. For example, when Jim has completed an evaluation, he sends it to Anita for downloading at a later time for inclusion in the chart. Anita can request additional information or provide updates on the patient's progress at any time, and Jim can access it at home, or by utilizing his portable computer when away.

Computers and the Handicapped

Small microcomputers offer great opportunities for people with a wide variety of disabling handicaps. In recent years, occupational therapy personnel have been collaborating with rehabilitation engineers to develop electronic systems that will permit the handicapped individual to achieve independence in areas never before thought possible.[10] This is a problem solving process, based

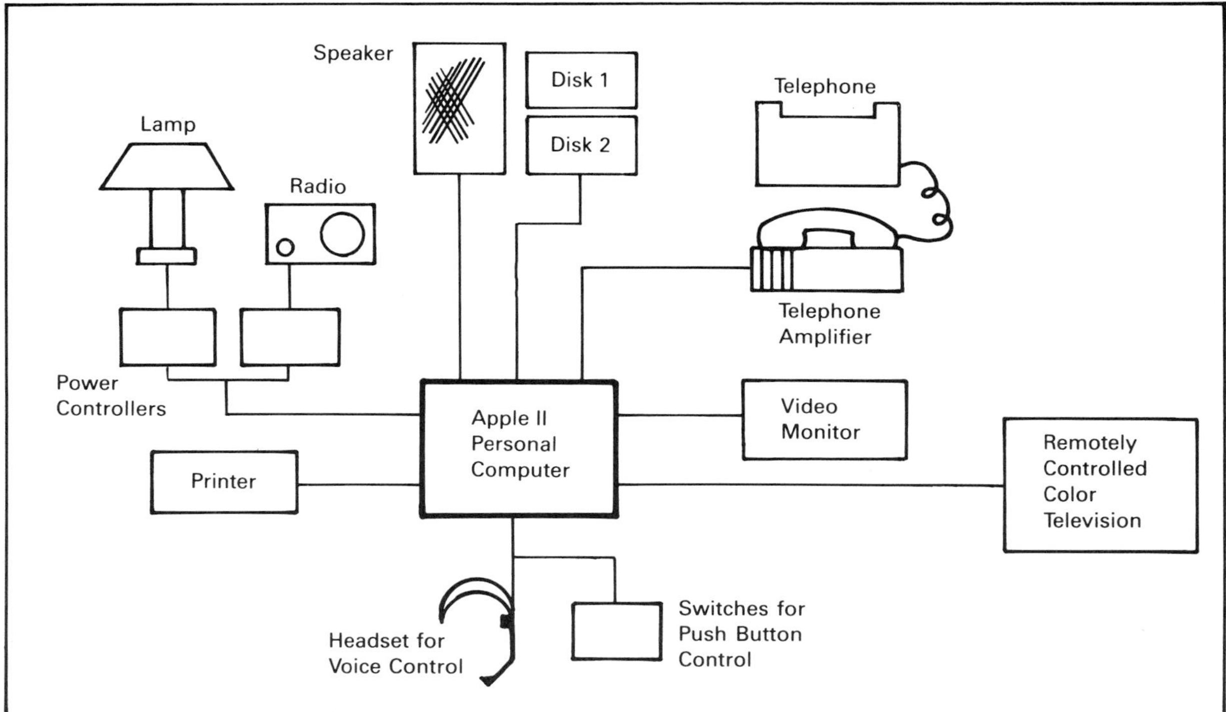

Figure 27-2. From Wambatt, JJ: Computer environmental control units for the severly disabled: A guide for the occupational therapist. Occup ther In Health Care, 4:156, 1984.

on a comprehensive needs assessment, that results in the design of a system or systems to provide patient-controlled decision making and solutions that assist in achieving such goals as:

1 Greater control of the living environment.
2 Enhanced communication skills.
3 Increased employment opportunities.
4 Development of new leisure pursuits.

Environmental Control

The *environmental control unit* (ECU) is an electronic system with sensors that monitor and perform a variety of tasks. This ever-changing technology usually includes a microcomputer and is capable of greatly increasing the independence of even the most severely handicapped individual. A person with a high spinal cord injury is now able to control the position of an electric bed or the operation of a television set, telephone, intercom system, light switches, and electronic door locks, as well as many other functions. Through the use of a properly designed ECU system, the patient can accomplish these tasks.

Instead of using the computer keyboard for input, a "suck and blow" tube may be connected that allows the user to send messages consisting of Morse code dots and dashes which are converted to a form that is recognized by the computer.[11] The computer then relays the message electronically and a task is performed such as dimming a lamp. Voice activated input systems are also available.

Environmental control systems can greatly enhance patients' independence as they no longer have to rely on another individual to carry out some of the daily tasks of living. In many instances they can remain in their own home instead of moving to a nursing home because around the clock care is no longer necessary. This increased independence results in renewed self-confidence and self-esteem.[12] Figure 27-2 illustrates the components of an ECU system.

Enhanced Communication Skills

The microcomputer, coupled with a voice synthesizer, can allow a stroke patient with expressive aphasia to speak. The person may use a software program that allows him or her to type in such statements as "I am hungry" or "I want to go to bed" and they will be spoken audibly by the synthesizer so they can be heard by others in the room. If an intercom system is in place, these messages can also be heard in other rooms. The voice level can be muted for conversations.

A voice synthesizer may also be used to facilitate communication for the blind. Braille "caps" can be placed over the keyboard keys and the written material is then typed one character at a time and relayed to the user audibly. A Braille printer may also be connected to the system to allow the blind person to go back and review work that has been completed.

Communication does not require use of the alphabet. A young child with cerebral palsy who is unable to spell can interact with others by using a special keyboard overlay that has symbols and pictures. Messages can be sent to the screen and the voice synthesizer by pressing just one key.

For the disabled person who has some knowledge of the alphabet, there are programs that allow complete sentences of up to 250 characters to be programmed and recalled with one or two key strokes. For example, a message that states "I would like to have a hamburger and french fries" could be assigned a simple letter code of "HF"; "I would like to go outside" could be assigned "GO."

Deaf people are able to overcome their communication handicaps by using a microcomputer and a speech analyzer device with a special microphone input system. This allows them to learn correct pronunciation, accent, and other subtleties of speech pattern. These speech training systems literally allow the user to see the words they are saying by producing a graph on the monitor. The person repeats the word and tries to duplicate the graph pattern. When the graph pattern has been reproduced exactly as it appears on the screen, correct pronunciation has been achieved. People who do not have hearing deficits are also using these programs to assist in learning foreign languages. Programs are also available that teach sign language.

Patients with amyotrophic lateral sclerosis (ALS), or Lou Gehrig disease, can become so disabled in the later stages that the only motor movements they are capable of performing are swallowing, eye rolling, and raising of the eyebrows. Through the development of an electronic eyebrow switch, mounted on a special headband that is connected to the microcomputer, the patient can communicate. A software program directs the cursor, also known as a position indicator, to scan a group of letters on the monitor screen. When the cursor is on the desired part of the screen, the switch is activated and becomes the first character in the message. While this is a time consuming process in the beginning, after some practice, the patient is able to reproduce several words per minute. It is possible for him or her to write informal messages, letters, or grocery lists and have them reproduced on the computer's printer.

These are but a few examples of the many applications possible. Every day, advances are being made that offer a great variety of both basic and complex communication aids and systems.

Increased Employment Opportunities

Handicapped people are finding that microcomputer skills are "door openers" in the employment market. The ability to use a simple word processing program has allowed the previouly unemployed to work at home as typists, freelance writers, and editors. The "spreadsheet" programs open up many opportunities for the handicapped to work in such areas as accounting, tax preparation, and financial planning. Skill in using file programs allows many to fill positions that involve management of inventory systems and other data processing tasks for business and industry. Others who are skilled in the use of graphics and creative applications are finding jobs with advertising agencies and public relations firms.

Shadick wrote about a woman with advanced multiple sclerosis who was able to continue her career as a loan investment advisor at home with a microcomputer, a printer, and a software program that had a spreadsheet and the capability of processing data to predict or forecast future trends.[13] Crystal provided a recent account of a deaf young man who had cystic fibrosis. He developed programming skills in seven different computer languages and is well on his way to a career as a freelance computer programmer.[14] A 1983 article in the *Washington Post* profiles a blind stock broker who uses a microcomputer with a synthetic voice system; *Information Thru Speech* (ITS) allows this account executive to carry out all of his job responsibilities.[15] As technological advances increase, so will the employment opportunities for the handicapped.

New Leisure Pursuits

The opportunities for developing new leisure time pursuits utilizing a microcomputer are virtually endless. The variety of games that involve one, two, or more players can provide many hours of entertainment and challenge. Programs such as bridge, chess, and conversational foreign languages offer education as well as entertainment. Creative abilities can be expressed through the use of word processing and graphics programs. For example, the learning disabled adolescent who would never have considered creative writing or drawing as a pastime is now able to use a word processing program and a graphics program to write and illustrate original poetry.

Computers in Occupational Therapy: Evaluation and Treatment

Occupational therapy personnel now have a challenging opportunity to use micorcomputers for evaluation and treatment of a wide variety of patients. The key to the successful use of computer activities is dependent on the skill of the therapists and assistants using them.[16] Care must be taken to match the best hardware, peripherals, adaptations, and software programs to the needs and goals of the individual patient. Costs must also be carefully considered, particularly when complex systems are required.

The following short case studies give some specific examples of the effective use of microcomputers in occupational therapy.

Case Study: Computer Assisted Rehabilitation for a Head Trauma Patient

A 26-year-old male received a closed head injury in a motor vehicle accident. After treatment in an acute care hospital he was transferred to a custodial facility with a diagnosis of severe vegetative state based on the *Glascow Coma Scale*.[17] Two years after injury, he was admitted to the University of Texas Medical Branch Adult Special Care Unit with left hemiparesis. The patient was then classified as Level 2 Severe Disability and was oriented to person but was disoriented to the environment. His attention span was less than 5 minutes, he was without problem solving skills, and he had severe left-sided neglect and exhibited an inability to cross the midline. He demonstrated lack of coordination, 1½ inches past pointing, poor dexterity, and all responses were severely delayed. He used a wheelchair for ambulation.

The occupational therapy program included peg and block designs, range of motion, perceptual tasks, right and left discrimination activities, orientation to time and environment, and self-care. Modalities were used to increase right upper extremity strength and to inhibit hypertonus of the left. The patient began to learn bathing, dressing, basic cooking, and laundry tasks. He was oriented to the hospital environment, played simple games, and joined in group activities.

Seven months later, computer generated tasks were added to the treatment plan. A stimulus/response and discrimination software program, which measures latency of response times in averages of computer cycles as well as variance and number of errors, was used for an evaluation tool because of its concrete database. The computer indicates correct responses with an auditory tone so that the patient can receive immediate feedback, and after 15 trials a cumulative score is given.

One discrimination task requires the patient to respond to a 1-inch yellow square and to inhibit a response when a blue square appears. The randomly presented stimuli require the patient to cross the midline visually and to scan the screen and eye-hand coordination to use the keyboard or the joystick. The patient was not trained on these programs to prevent over-learning and to ensure an objective evaluation tool.

The computer programs used for training were

Search,[18] *City Map*,[19] *Driver*,[20] *Sequential*,[21] *Baker's Dozen*,[22] and *Stars*.[23] The cognitive skills required for these programs involve planning, organization, decision making, simple problem solving, attention to details, logical thinking, and sequencing. The treatment goals focused on these areas.

On admission the patient had severe deficits in concentration and attention span which interfered with his functional performance and self-care activities. The computer programs selected for him provided a mechanism for developing his attention span and increasing coordination. A year and a half after admission, the patient was independent in bathing and dressing and required only stand-by assistance for transfers. He was able to integrate visual field information, move his wheelchair through an environment with distractions, and had marked improvement in his ability to delay gratification.

There are many computer programs available for training patients. The programs selected for this patient resulted in improvement in his activities of daily living as well as his cognitive and perceptual skills. Originally diagnosed as Severe Vegetative State, the patient was reclassified as between Severely and Moderately Disabled.[24]

Case study prepared by Ruth Garza, BS, COTA, OT Dep't, Univ. of Texas Medical Branch, Galveston, TX.

Editors Note: Please see the information presented in the section on Precautions for Computer Use in this chapter.

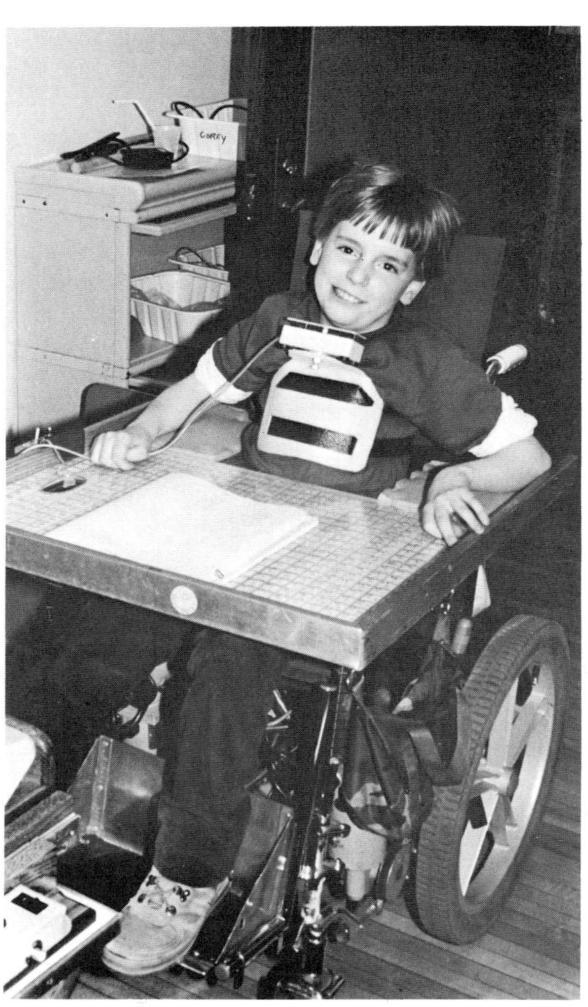

Figure 27-3

Case Study: Computer Assisted Learning for the Cerebral Palsy Child

Computer assisted learning was used with an 11-year-old boy with cerebral palsy. He is a quadriplegic athetoid who is completely dependent for all activities of daily living. His head control, trunk control, and graded movements are all poor. He is nonverbal and uses a Bliss communication system, pointing to the symbols with his index finger. His cognitive abilities are age appropriate and he is highly motivated. For mobility, he uses an electric powered wheelchair (see Figure 27-3).

To address his educational plan objective to "improve written communication skills," the child used a microcomputer, a word processing program, an interface for the computer, and a single switch. The interface converts the input from the switch into audible Morse code signals that provide feedback to the user. A brief activation of the switch results in a single "dot," or "short," of the code, heard as a one tone output. A longer activation results in a tone change, and the child can hear by the two tones that he has entered a "dash," or "long," of the Morse code. This code input is converted by the interface and displayed on the computer screen as keyboard characters.

Two types of switch placement have been used by the occupational therapist working with this child. One consists of a plate strapped to his chest, at the top of which, directly below his chin, the pressure switch is placed. He activates the switch by depressing his chin while his arms are secured to his lapboard to provide stability and limited extraneous movement. The other method uses the same switch mounted on his wheelchair lapboard. His right forearm is strapped to a board that elevates his hand approximately two inches to the same height as the surface of the switch. In this manner, flexion of the wrist operates the switch.

Formerly using a head pointer, keyguard, and keyboard input, the child was capable of inputing one word per minute with a large number of errors. Through the use of Morse code, he is now capable of four words per minute with few errors. It is anticipated that his performance will improve as he memorizes the Morse code, as switch operation is mastered, and as input simplification methods (through the use of special interface codes) are introduced.

Case study prepared by Mike Meyers, OTR, Michael Dowling School, Minneapolis, MN.

Precautions for Computer Use

Many individuals become so absorbed in the use of the computer that their extremities, trunk, and neck often remain in a static position for a considerable length of time; thus, it is necessary to make certain that work breaks are taken at frequent intervals and that proper positioning is maintained while the patient uses the computer. The computer and peripheral equipment should be placed on an adjustable height table to accommodate the individual needs of a variety of users. Failure to take these measures may result in patients experiencing general fatigue and eyestrain, as well as body aches, particularly in the neck and head.

According to Breines, care should be taken when using computer programs for patients with cognitive and perceptual disorders. *Overemphasis* on this treatment medium should be avoided. She has recommended further analysis and points to the problems inherent in using "a two-dimensional tool for the resolution of a problem which derives from a three-dimensional dysfunction requiring peripheral (vision) input."[25]

Breines also notes that further investigation is needed regarding the effects of computers on those individuals who are cataract prone or neurologically impaired. She has stated that since bifocal glasses are commonly used by the elderly, as well as others, special near-vision glasses may need to be substituted for these lenses when doing computer work.[25]

Summary

Computers are being used for numerous applications in occupational therapy departments. Once basic operations and related terminology are learned, the user finds that initial fears have been erased and new challenges have taken their place. The variety of input and output devices and software programs available offer numerous opportunities for occupational therapy personnel to utilize computer technology in administrative tasks, as well as patient evaluation and treatment activities. Word processors, databases, spreadsheets, and terminal programs offer ways to accomplish tasks in a much more efficient manner, thereby increasing the overall productivity of the department. Small microcomputers offer many new opportunities to individuals with a variety of disabling handicaps. They are often an important tool to enable patients to control elements of their environments, enhance their communication skills, increase their employment opportunities, and develop new leisure pursuits. A variety of computer systems and software is currently available. The Resource Guide at the conclusion of this chapter provides information on those sources that are useful in occupational therapy programs.

Because use of this computer technology is relatively new in the profession, care must be taken to exercise certain precautions, particularly with patients who have cognitive, neurological, or certain visual impairments. Research must be conducted to further validate the use of computers in rehabilitation in general and in occupational therapy specifically.

Resource Guide

Computers:

Apple Computer
Mail Stop 23-H
2525 Mariani Avenue
Cupertino, CA 95014

Heathkit Electronic Center
101 Shady Oak Road
Hopkins MN 55343

IBM Corporation
1001 Jefferson Plaza
Wilmington, DE 19801

Sensory Aids Corporation
205 W. Grand Avenue
Number 110
Bensenville, IL 60106

Sharp Electronic Corporation
1909 E. Cornell Street
Peoria, IL 61614

Tandy Corporation
Radio Shack Division
1400 One Tandy Center
Fort Worth, TX 76102

Access Equipment for the Handicapped:

Nonverbal:
Adaptive Communications Systems
P.O.Box 12440
Pittsburgh, PA 15231

Arctic Technologies
2234 Star Court
Auburn Heights, MI 48057

J. Jordan Associates
1127 Oxford Court
Neenah, WI 54956

Laureate Learning Systems
One Mill Street
Burlington, VT 05401

Street Electronics Corporation
1140 Mark Avenue
Carpenteria, CA 93013

Visually Impaired and Blind:
COPH-2
2030 West Irving Park Road
Chicago, IL 60618

Maryland Computer Services
2010 Rock Spring Road
Forest Hill, MD 21050

Sensory Aids Corporation
205 West Grand Avenue
Number 110
Bensenville, IL 60106

Telesensory Systems Inc.
455 N. Bernardo Avenue
Mountain View, CA 94043

Visualtek
1610 26th Street
Santa Monica, CA 90404

Multiple Handicaps:
Computability
Division of J.A. Preston
60 Page Road
Clifton, NJ O7012

Don Johnston Developmental
Equipment, Inc.
981 Winnetka Terrace
Lake Zurich, IL 60047

Intex Micro Systems
725 S. Adams Road
Suite L-8
Birmingham, MI 48011

Prentke Romich Company
8769 Township Road 513
Shreve, Ohio 44676

Sentient Systems Technology, Inc.
5001 Baum Boulevard
Pittsburgh, PA 15213

Scott Instruments
111 Willow Street
Denton, TX 76201

Softkey Systems, Inc.
4737 Hibiscus Drive
Edina, MN 55435

Zygo Industries, Inc.
P.O. Box 1008
Portland, OR 97201-1008

Software:

General:
To obtain information regarding basic general-use software programs for word processing, filing systems, spreadsheets and graphics, contact any of the companies listed in the preceding section on computers.

Special Education:
Borg-Warner Educational Systems
600 West University Drive
Arlington Heights, IL 60004

Curriculum Associates, Inc.
5 Esquire Road
North Ballerica, MA 01862

Dunamis, Inc.
3423 Fowler Boulevard
Laurenceville, GA 30245

Laureate Learning Systems
One Mill Street
Burlington, VT 05401

Learning Well
200 South Service Road
Roslyn Heights, NY 11577

Marble Systems
P.O Box 7012
Rochester, MN 55903

MCE, Inc.
175 South Kalamazoo Mall
Kalamazoo, MI 49007

Minnesota Educational Computing Corp.
3490 Lexington Avenue North
St. Paul, MN 55112

Science Research Association, Inc.
Rt. 4, Box 204
Detroit Lakes, MN 56501

IBM Special Education Programs
1001 Jefferson Plaza
Wilmington, DE 19801

Street Electronics Corporation
1140 Mark Avenue
Carpenteria, CA 93013

Sunburst Communications
1500 First Avenue N.E.
Rochester, MN 55904

Vocational and Life Skills:
Career Development Specialists
1625 Ninth Avenue S.E.
St. Cloud, MN 56301

Conover Company Ltd.
P.O. Box 155
Omro, WI 54963

Language:
Arctic Technologies
2234 Star Court
Auburn Heights, MI 48057

Laureate Learning Systems
One Mill Street
Burlington, VT 05401

Micro Video Corporation
314 North First Street
Ann Arbor, MI 48103

Science Research Association, Inc.
Route 4, Box 204
Detroit Lakes, MN 56501

Publications:

Computer Technology for the Handicapped. M Gergen, D Hagen, Editors. Closing the Gap, P.O. Box 68, Henderson, MN 56044.

Microcomputer Resource Book for Special Education. Delores Hagen. Closing the Gap, P.O. Box 68, Henderson, MN 56044.

Personal Computers and Special Needs. FBA, 1500 Massachusetts Avenue N.W., Number 138, Washington, DC 20005.

Proceedings of the Sixth Annual Conference on Rehabilitation Engineering, 1983 (proceedings of prior conferences also available). Rehabilitation Engineering Society of North America, 4405 East-West Highway, Bethesda, MD 20814.

Periodicals

Closing the Gap (bimonthly). P.O. Box 68, Henderson, MN 56044.

Cognitive Rehabilitation (bimonthly). B & B Publishing, P.O. Box 29344, Indianapolis, IN 46229.

Communication Outlook (quarterly). Communication Outlook, Artificial Language Laboratory, Michigan State University, East Lansing, MI 48824.

Database:

ABLEDATA is a database system offering product information on commercially available equipment, devices, and products for the handicapped including computer access equipment as well as software. It is funded by the National Institute of Handicapped Research and is located at the National Rehabilitation Information Center at the Catholic University of America. For more information, write to: ABLEDATA/NARIC, 4407 Eighth Street N.E., Washington, DC 20017.

References

1. Gerstenberger L: *The Apple Guide to Personal Computers in Education.* Cupertino, CA: Apple Computer, 1983.
2. Doerr C: *Microcomputers and the 3 Rs — A Guide for Teachers.* Rochelle Park, NJ: Hayden, 1979.
3. Edwards J, Ellis A, Richardson D: *Computer Applications in Instruction — A Teacher's Guide to Selection and Use.* Hanover, NH: Timeshare, 1978, p 13.
4. Sanders WB: *The Elementary Apple.* Chatsworth, CA: Datamost, 1983.
5. Poole I: *Apple Users Guide.* Berkeley, CA: Osborne/McGraw-Hill, 1981.
6. Robinson D: Word processing guide. *80 Micro Anniversary Issue.* 1983, p 28-31.
7. Keller W: The database explained. *80 Micro Anniversary Issue.* 1983, p 32.
8. Ahl D: What is a spreadsheet. *Creative Computing.* 10:S-2, 1984.
9. Glossbrenner A: *The Complete Handbook of Personal Computer Communications.* New York: St. Martin's Press, 1983.
10. Gordon RE, Kazole KP: Occupational therapy and rehabilitation engineering: A team approach to helping persons with severe physical disability to upgrade functional independence. *Occup Ther In Health Care.* 4:117, 1984.
11. Romich BA, Vagnini CB: Integrating communication, computer access, environmental control and mobility. In Gergen M, Hagen D, Eds:*Computer Technology for the Handicapped.* Henderson, MN: Closing The Gap, 1985, p 75.
12. Wambott JJ: Computer environmental control units for the severely disabled: A guide for the occupational therapist. *Occup Ther In Health Care.* 4:156, 1984.
13. Shadick M: Disease was her key to success. Call A.P.P.L.E. 10:66, 1983.
14. Crystal B: Computers help the deaf bridge the gap. In *Personal Computers and the Disabled - A Resource Guide.* Cupertino, CA: Apple Computers, 1984, p 7.
15. Williams JM: Blind broker takes stock with a talking computer. *The Washington Post.* July 18, 1983.
16. Wall N: Microcomputer activities and occupational therapy. *Developmental Disabilities Special Interest Section Newsletter.* Rockville, MD: American Occupational Therapy Association, 7:1, 1984.
17. Caronne JJ: The neurological examination. In Rosenthal M, et al (Eds): *Rehabilitation of the Head Injured Adult.* Philadelphia: FA Davis, 1983, p 59-73.
18. Anon: Search. *Cognitive Rehabilitation.* 4:26-27, 1983.
19. Anon: City map. *Cognitive Rehabilitation.* 2:24-26, 1984.
20. Anon: Driver. *Cognitive Rehabilitation.* 4:23-24, 1983.
21. Anon: Sequential. *Cognitive Rehabilitation.* 5:46-52, 1985.
22. Katz R: Baker's dozen. *Cognitive Rehabilitation.* 5:52-46, 1984.
23. Katz R: Stars. *Cognitive Rehabilitation.* 6:47-50, 1984.
24. Ben-Yishay Y: Cognitive remediation. In Rosenthal M, et al, (Eds): *Rehabilitation of the Head Injured Adult.* Philadelphia: FA Davis, 1983.
25. Breines E: Computers and the private practitioner in Occupational Therapy. *Occup Ther and Health Care.* 2:110-111, 1985.

Acknowledgments

Appreciation is also extended to John M. Bruen for his helpful content and editorial suggestions.

CHAPTER 28

Service Management

Robin A. Jones, COTA/L

Introduction

For the purpose of this chapter, *service management* is defined as a process that involves planning, organizing, and evaluating occupational therapy facilities and services. Primary responsibility for service management belongs with the department or program director; however, certain aspects of the management function will require the support of all occupational therapy personnel. The level of responsibility occupational therapy staff members assume for service management will be dependent upon the specific task involved and the level of training necessary to perform the task. The role of the certified occupational therapy assistant in service management will vary depending upon the type of agency or facility, specific policies and procedures, the amount of supervision available, the patient population being served, and the nature of the tasks to be performed.

The following components of service management will be discussed:

1 Scheduling;
2 Maintaining records and compiling and analyzing service data;
3 Preparation, maintenance and safety of the work setting;
4 Taking inventory and ordering supplies and equipment;
5 Reimbursement procedures;
6 Accreditation;
7 Program evaluation and quality assurance; and
8 Meetings.

In addition, continuing education, inservice training, public relations, and research will be addressed. Although these areas do not pertain specifically to service management, they are essential, related components for the continued growth and development of occupational therapy personnel and the profession of occupational therapy.

Service delivery is changing rapidly with the growth of outpatient clinics and other alternative treatment settings. Although methods given as examples in this chapter will need to be modified in order to accommodate changes in occupational therapy practice, it is important to ensure that all of the components are attended to.

Scheduling

Structuring the day to accommodate the demands made on one's time is an important aspect to consider under service management. The registered occupational therapist and the COTA should be able to establish priorities and utilize time management skills in order to plan effectively. Time needed to perform both direct and indirect patient care activities as well as to attend regularly scheduled meetings and conferences must be allotted. Schedules need to be clearly communicated and coordinated with all persons involved.

Under the category of direct patient care, occupational therapy personnel must take into account the frequency wth which a patient requires occupational therapy services, the level of care required, such as one-to-one or group, and the degree of supervision needed. In the majority of situations, this decision will be made initially by the supervising occupational therapist. Throughout the course of treatment, the patient's needs will be jointly reassessed and the COTA will adjust his or her schedule accordingly. The availability of personnel will significantly influence the time spent in direct patient care and will also be a factor in determining how patient care responsibilities are divided among the OTR and COTA staff members. Cost effectiveness will influence the manager's decision to utilize a COTA versus an OTR to perform certain direct patient care services.

Each facility or agency has a different policy for scheduling patient services. The type of setting and the population served influence the process. For example, in an acute care setting the therapist must take into consideration the fact that the patient's medical status is the primary focus and that occupational therapy treatment will be scheduled in accordance with the patient's medical needs. An illustration of this point is the individual with a spinal cord injury who is positioned on a Stryker frame and is able to work on self-feeding only when in a prone position. This situation requires coordination between the nursing staff and the occupational therapy personnel to schedule that patient's "turning times" so that they correspond to the times that meals are served. In a community setting, the schedule may vary daily according to the particular needs of of the OTR's and the COTA's patient population. The community setting offers less structure than the traditional medical setting and requires that occupational therapy personnel have the ability to function relatively independently. This can serve as a disadvantage because the occupational therapy staff often does not have control over the external factors which will influence the population they serve. Schedules must be coordinated with the family and other professionals involved with the patient's care and should accommodate the person's life style as much as possible. Community based programs in which COTAs may be involved include psychiatric day treatment centers, adult day care centers, vocational workshops, transitional living centers, and early intervention programs.

The availability of a patient or family financial reimbursement plan which includes coverage of occupational therapy services will influence the frequency and duration of the occupational therapy services received. The issue of reimbursement and how it affects service delivery will be discussed in more depth later in this chapter. Because an OTR's or a COTA's caseload may include several patients who require varying amounts of time for services, it is important that his or her time be managed accordingly. It is the responsibility of individual occupational therapy personnel, both OTRs and COTAs, to carefully examine each patient's individual needs when planning their time.

Occupational therapy personnel must also schedule time for indirect patient care activities, administrative tasks, and professional activities. Participation in departmental or patient-related meetings, supervision meetings (OTR and COTA), and patient documentation time must be considered. As a COTA becomes more experienced in an area of specialization, additional tasks may be assigned, such as participation in program development, research, and teaching. These professional activities will need to be planned in relation to other responsibilities. In most instances, occupational therapy personnel will find it difficult to incorporate additional responsibilities into their daily schedules and will need to decide what other tasks they are willing to do, if any, outside their regular working hours. Management may also be able to assist individual staff members in identifying ways to handle time more effectively, thus allowing more time for professional activities.

An area often neglected but very important to personal health and well-being is the need to allot

Table 28-1: Daily Schedule

Day of the week: TUESDAY 8:30 a.m.—A.M. dressing program with Mr. Smith (RM. 549)
9:00 a.m.—Feeding group on spinal cord unit
10:00 a.m.—DLS eval. with Mrs. Rose (RM. 762)
11:00 a.m.—Individual treatment session with Mr. Johnson; clinic
12:00 p.m.—Lunch
12:30 p.m.—Pt. care conference—Mrs. Rose and Mr. Smith
1:00 p.m.—Pt. care conference/documentation time
1:30 p.m.—Individual treatment session with Mr. Smith
2:00 p.m.—"X"
2:30 p.m.—Stroke group (community out-trip with th. rec.)
3:00 p.m.—"X"
3:30 p.m.—Staff inservice—infection control
4:00 p.m.—Documentation time: supervision meeting with Carol

time for lunch and periodic breaks. This is essential to a healthy mind and body, facilitates optimal performance, and is positive in terms of socialization, as well as providing a quiet time to think and reflect. It leads to increased job satisfaction and enhances working relationships, which indirectly increases productivity. These breaks contribute to maintaining the balance between work and leisure activities. They also promote professional and personal growth and development, which are essential aspects of quality care. A sample daily schedule for a COTA working in a rehabilitation setting is shown in Table 28-1. An "X" indicates that the previously listed activity extends into or fills the next time slot. This schedule does not reflect two 15- to 20-minute breaks, which are taken morning and afternoon.

Maintaining Records and Compiling and Analyzing Service Data

Maintenance of accurate records of patient performance, attendance, billing, and equipment ordered and received is an essential component of the management of an occupational therapy service program. In addition, service data are used by the administration as a means of evaluating program function in the process of internal quality assurance and efficiency studies as well as for research purposes.

Principles of Documentation

The most important aspect of record keeping is documentation of patient performance. Documentation of a patient's performance in occupational therapy will be utilized by other health professionals dealing with the patient's overall care. In addition, records of the treatment provided are often utilized to justify occupational therapy charges to third party payers such as private insurance companies, Medicare, and Medicaid. It is the responsibility of both the OTR and the COTA to enter information in the patient's medical record that accurately reflects the course of the treatment process. This includes the initial evaluation, a written plan of care, including long- and short-term goals, periodic progress notes, and a discharge evaluation. Written instructions given to the patient or family members concerning appropriate care after discharge from occupational therapy services must also be included. It is important that documentation of equipment that is issued include the functional purpose of the equipment and any training that was provided to insure proper use of the equipment. Other primary considerations are that continuity is evidenced in documentation and that the discharge summary relates directly to the functional status and goals identified at the time of the initial evaluation.

Terminology

Specific, accurate, and careful use of terminology is essential in documentation. An article written by the American Occupational Therapy Association (AOTA) Division of Practice in the *Occupational Therapy Newspaper* cites an example of terminology usage which would be unacceptable to Medicare. A statement which reads "teaching ADL" is not specific enough language. The article states that "training for independence in dressing skills" is acceptable. In the school setting, use of education related terminology is necessary. Goals should be stated so that they reflect enhancement of the educational program in order to establish the relationship between the educational process and occupational therapy.[1]

AOTA has developed the *Occupational Therapy Output Reporting System* and *Uniform Terminology for Reporting Occupational Therapy Services*, two documents which can assist occupational therapy personnel in establishing ways to document treatment. The latter has been reprinted in Appendix G. They were developed in order to keep pace with a movement within the health care field to use a uniform system for reporting costs and services. This has been helpful in educating third party payers as to what services occupational therapy service programs consistently provide nationwide.

Confidentiality

The administration of an agency or facility is responsible for establishing ways to document treatment that is consistent with the needs of confidentiality and professional standards of practice.

Confidentiality of patient care records is essential in order to maintain control over the dissem-

REHABILITATION INSTITUTE OF CHICAGO
Page 1 of 2
OCCUPATIONAL THERAPY DEPARTMENT

PROGRESS NOTE

[X] Team Conference [ ] Other______________

Key: ↓ Progress, ↑ Progress, — Status Quo, N/A Not Addressed

[X] Appropriate Box (Use Black Ball Point Pen Only)

Number of Days Seen 10

Period Covered From 6-24-85 To 7-8-85

Patient Name JS

RIC Number 010101

Physician

Date 7-8-85

[X] INPATIENT [ ] OUTPATIENT

OCCUPATIONAL THERAPY

II PSYCHOSOCIAL

	↓	↑	—	N/A
BEHAVIOR		X		
INTERPERSONAL RELATIONSHIPS			X	
SEXUAL ADJUSTMENT				X

III COGNITIVE/COMMUNICATIVE

	↓	↑	—	N/A
DEVELOPMENT				X
MENTATION				X
SENSORY/PERCEPTUAL				X
COMMUNICATION				X

IV FUNCTIONAL SKILLS

	↓	↑	—	N/A
MOTOR FUNCTION	X			
HAND FUNCTION	X			
MOBILITY			X	
A.D.L.				
FEEDING	X			
ORAL FACIAL	X			
BATHING			X	
COMMUNICATION			X	
TOILETING			X	
DRESSING			X	
HOMEMAKING			X	
COMMUNITY SKILLS			X	

PROBLEMS #______________
(Assoc. problems, respiration, equipment, comm. planning etc.)

PROB #	
	Page 1 of 2
II	Psychosocial: OBS. Patient's attendance to treatment sessions has been inconsistant. Patient reports that she has difficulty getting "motivated" in the morning. Patient continues to demonstrate limited knowledge of her disability and it's long term implications. She continues to have difficulty identifying realistic goals for her near future.
IV	Functional Skills: OBS.
	K) Motor Function: (L) UE P/ROM has increased from 145° to 160° shoulder flexion and from 150° to 175° shoulder abduction. (R) UE A/PROM continues to be limited secondary to clavicle fracture. Patient's endurance during performance of ADL activities has increased as demonstrated by her ability to tolerate increased resistance and perform increased number of repetitions with fewer rest periods.
	L) Hand Function: Patient recieved (L) wrist-driven flexor-hinge orthosis on 7-1-85. Patient is currently being trained it it's use. Patient is able to obtain a 7 pound palmar pinch with orthosis and is able to manipulate 2-3 inch weighted objects. Patient is able to don and doff orthosis independently. Patient will utilize the orthosis during self-care tasks, for self-catheterization process and vocational tasks.
	N) ADL: Patient is refusing to consistantly participate in self-care program on the nursing unit. Currently, she

PLAN/SHORT TERM GOAL/LONG TERM GOAL

(Continued on page 2)

THERAPIST ______________ 7-8-85 DATE

2-01359-10 (REV. 7/84)

MEDICAL RECORDS

Figure 28-1A Form has been reprinted with permission of the Rehabilation Institute of Chicago.

REHABILITATION INSTITUTE OF CHICAGO
Page 2 Of 2
OCCUPATIONAL THERAPY DEPARTMENT

PROGRESS NOTE

[X] Team Conference   [ ] Other__________

Key: ↑ Progress, ↓ Progress, — Status Quo, N/A Not Addressed

[X] Appropriate Box **(Use Black Ball Point Pen Only)**

Number of Days Seen 10

Period Covered From 6-24-85 To 7-8-85

Patient Name JS

RIC Number 010101

Physician

Date 7-8-85

[X] INPATIENT   [ ] OUTPATIENT

II PSYCHOSOCIAL

	↑	↓	—	N/A
BEHAVIOR		X		
INTERPERSONAL RELATIONSHIPS			X	
SEXUAL ADJUSTMENT				X

III COGNITIVE/COMMUNICATIVE

	↑	↓	—	N/A
DEVELOPMENT				X
MENTATION				X
SENSORY/PERCEPTUAL				X
COMMUNICATION				X

IV FUNCTIONAL SKILLS

	↑	↓	—	N/A
MOTOR FUNCTION	X			
HAND FUNCTION	X			
MOBILITY			X	
A.D.L.				
FEEDING	X			
ORAL FACIAL	X			
BATHING			X	
COMMUNICATION			X	
TOILETING			X	
DRESSING			X	
HOMEMAKING			X	
COMMUNITY SKILLS			X	

PROBLEMS #__________
(Assoc. problems, respiration, equipment, comm. planning etc.)

PROB #	
	Page 2 of 2
IV	Functional Skills: OBS (continued from page 1) is able to feed self I/S/E three meals a day. She requires assistance to open packages and cut food. Equipment includes a utensil cuff and bent utensils. Patient is able to change utensils independently. Patient is I/S/E with O/F hygiene requiring assistance to position self at sink and turn on the water due to limited mobility secondary to SOMI brace. She utilizes a utensil cuff to hold the toothbrush and is able to Independently apply toothpaste and clean-up. Patient is able to brush her hair using a brush with an adapted handle. She has difficulty reaching the Ⓡ side of her head due to ROM limitation.

PLAN/SHORT TERM GOAL/LONG TERM GOAL

1) Incorporate use of wrist driven flexor-hinge orthosis into daily self-care tasks.
2) Consistant performance of self-care tasks on nursing unit.
3) Decrease amount of set-up required for feeding and O/F hygiene.
4) I UE dressing

PLAN: Involve patient in a.m. program 5 times weekly. Provide adapted handles necessary for using wrist driven flexor-hinge orthosis during self-care tasks,

__________ THERAPIST   7-8-85 DATE

2-01359-10 (REV. 7/84)

MEDICAL RECORDS

OCCUPATIONAL THERAPY

Figure 28-1B

ination of the information contained therein. According to the American Hospital Association, confidential information in the medical record consists of reports based on examination, treatment, observation, or conversation with the patient.[2] Patient identification such as an address, dates of admission and discharge, names of spouse or nearest relative, and employer's name is considered nonconfidential information.[2] An institution or a hospital owns the medical record and may restrict removal of the record from the files or the premises and may determine who will have access to it or define the type of information that may be taken from it.[2] The patient has the right to examine his or her own medical record and may, for example, authorize release of the record for purposes of financial reimbursement, legal proceedings, or alternative medical opinions.[2]

The Problem Oriented Medical Record

One commonly used method of documentation which meets the requirements for documentation established by the Joint Commission on Accreditation of Hospitals (JCAH) and Medicare is referred to as the Problem-Oriented Medical Record (POMR).[1] It is often identified by the acronym SOAP, which represents components of the process—subjective, objective, assessment, and plan.[1] The subjective component of the POMR refers to the patient's disability and any symptoms or complaints. Any feelings or concerns expressed by the patient are also documented in this section. The objective component relates to the evaluation of the patient and includes present status and the therapist's and assistant's observations regarding progress or lack of progress. The assessment section deals with the patient's performance, the effectiveness of the current treatment plan, any expectation of changes in a given period of time, how the patient is reacting to treatment, as well as documentation of short- and long-term goals. The plan, which is the final component, identifies the patient's goals for each problem identified along with the planned treatment to achieve these goals. It is useful to incorporate the patient's own goals and his or her family's goals into this step. A statement regarding the need for continued or altered treatment as well as recommendations for additional testing or consultation by other team members should be included. Figure 28-1A and 28-1B presents an example of a Problem-Oriented Medical Record progress note. Figure 28-2 provides a compilation of problem areas which are printed on the reverse side of the progress note form. Figure 28-3A and 3B provides an example of a "generic" SOAP note form which can be used in a number of settings. The letter "L" with a circle around it means left, and "R" encircled means right; the abbreviation UE refers to the upper extremity. When using abbreviations, it is important to use only those approved by the facility.

OTR and COTA Documentation

The question of who is qualified to document in patient's charts is often asked. According to the *Entry-Level OTR and COTA Role Delineation* and the *Classification Standards for Occupational Therapy Personnel* published by AOTA, COTAs are qualified to document in patients' charts.[3] The countersignature of an OTR is not required but is recommended in some situations for the purposes of third party reimbursement. The following statement is reprinted from an article in the *Occupational Therapy Newspaper* which addressed the issue of countersignature requirements for COTAs: "COTAs work under the supervision of OTRs. It is the OTR's responsibility to evaluate and plan treatment programs. The COTA may then implement part or all of the program. If a COTA participates in the process of evaluation and planning and documents findings and recommendations, it is suggested that this note be co-signed by the OTR since these functions are ultimately the OTR's responsibility. In addition, co-signing is recommended in order to demonstrate compliance with the supervisory requirements of state and federal laws and regulations, and is necessary in order to receive reimbursement from third party payers."[3]

Preparation, Maintenance, and Safety of the Work Setting

Determining the utilization of space required to provide occupational therapy services as well as the equipment and supplies needed is a responsibility that rests primarily with the administrator of the department. The most effective system for developing and maintaining a given

Rehabilitation Institute of Chicago
Problem Oriented Medical Record
COMPILATION OF PROBLEM AREAS

I. Medical	
A. Medical Diagnosis	Primary medical, orthopedic, or neurological disorders (e.g., peripheral vascular disease, C-6 fracture, dislocation, right C.V.A., diabetes mellitus)
B. Impairment	Physical deficit (e.g., left hemiplegia, right B/K amputation, C-6 quadriplegia)
C. Associated Problems	Complications or secondary disorders related to primary medical diagnosis (for example, neurogenic bladder, dysphagia, respiratory status, infection, sacral decubitus, pain.)
II. Psychosocial	
D. Behavior	Disability adjustment, depression, anxiety, lability, denial, hostility
E. Interpersonal Relationships	Avocational, Recreational/Social activities, family, relationships
F. Sexual Adjustment	
III. Cognitive-Communicative	
G. Development	
H. Mentation	Orientation, intellectual dys., attention, judgement, impulsivity, calculation
I. Sensory/Perceptual Deficits	Visual motor, visual perception, proprioception
J. Communication	Speech, writing, reading, auditory comprehension
IV. Functional Skills	
K. Motor Function	Range of motion, strength, spasticity, coordination, endurance
L. Hand Function	Hand placement, prehension
M. Mobility	Bed, sitting-standing balance, transfers, wheelchair / ambulation, driving
N. ADL	Eating, dressing, O/F hygiene, toileting, homemaking
V. Vocational/Educational	
O. Planning	Vocational Diagnostic work-up, assets and liabilities for employment and/or training, testing and Work Evaluation results, vocational direction
P. Education-Training	Assets and liabilities for school or training, vocational plan, linkage and entry plan for proposed setting
Q. Job Placement	Placement plan, job interviews, type of work, employer, date hired and follow-up
VI. Community Planning	Preparation for community re-entry. Follow-up therapies, rechecks, housing, transportation; financial arrangements; equipment needs; architectural barrier, other community resources.

Figure 28-2 **Form has been reprinted with permission of the Rehabilation Institute of Chicago.**

work setting cannot be successful without the full cooperation and participation of all personnel who work in the area.

Environmental Considerations

The COTA and the OTR are responsible for identifying and communicating with the appropriate personnel regarding all issues and needs relevant to the patient population they serve. These may include, but are not limited to, issues relating to the treatment environment itself. For example, accessibility, lighting, noise levels, ventilation, maintenance, proper storage of equipment and supplies, as well as security measures, must all be considered. Identification of the type of treatment areas needed must be determined; some patients require a low stimulus rather than a high stimulus

NAME JB

Page 1 of 2

OCCUPATIONAL THERAPY

PROGRESS NOTES

PHYSICIAN

DATE	
7-1-85	S: Patient was oriented x3 today and was able to recall details of previous treatment session accurately. Patient's wife attended treatment session and reported that the patient actively participated in a card game with visitors the previous evening and required minimal verbal direction. Patient complained of fatique at start of treatment session but agreed to participate in 30 minute session. Patient requested that his wife be present during the treatment session.
	O: During the 30 minute treatment session the therapist reviewed A/PROM program with the patient and his wife. The wife assisted the patient with P/ROM of his Ⓛ UE. Nursing had reported that the patient was not carrying through with wearing his Ⓛ UE orthosis during the day or night. Instruction in the purpose and use of the patient's Ⓛ UE orthosis for positioning and to prevent further deformity was reviewed with the patient and his wife. Patient was observed during performance of his UE dressing. He required verbal and visual cueing to position his Ⓛ UE correctly. Once patient had extremities placed in the shirt sleeves correctly he was able to complete the task independently. Nursing was notified of patient's performance and instructed in the type of cueing needed. Patient shall perform UE dressing daily on the nursing unit.
	A: Patient appears to have adjusted to the hospital environment and become oriented to his situation. Patient responds well to treatment when instructions are given both verbally and visually and demonstrates retention of learned skills from treatment session to treatment session. No change is noted in Ⓛ UE function, however, patient was observed to be using the Ⓛ UE as a gross assist for

PROGRESS NOTES

Figure 28-3A

Page 2 of 2

OCCUPATIONAL THERAPY
PROGRESS NOTES

NAME JB

PHYSICIAN

DATE	
7-1-85	A: (continued from page 1) stabilization during UE dressing activity. Wife appears to be more comfortable with learning patient's care and was invited to attend treatment sessions whenever possible.
	P: 1) Continue daily A/PROM program to prevent contractures from non-use.
	2) Complete evaluation of functional abilities.
	3) Monitor patient performance of daily UE dressing and upgrade his a.m. program as indicated by patient performance.
	4) Refer patient and his wife to in-house educational program for stroke victims and their families.
	7-1-85

PROGRESS NOTES

Figure 28-3B

environment, while others may need an open rather than an isolated environment.

Space may be utilized for different purposes at different times of the day, a factor which will require coordination of schedules. Available space within a facility may be at a premium, and it is valuable if staff members can assist the administrator in developing creative ways to make use of space or identify alternative work areas. The goal is to utilize available space maximally for cost effectiveness, efficiency, and safety.

Continual monitoring of the work setting for evidence of worn out, broken, or depleted supplies and equipment is the responsibility of all occupational therapy personnel. A specific staff member, either an OTR or a COTA, may be assigned the responsibility of coordinating the repair or replacement of equipment and supplies. Many departments use nonprofessional staff, if available, for this function.

Safety Factors, Negligence and Malpractice Issues, and Infection Control

Safety awareness in the work setting is essential. Policies and procedures regarding the maintenance of a safe working environment are mandated by the majority of accrediting bodies. Safety includes such factors as the following:

1. Adherence of all staff members to infection control procedures.
2. Proper storage of toxic chemicals and flammable substances.
3. Use of proper clothing during the operation of certain equipment, such as power tools.
4. Knowledge of departmental and facility fire and other emergency plans.
5. Observance of precautions as they relate to specific diagnosis.

Risk management is the title given to the branch of management that deals with issues of liability. Negligence and malpractice are the primary liability areas that occupational therapy personnel need to be aware of in the work setting.

Negligence is a safety concern, and it refers to the failure to perform a task which would have been attended to properly under normal circumstances. It is often caused by heedlessness and carelessness.[4] Prevention is the key to maintaining a safe environment. All staff members should be aware of policies and practice them on a day-to-day basis. Examples include monitoring patients in reception areas and rest rooms and enforcing smoking regulations.

Malpractice relates to misconduct and lack of skill or care when performing professional duties. The COTA and the OTR can protect themselves from being named in a malpractice suit by adhering to a high standard of patient care, as dictated in the standards of practice for occupational therapy.[2] These standards have been reprinted in the Appendix. Both the OTR and the COTA engaged in practice should carry professional liability insurance. Most facilities maintain coverage for their personnel, but it is the responsibility of the individual practitioner to determine whether coverage is available and whether it is adequate. Related information appears in Chapter 30.

The proper storage of toxic chemicals and flammable substances is particularly important in the occupational therapy clinic owing to the presence of such items frequently used for avocational pursuits as well as the fabrication of orthotic devices and equipment. The use of proper protective clothing when using such substances and during the operation of power tools and equipment is essential. Face masks and gloves are recommended when working with toxic chemicals. Use of goggles to protect the face and eyes when operating power tools should be mandatory. Training and periodic review of the proper use of equipment and chemicals typically found in the department may be incorporated into the facility's orientation program for new staff members. It is also important that the facility provide thorough training for new employees in the specifics of both the departmental and the institutional procedures for fires and other emergencies.

A number of facilities require members of the staff to maintain current cardiopulmonary resuscitation (CPR) certificates and to provide periodic refresher courses. Knowledge of precautions as they relate to a given diagnosis is also essential as a preventative measure. Training in how to monitor a pulse rate or take a blood pressure reading, manage a seizure, or assist an individual who is choking is important for all occupational therapy personnel.

Infection control procedures have specific implications for occupational therapy departments because of the storage and utilization of food in the clinic setting. Proper storage and preparation of food are essential to minimizing the growth and spread of bacteria. Adherence to infection control procedures is of the utmost importance when working with a patient who is at risk for infecting others (e.g., herpes, hepatitis, and urinary tract and respiratory infections) as well as patients whose immune system is weakened secondary to their physical state.

Inventory, Supplies, and Equipment

Essential to the efficient operation of an occupational therapy program is an adequate supply of equipment and materials necessary to carry out treatment and operate the clinic efficiently. Responsibility for this particular function will vary within a given facility and must often be coordinated by the management body; however, the COTA may participate in some phase of this process.

In order to maintain an adequate supply of equipment and materials, some form of inventory system should be instituted. The complexity of the system will vary and be dependent upon such factors as:

1 Size of the occupational therapy department.
2 Quantity of supplies utilized during a given time period.
3 Availability and adequacy of storage space.
4 "Shelf life" of the materials.
5 Accessibility to vendors.
6 Delivery time for receiving ordered items.
7 Price of the items, including discounts given for quantity orders.

Well formulated inventory systems can greatly enhance the efficiency of re-ordering necessary supplies and equipment.

Large occupational therapy departments are often able to maintain a sizeable inventory of supplies and equipment which are issued to patients, while smaller departments may only be able to maintain an inventory of items for departmental use. As health care costs continue to escalate, administrators will be stressing the need to keep inventories as low as possible in order to decrease monies "tied up" and to maximize the use of storage space, possibly for other purposes. In addition, they will weigh any problems associated with the inability to provide equipment against the costs of processing purchasing orders. It is important that both the COTA and the OTR assist administration in identifying problems associated with maintaining an equipment supply and providing it for patient purchase, since they have direct contact with the consumer and can identify needs.

The departmental or institutional procedures for ordering equipment and supplies will influence the type of inventory system which is maintained. Information obtained through the inventory system will be used by the facility and departmental administration as well as staff members. One example of the way in which administration utilizes the occupational therapy department's inventory records is for the determination of the facility's total assets. Inventory records are also used as a basis for budget planning by administrators and may be utilized by occupational therapy personnel when determining the availability of equipment for patient issue or use.

An inventory system that may be used for recording equipment that is loaned temporarily to patients is referred to as a check-out system. The occupational staff member who loaned out the piece of equipment records the patient's name, a description of the equipment, the date loaned, the anticipated date of return, and the name of the responsible therapist or assistant on the appropriate form. When the equipment is no longer needed, the OTR or the COTA records the date that the equipment was returned on the original form and files it, and also checks the overall condition of the item. For example, suction cups might be missing from an adapted grab bar and need to be replaced before it is issued to another patient. This allows for an ongoing accounting and maintenance system of equipment in use as well as equipment available for use. More complex forms of inventory management may be utilized and the role of occupational therapy personnel will vary in maintaining these systems.

The specific procedures for ordering supplies and equipment will be determined by the administration and the department head in most cases.

It is important for all occupational therapy personnel to be aware of the many new products on the market through the review of professional journals, participation in continuing education activities, and attendance at the exhibits held at state and national conferences. A Resource Guide to equipment and supplies has been included in Appendix H to assist the occupational therapy assistant or therapist in identifying vendors that may provide occupational therapy services. Additional information may be obtained from the "Buyers Guide," published yearly in the the *American Journal of Occupational Therapy*. Specific information regarding small electronic devices and computers may be found in Chapters 26 and 27.

Reimbursement Procedures

Financial management of an occupational therapy department is the responsibility of the administrative staff. The department head establishes the budget and guidelines for expenditures, while the institutional management establishes the fees. Input into the development of the budget may be solicited from staff members in order to assist the director in determining monies needed for capital expenditures, such as major pieces of equipment and furniture, continuing education, and program development.

Occupational therapy is a revenue producing service in most settings, and it is the responsibility of individual therapists and assistants to submit accurate charges, either by units of time or for the specific cost of the occupational therapy service provided. Funding for occupational therapy services is obtained from both public and private sources. These may include the state and federal governments, private insurance companies, charities, foundations, endowments, and direct patient payment, depending on the facility.

Medicare and Medicaid

The major sources of public funding come from Medicare and Medicaid, which were established by Title XVII of the Social Security Act. They are federally funded insurance programs that provide medical benefits primarily for the aged, but benefits may also be received by persons who have been disabled for more than 24 months.[5] The standards for eligibility and services are established by the federal government. Previously, under this program, hospitals and other eligible health care facilities were reimbursed for their services under a cost-based reimbursement system whereby Medicare provided payment for services rendered based on what it cost the facility to provide a particular service.[6] Studies showed that the payments made for particular procedures or treatments were not consistent among service providers, and there was no apparent difference in the quality of care to account for the discrepancies.[6] This payment plan led to cost inflation in the health care field because there was no incentive for hospitals to operate more efficiently.

The Tax Equity and Fiscal Responsibility Act

The Tax Equity and Fiscal Responsibility Act of 1982 (TEFRA) was a major move toward changing hospital reimbursement under Medicare. This legislation included steps which placed limits on a hospital's inpatient charges. Adjustments were made to reflect each hospital's *case mix*, a term used to describe the types of disorders treated. In addition, it placed limits on the yearly rate of increase in total costs per patient treated and provided for incentive payments to be made to hospitals that were below the limits.[6] Historically, hospitals were reimbursed after a patient was discharged. Under the new system, reimbursement is determined prospectively.

Diagnostic Related Groups and Medicare

Further study by the Department of Health and Human Services resulted in the initiation of a new reimbursement procedure, based on the diagnosis of the patients treated, known as diagnostic related groups (DRGs). This system calls for a fixed price to be paid for each episode of illness regardless of the number of days that are spent in the hospital or the number of procedures performed.[6] Patients are classified according to 468 disease categories and conditions which include medical, surgical, psychiatric, and rehabilitation diagnoses. These categories were originally developed by researchers at Yale University and then utilized in the hospital reimbursement system of New Jersey, Maryland, and other states prior to use by Medicare.[5] DRGs are assigned to a Medicare patient upon discharge from a hospital based upon the following factors:[6]

1 The principal diagnosis.
2 The principle operating room procedure, if any.
3 Other diagnosis and procedures.
4 Age, sex, and discharge status.

Hospitals are paid a fixed rate for each Medicare patient regardless of what the actual cost of their treatment was. Provisions are available under the system to receive additional payment in cases in which there is an unusually long hospital stay and for patients who have accrued costs that exceed the DRG payment rate. These additional payments, however, must be reviewed by the Peer Review Organization established under the system. They will determine whether or not the additional costs are medically necessary and reasonable.

Currently, rehabilitation, psychiatric, children's, and long-term care hospitals as well as specific rehabilitation and psychiatric units within inpatient hospitals are exempt from the DRGs. A report was to be made to Congress by December 1985 regarding how these types of facilities can be phased into a DRG system.[7] The impact of the Medicare Diagnostic Related Groups on occupational therapy is not yet fully known. In light of the high cost of health care and restrictions imposed upon reimbursement for services, it is important that occupational therapy treatment be provided in the most efficient and cost effective manner possible. This will have a direct implication for staffing patterns, and more jobs will be available for the COTA. Increased emphasis is being placed on occupational therapy personnel in terms of productivity levels and the feasibility of increasing treatment times, while at the same time decreasing the length of time it takes to achieve goals. All occupational therapy practitioners should be familiar with reimbursement procedures and their impact on the services they provide.

Accreditation

Accreditation is the process by which an institution or facility is evaluated for its compliance with predetermined qualifications or standards by an agency or organization.[2] Most facilities are subject to regulations of some type. These facilities include acute care and rehabilitation hospitals, long-term care institutions, as well as mental health agencies and facilities. There are two major accrediting bodies that will be addressed in this chapter: the Joint Commission on Accreditation of Hospitals (JCAH) and the Commission on Accreditation of Rehabilitation Facilities (CARF).

JCAH is a private, voluntary, nonprofit organization comprised of representatives of the American Hospital Association, the American Medical Association, the American College of Physicians, and the American College of Surgeons.[2] Accreditation by JCAH has been used as a guideline and a requirement for certain public programs and funding agencies such as Medicare. By means of periodic on-site surveys, reviews of standards of care, methods of documentation, referrals, and management operations, data are gathered to support the decision to grant either full accreditation (three years) or provisional accreditation (one year).[2] Each department within a facility receives a request to present data which demonstrate their compliance with the standards set forth by the Joint Commission on Hospital Accreditation.

The Commission on Accreditation of Rehabilitation Facilities (CARF) is similar to JCAH except that it emphasizes the provision of rehabilitation services for the disabled population. Accreditation by CARF has become linked to funding agencies and public programs in much the same manner as JCAH has. Facilities may be accredited by more than one agency depending on the population they address and the services that they provide. For example, hospitals may provide both medical care and rehabilitation services. Individual states may require a process much the same as an accreditation process in order for a facility to receive a license to operate.

Program Evaluation and Quality Assurance

Program evaluation is an ongoing method of examining clinical outcomes and offers a factual, ready reference for both the staff and the consumer on what the program is accomplishing and how well it is being accomplished. The objective(s) of the program must be clearly established first, and then a set of measurable criteria can be

FIGURE 28-4. Program Evaluation: Quadriplegic Community Re-Entry Group*

*Please check appropriate response and comment, if so desired.

1. Do you feel that you have increased your awareness of how to plan for and actually get around in the community?
   ___ Yes ___ No
   Comment:

2. Do you feel that the information presented in this group related to your situation and/or needs?
   ___ Yes ___ No (If no, why not?)
   Comment:

3. Was there a particular program that you found to be:
   A. Most useful? (Why?)

   B. Least useful? (Why?)

4. Is there any additional information that you would like to see presented?

5. Do you feel that you will carry over the skills you learned in this group when in the community?
   ___ Yes ___ No
   Comment:

6. Do you feel that this group aided in your adjustment to your disability?
   ___ Yes ___ No
   Comment:

7. Please list any ideas you have that would improve this program.

8. Do you feel prepared to return to the community?
   ___ Yes ___ No
   Comment:

Thank you for taking time to complete this evaluation. The information will help us in improving the program for future participants.

Good luck and best wishes!!

*Developed by the Quadriplegic Community Re-entry Group Committee, 1984.
Reprinted with permission of Rehabilitation Institute of Chicago, Chicago, Illinois.

developed. If an area of the program demonstrates a decrease in its effectiveness, it may indicate that additional staff training is necessary or that changes or additions to the current program are needed. For example, if upon completion of a specialized program, patients are required to complete a program evaluation form that includes questions relating to areas of the program which did not meet their needs, then the program staff members will be able to examine the identified area or areas and take steps toward making improvements.

The Commission on Accreditation of Rehabilitation Facilities (CARF) places emphasis upon program evaluation in their accreditation process. Methods employed may include an interview with selected occupational therapy program participants or significant others, using a standard set of questions. An example of an individual program evaluation is shown in Figure 28-4.

The results of this form of program evaluation would be used to make ongoing changes in current programming. Four objectives can be met with program evaluation:[8]

1 Review of care provided to all patients.
2 Measurement of the outcomes achieved.
3 Reporting of treatment results on a regular basis.
4 Provision of feedback to the department regarding the achievement of goals.

In addition, program evaluation is an informational system that provides objective data that can be utilized in the decision making process, for research purposes, and to support program planning objectives. All levels of the staff are involved in the process of program evaluation. They may participate indirectly through providing feedback to administration and by maintaining accurate records of patient performance for evaluation purposes. As new programs are developed, a method of evaluation is also helpful in terms of justifying treatment outcomes to third party payers.

Quality assurance is another process which monitors patient care service delivery and its related components to assure that quality of care is maintained. Quality assurance programs are designed to utilize ongoing monitors in order to identify problems in the delivery of a service and to take steps toward remediating them. Focused studies may also be developed to demonstrate clinical outcomes. The Joint Commission on Accreditation of Hospitals requires that an effective quality assurance program be in place as a condition of accreditation.

The process of quality assurance involves five stages.[9] The initial stage is the process of identifying significant problems in patient care and prioritizing them. Stage two requires the application of some instrument for measuring the problem, such as standards of care. The third stage in the process is to produce plans which are directed toward improving the problem, and the fourth stage includes the actual implementation of a plan to improve a given problem. The fifth and final stage is the reassessment of the identified problem to determine whether the action has been effective. Documentation of these various steps must be kept and is reviewed during accreditation visits from JCAH.

Development of a quality assurance program is a management function. Staff members participate indirectly through identifying problem areas and reporting them to administration, by assisting administration in developing and implementing a plan which addresses the problem, and through ongoing feedback regarding the success or failure of the plan.

Meetings

Employee meetings are defined in the *Uniform Terminology for Reporting Occupational Therapy Services* as meetings of occupational therapy departmental staff members, both OTRs and COTAs, for the following purposes:[10]

1 Disseminating and receiving information.
2 Conveying information concerning the administrative policies of the institution and/or conditions of employment.
3 Discussing issues relevant to the management of the program.
4 Discussing issues relating to the development of the department and/or institution and its relationship to total health care.

Individual staff members are responsible for having knowledge and understanding of the policies and procedures of a given department and/or facility, and this information can be most effectively disseminated through such employee meetings. Attendance at these meetings is usually mandatory and should be considered a professional responsibility. Active participation in meetings of this nature is strongly recommended.

Program-related conferences are interdepartmental meetings which are held for the purpose of communicating issues relevant to the planning, development, and management of specific programs.[10] The COTAs report directly on issues relating to programs they are involved in or issues relevant to their role in the department.

Supervisory meetings between the OTR and COTA may be formal or informal depending upon the individual situation. The type of supervision available (close or general) and the needs of the individual COTA will influence the frequency of such meetings.

Continuing Education and Inservice Training

Regardless of experience, participation in continuing education and inservice training is a necessary part of professional life and required by most accrediting agencies. Inservice education refers to in-house seminars, regularly scheduled classes, and special training sessions that are provided within or outside of the facility.[10] It is the general purpose of such programs to provide an opportunity for personnel to enhance their knowledge, skills, and attitudes and for new staff to acquire basic skills. Programs may be related to clinical techniques, interpersonal skills, administrative issues, issues relevant to practice, supportive functions such as infection control, cardiopulmonary resuscitation and emergency procedures, or interdisciplinary sharing of expertise and services available (e.g., special programs, new equipment, demonstration of a treatment technique, clarification of roles).

Inservice educational opportunities allow for dissemination of information regarding programming, equipment demonstrations, research results, utilization of staff, and so forth and provide a good opportunity for staff to develop teaching skills. The COTA may be involved in the planning and implementation of such programming. The department as a whole should establish priorities for continuing education needs that address current trends in patient care. The frequency of departmental inservice programs will be determined by the individual facility and may be held jointly with other disciplines. Many larger institutions have designated staff positions for the planning and implementation of such programs, while others delegate this responsibility to clinical staff.

Continuing education refers to ongoing educational experiences beyond the basic educational level that enrich or enhance the individual's knowledge, skills, and attitudes toward his or her work performance.[10] Continuing education programs are designed to provide occupational therapy personnel with an opportunity to maintain or upgrade their knowledge, skills, and performance level. Mandatory participation in a continuing education program is not required currently by AOTA for maintenance of certification in occupational therapy as it is in some other professions such as nursing, medicine, and respiratory therapy. However, The American Occupational Therapy Association is currently exploring methods of incorporating requirements for continuing education into an annual recertification process. Regardless of whether continuing education is required, it remains the responsibility of both the COTA and the OTR to maintain a level of knowledge that incorporates the current trends of the profession. The COTA, for example, should keep informed through journal review, inservice education, and attendance at workshops and conferences.

The availability of funding for participating in continuing education programs may be limited in some facilities. The individual occupational therapy practitioner must be prepared to assume at least a portion of the costs associated with these programs. Money spent on continuing education is a tax deductible expense.

The limited availability of continuing education programs designed to meet the needs of the COTA has been a persistent problem for many years. Recent strides have been made to increase program offerings for COTAs at the AOTA national conference, and state associations have been strongly encouraged to promote continuing education programs for the COTA.

Public Relations

Increasing the public awareness of occupational therapy through marketing of services and publicity can increase the visibility of the profession and its services at a time when competition for health care is high. Occupational therapy is not yet a household word and often is misunderstood. It is necessary that the individual COTA and OTR working in the field promote his or her services. Included in the population to be educated are other health professions, third-party payers, legislators, consumers, and the public. A public relations program can serve a number of purposes, which include:[11]

1. Enhancing the role of the profession in the community.
2. Bringing available services to the attention of potential patients.
3. Increasing the visibility of occupational therapy within the practice setting.

4 Attracting potential students.
5 Demonstrating the value of services to society.

Public awareness of occupational therapy has increased in recent years. This is due in part to the heightened awareness of all occupational therapy personnel of the importance of educating the public about their services. Licensure has increased the visibility of occupational therapy on the state level while the work of the Government and Legal Affairs Division of AOTA has resulted in national attention. The Public Affairs Division of AOTA has developed a manual targeting occupational therapy in public relations activities which is available to the membership. It provides ideas and suggestions for the development of public relations strategies and materials. In addition, AOTA has a number of brochures, posters, and films available which may be used by the membership to promote occupational therapy.

Individual facilities may choose to develop their own plan for education and promotion. A variety of methods may be implemented, such as inservice training for other health professionals, development of a display which depicts occupational therapy procedures and services, sponsoring an open house in the occupational therapy department, development of audiovisual materials to be used for promotional purposes, providing tours of their clinics, and participating in local health fairs or career days.

Research

Research, as defined in the *Uniform Terminology for Reporting Occupational Therapy Services*, refers to the formalized investigation of activities for the purposes of improving the quality of occupational therapy patient care by means of recognized scientific methodologies and procedures.[10] Therapists and assistants have traditionally not been research oriented. Concern for the lack of attention given to research was the subject of a portion of an editorial written by Charles Christiansen, editor of *The Occupational Therapy Journal of Research*. He states that "research continues to be viewed commonly as an activity foreign to our clients (patients) and irrelevant to our practice."[12] Christiansen argues that we cannot remain competitive in a time of limited resources for health care dollars unless we have research to validate our claims of efficacy and value.[12] Research begins in the clinic. Therapists need to substantiate what they do and determine what is true and what is false.[13]

The American Occupational Therapy Foundation (AOTF) is a sister body to the American Occupational Therapy Association, and it has assumed much of the responsibility for guiding the research efforts of the profession. Through the foundation, a number of grants and educational funds have been made available for the pursuit of research activities. In addition, the Foundation maintains a resource library available to students, practitioners, and researchers, and publishes the *Occupational Therapy Journal of Research* (OTJR).

Research skills are usually taught at the Master's level of our profession. Professional level students generally are provided with basic principles and methods while technical level students receive minimal information. The clinic is an important site of research activities, and COTAs may assist in the development of the research question or questions through reporting observations and by identifying potential areas for research. In addition, they may also assist in the research process through compiling, posting, and recording specific data.

Summary

All COTAs should have a clear understanding of the service management functions in the facility or institution where they are employed. Knowledge of their roles in the areas of scheduling, record maintenance, preparation, and safe maintenance of the work area, inventory and ordering supplies is of the utmost importance. Accreditation procedures, program evaluation, and quality assurance activities all have components which directly involve the occupational therapy assistant. Although service management is primarily an administrative function, it is supported by all levels of personnel. Responsibilities and specific tasks will be assigned by the administration or the supervising occupational therapist. The *Entry-Level OTR and COTA Role Delineation*, which has been reprinted in Appendix E, provides a framework for the administrator, supervisor, and staff person to follow. As experience is gained,

COTAs may increase their participation and assume greater responsibility for service management functions.

Of equal importance is that the COTA recognize the value of meetings, continuing education, public relations, and research activities which relate to their overall growth as well as the growth of the profession and the facility where they are employed.

References

1. Division of Practice: I'm glad you asked. *Occup Ther Newspaper*, 37(October):13, 1983.
2. *Manual on Administration*. Rockville, MD: American Occupational Therapy Association, 1978.
3. Division of Practice: I'm glad you asked. *Occup Ther Newspaper*, 37(September):7, 1983.
4. Rowland H, Rowland B: *Hospital Administration Handbook*. Rockville, MD: Aspen Systems, 1984.
5. Levine R: Community health care The homebound patient. In: Hopkins H and Smith H, Eds: *Willard and Spackman's Occupational Therapy*, 6th Edition. Philadelphia: JB Lippincott, 1983, p 773.
6. Executive summary of the Department of Health and Human Services report to Congress on hospital prospective payment for Medicare. *Federal Report*. Rockville, MD: American Occupational Therapy Association, 83-5(May):3-7, 1983.
7. Medicare prospective payment. *Occup Ther Newspaper*, 38(October): 4, 1984.
8. Joe BE: Quality assurance consultants add program evaluation to repertoire. *Occup Ther Newspaper*, 38(April):5, 1984.
9. Ostrow PC: Quality assurance—Improving occupational therapy. In: Hopkins H and Smith H, Eds: *Willard and Spackman's Occupational Therapy*, 6th Edition. Philadelphia: JB Lippincott, 1983, p 862 .
10. *Uniform Terminology for Reporting Occupational Therapy Services*. Rockville, MD: American Occupational Therapy Association, 1979.
11. Publicity and professionalism. *Occup Ther Newspaper*, 37(December): 7, 1983.
12. Christiansen C: Research: An economic imperative. *Occup Ther J of Research*, 37:195-198, 1983.
13. Yerxa EJ: The occupational therapist as a researcher. In Hopkins H and Smith H, Eds: *Willard and Spackman's Occupational Therapy*, 6th Edition. Philadelphia: JB Lippincott, 1983, p 870.

Bibliography

Guide for supervision of occupational therapy personnel. *Reference Manual of the Official Documents of the American Occupational Therapy Association*. Rockville, MD: American Occupational Therapy Association, Chapter 5, 1983.

HCFA moves to implement medicare payment system. *Occup Ther Newspaper*, 37(August):3, 1983.

Acknowledgments

The author wishes to express sincere thanks and gratitude to Shari Intagiata, MS, MPA, OTR/L for her encouragement and persistence throughout the many phases of writing this chapter. The project could never have been completed without her guidance and support. Special appreciation is also extended to the author's many colleagues at the Rehabilitation Institute of Chicago for their support and understanding.

SECTION VI

Contemporary Issues and Trends

The theme for the final section of this text is recapitulation and integration. In other words, the goals of the authors, in part, are to restate, review and sum up various issues related to the education and practice of the certified occupational therapy assistant. Several concepts are combined and unified as a professional whole. The major focus is threefold.

Beginning with a review of the maturation process of the COTA in terms of intraprofessional relationships and socialization, the content builds to encompass principles of occupational therapy ethics as they relate to a variety of practice situations.

The concluding epilogue redefines the impact of social forces in relation to the culture of occupational therapy. Values are re-examined in terms of historical, current and future impact. Gilfoyle states, "Through transformation we will direct our future. The time for promotion of the idea 'health through doing' is now. It is the era where occupational therapy can proclaim its uniqueness as the therapeutic use of occupations to facilitate abilities so that individuals can influence the state of their own health."

CHAPTER **29**

Intraprofessional Relationships and Socialization: The Maturation Process

Toné F. Blechert, COTA
Marianne F. Christensen, OTR

Introduction

The process by which a certified occupational therapy assistant becomes socialized into the profession of occupational therapy includes a number of factors: acquisition of skills and knowledge to do the work of an occupation; the development and orientation of attitudes and behaviors needed for the specific role; and a commitment that motivates the person to pursue the occupation and feel accepted by the professional community.[1]

A student entering the field of occupational therapy has a partially developed value and belief system that has contributed to attitudes and behaviors that compelled the person to enter a health care field. Through the use of a process model, the steps in the development of socialization are outlined as shown in Figure 29-1. These steps include:

1 Mastery of entry-level knowledge and skills.
2 Practical application of technical knowledge and skills (*i.e.*, field work experiences).
3 Entry-level work experience.
4 Self-enhancement activities leading to new dimensions of knowledge, skill, and sensitivity.[2]
5 Commitment to life-long learning and to the profession: the socialized self.

Within this framework, patterns of supervision, team building strategies including intraprofessional and interprofessional relationships, and conflict management principles will be discussed.

Choosing a Career in Occupational Therapy

Women and men who begin to consider a career in occupational therapy at the professional or technical level are drawn from a diverse group

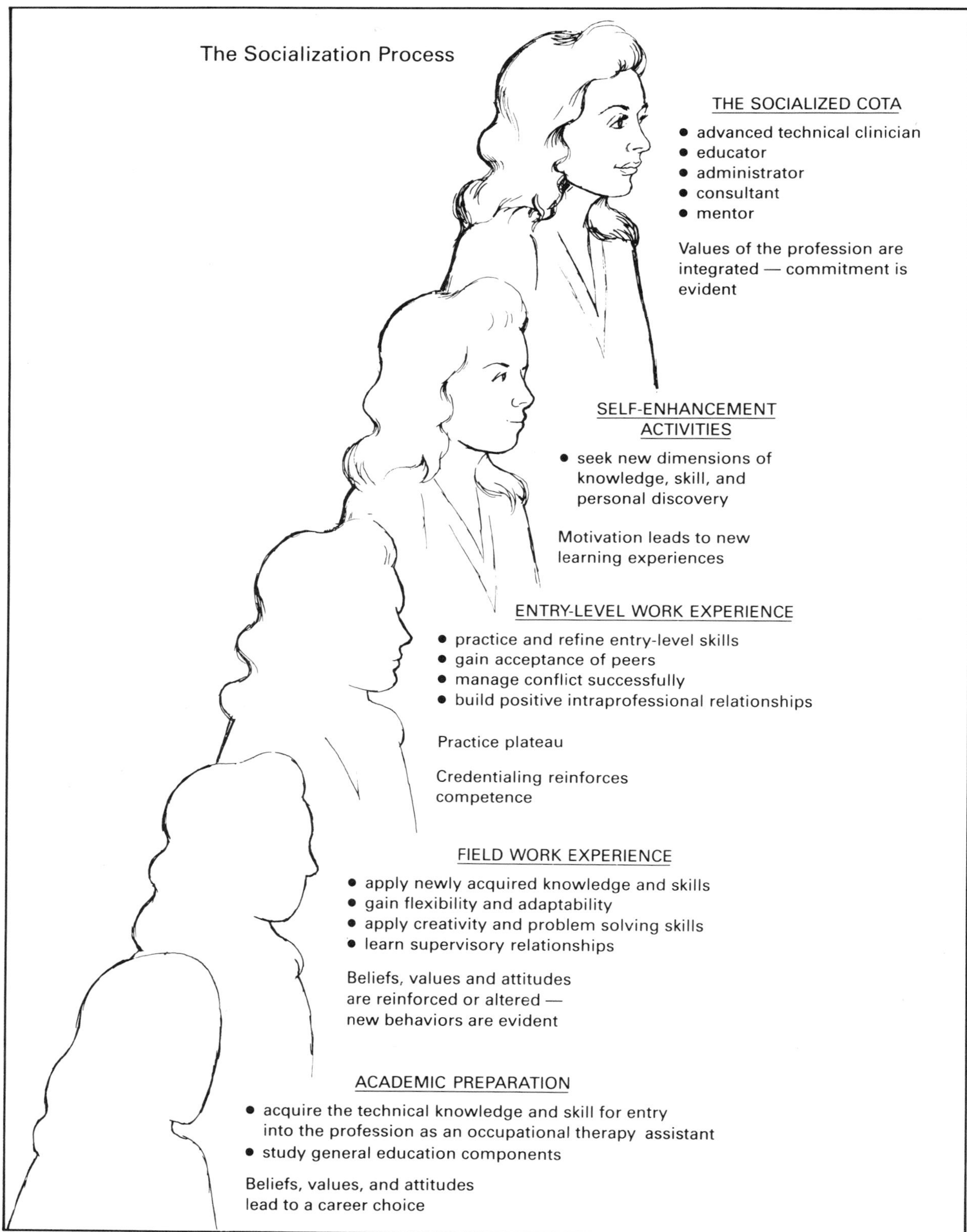
The Socialization Process
THE SOCIALIZED COTA
• advanced technical clinician
• educator
• administrator
• consultant
• mentor
Values of the profession are integrated — commitment is evident
SELF-ENHANCEMENT ACTIVITIES
• seek new dimensions of knowledge, skill, and personal discovery
Motivation leads to new learning experiences
ENTRY-LEVEL WORK EXPERIENCE
• practice and refine entry-level skills
• gain acceptance of peers
• manage conflict successfully
• build positive intraprofessional relationships
Practice plateau
Credentialing reinforces competence
FIELD WORK EXPERIENCE
• apply newly acquired knowledge and skills
• gain flexibility and adaptability
• apply creativity and problem solving skills
• learn supervisory relationships
Beliefs, values and attitudes are reinforced or altered — new behaviors are evident
ACADEMIC PREPARATION
• acquire the technical knowledge and skill for entry into the profession as an occupational therapy assistant
• study general education components
Beliefs, values, and attitudes lead to a career choice

Figure 29-1

representing a broad range of developmental needs, attitudes, values, and behaviors. However, studies have shown that one value held in common is the wish to contribute to the welfare of others.[3,4]

There are certain steps that the careful planner goes through in order to make career choices. These steps are as follows:

1 *Discovery*: The individual examines past accomplishments, present activities, and plans for the future. At this point usually some dissatisfaction can be noted which motivates the person to explore alternatives.

2 *Focus*: The individual spends time and energy searching for information related to possible alternatives. Exploration of levels of occupational therapy education should occur at this point. This early orientation process begins the socialization process.

3 *Validation*: In this stage, the planning and choices become more integrated, and the individual begins to share decisions with others in order to receive feedback and confirmation.

4 *Implementation*: This is the stage in which action toward the decision occurs. A time commitment is made and a school is selected, beginning a new phase of learning.[5]

Acquisition and Mastery of Entry-level Knowledge and Skills

Occupational therapy assistant education molds the student's orientation to his or her work. There are several basic frames of reference used in these curricula. Whichever frame of reference is favored, the curriculum must be tied to that framework which creates an organized body of knowledge. There are a variety of teaching methods used to convey this material. With close attention to the *Essentials of an Approved Educational Program for the Occupational Therapy Assistant* developed by the American Occupational Therapy Association, a curriculum design may include focus on principles and technical concepts in a variety of disability areas; fieldwork experiences to enhance that learning; opportunities to develop communication skills; and general education components. Involvement in this educational process may reinforce existing attitudes and values or allow them to change. Behaviors and even personalities may be altered. These changes occur as the student is exposed to the new concepts and experiences that the curriculum has to offer.

All students receive feedback during their education. The activities learned in the occupational therapy program provide unique opportunities for the student to receive feedback from nonhuman objects as well as instructors, clinical supervisors, patients, and peers. This ongoing feedback is the beginning of the student's ability to make critical changes in thinking and actions. As a result, students begin to perceive themselves as interpersonally and technically competent. This sense of mastery enables them to progress to higher levels of socialization.

Practical Application

Mastery of occupational therapy concepts and altered or reinforced beliefs and attitudes are the basis for the next step in the socialization process. It is here that the practical application of knowledge and skills occurs. In a professional or technical education program, fieldwork is the method used to provide this practical experience. During fieldwork, a student will not only apply acquired information but will also be exposed to new knowledge and methods. The problem solving skills gained during academic preparation are used as the student discovers possible alternatives in relating to patients and providing treatment. This also requires adaptability and flexibility on the part of the student.

Adaptability refers to the skill enabling one to easily and quickly conform to new and strange circumstances. Flexibility is the willingness and openness that one must have in order to be able to adapt. If a person is rigid or "set in his or her ways," there is less ability to adapt to new situations that arise. This may apply to new patient treatment techniques and approaches as well as relating to and interacting with new people, such as supervisors and coworkers.

Philosophies of treatment are changing in the health care field, and facilities and agencies vary in their styles and methods of treatment. The continuum may range from a predominant focus on prevention and the issues of health and wellness to the traditional medical model still found in many hospitals. Hopefully, the student can face these varied situations with a flexible attitude. One should be able to utilize the problem solving skills, creativity, and baseline of knowledge gained during classroom experiences to adapt to and meet new challenges.

Supervision

One necessary competence is that of acceptance of supervision. The relationships that are formed between students and supervisors are crucial in the socialization process. It is primarily the supervisor who defines the relationship between himself or herself and the student during a field work experience. It is the supervisor's behavior that signals to the student the dimensions of their relationship.

The sooner that a student can understand the social system and goals of a particular field work setting, the more likely the student is to have success. The idea of a psychological contract between an individual and a work place seems to have been originated in 1962 by Levinson, a clinical psychologist who became interested in mental health and work. As he studied workers entering a new company, Levinson observed a process of fulfilling mutual expectations and satisfying mutual needs in the relationship between a person and his or her work. Levinson described this process as reciprocation. Reciprocation is a process of carrying out a psychological contract between a person and company or any other institution where one works.[6]

According to Levinson's observations, an individual entering a work situation has certain expectations and needs, many of which are subconscious. Whether one is a student entering a fieldwork setting or a person beginning a new job, there is a hope that the work environment, the job itself, and relationships with supervisors and coworkers will fulfill these needs and expectations.

A fieldwork setting's expectations may be very clear and in writing as far as objectives and assignments are concerned, but where behavior is concerned, the expectations may be less clear. Whether the student is expected to be independent, warm, assertive, or distant with other therapists or the supervisor is seldom communicated formally. However, these expectations do exist and the student's ability to adapt quickly to the social system is a strong predictor of success. So it is in any work situation as the individual worker wants the work setting to satisfy his or her needs, and the work place wants the individual to satisfy its needs and help achieve its goals.

This is the psychological contract and its fulfillment depends on how well the reciprocity works. If the individual student or worker and the work place are able to satisfy each other's needs, the individual will tend to identify with the work place and consider his or her role appreciated and important.

The psychological contract identified by Levinson describes three needs which each person has to some degree when entering a work situation. These needs are for *ministration, mastery*, and *maturation*.[6]

Ministration needs for a student are needs for feeling close to others in the work setting and for support, guidance, and protection.[6] Of course, some students may need a significant amount of support in their work, while others may require very little. Students are not likely to tell a supervisor how much support is needed in order to function effectively; however, a supervisor will often sense these needs in the students' behavior. It is important for students to take responsibility for communicating any feelings of discomfort or lack of support. If the supervisor is unable to provide the support needed, he or she should be prepared to offer the students other sources of gratification. If the students' need for ministration is met, they are likely to perceive the work place as "caring."

The need for mastery is concerned with the desire to explore, understand, and, to some extent, control oneself and an environment.[6] A fieldwork supervisor who is sensitive to the student's need for mastery will provide the student with an appropriate measure of control early in the fieldwork experience. This may take the form of offering choices in assignments or patient groups, for instance. Supervisors usually appreciate a student's interest in achieving more independence; therefore, it is important to verbalize one's goals and needs. For the occupational therapy assistant student, important competencies to be achieved must include more than those relevant to patient treatment. For example, the ability to deal adequately with professionals from other departments

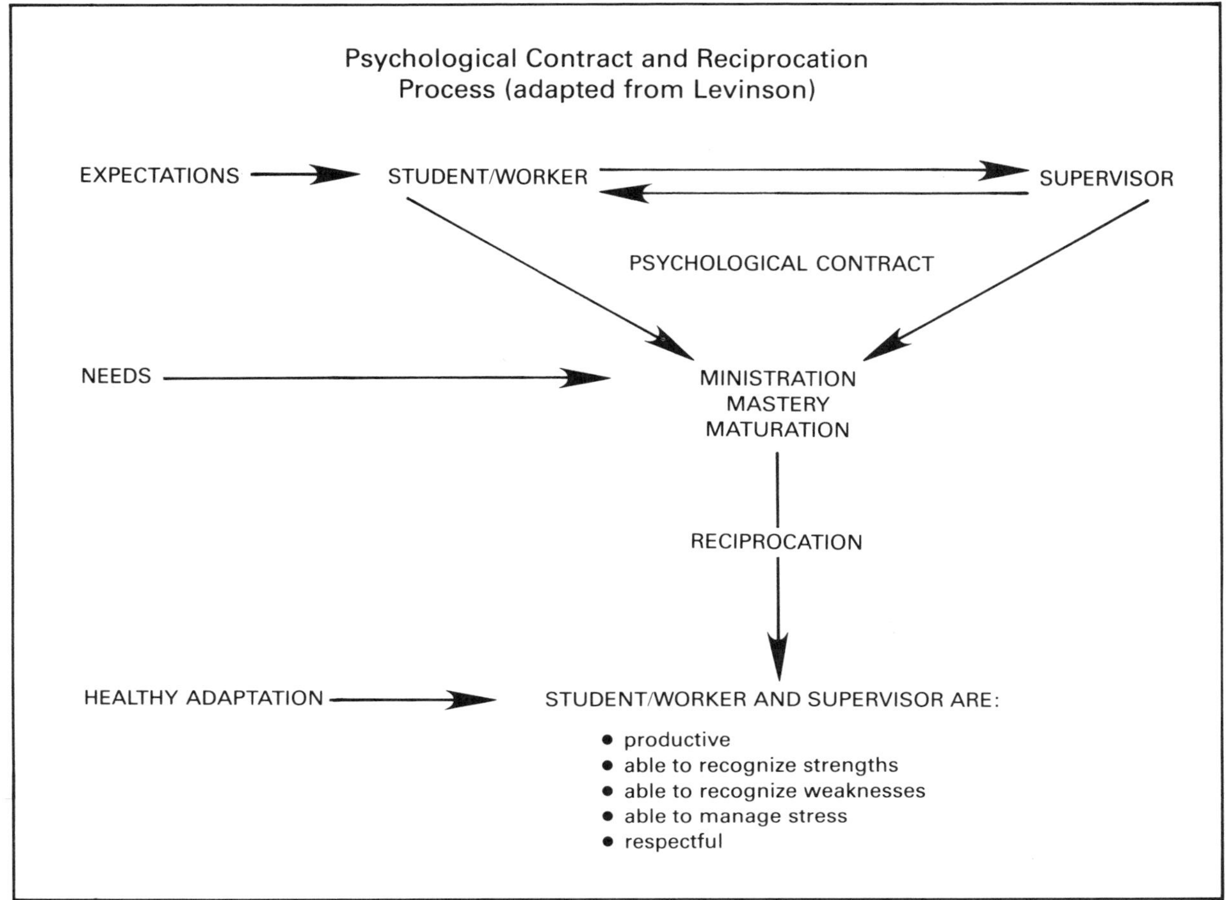

Figure 29-2

as well as other occupational therapy personnel should be an important goal.

If maturation needs are met, a person unfolds; if they are not, he or she vegetates.[6] Fieldwork provides reality testing opportunities for a student as concepts learned in school are applied in a real situation. This reality testing takes the form of feedback from supervisors and patients as a result of one's efforts. Feedback provides a student with the sense of growth necessary for some maturation to take place.

These concepts of the psychological contract and the reciprocation process as it is adapted to the interaction between fieldwork supervisor and students are summarized in Figure 29-2. Both supervisor and student bring expectations to the relationship. If the reciprocation process works, the student's needs will be satisfied and he or she will be able to perform at his best level. Just as the supervisor satisfies the student's needs so the student, though he or she doesn't have control of the relationship, can potentially satisfy the supervisor's needs, particularly for ministration and mastery, but not for maturation. The supervisor also has some need for closeness, warmth, and caring, as well as for mastery of the environment.

Entry Level Work Experience

Following the required fieldwork experiences, the student has fully completed the formal educational process and is ready to enter the work arena. Although there may be anxiety associated with leaving familiar environments to enter a new work environment, there is also a feeling of excitement and of competence which is then reinforced after successful completion of the certification examination.

As a COTA begins a first work experience, another phase in the maturing process begins. Many of the experiences, feelings, and behaviors that were initially and perhaps superficially developed during fieldwork will be enhanced and encountered in more depth during the first work experience. The new COTA will be meeting new challenges, practicing and refining skills, and continuing to gain acceptance from peers, patients, and the public.

Acceptance

Feeling accepted is a crucial phase in the socialization process of the COTA. If there isn't a feeling of respect and acceptance, particularly from the supervisor, it will be difficult to perform adequately and feel confident and satisfied. If dissatisfaction occurs, the motivation to achieve may decline. This is an indicator that ministration needs are not being met. It is at this point that the COTA may examine choices. If there is an investment in the profession and job because other satisfactions exist, there will be energy to remedy the situation. If other satisfactions or investments are not present, the COTA may choose a different path, such as a new job or different training.

There are many ways to remedy the situation and to gain acceptance if one chooses to try. First, it is important to enmesh oneself in the culture of the facility. Learning what is acceptable in terms of dress, language, and general expectations and establishing oneself as a member of a multidisciplinary team will strengthen one's connection with a particular work place. As a COTA begins to feel increased acceptance and respect, relationships will develop and the assistant will feel bonded to the setting. Four major aspects of work that encourage bonding are:[7]

1 The general nature of the work, its challenge, and the use it requires of one's talents.
2 Freedom to perform the work, to employ personal ideas, to feel vital in the efforts bringing about work accomplishment, and to make decisions about work.
3 Opportunities to grow and to develop through training, to receive feedback on performance, and to receive a reasonable variety of assignments.
4 Recognition of work achievement in a forthright, sincere, and timely manner.

The needs for ministration, mastery, and maturation also remain constant from the student role to that of an entry-level worker. As the ministration and mastery needs are met, maturation will occur. The work experience allows even more time for this process than the fieldwork experience because both work investment and time commitment are greater.

Team Building

Becoming a respected and accepted member of the team is an important goal. Effective team work can contribute to the welfare of patients, create high morale among staff members and foster an educational climate in the work setting.[8]

The term teamwork is often associated with morale. Morale refers to the attitudes of the employees in a department, whereas teamwork is the smoothly coordinated and synchronized action achieved by a closely knit group of employees.[8]

In an occupational therapy department effective teaming is built on the character and competencies of its members. Team efforts are strengthened as members improve their professional and personal abilities. For example, with practice and experience, an OTR or COTA team member may emerge as an expert in splinting techniques. Performance in this area may become so outstanding that no other team members could equal it. Another OTR or COTA may become an expert without equal in the use of effective group skills. One dynamic strength of teamwork is that it frees each member to do some of the things he or she is best at doing in the occupational therapy process.

Occupational therapy personnel who are satisfied, contributing team members are helpful to patients and each other. These individuals demonstrate a basic personal security. They are most often those who are confident of their knowledge and abilities and comfortable and honest about their limitations.

Among the necessary qualities of a successful occupational therapy assistant, there are several worthy of discussion as they relate to effective teamwork. These include the following areas:

Cooperation: Team members work together to achieve common goals. In this effort each individual must pay attention to details that make cooperation possible. The OTRs and COTAs on the team must be well informed of one another's activities. Cooperation allows the opportunity to teach and learn, to give and receive, and to increase the competence of all involved. A respectful attitude towards the other members of one's team is extremely important. As people work together more closely, they learn a great deal about each other. Team members must be discreet and avoid petty gossip. Cooperation is more difficult if trust is broken.

Flexibility: A successful team member sees change as a positive element. Changing approaches and methods must be met with an open and accepting mind. This openness to change encourages all team members to think creatively and express ideas freely.

Creativity: Occupational therapy personnel pride themselves on their creative abilities. Certainly one would hope for an atmosphere that encourages creativity among staff members. Creativity implies individuality but should never be construed as unrestrained liberty.[7] Teamwork demands an environment that is permissive enough to allow new ideas to develop and yet structured enough to provide order and direction for all members.

In addition to cooperation, flexibility, and creativity, one must also be aware of the purpose and philosophy of the work setting and understand his or her own duties and the duties of other department members. It is important for accurate and specific job descriptions to be available to all department members. A job description is a list of the tasks which one is expected to perform. A written copy of one's job description as well as those of co-workers should be available so that no misunderstandings occur.

Interdepartmental Teaming

The purpose of an interdepartmental treatment team is to provide the best possible service to the patient by the sharing of information and expertise and the coordination of services. The treatment team may be headed by a physician or other health professional depending upon the setting. The members of the team may include anyone who works with the patient in any capacity. Other team members may be from the physical therapy, therapeutic recreation, nursing, social service, vocational counseling, or dietary department. The following information describes the roles of these team members in various settings.

Physician: A physician is a medical doctor who practices the science and art of preventing and curing disease and preserving health. Occupational therapy personnel work with physicians who have varying specialty backgrounds. A *physiatrist* is a medical doctor who specializes in physical medicine. A *psychiatrist* specializes in mental illness. These two specialists often direct treatment teams in the hospital setting.

Clinical psychologist: The psychologist is not a medical doctor, although he or she may have a Ph.D. degree. A clinical psychologist functions in three areas: diagnosis, psychotherapy, and research. The psychologist administers diagnostic tests and interviews. Psychological tests are made up of a kind of standard situation in which varying reactions of different patients may be observed. Many people are reluctant to reveal their thoughts in an interview, but may show a characteristic way of thinking in response to tests. Psychotherapy may be done with individual patients or in patient groups, and families may be involved. Psychologists have a backgound in statistics and research methods and are prepared to assist staff members who wish to do research by helping to construct experimental procedures and interpret results.

Nursing service: The role of the nurse is to be aware of the total nursing needs of the patients. The nurse is responsible for seeing that these are fulfilled through preparing, administering, and supervising a patient care plan for each patient. This involves evaluation of the physical, spiritual, and emotional needs of the patient. The scientific basis for applying scientific principles in performing nursing procedures and techniques must be known. The nurse must be able to perform therapeutic measures prescribed and delegated by the physician and must be able to observe and evaluate patient symptoms, reactions, and progress.

Social service: The role of the social worker is to provide contact between the patient and the community, enabling one to make the best use of the resources available. Social workers may work in public or private hospitals, community settings such as welfare agencies, centers for emotionally disturbed children, corrections institutions and schools. In a private hospital, referrals come from the physicians for the discussion of such problems as lack of funds, placement of elderly patients in nursing homes, and similar community related needs. The patient is helped by referral to an appropriate agency.

Physical therapy: Physical therapy is the treatment of patients with disabilities resulting from disease or injury. Some of the modalities that are used in physical therapy include: light therapy, which involves ultraviolet and infrared light; electrotherapy, which may involve diathermy and electrical stimulation; hydrotherapy, which includes such things as the Hubbard tank, whirlpool and contrast baths; mechanical therapy, which involves massage, traction, and therapeutic exercise of various kinds; and thermotherapy, which involves heat such as paraffin baths and whirlpool. The purpose of the treatment may be to relieve pain, to increase function to a part by improving muscle strength and joint range of motion, or to teach patients to ambulate with the help of crutches, canes, and other ambulatory aides.

Therapeutic recreation: Therapeutic recreation is the use of free play, exercise, and other activity to meet treatment needs. Group recreation may encourage more positive relationships with others, improve the body image, allow an outlet for emotional release, aid circulation and other body functions, and provide enjoyment and relaxation. Some activities used in therapeutic recreation are swimming, music, games and contests, dancing, dramatics, special events, and outings. Leisure counseling is also provided.

Vocational counseling: The vocational counselor may be employed by a federal rehabilitation organization such as Vocational Rehabilitation or by the institution itself to test patients' vocational abilities. A patient may have to change occupations depending upon the extent of the illness or injury. For instance, a truck driver who has had a heart attack may need to find a less demanding job. The vocational counselor administers aptitude tests and does predischarge planning for special training and job placement. The OTR and COTA may work with the vocational counselor in evaluating the patient's work tolerance, coordination, and special skills. The vocational counselor is concerned with postdischarge plans of the patient.

Dietician: The function of the dietary department is to prepare and serve food for the patients. This includes planning and preparing many special diets. The occupational therapy assistant may be asked to be present at meal time to help the patient with physical disabilities, as following a stroke, to learn to feed himself again. The occupational therapy department must work with the dietary department in scheduling needs for various activities.

In summary, the COTA must understand the functions of other departments so as to encourage mutual respect and sound working relationships; recognize the importance of the other treatment procedures; communicate scheduling needs and changes; and cooperate in order to provide the best possible treatment.

Managing Conflict

Despite all of the positive aspects and efforts of teaming, it is inevitable that conflict will arise at some point. Conflict does not have to be a negative factor and can, in fact, improve situations and stimulate personal growth, if it is identified and dealt with in an appropriate way. It should be noted, however, that effective problem solving aimed at conflict resolution cannot take place without some conflicts over ideas and opinions.

Pre-existing conditions involving relationships and situations can lead to conflict. These conditions can include a conflict of interest between two people; physical, emotional, or time factors which lead to communication barriers; economic or emotional dependence of one person on another; or previous unresolved conflicts.[9]

These pre-existing conditions can lead to either perceived or actual conflict. *Perceived conflict* is that which is felt by a person that may or may not lead to actual conflict; *actual conflict* is that which does happen. It usually involves an awareness of disagreement and may involve personal hostilities.

The *manifest behavior* is the reaction of the individuals that occurs in response to conflict. This may be in the form of an argument, debate, or any type of confrontation. It may also be less overt but is evident in nonverbal body language between two people.

The *resolution* or *suppression* phase is perhaps the most crucial. If the conflict and related feelings are suppressed, the aftermath will only bring the cycle back to the beginning and more conflict will occur. It is important in this phase to find some way of resolving the conflict so that the outcome will lead to improved relationships.

There are several factors that are important during this phase that will make possible the resolution of conflict; however, the primary one is that both people must be willing to try to resolve things. If only one person is willing, no amount of effort will improve the situation. This can become frustrating for an individual so it is hoped that with proper understanding and communication, a willingness on the part of both people will develop.

As with the conflict process itself, there are many models for resolution. One such model is that of *integrative decision making*.[9] With this method, there are several steps which may be taken. First, the involved parties must identify and adjust any particular physical or situational factors that might be causing difficulty. For instance, the conflict might relate to a lack of office space which could be remedied by stating the problem to each other or to a supervisor who may be able to make different arrangements. If this isn't possible, perhaps a shift in scheduling would allow the two parties to share space more comfortably.

The next two steps that are important in this type of resolution are examination of each person's perceptions and attitudes: What is the other person feeling? Overburdened, insecure, moody, or inadequate? What are one's own feelings? Resentment, dependency, fear, or aggression? The next step would be for the two people to sit down and actually describe their perceptions to each other. It is important to own one's own feelings by using the personal pronoun and verb, "I feel. . . . Often it is at this point that a misunderstanding is clarified and the two people can easily remedy the situation. If the conflict still cannot be resolved, it is at least hopeful that a mutual understanding of each other's feelings and perceptions has occurred. This will then allow the problem to be identified.

Many times the actual problem is buried beneath negative feelings and is never accurately stated so that resolution can occur. Once the problem has been defined, a search process for solutions can begin. This should involve both people offering as many solutions as possible. Solutions from others may also be included. This search phase can include brainstorming, discussion groups, and surveys. Anything that can be looked at in an effort to resolve the problem should be considered. After this phase, a narrowing down process should begin until there is a mutual agreement by both people. During this evaluation and final stage, it is important to keep the original problem in mind as well as to be open about personal feelings so that they do not get in the way of reaching a satisfying solution.

Case Study

A new COTA is starting her first job in an activities department with a staff of two others and a supervisor. The supervisor and the two staff members have been employed at the facility for several years and have an established program, but an increase in caseload created the need for additional staffing. After a month of employment the assistant begins to feel comfortable with the supervisor but is having difficulty with the staff members regarding their choice of programming and their approach to patients. The COTA talks to the other staff members and expresses her concerns and new ideas but is met with resistance. Following this, the others become less friendly to her and continue with their routines, excluding her from any decision making.

At this point the pre-existing conditions are present, and both perceived and actual conflict have become manifest in behaviors. The COTA has several choices: ignore the situation and continue to feel uncomfortable and dissatisfied; quit the job; talk to the supervisor about it; or approach the staff members again in an effort to better resolve the situation.

If the COTA decides to talk with the other staff, it would first be helpful to express her feelings rather than to make suggestions. If the assistant can be open with her own feelings of frustration and perhaps rejection, this might enable the others to discuss their feelings. It is possible that they are feeling bored with the existing programming, yet threatened by a new staff member with new ideas. Once these feelings have been expressed, a problem can be defined more clearly. It may be a general programming problem that exists within the department.

If the emotions and feelings have been recognized, it will be easier and less threatening to re-

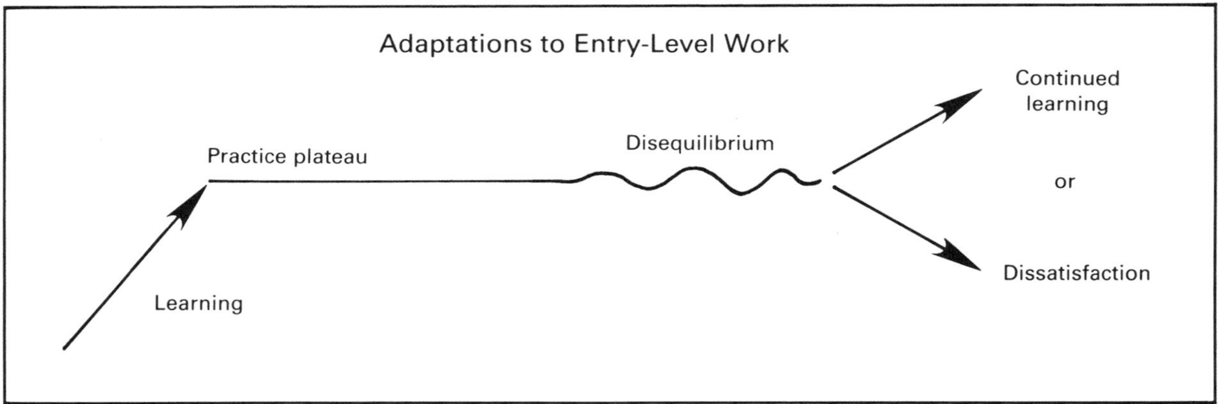

Figure 29-3

solve the problem together. The problem becomes less personalized and can be shared by all members of the department. In order to get new ideas to renew the old programs, books and periodicals may be consulted, other programs contacted, and so forth. With a pool of new ideas, the staff can decide together as a team what programming would best meet the needs of the patients.

In summary, the relationship with co-workers and supervisors depends largely on openness of communication, mutual respect and understanding, and cooperation instead of competition. If one should sense conflict or dissatisfaction, it is important to identify the problem and to proceed with necessary steps to resolve it; otherwise a weakened team structure may result.

Motivation

Entry-level work experience allows the COTA to practice and refine existing skills. A person will feel satisfied and comfortable for a period of time. Of course the mind is open to learn skills that relate to a particular work setting, but for a while new learning is essentially stopped. The COTA is on a practice plateau, making possible total integration of the technical knowledge and skills previously learned.

After some time has passed, and this differs for each individual, the COTA will desire to move off the plateau and begin a new learning experience. There is not always an intellectual awareness that this is happening. Instead, there may just be a desire operating on the will that causes one to act. This desire or motivation occurs because of a feeling of disequilibrium or a sense of dissatisfaction associated with the need to know or grow.

Many factors create this need to know, among which are newly emerging goals, competition or curiosity, a wish for success, a quest for novelty or change, and affiliation with a mentor. These motivators enable a person to move off the plateau and seek new learning experiences.

New learning takes several forms. Many people pursue increased specialization skills in occupational therapy. Others may seek knowledge in a totally different area to satisfy personal needs. Some may choose to pursue an education at the professional level to become an OTR. Whatever form the self-enhancement takes, it may serve as an example of healthy adaptation. If a person does not heed feelings of disequilibrium, a growing sense of dissatisfaction will occur. Relationships with peers and supervisors are likely to weaken and self-esteem will decrease. Figure 29-3 depicts this continuum.

Self-Enhancement

Continuing Education

Continuing education should be a life-long and self-directed process. The COTA who values and pursues life-long learning truly cares for himself or herself. The COTA's role is as a "caretaker of others." The most competent caretakers are those who continually care for and renew their own lives. Continuing education may be seen as a means of renewal and an investment in oneself, in the profession of occupational therapy, and in society in general.

One may continue to seek learning opportunities in order to enhance technical competence in occupational therapy or to gratify maturation needs through further study of other arts and sciences. The pursuit of learning in areas not directly related to one's profession helps to lay a firm foundation for occupational excellence.[2] Study or experience in diverse interest areas broadens one's perspectives and offers new insights into one's personal and work life. Self-directed learning is a pleasurable activity and provides restful change and relaxation to help one achieve a healthy balance.

Continued education goals related to maintaining competence in the profession may be set by state associations, licensure boards, or the individual. Such programs are offered through colleges, universities, technical schools, and health agencies. Many learning programs award the continuing education unit (CEU). CEUs are based on specific standards which assure some measure of quality to the learner. While not currently required, in the future, the American Occupational Therapy Association may choose to use CEUs as a means of measuring participation in continuing education. It is possible that this form of measurement will become one option in a recertification process.[10]

The AOTA and affiliated state associations also offer continuing education programs and resources to the membership. Conferences, workshops, seminars, programmed learning packets, and audiovisual materials are examples of offerings that assist practitioners in meeting their need for maintaining competence. Publications such as the *American Journal of Occupational Therapy* and the *Occupational Therapy Newspaper* offer pertinent articles and information that also contribute to life-long learning.

To become more fully socialized, however, one must expand on these concepts of continuing education. Most COTAs see the need for learning new theory and techniques that are directly applicable to a specific work role. More assistants must begin to recognize the learning potential related to volunteer activities such as participation on commissions, committees, and task forces to serve the local, state, and national occupational therapy associations.

The AOTA and the state affiliates draw their strength from each individual's contributions. These contributions are in the form of time, intellectual and emotional energy, and financial support. Active involvement in the association activities is absolutely essential if a COTA is to realize his or her full potential. Extended and expanded exposure to the practice of occupational therapy is only one part of becoming socialized into the profession. One must also experience an extended exposure to, and investment in, association activities. This investment offers multidimensional continuing education opportunities. Participation in association affairs aids the further development of communication and problem solving skills, for example. This work also contributes to an understanding of the whole of the profession and its central mission. Increased understanding leads to inquiry, action, as well as further learning, increased growth, and new challenges.

Volunteerism also leads to the development of professional and personal relationships outside of the work place. These relationships expand the support system, which is essential to the healthy practitioner. The wise COTA seeks social support as a means of preventing "burnout." Burnout is a term used to describe a state of mental fatigue that may be encountered during one's work life. Practitioners who suffer "burnout" experience an inability to generate energy for their job or to think creatively. Burnout can be disabling, and COTAs need to think in terms of prevention. Social support systems are an important part of any renewal plan in order to maintain a high energy level and motivation for learning.

The Socialized Self

A socialized person is involved in life-long learning as new personal goals continue to evolve. In addition, expectations of the profession and individuals within it increase significantly.[2] A COTA who has reached this level of maturation has a recognized area of expertise and is directing his or her efforts in expanding and sharing this expertise. There are a variety of ways that this is done, including teaching, specializing in a clinical area, managing, speaking, publishing, creating audiovisual tools, develping computer programs, consulting, or counselling others.

The COTA as Advanced Clinician

A majority of COTAs maintain their roles as clinicians; however, after reaching this level of maturation and socialization, they can be designated as advanced clinicians with a specialized area of expertise.

During the initial educational process, the focus was on general occupational therapy education with exposure to a variety of disability areas and problems. Students received a framework of knowledge and learned therapeutic application of purposeful activity as it related to these areas. This prepared a student to seek employment in a number of different settings. When a COTA seeks entry-level employment, he or she begins in one area and may remain there. Some COTAs choose to work in a variety of practice areas during their first few years of experience before they begin to specialize.

Whichever route one takes, there usually is a desire to seek additional training in a particular area. Some of this training may occur on the job, and some, obtained through continuing education methods previously discussed, may result in receiving a specialty certification from a particular agency. As experience increases, specialization permits a feeling of increased competence.[11] This feeling is an important source of self-gratification and mastery for the COTA and allows the patient to receive the best possible treatment.

Within one's area of expertise, it is important for each clinician to view that specialty as a part of the whole profession and not as a separate entity. Although terminology and techniques may vary, the philosophical base of occupational therapy remains central, and the connections to the profession and other clinicians must be maintained. For example, one COTA may be working in geriatrics while another specializes in psychiatry; however, the common base of activity should allow these COTAs to share problems, ideas, and goals. In addition to specialized skills, this ability to be an integral part of the total profession is a strength of a COTA who is an advanced clinician.

The COTA as Administrator

Proficient COTAs may seek new dimensions of work experience in a management or administrative position. Examples of these kinds of positions held by COTAs include director of activities in long term care settings, coordinator of volunteer services in community settings, and self-employed practitioners who manage others in offering supportive services to the elderly living at home.

Some individuals demonstrate a remarkable capacity to master management methods and principles through life and work experience. Others seek academic preparation to enhance their skills and knowledge. It has been said, however, that no program develops a manager; one develops oneself.[8] Educational programs, whether formal or informal, only assist a person in gaining awareness of strengths, limitations, and growth possibilities and then encourage self-directed learning. The motivation to acquire knowledge and ability in management must be strong within the individual.

The COTA as Educator

An ever increasing number of COTAs are becoming educators. They are fulfilling this role in both professional and technical level academic programs as well as functioning as fieldwork educators. In occupational therapy education, the primary goal is to prepare people to function as practitioners.[12] While there are many techniques that can be used in this preparation, a helpful one is to involve the learner as much as possible. This can be compared to one of the basic tenets of the occupational therapy profession, which is the "doing of purposeful activity."

It is important to view education as a facilitation process in which the learner is assisted toward the end goal of acquisition of skills and knowledge making possible independent functioning.[13] The steps of developing rapport or establishing a comfort level, setting learning objectives, and providing methods for the student to achieve these objectives are similar to those in any therapeutic interaction.

Some of the qualities that can assist an educator in facilitating the learning process include the following: keeping current in the subject; making ideas understandable and pertinent; using creativity to stimulate the students' desire to learn; and being open with the students and realizing that they also have knowledge to offer.[14]

Writing, Speaking, and Research

Whether a COTA chooses to become an educator, administrator, or advanced clinician, writing, speaking, and research are activities that permit further growth of the individual and the profession. Experienced COTAs are encouraged to share their knowledge in a formal way.

The purpose of writing and speaking is to communicate ideas and information in order to share knowledge or create change. COTAs contribute articles to professional journals and to state and national newspapers. They are involved in the development of pamphlets, scripts, and lessons for educational and public relations purposes. Speaking is a natural extension of writing. COTAs speak at national and state conferences, schools, seminars, and workshops. Writing and speaking are major forces in facilitating progress within the profession. Research is currently one of the focal points of the science of occupational therapy. If members of the profession become active consumers of research, the demand will increase and this, it is hoped, will cause the supply to expand.[15]

The role as consumer begins in the educational process with the studying and reading of information. It is hoped that the student will continue to read and study after graduation; however, this is not always the case. One method of encouraging continuing learning is to initiate a journal club among the staff where one is working. Journal clubs can assume a variety of formats, the basis being to read, share, and discuss current articles that are being published. This promotes the concepts of research and development within the profession in addition to providing new dimensions of knowledge to the members involved.

The role of contributor to research is often a more overwhelming thought, although it need not be. Contributing to research can begin in the simplest fashion by becoming a careful recorder of information. The complete recording of data such as patient ages, diagnoses, treatment techniques utilized, length of treatment, and responses to treatment can be a basis for developing research projects. The actual design and implementation of the project may require collaboration with an OTR or someone else with expertise; however, the compiling of data is the foundation of research.

Contributing to research is necessary in order to stimulate and validate the profession of occupational therapy as well as to allow all members of the profession to further their own growth. It is important for COTAs to seek out ways in which they can become actively involved in the research process.

The COTA as Consultant

The experienced and well informed COTA may be asked to serve as a consultant in an area of expertise. The main goal of consulting is to provide a service or resolve a problem. Consulting can occur formally or informally. Informally, it may be the sharing and offering of information to a colleague. Formally, it can be done in a more clearly defined job that involves conferring with other individuals or agencies on a regular basis to provide advice and guidance.

As advanced clinicians, administrators, and educators, COTAs have served as consultants in a variety of ways: consultants with directors of adult day care and senior citizen centers; designers of adaptive equipment; building planners regarding accessibility issues; and educators in existing and developing occupational therapy curricula.

The COTA as Role Model and Mentor

Role models are those people who stimulate and inspire others with their example and encouragement.[2] In this process, observing and copying are the primary methods of learning. The model may actively encourage; more often it is a passive role of influencing another.

Role modeling differs from the process of being a mentor. Mentorship involves much more of a commitment and sharing between two people. The word mentor is used to mean a wise and faithful counselor or guide and originated from Greek mythology.[16] There are different levels of involvement in being a mentor, depending upon the needs of the person who is seeking additional personal and professional growth experiences. The mentor can focus on academics, work, or involvement in professional activities. Acting as a mentor to others can be viewed as a form of ministration, which helps another person reach a higher level of maturity.

In order to be a mentor, certain qualities are necessary. These include the ability to provide direction; to be open and sensitive to another's needs; to recognize the potential strengths in others as well as realizing their limitations; to be responsive and available; and to desire to have some impact on the next generation.[16]

Some specific actions one can take in order to be a mentor may include inviting another COTA to work alongside oneself in any professional activity on a state or national level. While working with this person, one has the opportunity to introduce him or her to other members in the field. After working with this person, the next step would be to affirm strengths and identify areas for growth. Feedback and suggestions can be made to encourage growth.

The mentor can then begin to recommend his or her colleague to others. For example, one might nominate the individual for committee membership or chairmanship in the state association. The ultimate goal would be for the colleague to be self-motivating and able to seek out new challenges independently in order to become enmeshed in the professional organizations. When involvement has become integrated and comfortable, it is hoped that the person will consider mentorship of another.

Summary

Socialization is change or development toward increased maturity and responsibility. In general, the concept of socialization includes both the content that must be learned and the activities one must participate in to create potential for integration of learning and continued growth. The content in occupational therapy includes the norms, values, beliefs, and skills that are required for both the social integration of the person and the stability of the profession. Socialization can be said to be successful for both the individual and the profession if it provides for integration of the technician into the profession and mutual integration, understanding, and acceptance of both levels of occupational thearapy personnel into the health care community.[17] For COTAs to be truly socialized they must have extended exposure to the profession through education, practice, and involvement in professional activities. Experience gained in these formal and informal settings enables COTAs to recognize themselves and be recognized by others as competent, contributing members of the profession of occupational therapy.

References

1. Simpson I: *From Student to Nurse: A Longitudinal Study of Socialization.* New York: Cambridge University Press, 1979, p 6.
2. Houle C: *Continuing Learning in the Professions.* San Francisco: Jossey-Bass, 1980.
3. Holstrom E: Promising prospects: Students choosing therapy as a career. *Am J Occup Ther* 29:608-614, 1975.
4. Madigan, J: Characterisitics of students in occupational therapy educational programs. *Am J Occup Ther* 39:41-46, 1985.
5. Buck J, Daniels M, Harren V, Eds: *Facilitating Students' Career Development.* San Francisco: Jossey-Bass, 1981, p 7.
6. Levinson, et al: *Men, Management and Mental Health.* Cambridge, MA: Harvard University Press, 1962.
7. Terry G: *Principles of Management.* Homewood, IL: Richard Irwin, Inc., 1977.
8. Beggs D, Ed: *Team Teaching: Bold New Venture.* Indianapolis: United College Press, 1964.
9. Filley A: *Interpersonal Confict Resolution.* Glenview, IL: Scott Foresman and Co., 1975.
10. Robertson S, Martin E: Continuing education: A quality assurance approach. *Am J Occup Ther* 35:314-315, 1981.
11. Gillette N, Kielhofner G: The impact of specialization on the professionalization and survival of occupational therapy. *Am J Occup Ther* 33:20-28, 1979.
12. Shapiro D, Shanahan P: Methodology for teaching theory in OT basic professional education. *Am J Occup Ther* 30:217-224, 1976.
13. Bowen A: Carl Rogers' views of education. *Am J Occup Ther* 28:220-221, 1974.
14. Hansen E: Plain talk about good teaching. *Improving College and University Teaching.* 31:23-24, 1978.
15. Gilfoyle E: Caring: A philosophy for practice. *Am J Occup Ther* 34:517-521, 1980.
16. Rogers J: Sponsorship: Developing leaders for occupational therapy. *Am J Occup Ther* 36:309-313, 1982.
17. Gubrium J, Buckholdt D: *Toward Maturity.* San Francisco: Jossey-Bass, Inc., 1977, pp 126-144.

CHAPTER 30

Principles of Occupational Therapy Ethics

Sister Miriam Joseph Cummings, OTR

Ethics has to do with the rightness or wrongness of an action. It relates to what it is that "ought" to be done. Professional ethics, then, is the rightness or wrongness in relation to carrying out the duties and responsibilities of the profession.

What Are Ethical Principles? Primary Values

Ethics are usually stated in terms of principles, not in terms of rules. That is, there are basic attitudes and qualities that define what is ethical. All ethical principles are based on four values: prudence, temperateness, courage, and justice. These are important and essential values if registered occupational therapists and certified occupational therapy assistants are to be ethical persons and ethical professionals.

Prudence

Prudence means choosing the right means. This relates to using foresight and care in what must be done. Prudence is a basis for several of the ethical principles of occupational therapy. The opposite of prudence is negligence or recklessness. When therapists and assistants act with prudence, they are knowledgeable about what they are doing and use good judgment in evaluation and treatment planning and implementation. They are able to predict the consequences of what they do. For example, if COTAs use modalities that they were not educated to use, or engage in evaluation procedures that they do not have the background knowledge to carry out, they may be acting imprudently.

Temperance

Temperance refers to moderation. A regard for decency in behavior is another way of saying this. The opposite, cruelty or insensibility, helps to clarify what temperance means. Any behavior that treats the patient inhumanely, that discriminates against him or her, or that ridicules the person is an intemperate behavior.

Courage

Courage is a value that shows itself in patience. Being willing to do what is known to be right, in spite of difficulties or problems, is an example of how the value of courage relates to ethical principles. There are examples of occupational therapy personnel being discontinued in their work, or finding it necessary to leave their positions, because of taking action in circumstances of unethical behavior on the part of others. It takes courage to stand up for what is right when that action will have adverse effects, even to the point of depriving the therapist or the assistant of a position.

Justice

Justice requires that each person be treated with integrity and honesty. This is perhaps the most obvious value related to ethics. Any act that is dishonest is also unethical. Occupational therapy personnel owe their patients quality treatment, carefully planned and implemented, and accurately reimbursed. Giving persons their due is justice.

Secondary Values

There are other values that are basic to ethical behavior, such as reverence, fidelity, awareness of responsibility, truthfulness, and goodness. These sometimes seem abstract, but they are the foundation of ethical principles.

For instance, reverence calls for respect for each person. Fidelity relates to the patient and to the employer. Awareness of responsibility provides a framework for ethical behavior. Truthfulness is the hallmark of informed consent and of all relations with patients, families, colleagues, and other professionals. Goodness has to do with rightness, aptness, fitness, and excellence. These are obviously basic to ethics.

Professional Ethics

One of the hallmarks of a profession is that it has a set of ethical principles that it adheres to and a means of assuring that its practitioners behave ethically. For many years, the American Occupational Therapy Association had a statement in its bylaws that indicated all occupational therapists and assistants were bound by a code of ethics. The Association, however, did not have an established, clearly articulated code. In 1977, the Association adopted principles of occupational therapy ethics, and established these as a "guide to appropriate conduct of its members." The Standards and Ethics Commission of the Association, under the leadership of Carolyn Baum, studied the ethical principles of many other professions in developing those appropriate for occupational therapy. In 1980, guidelines were completed to accompany each of the ethical principles.

A system of enforcement has been developed also, so that the Association currently has principles, guidelines, and an enforcement procedure. These are always under study and possible revision, particularly the guidelines and the procedures.

Elements Essential to Ethics

Some of the elements that are essential to the ethical behavior for any professional, and therefore for the occupational therapist and the assistant, are identified as the following:

Universalism: Universalism means that the therapist and the assistant serve persons regardless of age, race, socioeconomic status, personality, likableness, or any other similar considerations. To be selective in who is treated, based on any reason other than professional judgment of ability of the person to benefit from treatment, is unethical.

Disinterest: An occupational therapist or an assistant should not be motivated by profit or self-interest. Treatment has to be the best that can be provided under the circumstances.

Cooperation: A truly ethical person cooperates with colleagues and is supportive of them. Sharing knowledge and advancements in theory and practice is one sign of cooperation.

Occupational Therapy Ethical Principles

Each of the principles of occupational therapy ethics can be considered in detail, and examples given of some of the ways that the particular principle can be carried out or violated. While this text focuses on the occupational therapy assistant, the ethical principles of the profession are stated in such a manner that both the therapist's and the assistant's roles and obligations in the delivery of services must be discussed. There are 13 principles, identified here by Roman numerals and phrases describing the content of the principle.

The AOTA document *Principles of Occupational Therapy Ethics* has been reprinted in Appendix J.

I. Principles Related to the Recipient of Service

This principle states that the good of the patient must always be kept in mind in planning and delivering service. A goal-directed relationship must be maintained. Respect for the person's rights governs treatment and relationships. Financial gain should never be foremost. Therapists and assistants are obligated to provide the highest quality treatment that they are capable of providing.

Some of the ways in which this principle may *not* be carried out include:

1 Continuing patient treatment after the patients have achieved maximum benefit from treatment.
2 Filling in time during the treatment with unrelated activities.
3 Treating too many patients at one time for greater income and therefore not being able to give the attention that each individual patient needs.
4 Performing inappropriate assessments and thereby establishing treatment goals that are unrealistically high or too low.
5 Avoiding treating patients who will be difficult to treat or who will not be able to respond quickly to therapeutic intervention efforts.
6 Failing to involve the patient directly in decisions about goals and treatment if the person is capable of participating.

The fact that occupational therapy personnel must be productive in the current health care climate is a fact which cannot be ignored. However, the therapist or assistant must be ethical in the process of being productive. Many of the examples listed might enable occupational therapy personnel to appear productive, but they would be a detriment to the patient.

The principle of universalism stated in previous discussion applies in this ethical statement. The therapist and the assistant must be willing to treat patients who are able to benefit from treatment without regard to such things as race, creed, sex, or handicap. To do otherwise would be to deny the patient the right to appropriate treatment and its benefits.

II. Principles Related to Competence

An occupational therapist has a high level of professional competence. An occupational therapy assistant has a high degree of technical competence. It is essential that each of these practitioners continue to increase competence. It is obvious that health care, in all of its aspects, is a constantly changing environment. To maintain skills at any one level is not sufficient; the therapist and assistant must improve skills to keep pace. This can be done in a number of ways such as further formal, academic education, self-study, participation in conferences, making use of a mentor, or through an experiential study in an occupational therapy treatment facility.

Competence must be represented accurately to other professionals, to the patient, the patient's family, and to the public. Occupational therapy personnel are called upon to do many things as a part of the health care team. Care must be taken not to allow others to presume capabilities that are not present.

Occupational therapy assistants need to be aware of what their abilities and skills are and what their education and background prepares them to do. They should not take on other professional duties which are not within their area of competence. In a competitive health care climate, there can be a drive to make individual personnel indispensable by having them do "all things." The supervising occupational therapist must use professional judgment to determine what may ethically be done by subordinate personnel, as well as what cannot be done by the personnel, or that which exceeds the parameters of the profession.

It is of great importance that occupational therapy assistants be aware of when the needs of the patient go beyond their ability to meet those needs. It may be necessary to refer the person to an occupational therapist who has the required skills; or it may be that the skills of someone in another profession are needed. There should be no hesitation in referring the patient to the person who will be best able to provide the services needed.

III. Principles Related to Records, Reports, Grades and Recommendations

Keeping records and writing and making reports are part of professional duties. The therapist as well as the assistant must conform to the legal requirements and to the policies of the institution or facility. It is an important part of treatment to actually record and report the process and result of treatment. Objective data should be used whenever appropriate. Subjective data may be valuable when based on sound professional judgment and on available objective data. It is important for the therapist to know what objective measurements are appropriate, to use these with skill, and to report and interpret the findings accurately. Generally, the occupational therapy assistant does not interpret such data, but should be skilled in the administration of structured assessment tools.

Falsifying records for reimbursement purposes is dishonest and unethical. Indicating on a record that a patient was treated when the person did not receive treatment is an example of falsifying records. Indicating that the occupational therapy assistant was supervised by a registered occupational therapist when treatment was provided, when such was not the case, is, of course, dishonest. Occupational therapy personnel must be alert to the pressures of producing income. While recognizing the need for adequate income to the facility or private practice group, it is never ethical to achieve this income through the falsification of records. When a therapist or assistant is asked to do such recording, it is necessary to report this fact to the next person in the channel of authority. In some instances, it may be necessary for the occupational therapy personnel involved to leave their position(s) because persons in authority require this behavior.

IV. Principles Related to Intraprofessional Colleagues

This principle focuses on the issue of respect that must be shown toward all occupational therapist and assistant colleagues that the individual works or deals with in any way. Each therapist and assistant represents the entire profession, and the quality of each one's service is a concern to all. The behavior of each one reflects on all members of the profession.

It is essential that occupational therapy personnel discuss with other intraprofessional colleagues only that information concerning patients which is necessary. Revealing data or information about a patient when it is not for the purpose of enhancing the treatment of the patient or advancing the knowledge of the profession is a breach of confidentiality. Data or information used in publications or papers presented should be given in such a way that the identity of the patient is protected. Occupational therapy students must be particularly aware of this when using progress reports or other patient records to fulfill assignments in their educational programs.

The reputation of colleagues also must be protected. Comments concerning the quality of treatment given should be carefully considered. Often, such evaluations are subjective and a matter of opinion. When information such as peer evaluations indicates a problem in the quality of treatment being provided, the matter should be handled with discretion. This does not mean that poor quality of treatment should be ignored, but rather that it should be handled through the proper channels.

When using work developed by others, it is essential that credit be given to the originators. It may happen that work which has been developed by many therapists and built on by the profession is then copyrighted by an individual. Since the work really belongs to the profession as a whole, this is not ethical. When a therapist or assistant makes a significant contribution to the work, revises, updates or changes it, then the person has the right to be identified with the work. It is always necessary to give credit to those who contributed substantially to the work.

One of the most difficult things for occupational therapy personnel to deal with is unethical behavior on the part of others. Upon becoming aware of possible unethical behavior on the part of others, the therapist or the assistant has an obligation to act. When possible, discussing and clarifying the situation with the person may be all that is necessary. It is possible for a therapist or assistant to be unaware that the behavior is not considered ethical or may be questionable. When such discussion is not possible or does not result in change, the next step is to report the situation to the appropriate body. This may be a standards and ethics committee of a district or state occupational therapy association if such exists, or it may be the Standards and Ethics Commission of the American Occupational Therapy Association.

Enforcement Procedures

Reporting an alleged violation of ethics to the

Standards and Ethics Commission is done by writing to the chairperson of the Commission describing the the situation. A form has been developed by the Commission, the use of which assures the inclusion of necessary information. The Commission will then make a preliminary review to determine if the situation described appears to be in the realm of unethical behavior. If so, a formal investigation is initiated.

The chairperson of the Commission appoints an investigation committee of one or more AOTA members. The individual involved is informed of the complaint and has the opportunity to reply in writing. The investigation committee can decide whether the matter should be investigated further, whether a hearing is necessary, or if sufficient information is available without a hearing. This committee reports to the Standards and Ethics Commission.

It is the role of the Standards and Ethics Commission to determine whether a formal charge of violation of ethics is to be made. If such a charge is made, all parties are notified. The president of the American Occupational Therapy Association receives all of the information needed for the charge and appoints a judicial council of three AOTA members. These individuals conduct a hearing and make a decision which they give to the president. The president then notifies the parties of the decision and any action which may follow. An appeal procedure is provided.

Although the procedure may appear to be cumbersome, it is important to protect the rights of all persons involved. Because of the need to do this, the time elements of the process are long. The total time may be over a year if the entire process, including appeal, is completed. Protection of the rights of the persons involved and of the profession, which means the protection of all therapists and assistants, is of paramount importance. Since this is a very serious matter, it is appropriate that the procedure not be rushed, and that adequate time for prudent decisions be allowed.

V. Principles Related to Other Personnel

It is very important for occupational therapists and assistants to understand the role and educational background of other persons involved in treating the patient. Respect for their role and service is a necessary part of ethical behavior. Occupational therapy personnel must be concerned with the quality of all services which the patient receives. Therefore, it is the concern of the therapist and the assistant if related health care personnel are not performing at a competent level.

One of the important aspects of this principle of ethics is the delegation of services to others. Occupational therapists must not delegate when the skills needed are those of occupational therapy. Therapists do work with many other persons, including the family of the patient, in providing services. However, professional judgment must be used regarding the aspects of the treatment that can be taught and delegated, and those which require the level of service of the therapist. When students are involved in providing treatment, the supervising therapist is responsible for determining the competency of the student to render the service.

VI. Principles Related to Employers and Payers

Honesty is the hallmark of all relations with employers and payers. These relations must be carried out with integrity in all areas. In accepting employment, therapists and assistants accept the job description, the policies, and the procedures of the facility. They are obligated then to follow these.

Such things as charging for services not rendered, engaging in "kickbacks" in purchasing materials, using favoritism in the choice of vendors, or using supplies and equipment without approval all constitute unethical behavior.

Because not all services needed by the patient are reimbursable by third party payers, there is a tendency to try to provide these services by charging them under a reimbursable service such as occupational therapy. The purpose of this practice is to lead the payers to believe that they are paying for a type of service that was not rendered. Looked at in this way, such a practice is dishonest. Unless there is a clear understanding that a related service is a part of occupational therapy and can be billed as such, it is unethical to do this.

Fees for service should reflect costs and be appropriate and justifiable. An appropriate profit may be built into a fee schedule.

VII. Principles Related to Education

A key role of an occupational therapist is to provide education for occupational therapy students, patients and their families, public and private agencies, and the public in general. Although it would be difficult to allege unethical behavior in relation to this principle, it is an important one. It should be looked at, as all of the principles should, from a positive point of view. Occupational therapy personnel have knowledge and skills that will assist others and have much to contribute. They should be willing to do so for the common good of those served.

VIII. Principles Related to Evaluation and Research

All members of the profession have a responsibility to advance the theory and practice of the profession. Research is the primary way that this is done. In conducting research, it is essential that the rights of the subjects be protected.

There are a number of codes that have been developed dealing with principles of ethical research. These usually include the following elements:

Informed, voluntary consent is absolutely essential. This means that the persons involved must have the capacity to understand the possible effects of participation in the research and must be free to choose to participate. This presents particular problems in relation to research with children, prisoners, persons with head trauma, or those with mental illness. Informed consent means that a complete explanation must be given to the persons who are being asked to participate, or to those who have the responsibility to make decisions for them.

Beneficial results must be anticipated from the research. In using human subjects, it is necessary that the results would not be possible to achieve by other means and that the anticipated results justify the inconvenience or risk to the persons.

Only qualified persons should conduct research. The persons participating need the assurance that the investigator knows proper procedure. There are many levels of research; thus, there are also many levels of qualification.

During a research project, a subject must be able to withdraw from the study. There cannot be any coercion to continue when the person chooses not to be involved further. If it becomes clear that the patient would benefit from a different treatment than that which is involved in a research project, the treatment of greatest benefit to the patient must be used.

The investigator must adhere to the policies and procedures of the facility in which the research is taking place. All facilities that conduct research have committees to review research design and the protection of the rights of human subjects. A facility, of course may have additional rules to govern the use of persons in studies.

It is important to report results accurately and to make known any reservation regarding the validity or reliability of the research studies. If preliminary results are being reported, particular care must be taken.

IX. Principles Related to the Profession

It is the responsibility of each therapist and assistant to know the principles of occupational therapy and to know the standards of the profession. The document *Standards of Practice for Occupational Therapy* published by AOTA has been reprinted in this book as Appendix E-1, Therapeutic Intervention—An Overview. The American Occupational Therapy Association develops, adopts and publishes these standards which should guide the performance of occupational therapists and assistants. It is essential that all occupational therapy personnel be aware of changes in the field. One important way of doing this is by reading professional journals. Involvement in local, state, and national associations also helps therapists and assistants not only to know the changes but also to participate in the development of the profession.

The actions of each therapist and assistant reflect upon the profession. How each behaves in carrying out professional duties will influence how the patient, the patient's family, and other professionals view the field of occupational therapy.

Occupational therapy personnel who never read a professional journal, never discuss development of the field, never are involved in the professional association, and never attend conferences or workshops cannot know the developments in the field and cannot treat patients adequately. It has often been said that some therapists and assistants have ten years' experience while others have one year of experience repeated ten times. Often occupational therapy personnel do not think of this behavior as being unethical, but the effect of this lack of currentness on the patient makes it literally unethical.

X. Principles Related to Advertising

In the past, one of the elements of a profession was that a profession did not advertise. In fact, it was considered unethical to advertise in any way. This is no longer the case, and advertising may be very appropriate. For example, in private practice, it would be very difficult to inform potential patients of the occupational therapy services available without advertising.

It is necessary, of course, to be truthful in advertising. Examples of dishonest advertising are: those which promise a result from treatment which cannot be guaranteed; those which mislead the public in regard to the qualifications of the person; and those which depreciate another therapist or service. Usually, an occupational therapy assistant will not advertise, but may be involved in a private practice which advertises.

XI. Principles Related to Law and Regulations

All things that are legal are not necessarily ethical, but usually things that are illegal are unethical. There are a number of laws that govern or relate to the delivery of health services. It is the duty of all occupational therapy personnel to be knowledgeable about those laws and to act in conformity to them.

Fraudulent billing to government programs such as Medicare and Medicaid is a major unethical practice. It is obviously both illegal and dishonest. The reflection on the profession and on all health professionals can be profound.

In recent years, there have been a number of instances in which health professionals have been accused of treating patients in an inhumane manner. This is particularly true in the treatment of those with emotional or mental disabilities. When patients are particularly vulnerable and cannot protect themselves, this kind of behavior takes on an exceptional seriousness. Ethical violations that have a direct effect on the patient, such as this type of behavior, are more serious than those which affect the profession or other therapists and assistants.

XII. Principles Related to Misconduct

Several of the principles of ethics previously discussed overlap with this principle. Any action which takes advantage of a patient's condition, any inhumane act, or anything that discriminates against a patient is an aspect of misconduct. Behavior which is not related to the responsibilities of the therapist or the assistant, but which is illegal, reflects on the profession and is unethical. Stealing, driving while intoxicated, and embezzlement of funds are possible illegal actions not directly related to professional duties, but nevertheless are unethical.

XIII. Principles Related to Bioethical Issues and Problems of Society

This is an example of a principle that has a positive implication. It calls the therapist and the assistant's attention to the fact that all members of the profession have responsibilities beyond the particular field of occupational therapy. Occupational therapy personnel need to be concerned about all health care issues and how such issues affect society.

There are many bioethical issues that are facing those in health care today. The defining of death, the allocation of scarce medical resources, the problems of informed consent for treatment, and psychosurgical procedures are among these issues. In addition, the prolongation of life or of dying, behavior control, and the selection of persons to receive treatment are some of the many problems being met daily in health care. It is essential that occupational therapy personnel keep informed concerning these issues.

Bioethical issues usually do not have a clear answer as to what is right or what is wrong. Some of the steps a therapist or an assistant can take to understand these issues and respond to them are:

Clarify the question: Often it is necessary to look at an issue from many different viewpoints in order to clarify what the basic question involved is. The question which appears on the surface may not be the real one. To begin to deal with the issue, it is important to be as clear and succinct in stating the question as possible.

Identify values: When the answer to a bioethical issue is not apparent or agreed upon by all, it is usually because there are competing values related to the issue. These may relate to the values of the individual, which vary from person to person, or they may relate to the values of society. Not all people may agree on what are relative values and what are absolute ones. Identifying and clarifying values involved will help to determine the decisions needed.

Explore world views: There are a number of ethical theories which determine how an issue will be approached and what will be an acceptable decision in relation to an issue. It is important to be clear in the implications of each. An individual's personal philosophy and religious beliefs will be important factors in world view and greatly influence how ethical issues will be resolved.

Examine data: It is essential to make use of all information that is available. Looking at the present situation with all the facts and knowledge applied will help to develop the possibilities and the alternatives in action.

Looking at bioethical issues from these views helps the professional to form a basis for decision making. Even if occupational therapy personnel are not directly involved in making a decision, it is important to clarify the aspects related to any bioethical issue and to assist society in understanding the basis of decision making.

Ethical behavior is essential to the occupational therapist and the occupational therapy assistant. Such behavior is often a matter of attitude and not of rule following. All principles of occupational therapy ethics are positive statements. It is important to view them as guidelines of positive behavior. It is apparent that the principles overlap each other. Often a particular unethical behavior will relate to two, three, or more principles. There is a problem in giving examples of unethical behavior, because whether a particular action is unethical or not depends upon a number of circumstances. The knowledge the person has, the intention, and the motivation may all contribute to a decision concerning the determination of what may in fact be unethical.

If occupational therapists and assistants always keep the good of the patient and the profession in the forefront of their considerations in making decisions concerning their behavior, those decisions, in all likelihood, will be ethical ones. Therapists and assistants, then, can be proud of their behavior and of their profession.

Summary

All ethical principles are based on the four values of prudence, temperance, courage, and justice. Secondary values related to ethical behavior include reverence, fidelity, awareness of responsibility, truthfulness, and goodness. One of the hallmarks of a profession is that it has a set of ethical principles that it adheres to as a means of assuring that its practitioners behave ethically. Elements that are essential to professional ethics are universalism, disinterest, and cooperation. The AOTA has adopted a code of occupational therapy ethics which outlines 13 principles that both occupational therapists and assistants must uphold. These relate to the recipient of service, competence, documentation, intraprofessional colleagues and other personnel, employers and payers, educational issues, evaluation and research, professional responsibility, advertising, laws and regulations, misconduct, and bioethical issues.

Ethical behavior is essential for all occupational therapy personnel. It is imperative that practitioners keep the good of the patient and the profession foremost so as to avoid possible unethical decisions or actions.

Bibliography

Ashley BM, O'Rourke KD: *Health Care Ethics*. St Louis: Catholic Hospital Association, 1978.

Fagothy A: *Right and Reason*. St. Louis: CV Mosby, 1967.

Munson R: *Intervention and Reflection: Basic Issues in Medical Ethics*. Belmont, CA: Wadsworth, 1979.

Principles of occupational therapy ethics. *Am J Occup Ther* 34:869-899, 1980.

Vollmer HM, Mills DL: *Professionalism*. Englewood Cliffs, NJ: Prentice-Hall, 1966.

EPILOGUE

The Future of Occupational Therapy: An Environment of Opportunity

Elnora M. Gilfoyle, OTR

Introduction

The social forces shaping health care systems in the 1980s and 1990s provide an environment of opportunity for occupational therapy. As a profession, we must realize that we are not helplessly dependent upon the forces of our environment; rather the environment is created by historical, social, political, and economic forces, and we can be part of the force. As a profession, we have an influence upon our environment as well as being affected by its forces. Because the influence of the environment upon the profession is a transactional process, occupational therapy personnel must work together to create opportunities that facilitate growth and development of the profession. By so doing, our profession will expand its services.

An awareness of social forces is a necessary beginning in providing occupational therapists and assistants with abilities to create opportunities for themselves. Contemporary social forces that have a direct impact upon the profession and its practitioners include:

1 Society's decline in allegiance to the biomedical model with its institutional care to an allegiance toward a model for "wellness" or the fullness of life and its subsequent concepts of "self-care."[2]
2 Society's use of high technology and the impact of that technology upon life, as well as upon work and leisure lifestyles.[3]
3 Society's decline in allegiance to male supremacy toward a healthier balance of female/male ideals and values.[4]
4 Legislative definitions and support for occupational therapy services in clinics, home health agencies, hospitals, and schools.[5]
5 Rapid growth of health care expenditures and resulting care funding patterns for reimbursement of services.[6]

The social forces just outlined provide an environment of opportunity from which occupational therapy can grow; however, the culture of occupational therapy must be modified to meet the needs of society. In the process of modification, social forces become the primary impetus for a change or shift in the profession's culture. Thus, a cultural shift is a response of social forces and is viewed as dynamic change or transformation. Transformation is a new seeing, insight, vision; it is a period of shift in ideas or new ways of thinking about old concepts. The original concepts and ideas that made the profession in the beginning are the historical force behind the success of its transformation.

History has witnessed an expansion of occupational therapy services that has evolved into a variety of specializations and the need for two levels of personnel. Professional diversity can exist and a diverse profession can continue to meet the demands of the environment and expand its services, as long as there is continuity in the profession's philosophy. The beliefs and values that make up the philosophy of occupational therapy provide continuity to the profession's practices, while social demands for our services promote diversity in practice. The strength of our philosophical base provides us with the security to react to social forces and create opportunities for ourselves.

Our profession's legacy has provided basic concepts, beliefs, and values that form the reality of occupational therapy. The profession's reality is in its culture, and culture's real existence lies in the hearts and minds of its people. Webster defines culture as "the integrated pattern of human behavior that includes thought, speech, action, and artifact . . . culture depends on man's capacity for learning and transmitting knowledge to succeeding generations."

Therefore, the growth and development of our profession are not only in the tools of scientific management but in the people who make the profession work. The culture of occupational therapy becomes a synthesis of objective and subjective contributions.[5]

Central to the culture of occupational therapy is "the science and art of the occupational process which facilitates meaning and order to the lives of persons with disabilities."[5] The therapeutic use of occupation to promote fullness of life is the basic value at the heart of our culture. During transformation, our value system will remain and our basic concepts and beliefs will expand into a science of occupation and an art of purposefulness.[5]

Through our transformation process, the roles and functions of occupational therapy personnel will change. Occupational therapists will assume independent health care professional roles with the majority of services being provided through consultation, monitoring, and supervision, and increasing numbers of OTRs being involved in research, theory development, education, and administration. Certified occupational therapy assistants will continue to provide direct patient care and work closely with OTRs in carrying out services; however, there will be an increase in COTA/OTR collaborative efforts with more opportunities for COTAs to carry out independent practices. The escalating costs of health care, as well as society's shift from the biomedical model will provide opportunities and dictate a need to change the current roles and functions of occupational therapy personnel. Change in roles and functions necessitates a change in educational preparation and professional regulations.

The Power of Values

Occupational therapy's value system is based upon basic concepts and beliefs. Values become the essence of our philosophy, as values state what it is that we believe and do. Therefore, our values communicate what is unique about occupational therapy.[7]

The rapidly changing society of the 1980s and consequences of future shock demand that accurate and logical choices be made. The most reliable guide for making logical choices is an awareness of our values. Bryan Hall states that clarification of values is not a skill that stands apart from science, but rather value clarification integrates the facts of science by bringing present knowledge into a more holistic focus.[8] Values are essential not only to the profession but also to each professional, as values are the integrating force that brings all elements of the profession into focus. Through the profession's clarification of its value system, we will declare the power and uniqueness of occupational therapy.[8]

Values involve an internal choosing by the profession, not an external giving or demand by society.[8] A profession must view itself as a subject freely controlling its own destiny, not as an object that is at the beck and call of others.[8] Hall proposed that controlling one's own destiny and becoming dependent upon others are alternative ways of conceptualizing oneself and are designated by the terms integration and adaptation.[8]

"Integration results from the capacity to adapt oneself to reality plus the critical capacity to make choices and transform that reality. To the extent that man loses his ability to make choices and is subjected to the choices of others, man is no longer integrated, rather, he has adapted; he has adjusted."

Hall goes on to state: "Passive obedience, conformity, external approval, and reliance on the directions of others characterize the adaptive person, while independence, creativity, self-confidence and self-directiveness are typical of the integrated person."[8] Occupational therapy must not succumb to being an adaptive profession; rather our future must be directed to the recognition of our value system so that we can clarify the power of our profession, direct choices, and transform the reality of occupational therapy toward a vital profession that can sustain a continual interactive process with society.

Through the transactional process of our profession and environment, there will be a shift in the reality of occupational therapy, including its concepts, beliefs, and values. A newly emerging value system will be defined in response to social forces and research findings, providing the profession with opportunities for expansion. Although a future value system is emerging, future and present are based upon the past. Therefore, an understanding of our historical roots is necessary for us to prepare for the future.

The Legacy of Our Value System

Our roots have been traced to Galen, 172 AD, in the statement:[9] "Employment is nature's best physician and is essential to human happiness." The early Egyptians and Greeks used music, games, and physical and mental activities to improve people's state of health. During the 18th and 19th centuries, reports of the use of occupations for restoration of mental health appeared in the literature, and the term "moral treatment" was introduced. In 1873, a Frenchman named Pinel wrote a book on moral treatment in which he discussed benefits of occupation for the mentally ill.[10] The idea of occupation or work for the mentally ill spread rapidly in Europe and to the United State.

Moral treatment continued to be popular in caring for the mentally ill until the time of the Civil War, after which the concept of moral treatment declined; however, in the early 1900s, Dr. Herbert Hall and nurse Susan E. Tracy rediscovered the idea of moral treatment and began to write about it.[11] Further writings proclaimed the value of occupation and in 1909 Haviland stated: "The therapeutic value of occupation for the insane is axiomatic and is based upon sound psychological laws."[5] Haviland's statement was one of the first to relate the therapeutic value of occupation with rudiments of theory.

In 1914, George Barton, speaking at a conference in Massachusetts, coined the term occupational therapy. Mr. Barton had been a patient at Clifton Springs Sanatorium where he helped his own recovery by engaging in manual work, primarily carpentry and gardening. He was so successful in influencing his own recovery that he became an advocate of the value of "doing" as a means to influence the individual's health. Barton's term occupational therapy was so descriptive of the value of occupation and the idea of "doing" that the term rapidly became popular, replacing early terms such as moral treatment and ergotherapy.[12]

Just as the legacy of our values can be traced to the early 1900s, the legacy of essential characteristics of occupational therapy personnel can be traced to a book written by Herbert Hall entitled *Occupational Therapy—A New Profession*.[13] Mr. Hall stated that occupational therapy is a well-paid and attractive new profession for educated young women! He also wrote that occupational therapy is a full-time job and demands health, energy, an attractive personality, an interest and facility in handicrafts, a desire to serve crippled humanity, and very special education. Mr. Hall declared: "The girl who undertakes training should be at least 20 years old. The age limit the other way is elastic—but few women over 35 should attempt the work."[13] The personal characteristics of occupational therapy personnel were established! Social transformation, particularly the feminist movement, has had a direct impact upon the essential characteristics of occupational therapy personnel.

In 1917, the National Society for the Promotion of Occupational Therapy was formed, objectives of the Association were developed, and statements of principles were put forth which adopted occupational therapy as a method of treatment by means of purposeful occupation.[10] Therefore, the early 1900s saw the emergence of the values of occupation and of the patient's "doing," characteristics of the people in occupational therapy being described, and the formation of an association to promote the ideas of occupational therapy.

Because of social forces, the early ideas of "occupation" and "doing" were modified by the demands of both World War I and World War II. Wounded soldiers needed rehabilitation, and early ideas of the use of games, handicrafts, and work evolved into values of exercise, constructive activities, and activities of daily living. Concepts of work simplification and training in the use of adaptive equipment and prosthetic and orthotic devices became the therapeutic media for occupational therapy, and the original values of occupation were modified. Medical technology expanded and specialization in medicine became a necessity; the concepts of "allied health fields" emerged. Occupational therapy identified itself with medicine and the profession's media and practices began to adopt biomedical ideals.

By the 1950s and 1960s, occupational therapy programs for persons with physical disabilities were based on sensorimotor rehabilitation techniques, borrowed from physical therapy. The concept of the therapeutic use of self in the treatment of psychiatric disorders was borrowed from psychology, and the therapeutic use of occupations was given less emphasis. By 1950, the profession's services and its educational preparation began to identify two areas of specialization—physical disabilities and psychosocial disabilities.

With further advances in medical technology, lifesaving techniques emerged, with more babies surviving birth trauma and congenital disorders. Knowledge regarding early development began to appear in the literature, and therapy based upon developmental concepts began to be reported. The recognition of a pediatric specialty for occupational therapists practice emerged.

By the 1960s and 1970s, the idea of "purposeful activity" was introduced and the term "occupation" dropped. The value of activity based on a neurobehavioral or occupational behavioral orientation or upon the biopsychosocial model became popular, and the need for theory became a professional issue.[14] Professionals began to cry for a unifying theory, and the concept of adaptation as the unifying or single theory for occupational therapy began to appear in the literature.[15,16] Kielhofner modified the early concepts of occupational behavior and proposed "human occupation" as the unifying force of the profession,[17] and occupational therapy personnel began, once again, to include "occupation" as a descriptive term.

During the past decade the change in the age of the population has had an impact on health care services, and occupational therapy has begun to expand its services in the area of gerontology. Current values and practices of occupational therapy as well as its educational preparation are based upon a false dichotomy of two diagnostic groups (physical and psychosocial) and the dichotomy of two age groups (pediatrics and gerontology). Diversity based upon two disabilities and two age groups does not provide the profession with a clear sense of its values or directions.

Another major development in our legacy was an official philosophy statement which the Association adopted in 1979. The statement was developed to describe our belief system and to declare our uniqueness.[18] Although the statement is an attempt to provide continuity to our culture, our philosophy does not appear to provide us with a certainty about our day-to-day practices, it does not give us convincing responses about the therapeutic value of occupation, and it does not provide a sense of direction for our services. Consequently, recent literature in occupational therapy communicates an internal debate about the efficacy and credibility of activities as therapeutic media.[19]

The 1980s finds occupational therapy as a profession which has uncertainty about its values, therapeutic media and methods, and dimensions of practice. The current uncertainty together with contemporary social forces must not become our pathologic way of thinking. Instead, they must be recognized as opportunity for change and a time to transform concepts about activity into new perspectives of occupation and occupational. A value system which is based upon the concept of occupation as action with the events of the environment and the dimension of occupational as the process of action in which the patient becomes the action agent or "doer" will be the unifying force that provides continuity in the philosophies and theories of occupational therapy.[5]

The following theoretical statements are presented as an attempt to summarize the profession's concepts and beliefs. The statements provide a framework for value clarification, research and theory development, as well as a framework for occupational therapy practice and educational preparation.

1 Human beings have the capacity to influence their own state of health.
2 Human beings can achieve a state of healthfulness through the processes of adaptation and integration.
3 Adaptation and integration occur through dynamic transactions of an individual with his or her biopsychosocial environment.
4 Transactions with one's biopsychosocial environment take place through human occupations.
5 Human occupations include self-care, play/leisure activities, work/school work, and rest.
6 Active processes of biopsychosocial transactions can influence a person's state of health as he or she functions as an open system.

Inherent in the above statements are core values which form the culture of occupational therapy. Core values are delineated as:

1 Human occupations as therapeutic media.
2 Active participation with biopsychosocial events as the occupational process.
3 Adaptation and integration as processes by which a person can influence his or her own state of health.
4 Therapists as action facilitators with the patient being the action agent.
5 Each patient as a unique individual.

Thus, concepts of "doing," "action," and "occupation" and the values of the patient as being unique and the "doer" or action agent are the integrating force that brings the science and art of purposeful occupation into focus as the heart of our culture.[5]

Through science, explanations and rational knowledge about the values of the profession will be identified and measured. Clarifying a value system provides direction for the profession's research efforts, while research measures the efficacy of concepts and values. Although science is primary in defining the uniqueness of occupational therapy, the art of therapy is also a powerful force which exemplifies our uniqueness. The art of therapy provides us with an awareness or intuitive knowledge. Therapeutic art is a relationship where the patient receives from the therapist, but it is the patient who has the capacity to influence his or her fulfillment of life. The value of occupational therapy therapeutic relationships is not in external giving by the therapist but in the internal receiving by the patient. "It is through internal receiving that occupational experiences become purposeful."[5] Through our scientific findings we will be able to predict and explain the uses of occupations as therapeutic media, but the purposefulness of the occupational process will remain as a value which cannot be explained through scientific measurements. As such, the purposefulness of occupation remains as our unique therapeutic art.

In summary, our legacy provided the basic concepts and beliefs that form the reality of occupational therapy. Through history, society's forces had an impact upon the growth and development of our ideas. Our basic values in occupation were modified and the media of therapy expanded. The biomedical model and theories of development influenced our practices. Our past provided a heritage, and change was gradual, whereas our present is one of rapid change and the demand to act quickly. "In this era, professions are presented with a need and the pressure to respond to that need without the necessary time to reflect on the knowledge and skills required to respond effectively."[1] Effective response is dependent upon the profession's abilities to make choices, and the profession's values are essential for accurate and logical choice making. A value system based upon the concepts of "occupation" and "occupational" will be the integrating force that brings the science and art of occupational therapy into cultural focus. A strong culture provides the profession with abilities to react to the present, integrate the past, and prepare for the future.

Dimensions of Practice: Diversity Within Community

A unifying value system provides occupational therapy with needed continuity so that logical diversity within its practices can emerge. Practice diversity must be complementary to philosophy; then diversity can add strength and power to the profession. Our early roots found occupational therapy personnel practicing in hospital settings and the medical model dictating practice diversity. Operating from the medical model, practice was defined as the "art of healing through guided prescription."[1] Dimensions of practice were hospital based, and occupational therapists were identified as members of treatment-oriented medical teams.[1] Diversity of practice was founded on diagnosis or disabilities. As medical technology expanded to lifesaving techniques and developmental theories influenced medicine, practice dimensions added diversity based upon age, but a focus on disability remained paramount. From the 1920s until the 1970s practice dimensions were based upon the medical model, with diversity among practitioners having no identification with philosophic continuity but with diagnosis and age.

Because our diversity was based upon disabilities, our profession diminished its values with our "unique perspective and focus on asset, abilities, competencies and satisfying performance in all areas of human existence."[19] However, in the 1970s and 1980s, social forces began to provide the opportunity for our profession to re-identify itself with human performance. Society began to lose its allegiance to medicine, and occupational therapy began to respond with a change in its focus from treatment orientation to one of health promotion. The cost of medical care, with increasing health problems of people, is a major factor influencing society's allegiance to the biomedical model.[2] These social forces provide an opportunity for occupational therapy to "call up" earlier concepts and values and adapt those to society's needs. Through integration of our past values with present practices, occupational therapy is evolving into a comprehensive health profession. Subsequently, our roles in health promotion and the prevention of disability are expanding.[1]

In 1978 Yerxa stated: "As occupational therapists, we are at home with mundane stuff of everyday living, but society does not yet value the commonplace, everyday activities of play, leisure, and self-maintenance."[20] Yerxa proposed that "society does need us but it has not yet found that out."[20] In her address, Yerxa challenged the profession to "reaffirm to ourselves and society the significance of the mundane stuff of daily living. If we can hold on, articulate and perpetuate the valuing of everyday activity, we can give society the opportunity to catch up with us. For what we value is what existence is about, finding meaning in all that we do."[20] In the present decade, society is beginning to catch up with occupational therapy and the opportunity for our profession to influence its own dimensions of practice is now. Diversity within our practice will no longer be based on disability but on the continuity of our value systems; thus dimensions of occupational therapy services will have logical diversity.

There are two economic and political forces which have had major ramifications upon our dimensions of practice: first, legislation in the late 1970s that delineated occupational therapy as an education-related service and not a medical service; and second, governmental decisions in 1983, which created the prospective payment system, resulting in economic influences upon which health services are provided.

The term "related service" has had influences upon changing dimensions of our practices. Education-related services cannot be limited to direct treatment approaches. Although most handicapping conditions serviced by occupational therapy personnel in the school systems can be described as medical in their origin, the effect and amelioration of the conditions are not through medical treatment, but are educational in nature.[5] Through opportunities to provide services in school environments, occupational therapists have expanded their practice. One example of the expansion of occupational therapy services created by social and political forces is the current re-establishment of our concepts and values related to work, vocational rehabilitation, and a person's rights for a productive and purposeful life.[21] Opportunities to identify our services with vocational readiness programs resulted from social forces placed upon the public educational system. Consumers advocated for education and community agencies to collaborate in efforts to provide programs that focus on students' transition from school systems to community systems. In the 1980s, the United

States Department of Education identified transition as a funding priority. Financial support has subsequently provided our profession with opportunities to provide continuing education programs that update knowledge and skills-related services.[22]

The future of education-related occupational therapy practices will see an increase in the need for consultation and supervision, participation in research and development of cost-effective services, as well as management of resources. Thus, the OTRs will increase their roles with indirect services, with direct therapist-student relationships carried out primarily by COTAs.

With the advent of prospective payment, concepts of acute medical care within medical environments are changing. An awareness of the importance of personal responsibility or self-care has emerged, and home health and other community programs are being developed in response to economic forces. With government stressing the need for cost containment, occupational therapy personnel are struggling with reimbursement issues for certain services.[21] In response to reimbursement issues, the Association authorized funding for efficacy studies to demonstrate the cost effectiveness of occupational therapy.[21] Cost containment issues have opened up new opportunities for occupational therapy personnel to provide services through home health and other community agencies. Identifying ourselves with cost-effective services that can be offered outside the domain of the hospital setting has complemented the profession's efforts to re-establish our values in the promotion of human performance.

Another example created by social and economic forces to return the disabled to productive life is the newly developed programs in work evaluation, work hardening, and work capacity. Social forces prevalent today provide advantages for our profession to proclaim human occupation as a therapeutic medium and the occupational process as a cost-effective method to promote healthfulness. In this decade, OTRs must become actively involved in research and management of cost-effective services. Thus, the future will see an increasing number of COTAs being employed in schools, home health, and community agencies with their roles in direct services being expanded.

Trends in Educational Preparation

As service delivery patterns expand and diversity of practice is determined by the system in which services are provided, the roles and functions of occupational therapy personnel must be altered to meet the evolving focus upon health promotion and prevention of disabilities. In response to transformation, the AOTA must re-examine the delineation of roles and functions of the OTR and the COTA. No longer must the delineation be solely determined by current practices; future trends must be recognized and the impact of those trends upon OTR and COTA practices considered. Through delineation of predicted roles of the entry-level therapist and assistant, knowledge, skills, and attitudes needed by each of the personnel groups must be identified. Then, appropriate educational preparation of the OTR and COTA can be implemented.

The demands for OTRs to assume roles in consultation and supervision, to conduct research, develop theories, and manage cost-effective programs will require knowledge and skills that are associated with graduate-level programs. The demands for COTAs to function more independently will require knowledge and skills about occupational therapy theory and practice as well as liberal arts courses. As stated by Pierce,[23] "liberal arts studies are necessary for occupational therapists to make the appropriate interconnections needed to develop a perspective that allows the therapist to be professionally competent." The degree of liberal arts preparation and needed knowledge, skills, and attitudes specific to the practice of occupational therapy require a minimum of four years of higher education. The upcoming years will see COTAs functioning more independently in the areas of evaluation, planning, and treatment. Independent practices require problem-solving abilities and skills to analyze and synthesize complex information. Thus, additional educational preparation will be necessary.

Summary

The future of occupational therapy will be influenced by the current environment of opportunity. Social, political, and economic forces are having an impact on occupational therapy health care services. Demands for cost-effective programs and concepts of health promotion, together with society's recognition of the importance of one's own responsibilities toward maintaining health, are factors that will promote an expansion of our services.

Our profession is in a period of transformation with the emergence of a value system based on occupation and the process of occupational therapy providing sensible continuity for practice. Dimensions of practice will include diversity of our services as offered through community, education, and medical systems. Philosophy and practice will transform treatment orientation into health promotion in which our services can focus on the patient's assets and abilities.

Occupational therapy personnel will modify their roles and functions to meet the demands for services. As roles change, so must the educational preparation for both the OTR and COTA.

Through transformation we will direct our own future. The time for promotion of the idea of "health through doing" is now. It is the era when occupational therapy can proclaim its uniqueness, and when the therapeutic use of occupations to facilitate abilities can allow individuals to influence their own states of health.

References

1. Jaffe E: Transition in health care: Critical planning for the 1990s. *Am J Occup Ther*, 39:431-435, 1985.

2. Capra F: *The Turning Point: Science, Society, and the Rising Culture*. Toronto, Ontario: Bantam Books, 1983.

3. Naisbit J: *Megatrends*. New York: Warner Books, 1982.

4. Ferguson M: *The Aquarian Conspiracy: Personal and Social Transformation in the 1980s*. Los Angeles, CA: JP Tarcher, 1980, p 221.

5. Gilfoyle E: Transformation of a profession. *Am J Occup Ther*, 38:578-582, 1984.

6. Mittelstadt P: The future of our nation's health care: Will rationing be needed? *Am J Occup Ther*, 39:229-232, 1985.

7. Deal TE, Kennedy AA: *Corporate Cultures: The Rites and Rituals of Corporate Life*. Reading, MA: Addison-Wesley, 1982, p 21-25.

8. Hall BP: *The Development of Consciousness: A Confluent Theory of Values*. New York: Paulist Press, 1976.

9. Willard H and Spackman C: *Occupational Therapy*. Philadelphia: JB Lippincott Co., 1947, p 1.

10. Kidner TB: *Occupational Therapy: The Science of Prescribed Work for Invalids*. Stuttgart, Germany: W Kohlhanne, 1930.

11. Licht S: The founding and founders of the American Occupational Therapy Association. *Am J Occup Ther*, 23: 269-277, 1967.

12. Barton GE: *Teaching the Sick: A Manual of Occupational Therapy and Re-education*. Philadelphia: WB Saunders, 1914, p 4.

13. Hall H: *Occupational Therapy—A New Profession*. Concord, NH: Rumford Press, 1923.

14. Hopkins H, Smith H: *Willard and Spackman's Occupational Therapy*, 6th Edition. Philadelphia: JB Lippincott, 1983, p 3.

15. King LJ: Toward a science of adaptive responses. *Am J Occup Ther* 32: 429-430, 1978.

16. Gilfoyle E, Grady A, Moore J: *Children Adapt*. Thorofare, NJ: Charles B. Slack, 1980, Chapter 3.

17. Kielhofner G, ed: *Health Through Occupation: The Theory and Practice of Occupational Therapy*. Philadelphia: FA Davis, 1983.

18. The Philosophical Base of Occupational Therapy. American Occupational Therapy Association, Resolution 531, April, 1979.

19. West W: A reaffirmed philosophy and practice of occupational therapy for the 1980s . *Am J Occup Ther* 38:15-23, 1984.

20. Yerxa E: The philosophical base of occupational therapy. In *Occupational Therapy: 2001 AD*. Rockville, MD: American Occupational Therapy Association, 1978, p 29.

21. Davy J: Status report on reimbursement for occupational therapy. *Am J Occup Ther*, 38:295-297.

22. *PIVOT*: Rockville, MD: American Occupational Therapy Association, 1985.

23. Pierce E: The liberal arts connection. *Am J Occup Ther*, 38:237.

Appendix A. Explanation of Data, People, and Things*

Much of the information in this publication is based on the premise that every job requires a worker to [relate] in some degree to Data, People, and Things. These relationships are identified and explained below. They appear in the form of three lists arranged in each instance from the relatively simple to the complex in such a manner that each successive relationship includes those that are simpler and excludes the more complex.[1] The identifications attached to these relationships are referred to as worker functions, and provide standard terminology for use in summarizing exactly what a worker does on the job.

A job's relationship to Data, People, and Things can be expressed in terms of the lowest numbered function in each sequence. These functions taken together indicate the total level of complexity at which the worker performs. The fourth, fifth, and sixth digits of the occupational code numbers reflect relationships to Data, People, and Things, respectively.[2] These digits express a job's relationship to Data, People, and Things by identifying the highest appropriate function in each listing as reflected by the following table:

DATA (4th digit)	PEOPLE (5th digit)	THINGS (6th digit)
0 Synthesizing	0 Mentoring	0 Setting-Up
1 Coordinating	1 Negotiating	1 Precision Working
2 Analyzing	2 Instructing	2 Operating-Controlling
3 Compiling	3 Supervising	3 Driving-Operating
4 Computing	4 Diverting	4 Manipulating
5 Copying	5 Persuading	5 Tending
6 Comparing	6 Speaking-Signaling	6 Feeding-Offbearing
	7 Serving	7 Handling
	8 Taking Instructions-Helping	

[1]As each of the relationships to People represents a wide range of complexity, resulting in considerable overlap among occupations, their arrangement is somewhat arbitrary and can be considered a hierarchy only in the most general sense.
[2]Only those relationships which are occupationally significant in terms of the requirements of the job are reflected in the code numbers. The incidental relationships which every worker has to Data, People, and Things, but which do not seriously affect successful performance of the essential duties of the job, are not reflected.

Definitions of Worker Functions

DATA: Information, knowledge, and conceptions, related to data, people, or things, obtained by observation, investigation, interpretation, visualization, and mental creation. Data are intangible and include numbers, words, symbols, ideas, concepts, and oral verbalization.

0 Synthesizing: Integrating analyses of data to discover facts and/or develop knowledge concepts of interpretations.
1 Coordinating: Determining time, place, and sequence of operations or action to be taken on the basis of analysis of data; executing determination and/or reporting on events.
2 Analyzing: Examining and evaluating data. Presenting alternative actions in relation to the evaluation is frequently involved.
3 Compiling: Gathering, collating, or classifying information about data, people, or things. Reporting and/or carrying out a prescribed action in relation to the information is frequently involved.
4 Computing: Performing arithmetic operations and reporting on and/or carrying out a prescribed action in relation to them. Does not include counting.
5 Copying: Transcribing, entering, or posting data.
6 Comparing: Judging the readily observable functional, structural, or compositional characteristics (whether similar to or divergent from obvious standards) of data, people, or things.

PEOPLE: Human beings; also animals dealt with on an individual basis as if they were human.

0 Mentoring: Dealing with individuals in terms of their total personality in order to advise, counsel, and/or guide them with regard to problems that may be resolved by legal, scientific, clinical, spiritual, and/or other professional principles.
1 Negotiating: Exchanging ideas, information, and opinions with others to formulate policies and programs and/or arrive jointly at decisions, conclusions, or solutions.
2 Instructing: Teaching subject matter to others, or training others (including animals) through explanation, demonstration, and supervised practice; or making recommendations on the basis of technical disciplines.
3 Supervising: Determining or interpreting work procedures for a group of workers, assigning specific duties to them, maintaining harmonious relations among them, and promoting efficiency. A variety of responsibilities is involved in this function.
4 Diverting: Amusing others. (Usually accomplished through the medium of stage, screen, television, or radio.)
5 Persuading: Influencing others in favor of a product, service, or point of view.
6 Speaking-Signaling: Talking with and/or signaling people to convey or exchange information. Includes giving assignments and/or directions to helpers or assistants.
7 Serving: Attending to the needs or requests of people or animals or the expressed or implicit wishes of people. Immediate response is involved.
8 Taking Instructions-Helping: Helping applies to "non-learning" helpers. No variety of responsibility is involved in this function.

THINGS: Inanimate objects as distinguished from human beings, substances or materials; machines, tools, equipment and products. A thing is tangible and has shape, form, and other physical characteristics.

0 Setting up: Adjusting machines or equipment by replacing or altering tools, jigs, fixtures, and attachments to prepare them to perform their functions, change their performance,

*U.S. Department of Labor, Employment and Training Administration. *Dictionary of Occupational Titles*, 4th Ed. Washington, D.C.: U.S. Government Printing Office, 1977, pp. 1369-1371.

or restore their proper functioning if they break down. Workers who set up one or a number of machines for other workers or who set up and personally operate a variety of machines are included here.

1 Precision Working: Using body members and/or tools or work aids to work, move, guide, or place objects or materials in situations where ultimate responsibility for the attainment of standards occurs and selection of appropriate tools, objects, or materials, and the adjustment of the tool to the task require exercise of considerable judgment.

2 Operating-Controlling: Starting, stopping, controlling, and adjusting the progress of machines or equipment. Operating machines involves setting up and adjusting the machine or material(s) as the work progresses. Controlling involves observing gages, dials, etc., and turning valves and other devices to regulate factors such as temperature, pressure, flow of liquids, speed of pumps, and reactions of materials.

3 Driving-Operating: Starting, stopping, and controlling the actions of machines or equipment for which a course must be steered, or which must be guided, in order to fabricate, process, and/or move things or people. Involves such activities as observing gages and dials; estimating distances and determining speed and direction of other objects; turning cranks and wheels; pushing or pulling gear lifts or levers. Includes such machines as cranes, conveyor systems, tractors, furnace charging machines, paving machines and hoisting machines. Excludes manually powered machines, such as handtrucks and dollies, and power assisted machines such as electric wheelbarrows and handtrucks.

4 Manipulating: Using body members, tools, or special devices to work, move, guide, or place objects or materials. Involves some latitude for judgment with regard to precision attained and selecting appropriate tool, object, or material, although this is readily manifest.

5 Tending: Starting, stopping, and observing the functioning of machines and equipment. Involves adjusting materials or controls of the machine, such as changing guides, adjusting timers and temperature gages, turning valves to allow flow of materials, and flipping switches in response to lights. Little judgment is involved in making these adjustments.

6 Feeding-Offbearing: Inserting, throwing, dumping, or placing materials in or removing them from machines or equipment which are automatic or tended or operated by other workers.

7 Handling: Using body members, handtools, and/or special devices to work, move or carry objects or materials. Involves little or no latitude for judgment with regard to attainment of standards or in selecting appropriate tool, object, or material.

Appendix B. Recreational Organizations for Disabled Persons

American Alliance for Health, Physical Education and Recreation for the Handicapped
Information and Research
Utilization Center
1201 16th Street, NW
Washington, D.C. 20036
Phone: 202-833-5547

American National Red Cross
Program of Swimming for the Handicapped
17th and D Streets, NW
Washington, D.C. 20006
Phone: 202-857-3542

Handicapped Boaters
P.O. Box 1134, Ansonia Station
New York, NY 10023
Phone: 212-377-0310

National Association of Sports for Cerebral Palsy
United Cerebral Palsy Association of Connecticut
One State Steet
New Haven, CT 06511
Phone: 203-772-2080

National Park Service
Department of Interior
18th and C Streets, NW
Washington, D.C. 20240
Phone: 202-343-6843

National Wheelchair Athletic Association
Nassau Community College
Garden City, NY 11530
Phone: 212-222-1245

National Wheelchair Softball Association
P.O. Box 737
Sioux Falls, SD 57101

North American Riding Association
P.O. Box 100
Ashburn, VA 22011
Phone: 703-777-3540

American Athletic Association of the Deaf
3916 Lantern Drive
Silver Spring, MD 20902
Phone: 301-942-4042

American Blind Bowling Association
150 N. Bellair Avenue
Louisville, KY 40206
Phone: 502-896-8039

American Wheelchair Bowling Association
2635 NE 19th Street
Pompano Beach, FL 33062
Phone: 305-941-1238

International Committee on the Silent Sports
Gallaudet College
Florida Avenue and 7th Street, NE
Washington, D.C. 20002
Phone: 202-331-1731 or 447-0360

National Association of the Physically Handicapped
76 Elm Street
London, OH 43140
Phone: 614-852-1664

National Inconvenienced Sportsmen's Association
3738 Walnut Avenue
Carmichael, CA 95608
Phone: 916-484-2153

National Therapeutic Recreation Society
1601 N. Kent Street
Arlington, VA 22209
Phone: 703-525-0606

National Wheelchair Basketball Association
110 Seaton Center
University of Kentucky
Lexington, KY 40506
Phone: 703-777-3540

People-to-People Committee for the Handicapped
LaSalle Building, Suite 610
Connecticut Avenue and L Street
Washington, D.C. 20036
Phone: 202-785-0755

The President's Committee on Employment of the Handicapped
Subcommittee on Recreation and Leisure
Washington, D.C. 20210

Travel Information Center
Moss Rehabilitation Hospital
12th Street and Tabor Road
Philadelphia, PA 19141

United States Deaf Skiers Association
Two Sunset Hill Road
Simbury, CT 06070
Phone: 203-244-3341

National Handicapped Sports and Recreation Association
Capital Hill Station
P.O. Box 18664
Denver, CO 80218

National Spinal Cord Injury Foundation (Marathon Racing)
369 Elliot Street
Newton Upper Falls, MA 02164

Rehabilitation-Education Center (Football)
University of Illinois
Oak Street at Stadium Drive
Champaign, IL 61820

Wheelchair Motorcycle Association
(All Terrain Vehicles)
101 Torrey Street
Brockton, MA 02410

Sports And Spokes
(W/C Sports Magazine)
5201 N. 19th Ave.
Phoenix, AZ 85015

The Riding School Inc.
275 South Avenue
Weston, MA 02193
Phone: 617-899-4555

S.I.R.E. Inc. (Self-Improvement Through Riding Education)
91 Old Bolton Road
Stow, MA 01775
Phone: 617-897-3396

Winslow Riding for the Handicapped
P.O. Box 100
Ashburn, VA 22011
Phone: 703-777-3540

Vinland National Center
3675 Ihduhapi Rd.
Loretto, MN 55357
Phone: 612: 479-3555

National Foundation of Wheelchair Tennis
3855 Birch Street
Newport Beach, CA 92660

National Recreation and Park Association
1601 N. Kent Street
Arlington, VA 22209

Disabled Sportsmen of America Inc.
P.O. Box 26
Vinton, VA 24179

Wheelchair Pilots Association
11018 102nd Ave. North
Largo, FL 33540

American W/C Pilots Association
4419 N. 27th St. Apt. 3
Phoenix, AZ 85105

Winter Park Recreational Association (Skiing)
Hal O'Leary, Director, Handicapped Programs
Box 313, Winter Park, CO 80482

Appendix C-1. Work Skill Assessment Form*

	Yes	No
1. Willingness to start the task		
Agrees to start task without arguing		
Shows enthusiasm about task		
Starts immediately after directions have been given		
2. Ability to follow directions		
Follows verbal directions correctly		
Follows written directions correctly		
3. Acceptance of supervision		
Accepts direction without showing resentment		
Accepts criticism from supervisor without arguing or becoming defensive		
4. Ability to sustain interest in the task		
Works continuously without becoming distracted		
Tolerates small frustrations without losing interest		
Facial expression and posture indicate interest		
5. Appropriate use of tools and materials		
Uses familiar equipment for appropriate purposes		
Handles equipment skillfully and safely		
Uses material without wasting it		
6. Appropriate rate of performance		
Accomplishes task successfully within time limit		
7. Acceptable level of neatness		
Keeps working area uncluttered		
Maintains personal neatness		
Cleans up when finished		
8. Appropriate attention to detail		
Doesn't spend too much time or energy on unimportant details		
Performs accurately when necessary		
9. Ability to organize tasks in a logical manner		
Makes sure directions are clear before starting		
Checks to see that all materials and supplies are ready before starting		
Performs steps in logical sequence		
10. Problem solving		
Recognizes when a problem exists		
Attempts to solve problems without asking for help		
Shows creativity in solving problems		
Finds practical solutions to problems		

*Adapted from Mosey, AC: *Activities Therapy*, Raven Press: New York, 1973, pp. 112-120.

Appendix C-2. Assessment of Social Skills Form*

Dyadic Skills	Yes	No	Skill Components	Comments
1.			Expresses ideas clearly	
2.			Demonstrates appropriate affect	
3.			Initiates conversation	
4.			Maintains eye contact	
5.			Greets and calls people by name	
6.			Manners/habits are acceptable	
7.			Responds when spoken to	
8.			Responds beyond "yes" or "no"	
9.			Expresses feelings verbally	
10.			Shows consideration to others	
11.			Remains in contact throughout conversation	
12.			Speaks audibly and clearly	
Group Skills				
1.			Participates in group discussion	
2.			Asks for information	
3.			Contributes information	
4.			Asks for opinions	
5.			Contributes opinions	
6.			Encourages others	
7.			Assumes leadership role	
8.			Suggests operating procedures	
9.			Is willing to compromise	
10.			Accepts praise comfortably	
11.			Accepts criticism graciously	
12.			Supportive of others' contributions	

*The assessment is taken from an unpublished manual, P. Babcock, with permission.

Appendix D. Sample Group Exercise

The following patients have been working on craft activities in a parallel group. After discussion with the OTR supervisor, it was decided that the COTA should plan a *project* level activity that would meet the needs of the individuals in this group.

Patient	Observation	Plan
Ms. Wisenheimer	Is not interested in crafts. Identifies with staff. Is sarcastic and irritable.	Improve self-esteem. Allow some authority.
Ms. Gloomy Thoughts	Slowed down physically and mentally. Expresses feelings of inadequacy. Has difficulty making decisions.	Increase rate of performance. Provide activities that are easily recognized as useful and have a minimal number of steps.
Ms. Jitterbug	Capable and willing to work, but is tense, agitated, and restless. Socializes well with others, but sometimes annoys others with interfering behavior. Needs immediate gratification.	Increase attention span. Provide tasks that are structured and short term. Provide for release of energy.
Ms. Detached	Offers minimal conversation. Appears sensitive to the needs of others. Usually chooses to sit by herself. Is unable to make decisions without help.	Develop personal identity and decision making skills.
Ms. Picky	Is cooperative, conscientious, and a perfectionist. Works slowly and is seldom satisfied with her work. Becomes irritated with the poor performance of others. Has trouble expressing her ideas.	Improve decision making skills. Provide tasks that are easily corrected if mistakes are made. Develop behavior that is more tolerant of others.
Ms. Finagle	Undependable and manipulative. Appears friendly but talks about the other patients. Very bright and capable.	Develop dependable behavior. Provide activities that are intellectually stimulating and absorbing.

These patients are middle class young adults. All but one have completed high school, and they all have had problems with chemical dependency. Using the information regarding *project groups* as a reference, respond to the following:

1. What activity could the COTA choose?
2. What steps are involved in the activity, and how much time would each take?
3. What tools and materials would be required to complete the activity?
4. The supervisor has also asked the COTA to develop *task* related behavioral goals for two of the patients: Ms. Gloomy Thoughts and Ms. Jitterbug.
5. What goals might be appropriate for these patients? Is there a specific part of the selected activity that could be assigned to each of these patients in order to develop the desired behavior?
6. How might the activity be introduced to the group?
7. How would the group goal be explained to the members?

Appendix E-1. Standards of Practice for Occupational Therapy*

STANDARDS OF PRACTICE FOR OCCUPATIONAL THERAPY

compiled by:

Doris J. Shriver, OTR
Mary Foto, OTR
Members, AOTA Commission on Practice

for:

AOTA Commission on Practice
John Farace, OTR, Chair

Preface

These standards will assist the AOTA members in the management of occupational therapy services and will serve as a minimum standard for occupational therapy practice that is applicable to all client populations and the programs in which clients are served.

These standards are for qualified occupational therapists (OTRs) that are currently certified or licensed where required by the state.

Standard I: Screening

1. Occupational therapists have the responsibility to identify clients who may present problems in occupational performance (work, self-care, and play/leisure) that would require an evaluation.
2. Occupational therapists screen independently or as members of a team.
3. Screening methods shall be appropriate to the client's age, education, cultural background, medical status, and functional ability.
4. Screening methods may include interviewing, observation, testing, and record review.
5. Occupational therapists shall communicate the screening results and recommendations to all appropriate individuals.

Standard II: Referral

1. A client is appropriately referred to occupational therapy for remediation, maintenance, or prevention when the client has, or appears to have, a dysfunction or potential for dysfunction in occupational performance (work, self-care, play/leisure) or the performance components (sensorimotor, cognitive, psychosocial).
2. Clients shall be referred to occupational therapy for evaluation, design construction of, or training in therapeutic adaptations that include, but are not limited to, the physical environment, orthotics, prosthetics, and assistive and adaptive equipment.
3. Occupational therapists respond to a request for service and enter a case at their own professional discretion and on their own cognizance, and then assume full responsibility for the determination of the appropriate type, nature, and mode of service.
4. When physician referral is necessary to meet regulations (facility, state, federal, Joint Commission for Accreditation of Hospitals, licensure) or is required for third-party payment, the registered occupational therapist enters a case at the request of a physician; assumes full responsibility for the occupational therapy assessment; and, in consultation with the physician, establishes the appropriate type, nature, and mode of service.
5. Registered occupational therapists shall refer clients to other appropriate re-

*Uniform Terminology for Reporting Occupational Therapy Services, adopted March 1979 by The Representative Assembly, AOTA.

Adopted April 1983 by the Representative Assembly, The American Occupational Therapy Association, Inc.

sources when, in the judgment of the occupational therapist, the knowledge and expertise of another professional is required.

6. Occupational therapists have the responsibility to teach appropriate persons how to make occupational therapy referrals.

Standard III: Evaluation

1. Occupational therapists shall evaluate the client's performance according to the Uniform Occupational Therapy Checklist (AOTA-Adopted 1981).
2. Initial occupational therapy evaluations shall consider the client's medical, vocational, educational, activity, social history, and personal/family goals.
3. The occupational therapy evaluation shall include assessment of the functional abilities and deficits as related to the client's needs in the following areas:
   a. Occupational Performance: work, self-care, and play/leisure.
   b. Performance Components: sensorimotor, cognitive, psychosocial.
   c. Therapeutic adaptations and prevention.
4. Initial occupational therapy evaluations shall be completed and results documented within the time frames established by facilities, government agencies, and accreditation programs.
5. All evaluation methods shall be appropriate to the client's age, education, cultural and ethnic background, medical status, and functional ability.
6. The evaluation methods may include observation, interview, record review, and the use of evaluation techniques or tools.
7. When standardized evaluation tools are used, the tests should have normative data for the client characteristics. If normative data are not available, the results should be expressed in a descriptive report.
8. Collected evaluation data shall be analyzed and summarized to indicate the client's current status.
9. Occupational therapists shall document evaluation results in the client's record and indicate the specific evaluation tools and methods used.
10. Occupational therapists shall communicate evaluation results to the appropriate persons in the facility and community.
11. If the results of the evaluation indicate areas that require intervention by other professionals, the occupational therapist should refer the client to the appropriate service or request consultation.

Standard IV: Individual Program Planning

1. Occupational therapists shall use the results of the evaluation to develop an individual occupational therapy program that is:
   a. Stated in measurable and reasonable terms appropriate to the client's needs and goals and expected prognosis.
   b. Consistent with current principles and concepts of occupational therapy theory and practice.
2. The planning process shall include:
   a. Identifying short- and long-term goals.
   b. Collaborating with client, family, other professionals, and community resources.
   c. Selecting the media, methods, environment, and personnel needed to accomplish goals.
   d. Determining the frequency and duration of occupational therapy services.
3. The initial program plan shall be prepared and documented within the time frames established by facilities, government agencies, and accreditation programs.

Standard V: Individual Program Implementation

1. Occupational therapists shall implement the program according to the program plan.

2. Occupational therapists shall formulate and implement program modifications consistent with changes in the client's occupational performance and performance components.
3. Occupational therapists shall periodically re-evaluate and document the client's occupational performance and performance components.
4. Occupational therapists shall document the occupational therapy services provided and the frequency of the services within time frames established by facilities, government agencies, and accreditation programs.

Standard VI: Discontinuation of Service

1. Occupational therapists shall discontinue services when the client has achieved the goals or has achieved maximum benefit from occupational therapy.
2. Occupational therapists shall formulate and implement program modifications consistent with changes in the client's occupational performance and performance components.
3. Occupational therapists shall prepare a discharge plan that is consistent with the occupational therapy, client, interdisciplinary team, family and goals, and the expected prognosis. Consideration should be given to appropriate community resources for referral and environmental factors or barriers that may need modification.
4. Occupational therapists shall allow sufficient time for the coordination of and the effective implementation of the discharge plan.
5. Occupational therapists shall document recommendations for follow-up or reevaluation.

Standard VII: Quality Assurance

1. The occupational therapist shall periodically and systematically review all aspects of individual occupational therapy programs for effectiveness and efficiency.
2. Occupational therapists shall periodically and systematically review the quality and appropriateness of total services delivered, using predetermined criteria that reflect professional consensus and recent development in research and theory.

Standard VIII: Indirect Services

1. Occupational therapists shall provide supervision of other personnel as assigned in accordance with the AOTA *Guide for Supervision* (AOTA-Adopted, 1981).
2. Occupational therapists shall maintain records to meet facility, government agency, and accreditation program requirements.
3. Occupational therapists shall maintain a level of professional knowledge and skills to assure continued competency.
4. Occupational therapists shall facilitate research as it applies to the active practice of occupational therapy.
5. Occupational therapists shall provide administration and management services that ensure the use of AOTA standards.
6. Occupational therapists shall provide consultation services in order to develop or coordinate occupational therapy services, provide in-service education, adapt environments, and promote preventive health care in the home, client care facility, or community.

Standard IX: Legal Ethical Components

1. Occupational therapists shall maintain current AOTA certification or licensure where required by the state.
2. Occupational therapists shall practice and manage occupational therapy programs as defined by federal and state laws and regulations.
3. Occupational therapists shall be familiar with and abide by the ethical practices of the specific facility or system in which the service is provided.

4. Occupational therapists shall observe the ethical practices as defined by The American Occupational Therapy Association, Inc., *Principles of Ethics* (AOTA, Revised 1980).
5. Occupational therapists shall provide all aspects of direct and indirect services according to Standards and Policies of The American Occupational Therapy Association, Inc.

Glossary

OCCUPATIONAL THERAPY ASSESSMENT—the process of determining the need for, nature of, and estimated time of treatment, determining the needed coordination with other persons involved, and documenting these activities.

EVALUATION—the process of obtaining and interpreting data necessary for treatment. This includes planning for and documenting the evaluation process and results. This data may be gathered through record review, specific observation, interview, and the administration of data collection procedures. Such procedures include, but are not limited to, the use of standardized tests, performance checklists, and activities and tasks designed to evaluate specific performance abilities.

MAINTENANCE OF FUNCTION—the process of preserving and supporting an individual's current abilities to engage in interpersonal relationships and to manipulate the nonhuman environment.

OCCUPATIONAL PERFORMANCE—life tasks (self-care, work, play/leisure) that are all those activities that individuals must perform to meet their own needs and to be contributing members of the community.

PERFORMANCE COMPONENTS—the skill areas (sensorimotor, cognitive, psychosocial) a person develops to facilitate carrying out self-care, work, and play/leisure.

PROGRAM PLANNING—the development of an individual client's treatment plan.

SCREENING—the review of the potential client's case to determine the need for evaluation and treatment.

THERAPEUTIC ADAPTATIONS—the design and restructuring of the physical environment to assist self-care, work, and play/leisure performance. This includes selecting, obtaining, fitting, and fabricating equipment, and instructing the client, family, and staff in proper use and care of equipment. It also includes minor repair and modification for correct fit, position, or use. Categories of therapeutic adaptations consist of: orthotics, prosthetics, and assistive and adaptive equipment.

Appendix E-2. Entry-Level OTR and COTA Role Delineation*

This role delineation is intended for internal use by the American Occupational Therapy Association, Inc. as a guide to assist members in the practice of their profession. The role delineation may be used to assist in the development of entry-level educational Essentials and certification criteria, but may not be used (except with the written permission of the AOTA) to draft legal documents of any kind such as licensure bills or private contracts.

The contents of this document are not to be construed as entirely original, but represent a compilation of resource materials and professional judgment. Resource documents used were:

1. AOTA Entry Level Functions of the Registered Occupational Therapist, Certified Occupational Therapy Assistant and Occupational Therapy Aide; AOTA; 1972.
2. Task Inventory for Entry Level Occupational Therapy Personnel in Direct Service Roles; NIH Contract No. 72-4172; AOTA; June 1973.
3. Phase 1-Delineation of the Role of Entry Level Occupational Therapy Personnel; Contract #231-76-0052; AOTA; July 1, 1976—February 1, 1978.
4. AOTA Standards of Practice for Occupational Therapy Services for the Developmentally Disabled Client; Clients with Physical Disabilities; in a Mental Health Program; and in a Home Health Program; AOTA; January 1979.
5. Essentials of an Accredited Educational Program for the Occupational Therapist; June 1972; and Essentials of an Approved Educational Program for the Occupational Therapy Assistant; April 1975.
6. AOTA Resolution #533-79 (Funding for 518-77), #535-79 (Role Delineation Concept and Use), #552-79 (Strategy to Educate Independent Health Professionals), #551-79 (Position on Proficiency Testing for Individuals Outside the Field of Occupational Therapy), and proposed Resolution "J"-1980 (Strategy for Determining the Place of the COTA in the Profession of Occupational Therapy).
7. Entry Level Study Committee Memo; AOTA; April 7, 1980.
8. Essentials Review Committee Report: Recommendation #1; AOTA; 1980.
9. Components and Interrelationships of a Competency Assurance System, Chart #1 and Management of the AOTA Competency Assurance System, Chart #2; AOTA; 1979.
10. *AOTA Uniform Terminology for Reporting Occupational Therapy Services;* AOTA; 1979.

The following principles/concepts were used in the development of the role delineation document:

1. OTRs must be able to do all COTA roles and functions.
2. The role delineation reflects present and future practice of occupational therapy.
3. The role delineation reflects entry-level practice only and may be used only for that level when used to develop educational Essentials or certification requirements.
4. Entry-level is defined as the first year of practice.
5. Entry-level COTAs must receive direct supervision by an OTR during the first year of occupational therapy practice. COTAs are encouraged to participate in continuing education programs provided by agencies and professional associations and to pursue other continuing education opportunities.
6. Entry-level OTRs are certified for general practice and are able to independently provide services. Entry-level OTRs are encouraged to pursue continuing education, consultation and other collaborative activities in their professional role.

7. Employers should provide appropriate personnel for the supervision of new graduates.
8. The role delineation addresses tasks and not "professional" behaviors that reflect ethical or value judgments.

Refer to the Role Delineation Glossary and AOTA *Uniform Terminology System for Reporting Occupational Therapy Services* for definitions of terms used in this document.

Entry-Level OTR And COTA Role Delineation

I. Referral: the initiation or acknowledgment of a referral may be before initial screening or after. A referral for occupational therapy service must be based upon the provisions as outlined in the AOTA Statement of Referral.

The Entry-Level OTR

A. Responds to request for service, whatsoever its source

B. Initiates referrals when appropriate

C. Supervises documentation and filing of referrals according tò department standards

D. Delegates case to COTA, as appropriate, according to standards of department and profession

The Entry-Level COTA

A. Responds to a request for service by relaying information or formal referral to supervising OTR

B. Initiates referrals for independent living/daily living skills intervention

C. Enters case as appropriate to standards of department and profession when authorized by supervising OTR

II. Occupational Therapy Assessment: Occupational therapy assessment refers to the process of determining the need for, nature of, and estimated time of treatment, determining the needed coordination with other persons involved, and documenting these activities.

The Entry-Level OTR

A. *Screening:* determine client's need for occupational therapy services: may occur before or after referral
   1. Collect data:
      a. identify type and sources of information that are needed
      b. obtain and review information and identify pertinent details about client; or plan and supervise data collection
      c. explain overall occupational therapy services to client, family, and significant others
      d. observe and interview client, family, and significant others to obtain general history and information
   2. Analyze data:
      a. organize data
      b. summarize data
      c. interpret data
   3. Formulate recommendations
   4. Document and report occupational therapy screening data, interpretation, and recommendations

B. *Evaluation:* obtain and interpret data necessary for treatment.This includes planning for and documenting the evaluation process and results. The OTR is responsible for the evaluation process.

The Entry-Level COTA

A. *Screening:* determine client's need for occupational therapy services in collaboration with OTR; may occur before or after referral
   1. Collect data:
      a. obtain and review information as determined by OTR and identify pertinent details about client
      b. explain overall occupational therapy services to client, family and significant others
      c. observe and interview client, family, and significant others *using a structured guide* to obtain general history and information
   2. Organize data:
      a. summarize *own* data
      b. record and report *own* data to OTR

B. *Evaluation:* The COTA contributes to the evaluation process under the supervision of the OTR.

The Entry-Level OTR	The Entry-Level COTA

1. Select appropriate area(s) to evaluate
   a. independent living/daily living skills
      (1) Physical Daily Living Skills
         (a) Grooming and Hygiene
         (b) Feeding/Eating
         (c) Dressing
         (d) Functional Mobility
         (e) Functional Communication
         (f) Object Manipulation
      (2) Psychological/Emotional Daily Living Skills
         (a) Self-concept/Self-identity
         (b) Situation Coping
         (c) Community Involvement
      (3) Work
         (a) Homemaking
         (b) Child Care/Parenting
         (c) Employment Preparation
      (4) Play/Leisure
   b. sensorimotor components
      (1) Neuromuscular
         (a) Reflex Integration
         (b) Range of Motion
         (c) Gross and Fine Coordination
         (d) Strength and Endurance
      (2) Sensory Integration
         (a) Sensory Awareness
         (b) Visual-Spatial Awareness
         (c) Body Integration
   c. cognitive components
      (1) Orientation
      (2) Conceptualization/Comprehension
         (a) Concentration
         (b) Attention Span
         (c) Memory
      (3) Cognitive Integration
         (a) Generalization
         (b) Problem Solving
   d. psychosocial components
      (1) Self-management
         (a) Self-expression
         (b) Self-control
      (2) Dyadic Interaction
      (3) Group Interaction
2. Plan evaluation methodology
3. Explain evaluation plan to client, family, significant others, and other health professionals
4. Interview client, family, and significant others for information about:
   a. medical history and current health status
   b. developmental milestones
   c. social and family history

COTA:

1. Assist OTR by interviewing client, family, and significant others *using a structured format* as determined by OTR for information about:
   a. family history
   b. self-care abilities

The Entry-Level OTR	The Entry-Level COTA
d. self-care abilities e. academic history f. vocational history g. play history h. leisure interests and experiences i. future plans and goals j. accessibility of home environment k. accessibility of work or school system l. accessibility of community support system	c. academic history d. vocational history e. play history f. leisure interests and experiences
5. Observe client while engaged in individual and/or group activity to collect data and report on (refer to areas in Section II.B.1 for specifics in each area): a. independent living/daily living skills b. sensorimotor skills c. cognitive skills d. psychosocial skills	2. Assist OTR by observing client while engaged in individual and/or group activity to collect general data and report on (refer to areas in Section II.B.1 for specifics in each area): a. independent living/daily living skills b. selected sensorimotor skills: (1) Gross and fine coordination (2) Strength and endurance (3) Tactile awareness c. cognitive skills d. psychosocial skills
6. Administer standardized and non-standardized assessments in the following areas (refer to areas in Section II.B.1 for specifics in each area): a. independent living/daily living skills and performance b. sensorimotor skills and performance c. cognitive skills and performance d. psychosocial skills and performance e. therapeutic adaptations (1) Orthotics (2) Prosthetics (3) Assistive/Adaptive Equipment	3. Administer *structured* tests as directed by the OTR to collect data on: a. independent living/daily living skills and performance b. sensorimotor skills and performance in the following areas of: (1) Gross and Fine Coordination (2) Tactile Awareness c. cognitive skills and performance in the area of orientation
7. Analyze and synthesize evaluation data: a. state evaluation findings b. analyze, interpret, and synthesize scores or results of tests and assessments c. state client's assets and deficits	
8. Document evaluation data and interpretation	4. Summarize, record and report *own* evaluation data to OTR supervisor
9. Report evaluation data	5. Report evaluation data as determined by OTR
10. Develop recommendations as to the continuation or discontinuation of occupational therapy services and/or referral to other type of service.	6. Make recommendations to the OTR supervisor as to the continuation or discontinuation of occupational therapy services and/or referral to other type of service.

The Entry-Level OTR	The Entry-Level COTA

III. Program Planning: Planning refers to the identification of achievable program goals and the methods to those goals.

The Entry-Level OTR

A. Develop long- and short-term goals (in collaboration with client, family, and significant others) to develop, improve, and/or restore the performance of necessary functions; compensate for dysfunction; and/or minimize debilitation, in the areas of (refer to areas in Section II.B.1 for specifics in each area):
   1. Independent living/daily living skills and performance
   2. Sensorimotor skills and performance
   3. Cognitive skills and performance
   4. Psychosocial skills and performance

B. Refer client to experienced OTR for specialized evaluation and services; examples of specialized evaluations are employment preparation, evaluation (prevocational testing), sensory integration evaluation, prosthetic evaluation, driver's training evaluation.

C. Select occupational therapy techniques/media, and determine sequence of activities to attain goals in all areas

D. Analyze components which make up tasks and activities

E. Adapt techniques/media to meet needs, capacities and roles of the client

F. Discuss occupational therapy goals and methods with client, family, significant others, and other staff

G. Document and report program plan

H. Coordinate the program with staff and other services

I. Determine point of termination

The Entry-Level COTA

A. Assist OTR with the development of long- and short-term goals (in collaboration with client, family, and significant others) to develop, improve, and/or restore the performance of necessary functions; compensate for dysfunction; and/or minimize debilitation, in the areas of:
   1. Independent living/daily living skills and performance
   2. Sensorimotor skills and performance in the following areas:
      a. gross and fine coordination
      b. strength and endurance
      c. range of motion
      d. tactile awareness
   3. Cognitive skills and performance
   4. Psychosocial skills and performance

B. Assist OTR in selecting occupational therapy techniques/media, and in determining sequence of activities to attain goals in areas designated above

C. Analyze activities in the following areas:
   1. Relevance to client's interests and abilities
   2. Major motor processes
   3. Complexity
   4. Steps involved
   5. Extent to which it can be modified or adapted

D. Adapt techniques/media, under the supervision of the OTR, to meet client needs

E. Discuss occupational therapy program goals and methods with client, family, significant others, and staff

F. Document and report program plan as directed by the OTR

IV. Occupational Therapy Treatment: Occupational therapy treatment refers to the use of specific activities or methods to develop, improve, and/or restore the performance of necessary functions; compensate for dysfunction; and/or minimize debilitation.

- In situations where patient conditions or treatment settings are complex (involving multiple systems) and where conditions change rapidly, requiring frequent or ongoing reassessment and modification of treatment plan, the COTA is required to have close supervision by the OTR.

The Entry-Level OTR

A. Engage client in purposeful activity, in conjunction with therapeutic methods, to achieve goals identified in the program in the following areas:

1. Independent living/daily living skills
   a. physical daily living skills
      (1) Grooming and Hygiene
      (2) Feeding/Eating
      (3) Dressing
      (4) Functional Mobility

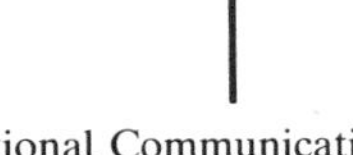

      (5) Functional Communication
      (6) Object Manipulation
   b. psychological/emotional daily living skills
      (1) Self-concept/Self-identity
      (2) Situational Coping
      (3) Community Involvement
   c. work
      (1) Homemaking
      (2) Child Care/Parenting
      (3) Employment Preparation
         (a) Work Process Skills and Performance
         (b) Work Product Quality
   d. play/leisure
2. Sensorimotor components
   a. neuromuscular
      (1) Reflex Integration
      (2) Range of Motion
      (3) Gross and Fine Coordination
      (4) Strength and Endurance
   b. sensory awareness
      (1) Sensory Awareness
      (2) Visual-Spatial Awareness
      (3) Body Integration
3. Cognitive components
   a. orientation
   b. conceptualization/comprehension
      (1) Concentration
      (2) Attention Span
      (3) Memory
   c. cognitive integration
      (1) Generalization
      (2) Problem Solving

The Entry-Level COTA

- In situations where patient conditions or treatment settings are more singular or stable so that decisions regarding program revision are required less frequently, the COTA may function independently as directed by the OTR.

A. Under the direction of the OTR, engage client in purposeful activity, in conjunction with therapeutic methods, to achieve goals identified in the program plan in the following areas:

1. Independent living/daily living skills
   a. physical daily living skills
      (1) Grooming and Hygiene
      (2) Feeding/Eating
      (3) Dressing
      (4) Functional Mobility:
         (a) Bed Mobility
         (b) Wheelchair Mobility
         (c) Transfers
         (d) Functional Ambulation
         (e) Public Transportation
      (5) Functional Communication
      (6) Object Manipulation
   b. psychological/emotional daily living skills
      (1) Self-concept/Self-identity
      (2) Situational Coping
      (3) Community Involvement
   c. work
      (1) Homemaking
      (2) Child Care/Parenting
      (3) Work Process Skills and Performance
   d. play/leisure
2. Sensorimotor components
   a. neuromuscular
      (1) Range of Motion
      (2) Gross and Fine Coordination
      (3) Strength and Endurance
   b. sensory integration
      (1) Tactile Awareness
      (2) Postural Balance
3. Cognitive components
   a. orientation
   b. conceptualization/comprehension
      (1) Concentration
      (2) Attention Span
      (3) Memory

The Entry-Level OTR	The Entry-Level COTA

The Entry-Level OTR

4. Psychosocial components
   a. self-management
      (1) Self-expression
      (2) Self-control
   b. dyadic interaction
   c. group interaction
5. Therapeutic adaptation
   a. orthotics
      (1) Static Splints
      (2) Slings
   b. assistive/adaptive equipment
6. Prevention
   a. energy conservation
   b. joint protection/body mechanics
   c. positioning
   d. coordination of daily living activities

B. Orient and instruct family, significant others and non-OT staff in activities which support the therapeutic program
C. Observe medical and safety precautions
D. Prepare and instruct a program with client, family, and significant others to implement at home
E. Monitor client's program
   1. Observe client's response to program
   2. Summarize and analyze client performance
   3. Document response to program
   4. Discuss client performance with client, family, significant others, and staff
   5. Reassess client's performance
   6. Modify goals
   7. Modify program
   8. Coordinate program modifications with other services

The Entry-Level COTA

4. Therapeutic adaptation
   a. orthotics
      (1) Static Splints
      (2) Slings
   b. assistive/adaptive equipment
5. Prevention
   a. energy conservation
   b. joint protection/body mechanics
   c. positioning
   d. coordination of daily living skills

B. Orient and instruct family and significant others in activities which support the therapeutic program
C. Observe medical and safety precautions
D. Assist in instruction of client, family, and significant others in implementation of home program developed by OTR
E. Monitor client's program
   1. Observe client's performance as directed by OTR
   2. Summarize client's performance as directed by OTR
   3. Document client's performance as directed by OTR
   4. Discuss client performance with client, family, significant others, and staff as directed by OTR
   5. Discuss need for reassessment with OTR
   6. Assist OTR in identifying program changes
   7. Coordinate program modifications with other services

V. Program Discontinuation: Program discontinuation refers to the termination of occupational therapy services when the client has achieved the program goals and/or has achieved maximum benefit from the services.

The Entry-Level OTR

A. Formulate, in collaboration with client, family, significant others, and staff, discharge and follow-up plan
B. Recommend termination of occupational therapy services
C. Prepare program for implementation at home
D. Recommend adaptations in client's everyday environment
E. Refer client and/or family to another occupational therapist or other service provider
F. Recommend community resources
G. Summarize and document outcome of the OT program
H. Terminate program

The Entry-Level COTA

A. Discuss need for program discontinuation with OTR
B. Assist OTR in preparing program for implementation at home
C. Assist OTR in recommending adaptations in client's everyday environment
D. Assist OTR in identifying community resources
E. Assist in summarizing and documenting outcome of the OT program

The Entry-Level OTR	The Entry-Level COTA

VI. Service Management: Service management refers to planning, leading, organizing, and controlling the occupational therapy facility and service.

The Entry-Level OTR

A. Maintain service
   1. Plan daily schedule according to assigned workload
   2. Prepare and maintain work setting, equipment, and supplies
   3. Order supplies and equipment according to established procedures
   4. Determine space, equipment, and supply needs
   5. Prepare and maintain records and budget
   6. Ensure safety and maintenance of program areas and equipment
   7. Compile and analyze data of OT service
   8. Follow reimbursement procedures
   9. Conduct and participate in employee meetings
   10. Participate in program-related conferences
   11. Receive supervision from immediate supervisor in order to enhance self-performance
   12. Comply with established standards and/or evaluate adherence to institutional policies
   13. Seek and use consultation

B. Recruit, select, orient, train, supervise, and evaluate:
   1. COTAs
   2. Support staff such as secretary, aide, transport personnel
   3. Volunteers

C. Plan, direct, coordinate, and evaluate service programs
D. Determine service and personnel needs
E. Assure collaboration, coordination, and communication
F. Develop and implement quality review program including:
   1. Standards of quality treatment/services
   2. Chart audit program
   3. Occupational therapy care review
   4. Inservice education programs
G. Participate in accrediting reviews
H. Supervise Level I fieldwork students, and non-OT students
I. Develop, through the use of statistics, the justification for having or increasing OT services

The Entry-Level COTA

A. Maintain service
   1. Plan daily schedule according to assigned workload
   2. Prepare and maintain work setting, equipment, and supplies
   3. Order supplies and equipment according to established procedures
   4. Maintain records according to department procedure
   5. Ensure safety and maintenance of program areas and equipment
   6. Assist with compiling and analyzing data of total OT service
   7. Follow reimbursement procedures
   8. Participate in employee meetings
   9. Participate in program-related conferences
   10. Receive supervision from immediate supervisor in order to enhance self-performance
   11. Comply with departmental standards and/or evaluate adherence to institutional policies

B. Assist with other personnel:
   1. Orient, supervise aides and assist in their training
   2. Recruit, select, orient, train, supervise, and evaluate volunteers under direction of OTR

C. Assist OTR with evaluation of service program

D. Participate in quality review program

E. Participate in accrediting reviews
F. Supervise Level 1 OTA fieldwork students as assigned by OTR

The Entry-Level OTR	The Entry-Level COTA
VII. Continued Education: Continued education refers to ongoing educational experiences beyond basic education.	
A. Participate in continuing education programs B. Participate in inservice programs C. Plan and provide inservice education	A. Participate in continuing education programs B. Participate in inservice programs C. Assist OTR in planning and providing inservice education
VIII. Public Relations: Public relations refers to promoting awareness and understanding of the profession of occupational therapy.	
A. Identify the need for and explain occupational therapy services and profession to public and professional groups B. Serve as a representative of the profession and the association	A. Explain occupational therapy services and profession to public groups B. Serve as a representative of the profession and the association

✓ Appendix E-3. Definitions

Independent living/daily living skills refer to the skill performance of physical and psychological/emotional self-care work and play/leisure activities to a level of independence appropriate to age, life-space, and disability. Life-space refers to an individual's cultural background, value orientation, and physical and social environment.

Physical daily living skills refer to the skill and performance of daily personal care, with or without adaptive equipment. It includes but is not limited to:

Grooming and hygiene refer to the skill and performance of personal health needs, such as bathing, toileting, hair care, shaving, and applying make-up.

Feeding/eating refers to the skill and performance of sequentially feeding oneself, including sucking, chewing, swallowing, and using appropriate utensils.

Dressing refers to the skill and performance of choosing appropriate clothing and dressing oneself in a sequential fashion, including fastening and adjusting clothing.

Functional mobility refers to the skill and performance of moving oneself from one position or place to another. It includes skills necessary for activities such as bed mobility, wheelchair mobility, transfers (bed, car, tub, toilet, chair), and functional ambulation, with or without adaptive aids. It also includes use of public and private travel systems, such as driving own automobile and using public transportation.

Functional communication refers to the skill and performance of using equipment or systems to enhance or provide communication, such as writing equipment, typewriters, letterboards, telephone, braille writers, artificial vocalization systems, and computers.

Object manipulation refers to the skill and performance of handling large and small common objects, such as calculators, keys, money, light switches, doorknobs, and packages.

Psychological/emotional daily living skills refers to the skill and performance of developing one's self-concept/self-identity, coping with life situations, and participating in one's organizational and community environment. It includes but is not limited to:

Self-concept/self-identity refers to the cognitive image of one's functional self. This includes but is not limited to:

- clearing perceiving other's needs, feelings, conflicts, values, beliefs, expectations, sexuality, and power
- realistically perceiving others' needs, feelings, conflicts, values, beliefs, expectations, sexuality, and power
- knowing one's performance strengths and limitations
- sensing one's competence, achievement, self-esteem, and self-respect
- integrating new experiences with established self-concept/self-identity
- having a sense of psychological safety and security
- perceiving one's goals and directions.

Situational coping refers to skill and performance in handling stress and dealing with problems and changes in a manner that is functional for self and others. This includes but is not limited to:

- setting goals and selecting, harmonizing, and managing activities of daily living to promote optimal performance
- testing goals and perceptions against reality
- perceiving changes and the need for changes in self and environment
- directing and redirecting energy to overcome problems
- initiating, implementing, and following through on decisions
- assuming responsibility for self and consequences of actions
- interacting with others, dyadic and group.

Community involvement refers to skill and performance in interacting within one's social system. This includes but is not limited to:

- understanding social norms and their impact on society

- planning, organizing, and executing daily life activities in relationship to society, including such activities as budgeting, time management, social role management, and using community resources
- recognizing and responding to needs of families and groups
- understanding and responding to organizational/community role expectations as both recipient and contributor.

Work refers to skill and performance in participating in socially purposeful and productive activities. These activities may take place in the home, employment setting, school, or community. They include but are not limited to:

Homemaking refers to skill and performance in homemaking and home management tasks, such as meal planning, meal preparation and cleanup, laundry, cleaning, minor household repairs, shopping, and use of household safety principles.

Child care/parenting refers to skill and performance in child care activities and management. This includes but is not limited to physical care of children and use of age-appropriate activities, communication, and behavior to facilitate child development.

Employment preparation refers to skill and performance in precursory job activities, including prevocational activities. This includes but is not limited to:

- job acquisition skills and performance
- organizational and team participatory skills and performance
- work process skills and performance
- work product quality.

Play/leisure refers to skill and performance in choosing, performing, and engaging in activities for amusement, relaxation, spontaneous enjoyment, and/or self-expression. This includes but is not limited to:

- Recognizing one's specific needs, interests, and adaptations necessary for performance
- Identifying characteristics of activities and social situations that make them play for the individual
- Identifying activities that contain those characteristics
- Choosing play activities for participation, such as sports, games, hobbies, music, drama, and other activities
- Testing out and adapting activities to enable participation
- Identifying and using community resources.

Sensorimotor components refer to the skill and performance of patterns of sensory and motor behavior that are prerequisites to self-care, work, and play/leisure performance. The components in this section include neuromuscular and sensory integrative skills, including perceptual motor skills.

Neuromuscular refers to the skill and performance of motor aspects of behavior. This includes but is not limited to:

Reflex integration refers to skill and performance in enhancing and supporting functional neuromuscular development through eliciting and/or inhibiting stereotyped, patterned, and/or involuntary responses coordinated at subcortical and cortical levels.

Range of motion refers to skill and performance in using maximum span of joint movement in activities with and without assistance to enhance functional performance. The standard levels of performance include:

- active range of motion: movement by patient, unassisted through a complete range of motion
- passive range of motion: movement performed by someone other than patient or by a mechanical device, requiring no muscle contraction on the part of the patient
- active-assistance range of motion: movement performed by the patient to the limit of his/her ability, and then completed with assistance.

Gross and fine coordination refers to skill and performance in muscle control, coordination, and dexterity while participating in activities. This includes:

- muscle control: skill and performance in directing muscle movement
- coordination: skill and performance in gross motor activities using several muscle groups
- dexterity: skill and performance in tasks using small muscle groups.

Strength and endurance refers to skill and performance in using muscular force within time periods necessary for purposeful task performance. This involves but is not limited to progressively building strength and cardiac and pulmonary reserve, increasing the length of work periods, and decreasing fatigue and strain.

Sensory integration refers to skill and performance in development and coordination of sensory input, motor output, and sensory feedback. This includes but is not limited to:

Sensory awareness refers to skill and performance in perceiving and differentiating external and internal stimuli, such as:

- tactile awareness: the perception and interpretation of stimuli through skin contact
- stereognosis: the identification of forms and nature of objects through the sense of touch
- kinesthesia: the conscious perception of muscular motion, weight, and position
- proprioceptive awareness: the identification of the positions of body parts in space
- ocular control: the localization and visual tracking of stimuli
- vestibular awareness: the detection of motion and gravitational pull as related to one's performance in functional activities, ambulation, and balance
- auditory awareness: the differentiation and identification of sounds
- gustatory awareness: the differentiation and identification of tastes
- olfactory awareness: the differentiation and identification of smells

Visual-spatial awareness refers to skill and performance in perceiving distances between and relationships among objects, including self. This includes but is not limited to:

- figure-ground: recognition of forms and objects when presented in a configuration with competing stimuli
- form constancy: recognition of forms and objects as the same when presented in different contexts
- position in space: knowledge of one's position in space relative to other objects

Body integration refers to skill and performance in perceiving and regulating the position of various muscles and body parts in relationship to each other during static and movement states. This includes but is not limited to:

- body schema: the perception of one's physical self through proprioceptive and interoceptive sensations
- postural balance: skill and performance in developing and maintaining body posture while sitting, standing, or engaging in activity
- bilateral motor coordination: skill and performance in purposeful movement that requires interaction between both sides of the body in a smooth refined manner
- right-left discrimination: skill and performance in differentiating right from left and vice versa
- visual-motor integration: skill and performance in combining visual input with purposeful voluntary movement of the hand and other body parts involved in an activity (includes eye-hand coordination)
- crossing the midline: skill and performance in crossing the vertical midline of the body
- praxis: skill and performance of purposeful movement that involves motor planning.

Cognitive components refer to the skill and performance of the mental processes necessary to know or apprehend by understanding. This includes but is not limited to:

Orientation refers to skill and performance in comprehending, defining, and adjusting oneself in an environment with regard to time, place, and person.

Conceptualization/comprehension refers to skill and performance in conceiving and understanding concepts or tasks, such as color identification, word recognition, sign concepts, sequencing, matching, association, classification, and abstracting. This includes but is not limited to:

Concentration refers to skill and performance in focusing on a designated task or concept

Attention span refers to skill and performance in focusing on a task or concept for a particular length of time

Memory refers to skill and performance in retaining and recalling tasks or concepts from the past.

Cognitive integration refers to skill and performance in applying diverse knowledge to environmental situations. This involves but is not limited to:

Generalization refers to skill and performance in applying specific concepts to a variety of related situations.

Problem solving refers to skill and performance in identifying and organizing solutions to difficulties. It includes but is not limited to:

- defining or evaluating the problem
- organizing a plan
- making decisions/judgments
- implementing a plan, including following through in logical sequence
- evaluating decision/judgment and plan.

Psychosocial components refer to skill and performance in self-management and dyadic and group interaction.

Self-management refers to skill and performance in expressing and controlling oneself in functional and creative activities.

Self-expression refers to skill and performance in perceiving one's feelings and interpreting and using a variety of communication signs and symbols. This includes but is not limited to:

- experiencing and recognizing a range of emotions
- having an adequate vocabulary
- having writing and speaking skills
- interpreting and using correctly an adequate range of nonverbal signs and symbols.

Self-control refers to skill and performance in modulating and modifying present behaviors, and in initiating new behaviors in accordance with situational demands. It includes but is not limited to:

- observing one's own and others' behavior
- conceptualizing problems in terms of needed behavioral changes or actions
- imitating new behaviors
- directing and redirecting energies into stress-reducing activities and behaviors.

Dyadic interaction refers to skill and performance in relating to another person. This includes but is not limited to:

- understanding social/cultural norms of communication and interaction in various activities and social situations
- setting limits on self and others
- compromising and negotiating
- handling competition, frustration, anxiety, success, and failure
- cooperating and competing with others
- responsibly relying on self and others.

Group interaction refers to skill and performance in relating to groups of three to six persons, or more. This includes but is not limited to:

- knowing and performing a variety of task and social/emotional role behaviors
- understanding common stages of group process
- participating in a group in a manner that is mutually beneficial to self and others.

Therapeutic adaptations refer to the design and/or restructuring of the physical environment to assist self-care, work, and play/leisure performance. This includes selecting, obtaining, fitting, and fabricating equipment and instructing the client, family, and/or staff in proper use and care of equipment. It also includes minor repair and modification for correct fit, position, or use. Categories of therapeutic adaptation consist of:

Orthotics refers to the provision of dynamic and static splints, braces, and slings for the purpose of relieving pain, maintaining joint alignment, protecting joint integrity, improving function, and/or decreasing deformity

Prosthetics refers to the training in use of artificial substitutes for missing body parts that augment performance of function

Assistive/adaptive equipment refers to the provision of special devices that assist in performance, and/or structural or positional changes, such as the installation of ramps and/or bars, changes in furniture heights, adjustments of traffic patterns, and modifications of wheelchairs.

Prevention refers to skill and performance in minimizing debilitation. It may include programs for persons in whom a predisposition to disability exists, as well as for those who have already incurred a disability. This includes but is not limited to:

Energy conservation refers to skill and performance in applying energy-saving procedures, activity restriction, work simplification, time management, and/or organization of the environment to minimize energy output.

Joint protection/body mechanics refers to skill and performance in applying principles or procedures to minimize stress on joints. Procedures may include the use of proper body mechanics, avoidance of static or deforming postures, and/or avoidance of excessive weight bearing.

Positioning refers to skill and performance in the placement of a body part in alignment to promote optimal functioning.

Coordination of daily living activities refers to skill and performance in selecting and coordinating activities of self-care, work, play/leisure, and rest to promote optimal performance of daily life tasks.

Reassessment refers to the process of obtaining and intepreting data necessary for updating treatment plans and goals. This frequently involves administering only portions of the initial evaluation, documenting results, and/or revising treatment.

Development of standards of quality treatment service refers to the development, implementation, evaluation, and documentation of departmental policy and procedures for the purpose of assuring standardized and quality treatment. This policy includes but is not limited to those procedures governing standards of occupational therapy practice, health and safety, infection control, and ethical behavior.

Chart audit refers to the evaluation of documentation based on criteria developed within the facility, the profession, health systems agency (Health Planning Act), and/or professional standards review organization for a specified geographical area.

Occupational therapy care review refers to the ongoing evaluation and documentation of the quality of care given. Three review programs may be included in the care review process: preadmission screening, concurrent review, and retrospective studies.

Inservice education refers to the participation of regularly employed occupational therapy personnel (e.g., OTR, COTA, OT Aide, or OT orderly) in regularly scheduled classes, inhouse seminars, and special training sessions, either in or outside the facility.

Accrediting reviews refer to those activities that are necessary to routinely document the meeting of the standards of a recognized accrediting body such as State Department of Health, Joint Commission on the Accreditation of Hospitals, Commission on Accreditation of Rehabilitation Facilities, or other accreditation procedures, voluntary or mandated by state or local law, and/or by the administration of a particular institution.

Appendix F-1. Job Analysis Categories: Physical Demands*

The physical demands listed in this publication serve as a means of expressing both the physical requirements of the job and the physical capacities (specific physical traits) a worker must have to meet those required by many jobs (perceiving by the sense of vision), and also the name of a specific capacity possessed by many people (having the power of sight). The worker must possess physical capacities at least in an amount equal to the physical demands made by the job.

The Factors

1. *Strength:* This factor is expressed in terms of *Sedentary, Light, Medium, Heavy,* and *Very Heavy*. It is measured by involvement of the worker with one or more of the following activities:
   a. Worker position(s):
      (1) *Standing:* Remaining on one's feet in an upright position at a workstation without moving about.
      (2) *Walking:* Moving about on foot.
      (3) *Sitting:* Remaining in the normal seated position.
   b. Worker movement of objects (including extremities used):
      (1) *Lifting:* Raising or lowering an object from one level to another (includes upward pulling).
      (2) *Carrying:* Transporting an object, usually holding it in the hands or arms or on the shoulder.
      (3) *Pushing:* Exerting force upon an object so that the object moves away from the force (includes slapping, striking, kicking, and treadle actions).
      (4) *Pulling:* Exerting force upon an object so that the object moves toward the force (includes jerking).

The five degrees of Physical Demands Factor No. 1 (strength) are as follows:

S Sedentary Work
Lifting 10 lbs. maximum and occasionally lifting and/or carrying such articles as dockets, ledgers, and small tools. Although a sedentary job is defined as one which involves sitting, a certain amount of walking and standing is often necessary in carrying out job duties. Jobs are sedentary if walking and standing are required only occasionally and other sedentary criteria are met.

L Light Work
Lifting 20 lbs. maximum with frequent lifting and/or carrying of objects weighing up to 10 lbs. Even though the weight lifted may be only a negligible amount, a job is in this category when it requires walking or standing to a significant degree, or when it involves sitting most of the time with a degree of pushing and pulling of arm and/or leg controls.

M Medium Work
Lifting 50 lbs. maximum with frequent lifting and/or carrying of objects weighing up to 25 lbs.

H Heavy Work
Lifting 100 lbs. maximum with frequent lifting and/or carrying of objects weighing up to 50 lbs.

V Very Heavy Work
Lifting objects in excess of 100 lbs. with frequent lifting and/or carrying of objects weighing 50 lbs. or more.

2. *Climbing and/or Balancing:*
   (1) Climbing: Ascending or descending ladders, stairs, scaffolding, ramps, poles, ropes, and the like, using the feet and legs and/or hands and arms.
   (2) Balancing: Maintaining body equilibrium to prevent falling when walking, standing, crouching, or running on narrow, slippery, or erratically moving surfaces; or maintaining body equilibrium when performing gymnastic feats.
3. *Stooping, Kneeling, Crouching, and/or Crawling:*
   (1) Stooping: Bending the body downward and forward by bending the spine at the waist.
   (2) Kneeling: Bending the legs at the knees to come to rest on the knee or knees.

*U.S. Department of Labor, Employment and Training Administration. *Selected Characteristics of Occupations Defined in the Dictionary of Occupational Titles.* Washington, D.C.: U.S. Government Printing Office, 1981, pp. 465-466.

(3) Crouching: Bending the body downward and forward by bending the legs and spine.

(4) Crawling: Moving about on the hands and knees or hands and feet.

4. *Reaching, Handling, Fingering, and/or Feeling:*
   (1) Reaching: Extending the hands and arms in any direction.
   (2) Handling: Seizing, holding, grasping, turning, or otherwise working with the hand or hands (fingering not involved).
   (3) Fingering: Picking, pinching, or otherwise working with the fingers primarily (rather than with the whole hand or arm as in handling).
   (4) Feeling: Perceiving such attributes of objects and materials as size, shape, temperature, or texture, by means of receptors in the skin, particularly those of the fingertips.

5. *Talking and/or Hearing:*
   (1) Talking: Expressing or exchanging ideas by means of the spoken word.
   (2) Hearing: Perceiving the nature of sounds by the ear.

6. *Seeing:* Obtaining impressions through the eyes of the shape, size, distance, motion, color, or other characteristics of objects. The major visual functions are: (1) acuity, far and near, (2) depth perception, (3) field of vision, (4) accommodation, and (5) color vision. The functions are defined as follows:
   (1) Acuity, far—clarity of vision at 20 feet or more. Acuity, near—clarity of vision at 20 inches or less.
   (2) Depth perception—three-dimensional vision. The ability to judge distance and space relationships so as to see objects where and as they acutally are.
   (3) Field of vision—the area that can be seen up and down or to the right or left while the eyes are fixed on a given point.
   (4) Accommodation—adjustment of the lens of the eye to bring an object into sharp focus. This item is especially important when doing near-point work at varying distances from the eye.
   (5) Color vision—the ability to identify and distinguish colors.

Appendix F-2. Environmental Conditions*

Environmental conditions are the physical surroundings of a worker in a specific job.

1. *Inside, Outside, or Both:*
   I Inside: Protection from weather conditions but not necessarily from temperature changes.
   O Outside: No effective protection from weather.
   B Both: Inside and outside.

A job is considered "inside" if the worker spends approximately 75 percent or more of the time inside, and "outside" if the worker spends approximately 75 percent or more of the time outside. A job is considered "both" if the activities occur inside or outside in approximately equal amounts.

2. *Extremes of Cold Plus Temperature Changes:*
   (1) Extremes of Cold: Temperature sufficiently low to cause marked bodily discomfort unless the worker is provided with exceptional protection.
   (2) Temperature Changes: Variations in temperature which are sufficiently marked and abrupt to cause noticeable bodily reactions.
3. *Extremes of Heat Plus Temperature Changes:*
   (1) Extremes of Heat: Temperature sufficiently high to cause marked bodily discomfort unless the worker is provided with exceptional protection.
   (2) Temperature Changes: Same as 2(2).
4. *Wet and Humid:*
   (1) Wet: Contact with water or other liquids.
   (2) Humid: Atmospheric condition with moisture content sufficiently high to cause marked bodily discomfort.
5. *Noise and Vibration:* Sufficient noise, either constant or intermittent, to cause marked distraction or possible injury to the sense of hearing, and/or sufficient vibration (production of an oscillating movement or strain on the body or its extremities from repeated motion or shock) to cause bodily harm if endured day after day.
6. *Hazards:* Situations in which the individual is exposed to the definite risk of bodily injury.
7. *Fumes, Odors, Toxic Conditions, Dust, and Poor Ventilation:*
   (1) Fumes: Smoky or vaporous exhalations, usually odorous, thrown off as the result of combustion or chemical reaction.
   (2) Odors: Noxious smells, either toxic or nontoxic.
   (3) Toxic Conditions: Exposure to toxic dust, fumes, gases, vapors, mists, or liquids which cause general or localized disabling conditions as a result of inhalation or action on the skin.
   (4) Dust: Air filled with small particles of any kind, such as textile dust, flour, wood, leather, feathers, etc., and inorganic dust, including silica and asbestos, which make the workplace unpleasant or are the source of occupational diseases.
   (5) Poor Ventilation: Insufficient movement of air causing a feeling of suffocation; or exposure to drafts.

*U.S. Department of Labor, Employment and Training Administration. *Selected Characteristics of Occupations Defined in the Dictionary of Occupational Titles.* Washington, D.C.: Government Printing Office, 1981.

Appendix F-3. Mathematical Development and Language Development (Training Time)*

Commonly referred to as "tool knowledges," these embrace those aspects of education (formal and informal) of a general nature that contribute to the acquisition of such skills but do not have a recognized, fairly specific, occupational objective ordinarily obtained in elementary, high school, or college environs and augmented by past experiences and self-study. They provide linkage between norms used for interpretation of the Basic Occupational Literacy Test (BOLT) scores and level requisites for DOT occupations. Following are the definitions and scale levels applicable to each:

a. Mathematical Developmental or Arithmetic Computation (M): The acquisition of basic mathematical skills, not specifically vocationally oriented, such as the ability to solve arithmetic, algebraic, and geometric problems ranging from fairly elemental to dealing with abstractions.
b. Language Development or Literacy Training (L): The acquisition of language skills, not specifically vocationally oriented, such as mastery of an extensive vocabulary; use of correct sentence structure, punctuation, and spelling; and an appreciation of literature.

Level	Mathematical Development	Language Development
6	Advanced calculus: Work with limits, continuity, real number systems, mean value theorems, and implicit function theorems. Modern algebra: Apply fundamental concepts of theories of groups, rings, and fields. Work with differential equations, linear algebra, infinite series, advanced operations methods, and functions of real and complex variables. Statistics: Work with mathematical statistics, mathematical probability, and applications, experimental design, statistical inference, and econometrics.	Reading: Read literature, book and play reviews, scientific and technical journals, abstracts, financial reports, and legal documents. Writing: Write novels, plays, editorials, journals, speeches, manuals, critiques, poetry, and songs. Speaking: Conversant in the theory, principles, and methods of effective and persuasive speaking, voice and diction, phonetics, and discussion and debate.
5	Calculus: Apply concepts of analytical geometry, differentiations and integration of algebraic functions with applications. Algebra: Work with exponents and logarithms, linear equations, quadratic equations, mathematical induction and binomial theorems, and permutations. Statistics: Apply mathematical operations to frequency distributions, reliability and validity of tests, normal curves, analysis of variance, correlation techniques, chi-square application and sampling theory, and factor analysis.	Same as level 6

*U.S. Department of Labor, Employment and Training Administration. *Selected Characteristics of Occupations Defined in Dictionary of Occupational Titles*. Washington, D.C.: U.S. Government Printing Office, 1981.

Level	Mathematical Development	Language Development
4	Algebra: Deal with system of real numbers; linear, quadratic, rational, exponential; logarithmic, angle, and circular functions, and inverse functions; related algebraic solution of equations and inequalities; limits and continuity, and probability and statistical inference. Geometry: Deductive axiomatic geometry, plane and solid; and rectangular coordinates. Shop Math: Practical application of fractions, percentages, ratio and proportion, mensuration, logarithms, slide rule, practical algebra, geometric construction, and essentials of trigonometry.	Reading: Read novels, poems, newspapers, periodicals, journals, manuals, dictionaries, thesauruses, and encyclopedias. Writing: Prepare business letters, expositions, summaries, and reports, using prescribed format, and conforming to all rules of punctuation, grammar, diction, and style. Speaking: Participate in panel discussions, dramatizations, and debates. Speak extemporaneously on a variety of subjects.
3	Compute discount, interest, profit, and loss; commission, markups, and selling price; ratio and proportion, and percentages. Calculate surfaces, volumes, weights, and measures. Algebra: Calculate variables and formulas, monomials and polynomials; ratio and proportion variables; and square roots and radicals. Geometry: Calculate plane and solid figures, circumference, area, and volume. Understand kinds of angles, and properties of pairs and angles.	Reading: Read a variety of novels, magazines, atlases, and encyclopedias. Read safety rules, instructions in the use and maintenance of shop tools and equipment, and methods and procedures in mechanical drawing and layout work. Writing: Write reports and essays with proper format, punctuation, spelling, and grammar, using all parts of speech. Speaking: Speak before an audience with poise, voice control, and confidence, using correct English and well-modulated voice.
2	Add, subtract, multiply, and divide all units of measure. Perform the four operations with like common and decimal fractions. Compute ratio, rate, and percent. Draw and interpret bar graphs. Perform arithmetic operations involving all American monetary units.	Reading: Passive vocabulary of 5,000-6,000 words. Read at rate of 190-215 words per minute. Read adventure stories and comic books, looking up unfamiliar words in dictionary for meaning, spelling, and pronunciation. Read instructions for assembling model cars and airplanes. Writing: Write compound and complex sentences, using cursive style, proper end punctuation, and employing adjectives and adverbs. Speaking: Speak clearly and distinctly with appropriate pauses and emphasis, correct pronunciation, variations in word order, using present, perfect, and future tenses.
1	Add and subtract two digit numbers. Multiply and divide 10's and 100's by 2, 3, 4, 5. Perform the four basic arithmetic operations with coins as part of a dollar. Perform operations with units such as cup, pint, and quart; inch, foot, and yard; and ounce and pound.	Reading: Recognize meaning of 2,500 (two- or three-syllable) words. Read at a rate of 95-120 words per minute. Compare similarities and differences between words and between series of numbers. Writing: Print simple sentences containing subject, verb, and object, and series of numbers, names, and addresses. Speaking: Speak simple sentences, using normal word order, and present and past tenses.

Appendix F-4. Specific Vocational Preparation (Training Time)*

This represents the amount of time required to learn the techniques, acquire information, and develop the facility needed for average performance in a specific job-worker situation. The training may be acquired in a school, work, military, institutional, or a vocational environment. It does not include orientation training required of even every fully qualified worker to become accustomed to the special conditions of any new job. Specific vocational training includes training given in any of the following circumstances:

a. Vocational education (such as high school commercial or shop training, technical school, art school, and that part of college training which is organized around a specific vocational objective);
b. Apprentice training (for apprenticeable jobs only);
c. In-plant training (given by an employer in the form of organized classroom study);
d. On-the-job training (serving as learner or trainee on the job under the instruction of a qualified worker);
e. Essential experience in other jobs (serving in less responsible jobs which lead to the higher grade job or serving in other jobs that qualify).

The following is an explanation of the various levels of specific vocational preparation.

Short demonstration.

Level	Time
1	Short demonstration.
2	Anything beyond short demonstration up to and including 30 days.
3	Over 30 days up to and including 3 months.
4	Over 3 months up to and including 6 months.
5	Over 6 months up to and including 1 year.
6	Over 1 year up to and including 2 years.
7	Over 2 years up to and including 4 years.
8	Over 4 years up to and including 10 years.
9	Over 10 years.

*U.S. Department of Labor, Employment and Training Administration. *Selected Characteristics of Occupations Defined in the Dictionary of Occupational Titles.* Washington, D.C.: U.S. Government Printing Office, 1981.

Appendix F-5. Occupational Aptitude Patterns*

This listing represents the 1979 revision of the Occupational Aptitude Pattern (OAP) structure and is extracted from the *Manual for the USES General Aptitude Test Battery*. It consists of 66 OAP's that closely relate to 59 of the Work Groups of the *Guide for Occupational Exploration,* identifies the most important aptitudes for Work Groups to which each OAP applies, and establishes the limits of specific occupational coverage for each OAP. Development of the OAP structure is described in Section II A of the *Manual for the USES General Aptitude Test Battery*.

Aptitudes Measured by the GATB

The nine aptitudes measured by the GATB are listed below. The letter used as the symbol to identify each aptitude and the part or parts of the GATB measuring each aptitude are also shown.

Aptitude	Tests
G—Intelligence	Part 3—Three-Dimensional Space Part 4—Vocabulary Part 6—Arithmetic Reason
V—Verbal Aptitude	Part 4—Vocabulary
N—Numerical Aptitude	Part 2—Computation Part 6—Arithmetic Reason
S—Spatial Aptitude	Part 3—Three-Dimensional Space
P—Form Perception	Part 5—Tool Matching Part 7—Form Matching
Q—Clerical Perception	Part 1—Name Comparison
K—Motor Coordination	Part 8—Mark Making
F—Finger Dexterity	Part 11—Assemble Part 12—Disassemble
M—Manual Dexterity	Part 9—Place Part 10—Turn

The following are the definitions of the nine aptitudes measured by the GATB:

G—Intelligence.—General learning ability. The ability to "catch on" or understand instructions and underlying principles; the ability to reason and make judgments. Closely related to doing well in school.

V—Verbal Aptitude.—The ability to understand meaning of words and to use them effectively. The ability to comprehend language, to understand relationships between words and to understand meanings of whole sentences and paragraphs.

N—Numerical Aptitude.—Ability to perform arithmetic operations quickly and accurately.

S—Spatial Aptitude.—Ability to think visually of geometric forms and to comprehend the two-dimensional representation of three-dimensional objects. The ability to recognize the relationships resulting from the movements of objects in space.

P—Form Perception.—Ability to perceive pertinent detail in objects in pictorial or graphic material. Ability to make visual comparisons and discriminations and see slight differences in shapes and shadings of figures and widths and lengths of lines.

Q—Clerical Perception.—Ability to perceive pertinent detail in verbal or tabular material. Ability to observe differences in copy, to proofread words and numbers, and to avoid perceptual errors in arithmetic computation. A measure of speed of perception which is required in many industrial jobs even when the job does not have verbal or numerical content.

K—Motor Coordination.—Ability to coordinate eyes and hands or fingers rapidly and accurately in making precise movements with speed. Ability to make a movement response accurately and swiftly.

F—Finger Dexterity.—Ability to move the fingers, and manipulate small objects with the fingers, rapidly or accurately.

M—Manual Dexterity.—Ability to move the hands easily and skillfully. Ability to work with the hands in placing and turning motions.

*U.S. Department of Labor, Employment and Training Administration. *Selected Characteristics of Occupations Defined in the Dictionary of Occupational Titles*. Washington, D.C.: U.S. Government Printing Office, 1981.

Appendix F-6. Interest Factors*

An interest is a tendency to become absorbed in an experience and to continue it, while an aversion is a tendency to turn away from it to something else.

The Interest Factors

The Interest Factors are as follows:

1*a*.	A preference for activities dealing with things and objects.	*vs*.	1*b*.	A preference for activities concerned with the communication of data.
2*a*.	A preference for activities involving business contact with people.	*vs*.	2*b*.	A preference for activities of a scientific and technical nature.
3*a*.	A preference for activities of a routine, concrete, organized nature.	*vs*.	3*b*	A preference for activities of an abstract and creative nature.
4*a*.	A preference for working for the presumed good of people.	*vs*.	4*b*.	A preference for activities that are carried on in relation to processes, machines, and techniques.
5*a*.	A preference for activities resulting in prestige or the esteem of others.	*vs*.	5*b*.	A preference for activities resulting in tangible, productive satisfaction.

*U.S. Department of Labor, Manpower Administration. *Handbook for Analyzing Jobs*. Washington, D.C.: U.S. Government Printing Office, 1972, p. 317.

Appendix F-7. Temperaments*

Temperaments are defined as the adaptability requirements made on the worker by specific types of job-worker situations.

D—DCP
Adaptability to accepting responsibility for the direction, control, or planning of an activity.

F—FIF
Adaptability to situations involving the interpretation of feelings, ideas, or facts in terms of personal viewpoint.

I—INFLU
Adaptability to influencing people in their opinions, attitudes, or judgments about ideas or things.

J—SJC
Adaptability to making generalizations, evaluations, or decisions based on sensory or judgmental criteria.

M—MVC
Adaptability to making generalizations, judgments, or decisions based on measurable or verifiable criteria.

P—DEPL
Adaptability to dealing with people beyond giving and receiving instructions.

Consider jobs for this factor when the worker must relate to people in situations involving more than giving or receiving instructions.

R—REPCON
Adaptability to performing repetitive work, or to continuously performing the same work, according to set procedures, sequence, or pace.

S—PUS
Adaptability to performing under stress when confronted with emergency, critical, unusual, or dangerous situations; or in situations in which working speed and sustained attention are make or break aspects of the job.

T—STS
Adaptability to situations requiring the precise attainment of set limits, tolerances, or standards.

V—VARCH
Adaptability to performing a variety of duties, often changing from one task to another of a different nature without loss of efficiency or composure.

*U.S. Department of Labor, Manpower Administration. *Handbook for Analyzing Jobs.* Washington, D.C.: U.S. Government Printing Office, 1972, pp. 297-313.

Appendix G. Uniform Terminology for Reporting Occupational Therapy Services*

Adopted March 1979 by The Representative Assembly, AOTA

Introduction

August 1978, the American Occupational Therapy Association Executive Board charged the Commission on Practice to form a Task Force to 1) review the existing occupational therapy terminology and relative value reporting systems, and 2) develop a proposal for a national occupational therapy product output reporting system.

At the time Public Law 95-142 was passed, no national system for reporting productivity of hospital based occupational therapy services existed. The American Occupational Therapy Association Commission on Practice OT Uniform Reporting System Task Force was created in August 1978 to develop a proposal for a national system. Sylvia Harlock, OTR (Washington), member of the AOTA Commission on Practice, was appointed by the Commission Chair, John Farace, OTR, to chair the Task Force. Members selected to serve on the Task Force were:

Mary Lou Hymen, OTR	California
Kathy McFarland, OTR	Washington
Kathy Saunders, OTR	Wisconsin
Louise Thibodaux, OTR	Alabama
Carole Hays, OTR	Division on Practice, AOTA National Office

A bound copy, containing both the *Occupational Therapy Product Output Reporting System* and *Uniform Terminology for Reporting Occupational Therapy Services*, is available from the Distribution Center, AOTA, 1383 Piccard Dr., Rockville, MD 20850.

Description of Occupational Therapy Services. Given the diversity of services provided by occupational therapy, the multiplicity of evaluation and treatment procedures which may often be used to achieve the same treatment outcomes, and the lack of a uniformly used description of occupational therapy service delivery, including definitions of terminology, the Task Force first developed the Description of Occupational Therapy Services. In selecting items and defining terms, the following criteria were taken into consideration:

1. Emphasis on description of treatment outcomes rather than treatment procedures.
2. Reflection of Medicare and Medicaid guidelines in terminology and category selection and definition.
3. Comprehensive description of occupational therapy services/product.
4. Reflection of the uniqueness of occupational therapy services/product in comparison with the services of other professions.
5. Coverage of recognized occupational therapy role in medical practice rather than all possible occupational therapy roles.

*Commission on Practice, the American Occupational Therapy Association, Inc.

OCCUPATIONAL THERAPY SERVICES

I. *OCCUPATIONAL THERAPY ASSESSMENT*

Occupational therapy assessment refers to the process of determining the need for, nature of, and estimated time of treatment, determining the needed coordination with other persons involved, and documenting these activities.

A. *Screening*

Screening refers to the review of potential patient's/client's case to determine the need for evaluation and treatment. It includes discussion with other professionals and/or patient advocate, and patient/client interview or administration of screening tool.

B. *Patient-Related Consultation*

Patient-related consultation refers to the sharing of relevant information with other professionals of patients/clients who are not currently referred to occupational therapy. This may include but is not limited to discussion, chart review, treatment recommendation, and documentation.

C. *Evaluation*

Evaluation refers to the process of obtaining and interpreting data necessary for treatment. This includes planning for and documenting the evaluation process and results. These data may be gathered through record review, specific observation, interview, and the administration of data collection procedures. Such procedures include but are not limited to the use of standardized tests, performance checklists, and activities and tasks designed to evaluate specific performance abilities. Categories of occupational therapy evaluation include independent living, daily living skills and performance and their components.

1. Independent Living/Daily Living Skills and Performance (see II A).
2. Sensorimotor Skill and Performance Components (see II B).
3. Cognitive Skill and Performance Components (see II C).
4. Psychosocial Skill and Performance Components (see II D).
5. Therapeutic Adaptations (see II E).
6. Specialized Evaluations.

   Specialized evaluations refer to evaluations or tests requiring specialized training and/or advanced education to administrate and interpret. Examples of specialized evaluations are employment preparation, evaluation (prevocational testing), sensory integration evaluation, prosthetic evaluation, driver's training evaluation.

D. *Reassessment*

Reassessment refers to the process of obtaining and interpreting data necessary for updating treatment plans and goals. This frequently involves administering only portions of the initial evaluation, documenting results, and/or revising treatment.

II. *OCCUPATIONAL THERAPY TREATMENT*

Occupational therapy treatment refers to the use of specific activities or methods to develop, improve, and/or restore the performance of necessary functions: compensate for dysfunction; and/or minimize debilitation; and the planning for and documenting of treatment performance. The necessary functions treated in occupational therapy are the following:

A. *Independent Living/Daily Living Skills*

Independent living/daily living skills (including self-care) refer to the skill and performance of physical and psychological/emotional self-care, work, and play/leisure activities to a level of independence appropriate to age, life-space, and disability. Life-space refers to an individual's cultural background, value orientation, and physical and social environment.

1. *Physical Daily Living Skills*

   Physical daily living skills refer to the skill and performance of daily personal care, with or without adaptive equipment. It includes but is not limited to:

a. *Grooming and Hygiene*
Grooming and hygiene refer to the skill and performance of personal health needs, such as bathing, toileting, hair care, shaving, applying make-up.

b. *Feeding/Eating*
Feeding/eating refers to the skill and performance of sequentially feeding oneself, including sucking, chewing, swallowing, and using appropriate utensils.

c. *Dressing*
Dressing refers to the skill and performance of choosing appropriate clothing, dressing oneself in a sequential fashion, including fastening and adjusting clothing.

d. *Functional Mobility*
Functional mobility refers to the skill and performance in moving oneself from one position or place to another. It includes skills necessary for activities such as bed mobility, wheelchair mobility, transfers (bed, car, tub, toilet, chair), and functional ambulation, with or without adaptive aids. It also includes use of public and private travel systems, such as driving own automobile and using public transportation.

e. *Functional Communication*
Functional communication refers to the skill and performance in using equipment or systems to enhance or provide communication, such as writing equipment, typewriters, letterboards, telephone, braille writers, artificial vocalization systems and computers.

f. *Object Manipulation*
Object mainpulation refers to the skill and performance in handling large and small common objects, such as calculators, keys, money, light switches, doorknobs, and packages.

2. *Psychological/Emotional Daily Living Skills*
Psychological/emotional daily living skills refer to the skill and performance in developing one's self-concept/self-identity, coping with life situations, and participating in one's organizational and community environment. It includes but is not limited to:

a. *Self-concept/Self-identity*
Self-concept/self-identity refers to the cognitive image of one's functional self. This includes but is not limited to:
(1) clearly perceiving one's needs, feelings, conflicts, values, beliefs, expectations, sexuality, and power
(2) realistically perceiving others' needs, feelings, conflicts, value, beliefs, expectations, sexuality, and power
(3) knowing one's performance strengths and limitations
(4) sensing one's competence, achievement, self-esteem, and self-respect
(5) integrating new experiences with established self-concept/self-identity
(6) having a sense of psychological safety and security
(7) perceiving one's goals and directions

b. *Situational Coping*
Situational coping refers to skill and performance in handling stress and dealing with problems and changes in a manner that is functional for self and others. This includes but is not limited to:
(1) setting goals, selecting, harmonizing, and managing activities of daily living to promote optimal performance
(2) testing goals and perceptions against reality
(3) perceiving changes and need for changes in self and environment
(4) directing and redirecting energy to overcome problems
(5) initiating, implementing, and following through on decisions

(6) assuming responsibility for self and consequences of actions
(7) interacting with others, dyadic and group

c. *Community Involvement*
Community involvement refers to skill and performance in interacting within one's social system. This includes but is not limited to:
(1) understanding social norms and their impact on society
(2) planning, organizing, and executing daily life activities in relationship to society, including such activities as budgeting, time management, social role management, arranging for housing, nutritional planning, assessing and using community resources
(3) recognizing and responding to needs of families, groups, and complex social units
(4) understanding and responding to organizational/community role expectations as both recipient and contributor.

3. *Work*
Work refers to skill and performance in participating in socially purposeful and productive activities. These activities may take place in the home, employment setting, school, or community. They include but are not limited to:
a. *Homemaking*
Homemaking refers to skill and performance in homemaking and home management tasks, such as meal planning, meal preparation and clean-up, laundry, cleaning, minor household repairs, shopping, and use of household safety principles.
b. *Child Care/Parenting*
Child care/parenting refers to skill and performance in child care activities and management. This includes but is not limited to physical care of children, and use of age-appropriate activities, communication, and behavior to facilitate child development.
c. *Employment Preparation*
Employment preparation refers to skill and performance in precursory job activities (including prevocational activities). This includes but is not limited to:
(1) job acquisition skills and performance
(2) organizational and team participatory skills and performance
(3) work process skills and performance
(4) work product quality

4. *Play/Leisure*
Play/leisure refers to skill and performance in choosing, performing, and engaging in activities for amusement, relaxation, spontaneous enjoyment, and/or self-expression. This includes but is not limited to:
a. Recognizing one's specific needs, interests, and adaptations necessary for performance.
b. Identifying characteristics of activities and social situations that make them play for the individual.
c. Identifying activities that contain those characteristics.
d. Choosing play activities for participation, such as sports, games, hobbies, music, drama, and other activities.
e. Testing out and adapting activities to enable participation.
f. Identifying and using community resources.

B. *Sensorimotor Components*
Sensorimotor components refer to the skill and performance of patterns of sensory and motor behavior that are prerequisites to self-care, work, and play/leisure performance. The components in this section include neuromuscular and sensory integrative skills, including perceptual motor skills.
1. *Neuromuscular*
Neuromuscular refers to the skill and performance of motor aspects of behavior. This includes but is not limited to:

a. *Reflex Integration*
Reflex integration refers to skill and performance in enhancing and supporting functional neuromuscular development through eliciting and/or inhibiting stereotyped, patterned, and/or involuntary responses coordinated at subcortical and cortical levels.

b. *Range of Motion*
Range of motion refers to skill and performance in using maximum span of joint movement in activities with and without assistance to enhance functional performance. The standard levels of performance include:
(1) active range of motion: movement by patient, unassisted through a complete range of motion
(2) passive range of motion: movement performed by someone other than patient or by a mechanical device, requiring no muscle contraction on the part of the patient
(3) active-assistive range of motion: movement performed by the patient to the limit of his/her ability, and then completed with assistance

c. *Gross and Fine Coordination*
Gross and fine coordination refers to skill and performance in muscle control, coordination, and dexterity while participating in activities.
(1) *muscle control*
muscle control refers to skill and performance in directing muscle movement
(2) *coordination*
coordination refers to skill and performance in gross motor activities using several muscle groups
(3) *dexterity*
dexterity refers to skill and performance in tasks using small muscle groups

d. *Strength and Endurance*
Strength and endurance refers to skill and performance in using muscular force within time periods necessary for purposeful task performance. This involves but is not limited to progressively building strength and cardiac and pulmonary reserve, increasing the length of work periods, and decreasing fatigue and strain.

2. *Sensory Integration*
Sensory integration refers to skill and performance in development and coordination of sensory input, motor output, and sensory feedback. This includes but is not limited to:

a. *Sensory Awareness*
Sensory awareness refers to skill and performance in perceiving and differentiating external and internal stimuli, such as:
(1) tactile awareness: the perception and interpretation of stimuli through skin contact
(2) stereognosis: the identification of forms and nature of objects through the sense of touch
(3) kinesthesia: the conscious perception of muscular motion, weight, and position
(4) proprioceptive awareness: the identification of the positions of body parts in space
(5) ocular control: the localization and visual tracking of stimuli
(6) vestibular awareness: the detection of motion and gravitational pull as related to one's performance in functional activities, ambulation, and balance
(7) auditory awareness: the differentiation and identification of sounds
(8) gustatory awareness: the differentiation and identification of tastes
(9) olfactory awareness: the differentiation and identification of smells

b. *Visual-Spatial Awareness*
Visual-spatial awareness refers to skill and performance in perceiving distances between and relationships among objects, including self. This includes but is not limited to:
(1) figure-ground: recognition of forms and objects when presented in a configuration with competing stimuli
(2) form constancy: recognition of forms and objects as the same when presented in different contexts
(3) position in space: knowledge of one's position in space relative to other objects

c. *Body Integration*
Body integration refers to skill and performance in perceiving and regulating the position of various muscles and body parts in relationship to each other during static and movement states. This includes but is not limited to:
(1) *body schema*
body schema refers to the perception of one's physical self through proprioceptive and interoceptive sensations
(2) *postural balance*
postural balance refers to skill and performance in developing and maintaining body posture while sitting, standing, or engaging in activity
(3) *bilateral motor coordination*
bilateral motor coordination refers to skill and performance in purposeful movement that requires interaction between both sides of the body in a smooth, refined manner
(4) *right-left discrimination*
right-left discrimination refers to skill and performance in differentiating right from left and vice versa
(5) *visual-motor integration*
visual-motor integration refers to skill and performance in combining visual input with purposeful voluntary movement of the hand and other body parts involved in an activity. Visual-motor integration includes eye-hand coordination
(6) *crossing the midline*
crossing the midline refers to skill and performance in crossing the vertical midline of the body
(7) *praxis*
praxis refers to skill and performance of purposeful movement that involves motor planning

C. *Cognitive Components*
Cognitive components refer to skill and performance of the mental processes necessary to know or apprehend by understanding. This includes but is not limited to:

1. *Orientation*
Orientation refers to skill and performance in comprehending, defining, and adjusting oneself in an environment with regard to time, place, and person.

2. *Conceptualization/Comprehension*
Conceptualization/comprehension refers to skill and performance in conceiving and understanding concepts of tasks such as color identification, word recognition, sign concepts, sequencing, matching, association, classification, and abstracting. This includes but is not limited to:
a. *Concentration*
Concentration refers to skill and performance in focusing on a designated task or concept.
b. *Attention Span*
Attention span refers to skill and performance in focusing on a task or concept for a particular length of time.
c. *Memory*
Memory refers to skill and performance in retaining and recalling tasks or concepts from the past.

3. *Cognitive Integration*
Cognitive integration refers to skill and performance in applying diverse

knowledge to environmental situations. This involves but is not limited to:

a. *Generalization*
Generalization refers to skill and performance in applying specific concepts to a variety of related situations.

b. *Problem Solving*
Problem solving refers to skill and performance in identifying and organizing solutions to difficulties. It includes but is not limited to:
(1) defining or evaluating the problem
(2) organizing a plan
(3) making decisions/judgments
(4) implementing plan, including following through in logical sequence
(5) evaluating decision/judgment and plan

D. *Psychosocial Components*
Psychosocial components refer to skill and performance in self-management, dyadic and group interaction.

1. *Self-management*
Self-management refers to skill and performance in expressing and controlling oneself in functional and creative activities.

a. *Self-expression*
Self-expression refers to skill and performance in perceiving one's feelings and interpreting and using a variety of communication signs and symbols. This includes but is not limited to:
(1) experiencing and recognizing a range of emotions
(2) having an adequate vocabulary
(3) having writing and speaking skills
(4) interpreting and using correctly an adequate range of nonverbal signs and symbols

b. *Self-control*
Self-control refers to skill and performance in modulating and modifying present behaviors, and in initiating new behaviors in accordance with situational demands. It includes but is not limited to:
(1) observing own and others' behavior
(2) conceptualizing problems in terms of needed behavioral changes or action
(3) imitating new behaviors
(4) directing and redirecting energies into stress-reducing activities and behaviors

2. *Dyadic Interaction*
Dyadic interaction refers to skill and performance in relating to another person. This includes but is not limited to:
a. Understanding social/cultural norms of communication and interaction in various activity and social situations.
b. Setting limits on self and others.
c. Compromising and negotiating.
d. Handling competition, frustration, anxiety, success, and failure.
e. Cooperating and competing with others.
f. Responsibly relying on self and others.

3. *Group Interaction*
Group interaction refers to skill and performance in relating to groups of three to six persons, or larger. This includes but is not limited to:
a. Knowing and performing a variety of tasks and social/emotional role behaviors.
b. Understanding common stages of group process.
c. Participating in a group in a manner that is mutually beneficial to self and others.

E. *Therapeutic Adaptations*
Therapeutic adaptations refer to the design and/or restructuring of the physical environment to assist self-care, work, and play/leisure performance. This includes selecting, obtaining, fitting, and fabricating equipment, and instructing the client, family, and/or staff in proper use and care of equipment. It also includes minor repair and modification for correct fit, po-

sition, or use. Categories of therapeutic adaptations consist of:

1. *Orthotics*
   Orthotics refers to the provision of dynamic and static splints, braces, and slings for the purpose of relieving pain, maintaining joint alignment, protecting joint integrity, improving function, and/or decreasing deformity.
2. *Prosthetics*
   Prosthetics refers to the training in use of artificial substitutes of missing body parts, which augment performance of function.
3. *Assistive/Adaptive Equipment*
   Assistive/adaptive equipment refers to the provision of special devices that assist in performance, and/or structural or positional changes such as the installation of ramps, bars, changes in furniture heights, adjustments of traffic patterns, and modifications of wheelchairs.

F. *Prevention*
Prevention refers to skill and performance in minimizing debilitation. It may include programs for persons where predisposition to disability exists, as well as for those who have already incurred a disability. This includes but is not limited to:

1. *Energy Conservation*
   Energy conservation refers to skill and performance in applying energy-saving procedures, activity restriction, work simplification, time management, and or organization of the environment to minimize energy output.
2. *Joint Protection/Body Mechanics*
   Joint protection/body mechanics refers to skill and performance in applying principles of procedures to minimize stress on joints. Procedures may include the use of proper body mechanics, avoidance of static or deforming postures, and/or avoidance of excessive weight bearing.
3. *Positioning*
   Positioning refers to skill and performance in the placement of a body part in alignment to promote optimal functioning.
4. *Coordination of Daily, Living Activities*
   Coordination of daily living activities refers to skill and performance in selecting and coordinating activities of self-care, work, play leisure, and rest to promote optimal performance of daily life tasks.

III. *PATIENT/CLIENT-RELATED CONFERENCES*
Patient/client-related conferences include participating in meetings to discuss and identify needs, treatment program, and future plans of referred client, and documenting such participation. Patient/client may or may not be present. Categories of conferences include:

A. *Professional Conferences*
Professional conferences refers to participating in meetings with a group or individual professionals to discuss patient/client's status, and to advise consult regarding treatment needs. Synonymous terms for professional conferences include initial conference, interim review, discharge planning, case conference, and others.

B. *Agency Conferences*
Agency conferences refer to participating in meetings with vocational, social, religious, recreational, health, educational, and other community representatives to assess, implement, or coordinate the use of services.

C. *Client-Advocate Conferences*
Client-advocate conferences refer to participating in meetings with client advocate (e.g., family, guardian, or others responsible for patient/client) to assess patient/client's situation, set goals, plan treatment and/or discharge; and or to instruct client advocate to support or carry out treatment program.

IV. *TRAVEL PATIENT-TREATMENT RELATED*
Travel; patient-treatment related refers to travel by therapists, with or without patient; that is, related to direct patient treatment.

THE FOLLOWING ITEMS DO NOT INVOLVE DIRECT PATIENT CARE

V. *SERVICE MANAGEMENT*
Service management refers to planning, leading, organization, and controlling the occupational therapy facility and service.

A. *Quality Review/Maintenance of Quality*
Quality review/maintenance of quality refers to those phases of departmental management that serve to assure and document normative standards of occupational therapy service.

1. *Development of Standards of Quality Treatment/Services*
Development of standards of quality treatment/service refers to the development, implementation, evaluation, and documentation of departmental policy and procedures for the purpose of assuring standardized and quality treatment. This policy includes but is not limited to those procedures governing standards of occupational therapy practice, health and safety, infection control, and ethical behavior.

2. *Chart Audit*
Chart audit refers to the evaluation of documentation based on criteria developed within the facility, the profession, Health Systems Agency (Health Planning Act), and/or Professional Standards Review Organizations for a specified geographical area.

3. *Accrediting Reviews*
Accrediting reviews refer to those activities that are necessary to routinely document the meeting of the standards of a recognized accrediting body such as State Department of Health, Joint Committee on the Accreditation of Hospitals, Commission on Accreditation of Rehabilitation Facilities, or other accreditation procedures, voluntary or mandated by state or local law, and/or by the administration of a particular institution.

4. *Occupational Therapy Care Review*
Occupational therapy care review refers to the ongoing evaluation and documentation of the quality of care given. Three review programs may be included in the care review process: preadmission screening, concurrent review, and retrospective studies.

5. *Inservice Education*
Inservice education refers to the participation of regularly employed occupational therapy personnel (e.g., OTR, COTA, OT aide, or OT orderly) in regularly scheduled classes, in-house seminars, and special training sessions, either in or outside the facility.

B. *Departmental Maintenance*
Departmental maintenance refers to activities to maintain the physical environment of the occupational therapy department so as to assure the health and safety of patients and staff. Some of these activities are mandated by accrediting agencies, state or local law, or administration of the facility, whereas others may be developed by the occupational therapy service.

C. *Employee Meetings*
Employee meetings refer to meetings of occupational therapy departmental staff for the purpose of disseminating and receiving information, conveying information concerning the administrative policies of the institution and/or conditions of employment, and discussing issues relevant to the management of the program, the development of the department, and/or institution, and its relationship to total health care.

D. *Program-Related Conferences*
Program-related conferences refer to interdepartmental meetings for the purpose of disseminating and receiving information and discussing issues relevant to program planning, developing, and management.

E. *Supervision*
Supervision refers to activities to enhance the performance of departmental employees through appraisal of their effectiveness, evaluation of their conformance to departmental standards, and/or evaluation of their adherence to specific institutional policies.

VI. *EDUCATION*

Education refers to the dissemination and collection of knowledge pertaining to occupational therapy and health care by means of lecture, demonstration, observation, or direct participation.

A. *Occupational Therapy Clinical Education: Occupation Therapy Students*

Occupational therapy clinical education: occupational therapy students refer to the orientation, instruction, supervision of student involvement in the occupational therapy program. This may include preclinical, field-work professional, and/or technical level occupational therapy students.

B. *Occupational Therapy Clinical Education: Others*

Occupational therapy clinical education: others refer to the orientation of nonoccupational therapists to occupational therapy treatment principles and theories and to interprofessional working relationships by occupational therapy departmental staff.

C. *Occupational Therapy Clinical Education: Continuing Education*

Occupational therapy clinical education: continuing education refers to ongoing educational experiences beyond basic education. The purpose of continuing education is to enrich or improve the occupational therapist's knowledge, skills, and attitudes in his/her work performance. Continuing education is designed for therapists interested in maintaining and updating themselves in the field of occupational therapy and in its related aspects such as research, consultation, education, administration, and supervision.

VII. *RESEARCH*

Research refers to formalized investigative activities for the purpose of improving the quality of occupational therapy patient care by means of recognized scientific methodologies and procedures.

Appendix H. Resource Guide for Equipment

Adaptive Equipment (Self-care, Communication, and Homemaking):

Achievement
Products, Inc.
P.O. Box 547
Mineola, NY 11501

Ali Med, Inc.
70 Harrison Avenue
Boston, MA 02111

Bradley Company
P.O. Box 2186
Madison, WI 53701

Cleo Living Aids
3957 Mayfield Road
Cleveland, OH 44121

Equipment Shop, Inc.
P.O. Box 33
Bedford, MA 01730

FashionAble
Box S
Rocky Hill, NJ 08553

Maddak, Inc.
6 Industrial Road
Pequannock, NJ 07440

Medical Equipment
Distributors, Inc.
1701 South First Ave.
Maywood, IL 60153

OMED
777 Alpha Drive
Cleveland, OH 44143

Ortho-Kinetics, Inc.
W220 N507 Springdale
Waukesha, WI 53187

J.A. Preston Corp.
60 Page Road
Clifton, NJ 07012

Raymo Products, Inc.
212 South Blake St.
Olathe, KS 66061

Rehabilitation
Products
6302 Odana Road
Madison, WI 53719

Rifton Equipment
Route 213
Rifton, NY 12471

Fred Sammons, Inc.
Box 32
Brookfield, IL 60513

Sears, Roebuck Co.
Department 608 J
2 North Lasalle
Chicago, IL 60602

Skill Development
Equipment
P.O. Box 6300
Anaheim, CA 92806

Therafin Corporation
3800 South Union Ave.
Steger, IL 60475

Therapeutic React
268 Norwood Ave.
Buffalo, NY 14222

T.R.S., Inc.
1280 28th Street, #3
Boulder, CO 80303

Bathroom and Toileting Equipment:

Achievement
Products, Inc.
P.O. Box 547
Mineola, NY 11501

Activeaid, Inc.
501 East Tin Street
Redwood Falls, MN
56283

Alimed, Inc.
70 Harrison Avenue
Boston, MA 02111

Cleo Living Aids
3957 Mayfield Road
Cleveland, OH 44121

Everest & Jennings,
Inc.
3233 East Mission
Oaks Blvd.
Camarillo, CA 93010

FashionAble
Box S
Rocky Hill, NJ 08553

Garelick Mfg. Co.
644 Second Street
St. Paul Park, MN
55071

Guardian Products,
Inc.
780 Easy Street
Simi Valley, CA
93062

Invacare Corporation
899 Cleveland Street
Elyria, OH 44036

Lumex
100 Spence Street
Bay Shore, NY
11706

Maddak, Inc.
6 Industrial Road
Pequannock, NJ
07440

Medical Equipment
Distributors
1701 South First Ave.
Maywood, IL 60153

Mobility Plus, Inc.
P.O. Box 391
Santa Paula, CA
93060

Motor Development
Corporation
P.O. Box 4054
Downey, CA 92041

J.E. Nolan & Co.,
Inc.
1826 Laser Lane
Louisville, KY 40299

J.A. Preston Corp.
60 Page Road
Clifton, NJ 07012

Rehabilitation
Equipment
1823 West Moss Ave.
Peoria, IL 61606

Fred Sammons, Inc.
Box 32
Brookfield, IL 60513

Avocational Activities, Equipment and Supplies:

Bailey Manufact. Co.
118 Lee Street, Dept. J.
Lodi, OH 44254

Berman Leathercraft
145 South Street
Boston, MA 02111

Boin Arts and Crafts
91 Morris Street
Morristown, NJ 07960

Chaselle Inc.
9645 Gerwig Lane
Columbia, MD 21046

Cleo, Inc.
3957 Mayfield Road
Cleveland, OH 44121

Creative Crafts International
Essex Industrial Park
Centerbrook, CT 06409

LeisureCrafts
306 Maria Street, P.O. Box 330
Rancho Dominguez, CA 90224

Nasco
901 Janesville Ave.
Fort Atkinson, WI 53538

OMED
777 Alpha Drive
Cleveland, OH 44143

Sax Arts & Crafts, Inc.
316 North Milwaukee Street
P.O. Box 2002
Milwaukee, WI 53201

School Arts Magazine
50 Portland Street
Worcester, MA 01608

Curriculum Resources, Inc.
Box 923
Fairfield, CT 06430

Earth Leather Corp.
10883 Big Bone Rd.
Union, KY 41091

Flaghouse, Inc.
18 West 18th Street
New York, NY 10011

Dick Blick Hortoncraft
Box 330
Farmington, CT 06032

Skill Development Equipment
P.O. Box 6300
Anaheim, CA 92806

S & S Arts and Crafts
Norwich Avenue
Colchester, CT 06415

Tandy Leather Co.
P.O. Box 2934, Dept. BG-TI
Fort Worth, TX 76113

Vanguard Crafts, Inc.
1701 Utica Avenue
Brooklyn, NY 11234

Veteran Leather Co.
204 25th Street
Brooklyn, NY 11232

Appendix I. Roles and Functions of Occupational Therapy in Long-Term Care: Occupational Therapy and Activity Programs*

by:
Joan C. Rogers, Ph.D., OTR, FAOTA

for:
AOTA Commission on Practice

John Farace, OTR, Chair

The American Occupational Therapy Association, Inc. (AOTA), submits this paper to reaffirm and illustrate the role of occupational therapy in the promotion of health and the prevention of disability for individuals requiring long-term care.

Occupational therapy facilitates the functional independence of individuals needing long-term care through the use of self-care, play/leisure, and work occupations. Occupational therapy services range from the selection of therapeutic activities to restore, maintain, and enhance function, to the implementation of planned activities to arouse, stimulate, and sustain interests and activity levels. In providing these services, occupational therapy personnel may serve as providers of occupational therapy, as coordinators or directors of activities programs, or as indirect service providers.

The purpose of this paper is to distinguish between the use of activities in occupational therapy and in activities programs, and to clarify the functions of the occupational therapist, registered (OTR), and the certified occupational therapy assistant (COTA) in regard to these services.

Individuals experiencing problems in daily living as a result of developmental disabilities, the aging process, or medical problems are served by occupational therapy in long-term care programs. The independence and quality of life of these individuals may be threatened by chronic disability as well as by immobility and restricted environmental stimulation. Long-term care may be provided in institutional and community settings such as skilled and intermediate care facilities, adult day care centers, half-way houses, congregate living facilities, and private residences.

Philosophical Base of Occupational Therapy

The philosophical base for the practice of occupational therapy, adopted in 1979 (1), identifies the contribution occupational therapy makes to health care through its accent on human activity as a health determinant.

"Man is an active being, whose development is influenced by the use of purposeful activity. Using their capacity for intrinsic motivation, human beings are able to influence their physical environment through purposeful activity. Human life includes a process of continuous adaptation. Adaptation is a change in function that promotes survival and self-actualization. Biological, psychological, and environmental factors may interrupt the adaptation process at any time throughout the life cycle. Dysfunction may occur when adaptation is impaired. Purposeful activity facilitates the adaptive process."

Occupational therapy is based on the belief that purposeful activity (occupation), including its interpersonal and environmental components, may be used to prevent and mediate dysfunction and elicit maximum adaptation. Activity, as used by the Occupational Therapist, includes both an intrinsic and a therapeutic purpose.

Definitions

Occupational Therapy: Occupational therapy is the application of occupation or goal-directed activity to achieve optimum function, to prevent dysfunction, and to promote health. The term *occupation,* as used in occupational therapy, refers to any activity engaged in for evaluating, specifying, and treating problems interfering with functional performance (2).

Activities Programs: Activities programs consist of planned events and tasks designed to provide incentive and opportunity to engage in continuing

*Reprinted with the permission of The American Occupational Therapy Association, Inc., copyright holder. © Copyright 1983, *The American Journal of Occupational Therapy.* December 1983, Volume 38, Number 12, pp. 799-802.

life experiences and, hence, to satisfy interests and meet general activity needs. Activities programs contribute to the prevention of deterioration of mental, physical, and social abilities (3).

History/Legal: The involvement of occupational therapy in long-term care may be traced to the early 1900s when occupational therapy programs were introduced in psychiatric hospitals and tuberculosis sanitoriums to counteract the deleterious effects of inactivity and idleness. The role of occupational therapy in long-term care was extended in 1965 by the passage of the Medicare legislation that provides coverage for restorative inpatient services while on part A coverage, and home health occupational therapy as an adjunctive service. The Omnibus Reconciliation Act of 1981 enables clients to receive occupational therapy under the home health benefit even after their need for skilled nursing, physical therapy, or speech therapy ends. States have the option to provide home health services, including occupational therapy, as part of their Medicaid provisions. Activities programs are included as part of the routine care provided for residents in institutional settings.

Occupational Therapy and Activities Programs: Occupational therapy and activities programs differ in: (a) the purpose for which activity is used, (b) the process of selecting activity, (c) the role of interests in the selection process, and (d) the scope of services.

Both occupational therapy and activities programs make use of self-care, play/leisure, and work activities. However, these activities are used for different purposes. In occupational therapy, activities are used to alleviate present or potential functional problems resulting from medical or developmental conditions or restricted environmental stimulation. Once a client's maximum functional capacity has been achieved and discharge plans have been instituted to maintain function, occupational therapy is discontinued. In activities programs, activities are introduced to provide an adequate level and balance of normal activity to promote and maintain health. Individuals requiring long-term care may need assistance in using their abilities because of their functional limitations. Assistance may also be needed because many normal daily activities are not easily carried out in long-term care settings. In contrast to occupational therapy that is problem-specific and time-limited, activities programs serve normal activity needs and are ongoing. In occupational therapy, for instance, a client may learn how to overcome arthritic hand deformities in order to do ceramic sculpture. Once the skill has been learned, however, the activities program would provide opportunities for using that skill.

In both occupational therapy and activities programs, the selection of activity is based on an individualized assessment of the client's needs and interests. For activities programs, the primary objective of assessment is to describe the tasks and events the client wants and is able to participate in. These data are used to judge the adequacy of the client's general activity level and to plan individual and group activities that provide a variety of physical, mental, and social stimulation. In occupational therapy, the selection of activity relies on problems discerned in self-care, play/leisure, and work occupations, and on a detailed assessment of the client's sensorimotor, cognitive, and psychosocial abilities. Comprehensive assessment is needed to discern functional limitations that are amenable to treatment, and to institute the appropriate kind of remedial, maintenance, or preventive activity. The choice of therapeutic activity depends on an in-depth analysis of the characteristics of the activity as well as of the client, and a thorough understanding of associated disease process. For example, for persons with thought disorders, such as those associated with Alzheimer's disease or schizophrenia, occupational therapy may use a structured activity requiring few repetitive steps (e.g., one color tile trivet) and progress to that requiring a sequence of steps and more flexibility (e.g., a mosaic design using several colors and textures) if the client improves.

In activities programs, the client's interests serve as a primary determinant in meeting general activity needs. Although client interests are accommodated in occupational therapy, they must serve the therapeutic goal. For instance, if a client needed practice in picking up and placing objects to increase hand dexterity, checkers or a tile project would be selected in occupational therapy, rather than a book discussion group, regardless of interest.

In addition to the use of self-care, play/leisure, and work, occupational therapy also incorporates therapeutic procedures that do not overlap with activities programs. These procedures include splinting, body mechanics, positioning, the prescription of self-help devices, neuromuscular facilitation, joint protection, facilitation of sensory integration, and time management.

Education—OTR and COTA

The theoretical base for occupational therapy is drawn from the medical, biological, and behavioral sciences. Productivity and self-reliance are viewed as a function of the interaction between an individual and the surrounding physical and social environment. The occupational therapy curriculum concentrates on three major areas. The first is normal human development over the life span. Emphasis is on the biological, psychological, social, and architectural factors required for competence in daily living skills. The second area is the functional disabilities associated with disease, trauma, developmental disorders, the aging process, and environmental deprivation. The third is the occupational therapy process, and provides knowledge of the evaluation, remediation, and prevention of functional disabilities through occupation. In each of the three curricular areas the knowledge and skills of the professionally educated therapist (OTR) are more complex and comprehensive than those of the occupational therapy assistant (COTA). The educational program for the registered therapist (OTR) prepares them for independent practice in occupational therapy, whereas that of the certified assistant (COTA) prepares them to practice occupational therapy under the supervision of an OTR. The OTR maintains supervisory responsibility for all tasks delegated to the COTA, although the COTA may function independently in conducting activities programs.

The employment of an OTR or a COTA as an activities coordinator does not convert an activities program into occupational therapy. However, the educational background of the OTR and COTA, especially with regard to normal human development, medical pathology, and activity analysis, allows activities programs conducted under their supervision to have a more rehabilitative quality than those conducted by personnel without this educational background. Knowledge of functional skills and medical pathology is used by the OTR or COTA to guide the selection of activities appropriate for the client's needs and abilities. Knowledge of adapting tasks, of positioning clients, and of modifying equipment to compensate for functional limitations is used to increase the involvement of clients, to facilitate safe performance, and to promote success. In the case of severely disabled clients, the knowledge and skills of the OTR or COTA may enable participation that otherwise may have been precluded. The educational preparation of the OTR and COTA also includes knowledge of activities that are contraindicated for certain medical conditions.

Occupational Therapy: Direct Client Care

Occupational therapy provides restorative, supportive, and preventive services, which aid clients to achieve the highest possible degree of functional independence. Therapy is based on a screening and assessment process.

Screening:

Screening to identify problems in daily functioning is done by the OTR or COTA. The need for evaluation is based on an appraisal of the client's life style and general functional capacity in self-care, play/leisure, and work occupations. Screening is generally accomplished through observation, interview, and a review of medical records.

Assessment:

The OTR evaluates the client to determine the nature of the functional problems. The work appraisal covers household management (cooking, shopping, and cleaning), volunteer work, and paid jobs. The leisure assessment considers the client's ability to participate in recreational, educational, and cultural events. The self-care assessment includes feeding, dressing, hygiene, and mobility. The assessment extends to the underlying subcomponents of these functional skills, such as motivation, cognition, muscular strength, and coordination. Environmental factors that hinder function are also evaluated. Observing, interviewing, and testing are used to evaluate the client. Information may also be gathered from family, friends, and other health care providers. These evaluative data are used to formulate treatment goals consistent with the needs of, and acceptable to, the individual or responsible person.

Treatment:

The treatment plan is developed by the OTR and implemented by the OTR or the COTA under OTR supervision. The treatment program may be directed toward restoration of function, maintenance of function, or prevention of dysfunction. The restorative program focuses on the correction of disability whether physical or psychosocial. Such correction may be achieved through remediation or compensation. For example, an elderly person with a right upper-extremity hemiparesis may be retrained in using the right hand (remedial), or may be trained to use the left hand in a skilled fashion (compensatory), or a combination of both. Specific treatment procedures are based on the factor interfering with function. Clients, for instance, may not dress themselves because they lack adequate muscular strength, because they cannot recall the dressing sequence, or because they see no reason to dress. Although the end result is the same, each causal factor requires a different treatment approach. In addition to intervening with the client, treatment may also require environmental adaptations to encourage and support functional skills. Programs focused on maintaining function are instituted for clients who have reached their highest level of function and require assistance in retaining their abilities. Maintenance programs provide practice in the functional skills acquired through restorative programs. Preventive programs are directed toward the prevention of functional disabilities. They are begun at the first signs of difficulty in performing daily life tasks and are designed to assist clients to develop adaptive patterns conducive to long-term function.

Activities Programs: Direct Client Care

The activities program is designed to provide physical, intellectual, social, spiritual, and emotional challenges much the same as in everyday life. Participation is based on an assessment of interests and activity needs.

Assessment:

The OTR or COTA as activities coordinator assesses the interests of each client to determine the activity needs and preferences. The interest survey may be done by observing, interviewing, or testing. Family members, friends, and staff may also be contacted for information.

Activities Plan:

An activities plan is developed for each client. The plan identifies the client's interests and general activity needs, states goals, and gives the activities to be used to achieve these goals. The client's needs are reassessed regularly and the activities plan is adjusted accordingly.

Activities Program:

The OTR or COTA, as activities coordinator, collaborates with the clients to plan, execute, and evaluate a diversified program suited to identified needs and interests. Programs are planned to provide a balance of activities perceived by the participants as useful work and service, and activities viewed as recreational, spiritual, and educational. Activities programs are varied so that individual as well as group activities are offered. The OTR or COTA as activities coordinator routinely evaluates the effectiveness of the activities program.

Occupational Therapy and Activities Programs: Functions Related to Client Care

Indirect services, such as management and supervision, education, and consultation, facilitate the provision of client care.

Management Role: Occupational therapy personnel support the premise that good management results in the effective care of the client. Management responsibilities include but are not limited to: documentation, program administration and development, and committee or team participation.

Documentation refers to the written record of information to ensure the continuity of care of clients. Documentation includes information on each client's problems and goals. Revisions of the occupational therapy program or activities plans and the effects these changes have on clients' performance are recorded. Records are completed in accordance with the policies and procedures of the long-term care setting. Documentation of overall effectiveness of the service is also required.

Program administration refers to the planning, organizing, directing, and coordinating functions needed to carry out the occupational therapy or activities programs. Responsibility is assumed for the efficient management of material and human resources, including staff, students, and volunteers to achieve program goals.

Committee or team participation refers to involvement in meeting with other health care team members to coordinate the client's overall health plan. Participation on committees, such as discharge planning, budget, or utilization and review, permits occupational therapy personnel to address the occupational needs of clients.

Educational Role: In conjunction with the educational role, family members, friends, and staff are educated in the promotion of health through activity. Providing fieldwork experiences for students in occupational therapy and other health fields also provides a mechanism for participating in the education of personnel for long-term care.

Consultant Role: Consultation is the process by which expertise is transmitted for the purpose of solving existing or potential problems. Consultation is provided to individuals, families, or program staff serving those with long-term care needs. The consultant collaborates with the administrator to develop the plan and objectives of consultation.

Examples of tasks undertaken by the consultant include: instructing staff in technical skills, advising the management team on program development, and diagnosing problems in program management. A request for consultation is often initiated by the desire to upgrade the activities program or by code requirements for consultation.

The consultant functions within federal and state codes that address the qualifications of staff, program content, physical facilities, and practice. The consultant must be aware of the code requirements as well as related professional standards. Occupational therapy philosophy and theory are particularly appropriate for the delivery of long-term care based on a wellness rather than a medical model. Hence, occupational therapy consultation is well suited to program developments aimed at such services as functional assessment, preventing premature institutionalization, re-integration into community living, palliative care of the dying, and increasing vocational performance of those needing supportive care.

Summary

There is a difference between occupational therapy and activities programs. The nature of the services provided are different as well as the qualifications of the personnel who provide them.

References

1. The Philosophical Base of Occupational Therapy, The American Occupational Therapy Association, Inc., Approved by the AOTA Representative Assembly, 1979.
2. AOTA Representative Assembly; Minutes. *Am J Occup Ther* 31:599, 1977.
3. Crepeau EL: *Activities Programming,* Durham, NH: New England Gerontology Center, 1980.

Bibliography

Bengson, E: Training Programs for Activity Directors. *Am J Occup Ther* 28:103, 1974.

Crawford, J and Strehlow, H: OT in Homes for the Aged. *Am J Occup Ther* 25:160, 1971.

Diamond, M, et al: The Role of the OT in the Care of the Geriatric Patient. *Am J Occup Ther* 25:139, 1971.

Jackson, BA: The OT as Consultant to the Aged. *Am J Occup Ther* 24(8):573, 1970.

Kaplan J: The Social Care of Older Persons in Nursing Homes. *Am J Occup Ther* 11:240, 1957,

Schroepfer, M: A State OT Program for the Aged. *Am J Occup Ther* 25:145, 1971.

Ward, R: Review of Research Related to Work Activities, etc. *Am J Occup Ther* 25:348, 1971.

Adopted April 1983 by the Representative Assembly, The American Occupational Therapy Association, Inc.

Appendix J. Principles of Occupational Therapy Ethics*

Adopted April 1977; Adopted, Revised, April 1979

PREAMBLE:

The American Occupational Therapy Association (AOTA) and its component members are committed to furthering man's ability to function fully within his total environment. To this end the occupational therapist renders service to clients in all stages of health and illness, to institutions, other professionals, colleagues, students, and to the general public.

In furthering this commitment the American Occupational Therapy Association has established the Principles of Occupational Therapy Ethics. The Principles are intended for use by all occupational therapy personnel, including practitioners in all settings, administrators, educators, and students. Licensure laws and regulations should reflect and support these Principles, which are intended to be action oriented, guiding and preventive rather than negative or merely disciplinary. The Principles, likewise, should influence the consulting, planning, and teaching of occupational therapists.

It should be noted that these Principles are intended only for internal use by the American Occupational Therapy Association as a guide to appropriate conduct of its members. The Principles are not intended to define a standard of care for patients or clients of a particular community.

Professional maturity will be demonstrated in applying these basic Principles while exercising the large measure of freedom which they provide and which is essential to responsible and creative occupational therapy service.

For the purpose of continuity the following definitions will support information in this document: Occupational therapist includes registered occupational therapists, certified occupational therapy assistants, occupational therapy students; clients include patients, students, and those to whom occupational therapy services are delivered.

I. Related to the Recipient of Service

The occupational therapist demonstrates a beneficent concern for the recipient of services and maintains a goal-directed relationship with the recipient which furthers the objectives for which it is established. Services are evaluated against objectives and accountability is maintained therefore. Respect shall be shown for the recipients' rights and the occupational therapist will preserve the confidence of the client relationship.

Guidelines: Recipients of occupational therapy services refer to clients, patients, students, and the employers of occupational therapists, i.e., agencies, facilities, institutions, etc.

It is the professional responsibility of occupational therapists to provide services for clients without regard to race, creed, national origin, sex, handicap or religious affiliation. Occupational therapists recognize each client's individuality and worth as a unique person.

Services provided should be planned in concert with clients' involvement in goal-directed activities, in accordance with the overall habilitation or rehabilitation plan. Treatment objectives and the therapeutic process must be measurable to insure professional accountability.

Clients' and students' rights are to be protected as stipulated in the Federal Privacy Act of 1974, in addition to any specified rules, regulations, or procedures as may be required by the employer.

The financial gain of occupational therapists should never by paramount to the delivery of services. Those occupational therapists who are compensated by virtue of being a direct service provider or vendor have the right to assess reasonable fees for profit.

Occupational therapists are obligated to provide the highest quality of service to the recipient. If further services would be beneficial to the client, the referring practitioner should be informed. It is also incumbent upon occupational therapists to recommend termination of services when established goals have been met, or when further services would not produce improved recipient performance.

*Reprinted with the permission of The American Occupational Therapy Association, Inc., copyright holder. © Copyright 1983, *The American Journal of Occupational Therapy*. December 1983, Volume 37, Number 12, pp. 807-810.

Occupational therapy educators are obligated to provide the highest quality educational services supporting the AOTA "Essentials" and the current theory that supports service delivery.

II. Related to Competence

The occupational therapist shall actively maintain and improve one's professional competence, represent it accurately, and function within its parameters.

Guidelines: Occupational therapists recognize the need for continuing education and, where relevant, they obtain training, experience, self-study, or counsel to assure competent occupational therapy services.

Occupational therapists accurately represent their competence, education, training, and experience. Occupational therapists must accurately represent their skills and should not provide services or instructions, either for pay or in a voluntary capacity, that are not within their demonstrated competencies.

Occupational therapists must recognize the skills necessary to manage a client or a position. If client needs exist that the therapist cannot effectively manage, the therapist should seek consultation or refer the client to an occupational therapist or another professional who can provide the required service.

III. Related to Records, Reports, Grades and Recommendations

The occupational therapist shall conform to local, state, and federal laws and regulations, and regulations applicable to records and reports. The occupational therapist abides by the employing institution's rules. Objective data shall govern subjective data in evaluations, grades, recommendations, records and reports.

Guidelines: Occupational therapists realize that reports are a required function of any position. Occupational therapists accurately record information and report information as required by AOTA standards, facility standards, and state and national laws.

Occupational therapists fulfilling a teaching role utilize objective data in determining student grades.

All data recorded in permanent files or records should be supported by the occupational therapist's observations or by objective measures of data collection.

Students' records can only be divulged as authorized by law or the student's consent for release of information.

IV. Related to Intra-professional Colleagues

The occupational therapist shall function with discretion and integrity in relations with other members of the profession and shall be concerned with the quality of their services. Upon becoming aware of objective evidence of a breach of ethics or substandard service, the occupational therapist shall take action according to established procedure.

Guidelines: Information gained or data gathered on a client shall only be divulged as expedient to other professional colleagues, students, referring practitioner, and employer. This includes data used in the course of in-service programs, professional meetings, prepared papers of presentation or publication, and educational materials. Undue invasion of privacy should be of utmost concern. Any reference to quality or service rendered by, or the integrity of, a professional colleague will be expressed with due care to protect the reputation of that person.

It is the obligation of occupational therapists with first-hand knowledge of a breach of the ethical principles of this Association, by a colleague or student, to attempt to rectify the situation. If informal attempts fail, such activities or incidents against the ethical principles of this Association should immediately be brought to the attention of the appropriate local, regional, or national Association committee/commission on ethical standards. Designated procedures should be followed, and at all times the confidentiality of the information must be respected to protect the alleged party.

Practices by an employer which are in conflict with the ethical principles of this Association should also be brought to the immediate attention of the appropriate body(ies).

Information gained in peer review procedures should be held within the realm of confidentiality and be dealt with according to established procedures.

Publication credit for material developed by colleagues must be given. Also, credit for materials used in the classroom, manuals, in-service training, and oral or written reports, for example, should acknowledge the name of the individual or group who developed the material.

V. Related to Other Personnel

The occupational therapist shall function with discretion and integrity in relations with personnel and cooperate with them as may be appropriate. Similarly, the occupational therapist expects others to demonstrate a high level of competence. Upon becoming aware of objective evidence of breach of ethics or substandard service, the occupational therapist shall take action according to established procedure.

Guidelines: Occupational therapists understand the scope of education and practice of related professions, and make full use of all professional, technical, and administrative resources that best serve the interests of consumers.

Occupational therapists do not delegate to other personnel those client related services where the clinical skills and expertise of an occupational therapist is required. Other personnel or students may support treatment or educational goals, but must have demonstrated competency in each aspect of service to the occupational therapist before the responsibility can be delegated.

Occupational therapists who employ or supervise other professionals or technicians, or professionals or technicians in training, accept the obligation to facilitate their further development by providing suitable working conditions, consultation, and experience opportunities.

Occupational therapists protect the privacy of all persons with whom professional collaboration occurs. If, however, an occupational therapist has first-hand knowledge of a colleague's performance which is in conflict with ethical standards, the therapist shall attempt to rectify the situation. Failing an informal solution, the occupational therapist shall utilize procedures established within the facility or agency, or call the behavior to the attention of management, or utilize procedures established by the profession to handle such situations. Under no circumstances should the occupational therapist remain silent when a client, student, or facility's status is in jeopardy.

VI. Related to Employers and Payers

The occupational therapist shall render service with discretion and integrity and shall protect the property and property rights of the employers and payers.

Guidelines: Occupational therapists function within the parameter of the job description or the goals established mutually between the employer or agency, and the occupational therapist. Occupational therapists use the utmost integrity in all dealings with the facility, university/college, or contracting agency. Established procedures are followed regarding purchasing and bids.

Occupational therapists recommend appropriate fees for services and gain necessary acceptance for fees from the facility, agency, and payers. Fees must be based upon cost analysis or a factor that can be justified upon request.

Occupational therapists shall not use the property, such as supplies and equipment, of the employer for their own personal use and aggrandizement.

VII. Related to Education

The occupational therapist implements a commitment to the education of society and the consumer of health services as well as to the education of health personnel on matters of health which are within the purview of occupational therapy.

Guidelines: Occupational therapists do not only provide direct service to alleviate specific problems with clients, programs, or a community, but in addition include education of all phases of services which can be provided to the public. This should include education of situations and conditions for which the competency of occupational therapists is recognized to assist in alleviating barriers limiting a person's ability to function socially, emotionally, cognitively, or physically.

The public includes not only individuals concerned with the well-being of a member of their family, but also federal, state, and local governmental agencies, educational systems, and social agencies dealing with the health and well-being of the public.

VIII. Related to Evaluation and Research

Occupational therapists shall accept responsibility for evaluating, developing, and refining service and the body of knowledge and skills which underlie the education and practice of occupational therapy and at all times protects the rights of subjects, clients, insitutions, and collaborators. The work of others shall be acknowledged.

Guidelines: Clients' families have the right to have, and occupational therapists have the responsibility to provide, explanations of the nature, purposes, and results of the occupational therapy services unless, as in some employment or treatment settings, there is an explicit exception to this right agreed upon in advance.

In reporting test results, occupational therapists indicate any reservations regarding validity of reliability resulting from testing circumstances or inappropriateness of the test norms for the person tested.

In performing research and reporting research results, occupational therapists must use accepted scientific methodology.

IX. Related to the Profession

The occupational therapist shall be responsible for gaining information and understanding of the principles, policies, and standards of the profession. The occupational therapist functions as a representative of the profession.

Guidelines: Occupational therapists should provide accurate information to the public about the profession and the services that can be provided. Occupational therapists should remain informed about changes in the profession and represent the profession accurately to the consumer.

Occupational therapists should conduct themselves in a manner befitting professionals. The profession is judged in part by the conduct of its members as they carry out their functions.

Occupational therapists should show support and loyalty to the Association by cooperating with the Representatives in collecting information regarding proposed Association policy, replying to official requests for information, and supporting the policies of the Association. It is the member's duty if he disagrees with an Association policy to work through existing channels to effect change.

Occupational therapists who engage in work or volunteer activities in addition to professional occupational therapy responsibilities shall not violate the ethical principles of the Association in such activities.

X. Related to Advertising

Advertising by therapists under their professional title shall be in accordance with propriety and precedent in health professions.

Guidelines: Occupational therapists may provide information to the public about available services through procedures established by the employing facility or contracting agency. If an occupational therapist provides an independent service, it is appropriate to advertise those services.

The occupational therapist shall not use, or participate in the use of, any form of communication containing a false, fraudulent, misleading, deceptive, self-laudatory, or unfair statement or claim. Testimonials or statements which promise a favorable result shall be avoided.

XI. Related to Law and Regulations

The occupational therapist shall seek to acquire information about applicable local, state, federal, and institutional rules and shall function accordingly thereto.

Guidelines: Occupational therapists are obligated to function professionally as a practitioner within the limits of all laws related to the delivery of health services, and applicable to the practice of occupational therapy. Occupational therapists will not engage in any cruel, inhumane, or degrading practices in the treatment of clients or in the education of students, or in supervision of others or in peer relationships with other individuals.

It is the responsibility of occupational therapists to make known to their employers, employees, and colleagues those laws applicable to the practice of occupational therapy and education of occupational therapists.

XII. Related to Misconduct

The occupational therapist shall not appear to act with impropriety or engage in illegal conduct involving moral turpitude and will not circumvent the principles of occupational therapy ethics through actions of another.

Guidelines: As employees, occupational therapists refuse to participate in practices inconsistent with legal, moral, and ethical standards regarding the treatment of employees or the public. For example, occupational therapists will not condone practices that are inhumane, or that result in illegal or otherwise unjustifiable discrimination on the basis of race, age, sex, religion, handicap, or national origin in hiring, promotion, or training.

In providing occupational therapy services, occupational therapists avoid any action that will violate or diminish the legal and civil rights of clients or of others who may be affected.

As practitioners and educators, occupational therapists keep abreast of relevant federal, state, local, and agency regulations and American Occupational Therapy Association Standards of Practice and education essentials concerning the conduct of their practice. They are concerned with developing such legal and quasi-legal regulations that support the interests of the public, students, and the profession.

XIII. Related to Bioethical Issues and Problems of Society

The occupational therapist seeks information about the major health problems and issues to learn their implications for occupational therapy and for one's own services.

Guidelines: The principle is a philosophical statement that encourages occupational therapists to be global in their views in relationship to society.

Enforcement Procedures are available from the Division of Practice, 1383 Piccard Drive, Rockville, MD 20850. Complaints should be addressed to the Standards and Ethics Chair, 1383 Piccard Drive, Rockville, MD 20850.

Appendix K. Essentials of an Approved Educational Program for the Occupational Therapy Assistant*

Established and Adopted by
THE AMERICAN OCCUPATIONAL THERAPY ASSOCIATION, INC.

(Initially adopted 1958; revised 1962, 1967, 1970, 1975, 1983)

PREAMBLE

Objective:

These ESSENTIALS are the minimum requirements for the education of the entry-level occupational therapy assistant, i.e., certificate or associate degree programs. The sponsoring institution offering a technical education program assumes responsibility for ensuring that the established ESSENTIALS contained herein will be met and maintained. Surveys are made by the appropriate recognized body and lists of approved programs are published for public information.

Description of Occupational Therapy

Occupational therapy is the art and science of directing man's participation in selected tasks to restore, reinforce, and enhance performance, facilitate learning of those skills and functions essential for adaptation and productivity, diminish or correct pathology, and to promote and maintain health. Reference to occupation in the title is in the context of man's goal-directed use of time, energy, interest, and attention. Its fundamental concern is the development and maintenance of the capacity throughout the life span to perform with satisfaction to self and others those tasks and roles essential to productive living and to the mastery of self and the environment.

Since the primary focus of occupational therapy is the development of adaptive skills and performance capacity, its concern is with factors which serve as barriers or impediments to the individual's ability to function, as well as those factors which promote, influence, or enhance performance.

Occupational therapy provides service to those individuals whose abilities to cope with tasks of living are threatened or impaired by developmental deficits, the aging process, poverty and cultural differences, physical injury or illness, or psychological and social disability.

Occupational therapy serves a diverse population in a variety of settings such as hospitals and clinics, rehabilitation facilities, long-term care facilities, extended care facilities, sheltered workshops, schools and camps, private homes, housing projects, and community agencies and centers. Occupational therapists both receive from and make referrals to the appropriate health, educational, or medical specialists. Delivery of occupational therapy services involves several levels of personnel including the registered occupational therapist, the certified occupational therapy assistant, and aides.

Entry-level occupational therapy technical education programs prepare the individual to:

1. Collaborate in providing occupational therapy services with appropriate supervision to prevent deficits and to maintain or improve function in daily living skills and in underlying components, e.g., sensorimotor, cognitive, and psychosocial.
2. Participate in managing occupational therapy service.
3. Direct activity programs.
4. Incorporate values and attitudes congruent with the profession's standards and ethics.

The American Occupational Therapy Association maintains an entry-level role delineation.

NOTE: In the following sections the ESSENTIALS are in upper case, the guidelines in lower case.

I. SPONSORSHIP

A. AN OCCUPATIONAL THERAPY TECHNICAL EDUCATION PROGRAM SHALL BE LOCATED IN A POST-SECONDARY EDUCATION INSTITUTION.

B. IN PROGRAMS WHERE THE ACADEMIC AND FIELDWORK PHASES ARE PROVIDED IN TWO OR MORE INSTITUTIONS, APPROVAL WILL BE GRANTED TO THE SPONSORING INSTITUTION OR THE INSTITUTION THAT ASSUMES PRIMARY RESPONSIBILITY FOR CURRICULUM PLANNING AND SELECTION OF COURSE CONTENT, COORDINATES CLASSROOM TEACHING AND SUPERVISED FIELDWORK, APPOINTS FACULTY TO THE PROGRAM, RECEIVES AND PROCESSES APPLICATIONS FOR ADMISSION, AND GRANTS THE DEGREE OR CERTIFICATE DOCUMENTING COMPLETION OF THE PROGRAM. THE SPONSORING INSTITUTION SHALL BE RESPONSIBLE FOR ASSURING THAT THE ACTIVITIES ASSIGNED TO STUDENTS IN FIELDWORK ARE EDUCATIONAL.

C. INSTITUTIONS INVOLVED IN THE EDUCATIONAL PROCESS SHALL BE RECOGNIZED

1. AN EDUCATIONAL INSTITUTION SHALL MEET ITS APPLICABLE APPROVAL PROCEDURES.
2. FIELDWORK CENTERS SHALL BE APPROVED BY RECOGNIZED ACCREDITING AGENCIES OR MEET STANDARDS ESTABLISHED BY THE EDUCATIONAL PROGRAM.

D. RESPONSIBILITIES OF THE SPONSORING INSTITUTION AND EACH FIELDWORK EDUCATION CENTER SHALL BE CLEARLY DESCRIBED IN WRITTEN DOCUMENTS.

Examples of such documents include letters, contracts, educational objectives, or informational forms.

Provision should be made for periodic review of same.

II. EDUCATIONAL PROGRAM

A. THE STATEMENT OF THE MISSION AND PURPOSE OF THE OCCUPATIONAL THERAPY ASSISTANT PROGRAM SHALL BE CONSISTENT WITH THAT OF THE SPONSORING INSTITUTION.

B. THE STATEMENT OF PHILOSOPHY OF THE OCCUPATIONAL THERAPY ASSISTANT PROGRAM SHALL REFLECT THE PHILOSOPHY OF THE PROFESSION OF OCCUPATIONAL THERAPY.

C. A CURRICULUM DESIGN SHALL BE BASIC TO THE DEVELOPMENT, IMPLEMENTATION, AND CONTINUING EVALUATION OF THE PROGRAM AND SHALL

1. DESCRIBE THE BASIS FOR THE SELECTION OF CONTENT, SCOPE, AND SEQUENCE.
2. IDENTIFY GENERAL OBJECTIVES.
3. EXPLAIN CONTENT SEQUENCING AS IT RELATES TO CURRICULUM DESIGN.

A wide variety of curriculum patterns may serve as effective means of organizing the technical education program.

D. THE LENGTH OF THE EDUCATIONAL PROGRAM SHALL BE SUFFICIENT TO MEET

1. THE PROFESSION'S REQUIREMENTS.
2. THE REQUIREMENTS OF THE SPONSORING INSTITUTION AT THE

CERTIFICATE OR
ASSOCIATE DEGREE LEVEL

The profession's requirements refer to sufficient content for achievement of entry-level competencies and requirements for certification.

E. CONTENT REQUIREMENTS SHALL INCLUDE LIBERAL AND TECHNICAL EDUCATION.

Documentation should include instructional objectives, outlines, methods, and learning experiences.

1. GENERAL EDUCATION PREREQUISITE TO OR CONCURRENT WITH TECHNICAL EDUCATION ARE THOSE STUDIES WHICH INCLUDE
   a. ORAL AND WRITTEN COMMUNICATION SKILLS.
   b. SOCIO-CULTURAL SIMILARITIES AND DIFFERENCES.
      Course work should meet requirements of the institution and educational program as well as the student's personal and academic needs.
2. BIOLOGICAL, BEHAVIORAL, AND HEALTH SCIENCES
   a. BASIC STRUCTURE AND FUNCTION OF THE NORMAL HUMAN BODY.
   b. BASIC DEVELOPMENT OF PERSONALITY TRAITS AND LEARNING SKILLS.
   c. ENVIRONMENTAL AND COMMUNITY EFFECTS ON THE INDIVIDUAL.
   d. BASIC INFLUENCES CONTRIBUTING TO HEALTH.
   e. DISABLING CONDITIONS COMMONLY REFERRED FOR OCCUPATIONAL THERAPY.
3. OCCUPATIONAL THERAPY CONCEPTS AND SKILLS
   a. HUMAN PERFORMANCE

      LIFE TASKS AND ROLES AS RELATED TO THE DEVELOPMENTAL PROCESS FROM BIRTH TO DEATH.
   b. ACTIVITY PROCESSES AND SKILLS
      (1) PERFORMANCE OR SELECTED LIFE TASKS AND ACTIVITIES, INCLUDING SELF-CARE, WORK, PLAY, AND LEISURE.
      (2) ANALYSIS AND ADAPTATION OF ACTIVITIES.

         Activity analysis should relate to relevance of activity to patient/client interests and abilities, major motor processes, complexity, the steps involved, and the extent to which it can be modified and adapted.
      (3) INSTRUCTION OF INDIVIDUALS AND GROUPS IN SELECTED LIFE TASKS AND ACTIVITIES.
   c. CONCEPTS RELATED TO OCCUPATIONAL THERAPY PRACTICE INCLUDING
      (1) THE IMPORTANCE OF HUMAN OCCUPATION AS A HEALTH DETERMINANT.
      (2) THE USE OF SELF, INTERPERSONAL, AND COMMUNICATION SKILLS.
   d. USE OF OCCUPATIONAL THERAPY CONCEPTS AND SKILLS
      (1) DATA COLLECTION
         STRUCTURED OBSERVATION AND INTERVIEWS
         HISTORY
         STRUCTURED TESTS
      (2) PARTICIPATION IN PLANNING AND IMPLEMENTATION
         (a) THERAPEUTIC INTERVENTION RELATED TO DAILY LIVING SKILLS AND SENSORIMOTOR, COGNITIVE, AND PSYCHOSOCIAL COMPONENTS.

            Sensorimotor should include gross and fine motor coordination, strength and endurance, range of motion, and tactile awareness.

(b) THERAPEUTIC ADAPTATION INCLUDING METHODS OF ACCOMPLISHING DAILY LIFE TASKS, ENVIRONMENTAL ADJUSTMENTS, ORTHOTICS, AND ASSISTIVE DEVICES AND EQUIPMENT.

(c) HEALTH MAINTENANCE INCLUDING MENTAL HEALTH TECHNIQUES, ENERGY CONSERVATION, JOINT PROTECTION, BODY MECHANICS, AND POSITIONING.

(d) PREVENTION PROGRAMS TO FOSTER AGE-APPROPRIATE BALANCE OF SELF-CARE, WORK, AND PLAY/LEISURE.

(3) PARTICIPATION IN TERMINATION

PROGRAM TERMINATION INCLUDING ASSISTING IN RE-EVALUATION, SUMMARY OF OCCUPATIONAL THERAPY OUTCOME, AND APPROPRIATE RECOMMENDATIONS TO MAXIMIZE TREATMENT GAINS.

(4) DOCUMENTATION

Content should include professional terminology, and structured recording and reporting methods.

e. PARTICIPATION IN MANAGEMENT OF OCCUPATIONAL THERAPY SERVICE

(1) DEPARTMENTAL OPERATIONS: SCHEDULING, RECORD KEEPING, SAFETY, AND MAINTENANCE OF SUPPLIES AND EQUIPMENT.

(2) PERSONNEL TRAINING AND SUPERVISION: AIDES, VOLUNTEERS, AND LEVEL I OTA STUDENTS.

(3) DATA COLLECTION FOR QUALITY ASSURANCE

f. DIRECTIONS OF ACTIVITY PROGRAMS

(1) ASSESSMENT OF INDIVIDUAL NEEDS, FUNCTIONAL SKILLS, AND INTERESTS.

(2) PLANNING AND IMPLEMENTATION OF PROGRAMS TO PROMOTE HEALTH, FUNCTION, AND QUALITY OF LIFE.

(3) MANAGEMENT OF ACTIVITY SERVICE.

4. VALUES, ATTITUDES, AND BEHAVIORS CONGRUENT WITH

a. THE PROFESSION'S STANDARDS AND ETHICS.

b. INDIVIDUAL RESPONSIBILITY FOR CONTINUED LEARNING.

c. INTERDISCIPLINARY AND SUPERVISORY RELATIONSHIPS WITHIN THE ADMINISTRATIVE HIERARCHY.

d. PARTICIPATION IN THE PROMOTION OF OCCUPATIONAL THERAPY THROUGH PROFESSIONAL ORGANIZATIONS, GOVERNMENTAL BODIES, AND HUMAN SERVICE ORGANIZATIONS.

e. UNDERSTANDING OF THE IMPORTANCE OF OCCUPATIONAL THERAPY RESEARCH, PUBLICATION, PROGRAM EVALUATION, AND DOCUMENTATION OF SERVICES.

5. FIELDWORK EDUCATION

a. SUPERVISED FIELDWORK SHALL BE AN INTEGRAL PART OF THE TECHNICAL EDUCATION PROGRAM.

(1) THERE SHALL BE COLLABORATION BETWEEN ACADEMIC AND FIELDWORK EDUCATORS.

Collaboration may be fostered by on-site visits, written and oral communication, reports from students, a fieldwork council, and other mechanisms for communication.

(2) OBJECTIVES FOR EACH PHASE OF FIELDWORK SHALL BE

(a) DEVELOPED COLLABORATIVELY BY ACADEMIC AND FIELDWORK EDUCATORS.

(b) DOCUMENTED.

(c) KNOWN TO THE STUDENT.

(3) FIELDWORK SHALL BE CONDUCTED IN SETTINGS APPROVED BY THE PROGRAM AS PROVIDING EXPERIENCES APPROPRIATE TO THE LEARNING NEEDS OF THE STUDENT AND AS MEETING THE OBJECTIVES OF FIELDWORK.

b. LEVEL I FIELDWORK SHALL BE PROVIDED.

Level I Fieldwork includes those experiences designed as an integral part of didactic courses for the purpose of directed observation and participation in selected field settings. These experiences are not expected to emphasize independent performance or to be considered substitutes for or part of the sustained Level II Fieldwork.

c. LEVEL II FIELDWORK SHALL BE REQUIRED. IT SHALL

(1) INCLUDE A MINIMUM OF TWO MONTHS' PRACTICE.

(2) EMPHASIZE THE APPLICATION OF AN ACADEMICALLY ACQUIRED BODY OF KNOWLEDGE.

The purpose of Level II Fieldwork is to provide an in-depth experience in delivering occupational therapy services to clients with a variety of ages and conditions. These experiences should be specific to the role and functions expected of an entry-level occupational therapy assistant. Although a minimum of two one-month practicums (40 full-time work days) is recommended, longer fieldwork placements offer more experiences toward integration of academic learning and actual practice. Length and type of Level II Fieldwork assignment depend somewhat on the type and amounts of Level I Fieldwork integrated within the academic portions of the training program.

If equivalent time is used, it should be appropriate to the settings selected, student needs, and continuity of client services, e.g., consecutive half days. To ensure continuity and meaningful application of academic learning, all fieldwork experiences should be completed no later than 12 months following completion of academic preparation.

F. EVALUATION OF THE EDUCATIONAL PROGRAM SHALL BE CONDUCTED, INCLUDING

1. STUDENT LEARNING.

Methods for evaluation of student learning should be consistent with course objectives and methods of instruction. Prior to evaluation, the student should be made aware of the criteria, methods, and weight of measures to be used.

2. INSTRUCTOR AND COURSE EFFECTIVENESS.

3. CURRICULUM.

A variety of methods, procedures, and instruments may be used to obtain information on all aspects of instruction, e.g., instructor effectiveness, curriculum design, sequence, and relevance.

Information from student, instructor, and course evaluation should be used to make needed adjustments.

III. RESOURCES

RESOURCES SHALL BE PROVIDED TO MEET THE PURPOSE AND OBJECTIVES OF THE EDUCATIONAL PROGRAM.

A. PROGRAM DIRECTOR

1. THE DIRECTOR OF THE EDUCATIONAL PROGRAM SHALL BE A REGISTERED OCCUPATIONAL THERAPIST WHO HAS RELEVANT OCCUPATIONAL THERAPY EXPERIENCE IN ADMINISTRATION, TEACHING, AND DIRECT SERVICE AND WHO HOLDS THE BACCALAUREATE OR MASTER'S DEGREE.

   Work experience with certified occupational therapy assistants is recommended.

2. THE DIRECTOR OF THE EDUCATIONAL PROGRAM SHALL BE RESPONSIBLE FOR THE ORGANIZATION, ADMINISTRATION, EVALUATION, CONTINUED DEVELOPMENT, AND GENERAL EFFECTIVENESS OF THE PROGRAM.

   Administration should include such functions as budget development and control and faculty selection, development, and retention as congruent with institutional policy.

B. INSTRUCTIONAL STAFF

1. THE FACULTY SHALL INCLUDE EITHER REGISTERED OCCUPATIONAL THERAPISTS OR CERTIFIED OCCUPATIONAL THERAPY ASSISTANTS.
2. THE FACULTY SHALL BE QUALIFIED, KNOWLEDGEABLE, AND EFFECTIVE IN TEACHING THE CONTENT ASSIGNED.

   Selection of faculty should assure expertise in keeping with the content inherent in an occupational therapy curriculum. Faculty should meet the standards of the sponsoring institution for their academic preparation.

3. FACULTY RESPONSIBILITIES SHALL BE CONSISTENT WITH THE MISSION OF THE SPONSORING INSTITUTION.

   Faculty responsibilities may include teaching, community service, research, student advising, and participation in institutional activities.

4. THE FACULTY/STUDENT RATIO SHALL
   a. PERMIT THE ACHIEVEMENT OF THE PURPOSE AND THE STATED OBJECTIVES OF THE PROGRAM.
   b. BE COMPATIBLE WITH ACCEPTED PRACTICES OF THE INSTITUTION.
5. CONTINUING PROFESSIONAL DEVELOPMENT FOR FACULTY SHALL INCLUDE
   a. A PLAN FOR AND COMMITMENT BY FACULTY.
   b. SUPPORT FOR THE IMPLEMENTATION OF THE PLAN BY THE INSTITUTION.

   The plan should be documented and may be accomplished using institutional resources. This may include opportunities for participation in educational programs and workshops, research in the area of specialty, consultative appointments, and direct involvement with delivery of occupational therapy services. Support may include released time, funding, and recognition.

C. FIELDWORK EDUCATORS

1. THE RATIO OF FIELDWORK EDUCATORS TO STUDENTS SHALL BE SUCH AS TO ENSURE QUALITY EXPERIENCE AND MAXIMAL LEARNING.
2. LEVEL I FIELDWORK SHALL BE SUPERVISED BY QUALIFIED PERSONNEL.

   Qualified personnel may include occupational therapy personnel and other appropriate personnel such as teachers, social workers, public health nurses, ministers, probation officers, and physical therapists.

3. LEVEL II FIELDWORK SHALL BE THE RESPONSIBILITY OF A REGISTERED OCCUPATIONAL THERAPIST. SUPERVISION SHALL BE PROVIDED BY AN OTR OR A COTA WHO SHALL
   a. COLLABORATE WITH ACADEMIC FACULTY.
   b. HAVE A MINIMUM OF ONE YEAR OF EXPERIENCE.

D. SUPPORT SERVICES

SUPPORT SERVICES SHALL BE PROVIDED TO MEET PROGRAM AND ADMINISTRATIVE REQUIREMENTS.

E. FINANCIAL RESOURCES

A BUDGET OF REGULAR INSTITUTIONAL FUNDS SHALL BE SUFFICIENT TO DEVELOP AND MAINTAIN THE PROGRAM.

F. PHYSICAL RESOURCES

1. CLASSROOMS, LABORATORIES, OFFICES, AND OTHER FACILITIES SHALL BE PROVIDED.

   Assigned space should be consistent with the program's educational objectives and teaching methods.

   a. LABORATORY SPACE SHALL BE ASSIGNED TO THE OCCUPATIONAL THERAPY PROGRAM ON A PRIORITY BASIS.

      Space should be provided in the laboratory area to adequately store and secure equipment and supplies.

   b. FACULTY, STAFF, AND ADMINISTRATIVE OFFICES SHALL ALLOW FOR EFFICIENT OPERATION OF THE PROGRAM.
   c. SPACE SHALL BE AVAILABLE FOR PRIVATE ADVISING OF STUDENTS.

2. EQUIPMENT AND SUPPLIES CONSISTENT WITH PROGRAM OBJECTIVES AND TEACHING METHODS SHALL BE AVAILABLE.
3. A LIBRARY SHALL BE ACCESSIBLE, CONTAINING CURRENT STANDARD TEXTS, SCIENTIFIC BOOKS, PERIODICALS, AND OTHER REFERENCE MATERIALS RELEVANT TO THE PROGRAM.

   "Accessible" refers to convenient location, operating hours, and particular library policies, e.g., borrowing, reserve. There should be adequate budgetary provision for purchase of pertinent reference materials to support occupational therapy education.

IV. STUDENTS

A. PROGRAM DESCRIPTION

1. A DESCRIPTION OF THE PROGRAM AND ITS CONTENT SHALL BE MADE AVAILABLE TO THE STUDENT.
2. REQUIREMENTS FOR SUCCESSFUL COMPLETION OF THE ACADEMIC AND FIELDWORK SEGMENTS OF THE PROGRAM, AND FOR GRADUATION, SHALL BE MADE AVAILABLE TO EACH STUDENT.

B. SELECTION

SELECTION OF STUDENTS SHALL BE MADE IN ACCORDANCE WITH GENERALLY ACCEPTED PRACTICES OF THE INSTITUTION. THESE PRACTICES SHALL BE DEFINED AND PUBLISHED.

The selection of students to the program and their retention should be a joint responsibility of the Director, the faculty of the program, and the appropriate administrative officials.

C. ADVISING

1. ADVISING RELATED TO PROFESSIONAL COURSE WORK AND FIELDWORK EDUCATION

SHALL BE THE RESPONSIBILITY OF THE OCCUPATIONAL THERAPY FACULTY.

2. ADVISING DURING AND PERTAINING TO FIELDWORK EXPERIENCE SHALL BE A COLLABORATIVE PROCESS BETWEEN THE FACULTY AND THE FIELDWORK EDUCATORS.

D. RIGHTS AND APPEAL MECHANISMS

STUDENTS' RESPONSIBILITIES AND RIGHTS, INCLUDING APPEAL MECHANISMS, SHALL BE PUBLISHED AND MADE AVAILABLE. THESE SHALL RELATE TO BOTH THE ACADEMIC AND FIELDWORK COMPONENTS OF THE PROGRAM.

E. RECORDS

RECORDS SHALL BE MAINTAINED IN ACCORDANCE WITH INSTITUTIONAL POLICIES FOR STUDENT ADMISSION, HEALTH, ATTENDANCE, ACHIEVEMENT, AND EVALUATION.

V. OPERATIONAL POLICIES

A. AN OFFICIAL PUBLICATION INCLUDING A CURRENT DESCRIPTION OF THE EDUCATIONAL PROGRAM SHALL BE PROVIDED.

B. THERE SHALL BE ACCURATE AND AVAILABLE PUBLISHED STATEMENTS OF FAIR PRACTICE THAT HAVE AS THEIR PURPOSE THE PROTECTION OF THE RIGHTS, PRIVILEGES, AND RESPONSIBILITIES OF THE STUDENT, FACULTY, AND INSTITUTION, AS FOLLOWS

1. NONDISCRIMINATION POLICIES AS THEY RELATE TO STUDENT ADMISSION, MATRICULATION, AND FACULTY RECRUITMENT.
2. FEE AND TUITION COSTS FOR ALL REQUIREMENTS OF THE EDUCATIONAL PROGRAM.
3. POLICIES AND PROCEDURES REGARDING DISCONTINUANCE, WITHDRAWAL, AND REFUNDS OF TUITION AND FEES.
4. SEPARATE MECHANISMS FOR GRADUATION AND CREDENTIALING.

Certification with The American Occupational Therapy Association and licensure with the state are credentialing mechanisms separate from program completion.

VI. CONTINUING PROGRAM EVALUATION

THERE SHALL BE SYSTEMATIC AND PERIODIC PROGRAM EVALUATION.

Program evaluation should include data from faculty, fieldwork centers, students, graduates, employers, sponsoring institution, and professional associations. Such information should contribute to on-going program development and modifications. (Sometimes referred to as a Self-study.)

VII. MAINTAINING APPROVAL

A. THE ANNUAL REPORT FORM PROVIDED BY THE AMERICAN OCCUPATIONAL THERAPY ASSOCIATION SHALL BE COMPLETED, SIGNED BY AN APPROPRIATE OFFICIAL, AND RETURNED BY THE ESTABLISHED DEADLINE.

B. IF THE PROGRAM DIRECTOR OF AN APPROVED PROGRAM IS CHANGED, PROMPT NOTIFICATION SHALL BE SENT TO THE ACCREDITATION SECTION, THE AMERICAN OCCUPATIONAL THERAPY ASSOCIATION. A CURRICULUM VITAE OF THE NEW PROGRAM OFFICIAL, GIVING DETAILS OF EDUCATION AND EXPERIENCE IN THE FIELD, SHALL BE PROVIDED.

C. THE AMERICAN OCCUPATIONAL THERAPY ASSOCIATION ACCREDITATION COMMITTEE MAY WITHDRAW APPROVAL WHENEVER THE EDUCATIONAL PROGRAM IS NOT MAINTAINED IN SUBSTANTIAL COMPLIANCE WITH THE ESSENTIALS OR THERE ARE NO STUDENTS IN THE PROGRAM FOR TWO CONSECUTIVE YEARS.

D. APPROVAL SHALL BE WITHDRAWN ONLY AFTER NOTICE HAS BEEN GIVEN TO THE CHIEF EXECUTIVE OFFICER OF THE INSTITUTION THAT SUCH ACTION IS CONTEMPLATED, WITH REASONS FOR SAME, AND WITH SUFFICIENT TIME TO PERMIT A CONSIDERED RESPONSE. ESTABLISHED PROCEDURES FOR APPEAL AND REVIEW SHALL BE AVAILABLE.

The sponsoring institution should provide students with notification of substantial noncompliance with ESSENTIALS that may jeopardize approval of the educational program.

ADMINISTRATION OF APPROVAL

1. Application for approval of a program should be made to:

   Accreditation Section
   The American Occupational Therapy Association
   1383 Piccard Drive
   Rockville, MD 20850

2. The evaluation and approval of a program can be initiated only at the written request of the chief executive officer of the sponsoring institution or an officially designated representative.
3. A sponsoring institution may withdraw its request for initial approval at any time (even after the site visit) prior to final action.
4. The program being evaluated is given the opportunity to review the factual report of the visiting survey team and to comment on its accuracy before final action is taken.
5. The Accreditation Committee, The American Occupational Therapy Association, will periodically resurvey educational programs for continued approval.
6. The chief executive officer of the sponsoring institution may request that a return on-site evaluation be made in the event of significant deficiencies in the performance of an earlier evaluation team.
7. Adverse approval decisions may be appealed by writing to The American Occupational Therapy Association. Due process will be followed.

Appendix L.

SELECTED DEVELOPMENTAL SUMMARY

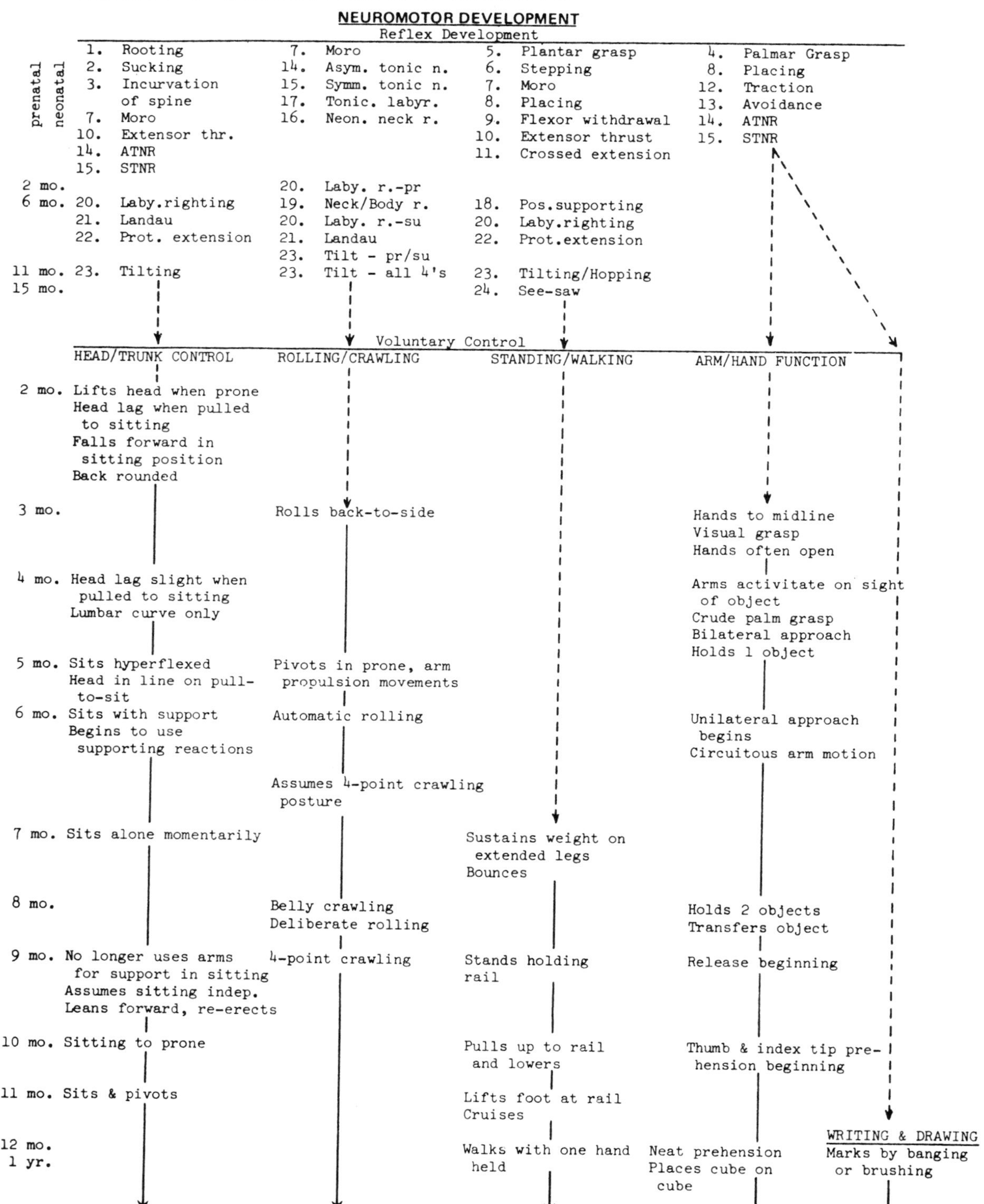

NEUROMOTOR DEVELOPMENT
Reflex Development
prenatal
neonatal
1. Rooting
2. Sucking
3. Incurvation of spine
7. Moro
10. Extensor thr.
14. ATNR
15. STNR
7. Moro
14. Asym. tonic n.
15. Symm. tonic n.
17. Tonic. labyr.
16. Neon. neck r.
5. Plantar grasp
6. Stepping
7. Moro
8. Placing
9. Flexor withdrawal
10. Extensor thrust
11. Crossed extension
4. Palmar Grasp
8. Placing
12. Traction
13. Avoidance
14. ATNR
15. STNR
2 mo.
6 mo.
20. Laby.righting
21. Landau
22. Prot. extension
20. Laby. r.-pr
19. Neck/Body r.
20. Laby. r.-su
21. Landau
23. Tilt - pr/su
23. Tilt - all 4's
18. Pos.supporting
20. Laby.righting
22. Prot.extension
11 mo.
15 mo.
23. Tilting
23. Tilting/Hopping
24. See-saw
Voluntary Control
HEAD/TRUNK CONTROL
ROLLING/CRAWLING
STANDING/WALKING
ARM/HAND FUNCTION
2 mo. Lifts head when prone
Head lag when pulled to sitting
Falls forward in sitting position
Back rounded
3 mo.
Rolls back-to-side
Hands to midline
Visual grasp
Hands often open
4 mo. Head lag slight when pulled to sitting
Lumbar curve only
Arms activitate on sight of object
Crude palm grasp
Bilateral approach
Holds 1 object
5 mo. Sits hyperflexed
Head in line on pull-to-sit
Pivots in prone, arm propulsion movements
6 mo. Sits with support
Begins to use supporting reactions
Automatic rolling
Unilateral approach begins
Circuitous arm motion
Assumes 4-point crawling posture
7 mo. Sits alone momentarily
Sustains weight on extended legs
Bounces
8 mo.
Belly crawling
Deliberate rolling
Holds 2 objects
Transfers object
9 mo. No longer uses arms for support in sitting
Assumes sitting indep.
Leans forward, re-erects
4-point crawling
Stands holding rail
Release beginning
10 mo. Sitting to prone
Pulls up to rail and lowers
Thumb & index tip prehension beginning
11 mo. Sits & pivots
Lifts foot at rail
Cruises
12 mo.
1 yr.
Walks with one hand held
Neat prehension
Places cube on cube
WRITING & DRAWING
Marks by banging or brushing

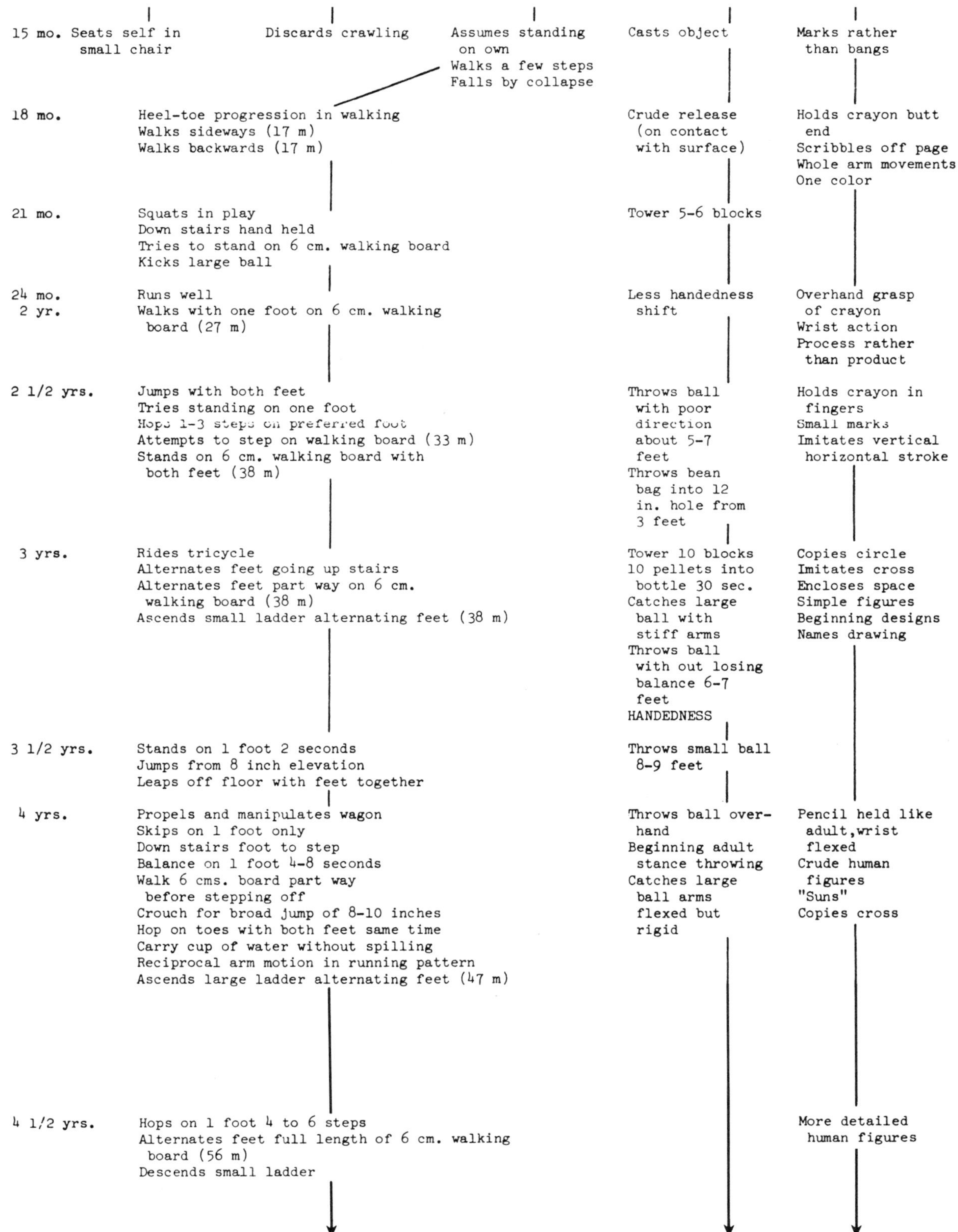

Age					
15 mo.	Seats self in small chair	Discards crawling	Assumes standing on own Walks a few steps Falls by collapse	Casts object	Marks rather than bangs
18 mo.	Heel-toe progression in walking Walks sideways (17 m) Walks backwards (17 m)			Crude release (on contact with surface)	Holds crayon butt end Scribbles off page Whole arm movements One color
21 mo.	Squats in play Down stairs hand held Tries to stand on 6 cm. walking board Kicks large ball			Tower 5-6 blocks	
24 mo. 2 yr.	Runs well Walks with one foot on 6 cm. walking board (27 m)			Less handedness shift	Overhand grasp of crayon Wrist action Process rather than product
2 1/2 yrs.	Jumps with both feet Tries standing on one foot Hops 1-3 steps on preferred foot Attempts to step on walking board (33 m) Stands on 6 cm. walking board with both feet (38 m)			Throws ball with poor direction about 5-7 feet Throws bean bag into 12 in. hole from 3 feet	Holds crayon in fingers Small marks Imitates vertical horizontal stroke
3 yrs.	Rides tricycle Alternates feet going up stairs Alternates feet part way on 6 cm. walking board (38 m) Ascends small ladder alternating feet (38 m)			Tower 10 blocks 10 pellets into bottle 30 sec. Catches large ball with stiff arms Throws ball with out losing balance 6-7 feet HANDEDNESS	Copies circle Imitates cross Encloses space Simple figures Beginning designs Names drawing
3 1/2 yrs.	Stands on 1 foot 2 seconds Jumps from 8 inch elevation Leaps off floor with feet together			Throws small ball 8-9 feet	
4 yrs.	Propels and manipulates wagon Skips on 1 foot only Down stairs foot to step Balance on 1 foot 4-8 seconds Walk 6 cms. board part way before stepping off Crouch for broad jump of 8-10 inches Hop on toes with both feet same time Carry cup of water without spilling Reciprocal arm motion in running pattern Ascends large ladder alternating feet (47 m)			Throws ball over-hand Beginning adult stance throwing Catches large ball arms flexed but rigid	Pencil held like adult, wrist flexed Crude human figures "Suns" Copies cross
4 1/2 yrs.	Hops on 1 foot 4 to 6 steps Alternates feet full length of 6 cm. walking board (56 m) Descends small ladder				More detailed human figures

5 yrs.	Roller skates, ice skates and rides small bicycle (5 or 6 yrs.) Skips alternating feet Stand indefinitely on 1 foot Hop a distance of 16 feet Walks long distance on tip toes Walks length of 6 cm. walking board in 6-9 seconds (60 m) Running broad jump 28 to 35 inches Runs 11.5 feet per second Descends large ladder	Adult posture distance throwing Boys 24 feet Girls 15 feet Catches ball hands more than arms, misses Bounces large ball	Buildings & houses Animals Idea before starting Copies triangle
6 yrs.	Stand on each foot alternately with eyes closed Walk a 4 cm. walking board in 9 seconds with one error Jump down from 12 inches landing on toes only Standing broad jump of 38 inches Running broad jump 40 to 45 inches Hop 50 feet in 9 seconds	Reach, grasp, release & body movement smooth Catch ball 1 hand *Grip strength Boys 11.3 lbs. Girls 3.2 lbs.	Finger & wrist movement Copies diamond
7 yrs.	MOTOR PERFORMANCE CONTINUES TO BECOME MORE REFINED (Running, jumping, balancing, etc.) Strength increases Learns to inhibit motor activity	*Grip strength Boys 18.5 lbs. Girls 8.7 lbs.	
8 yrs.	Runs 5 yards per second Standing broad jump of 45 inches	*Grip strength Boys 26 lbs. Girls 14.4 lbs.	
9 yrs.		Distance throw Boys 60 feet Girls 35 feet	3-dimensional geometric figures
10 yrs.			Linear perspective
11 yrs.	Runs 6 yards per second Standing broad jump of 60 inches	*Grip strength Boys 45.2 lbs. Girls 33.8 lbs. Distance throw Boys 95 feet Girls 60 ft.	
14 yrs.	Boys standing broad jump 76 inches Girls standing broad jump 63 inches Boys run 6 yards 8 inches per second Girls run 6 yards 3 inches per second	*Grip strength Boys 71.2 lbs. Girls 46.2 lbs.	
17 yrs.	Boys run 7 yards per second Boys standing broad jump 90 inches	Boys distance throw 150 feet	

*Dynamometer norms for dominant hand (average/mean) (unpublished) Scottish Rite Hospital for Crippled Children Dallas, Texas

SELECTED DEVELOPMENTAL SUMMARY
(continued)

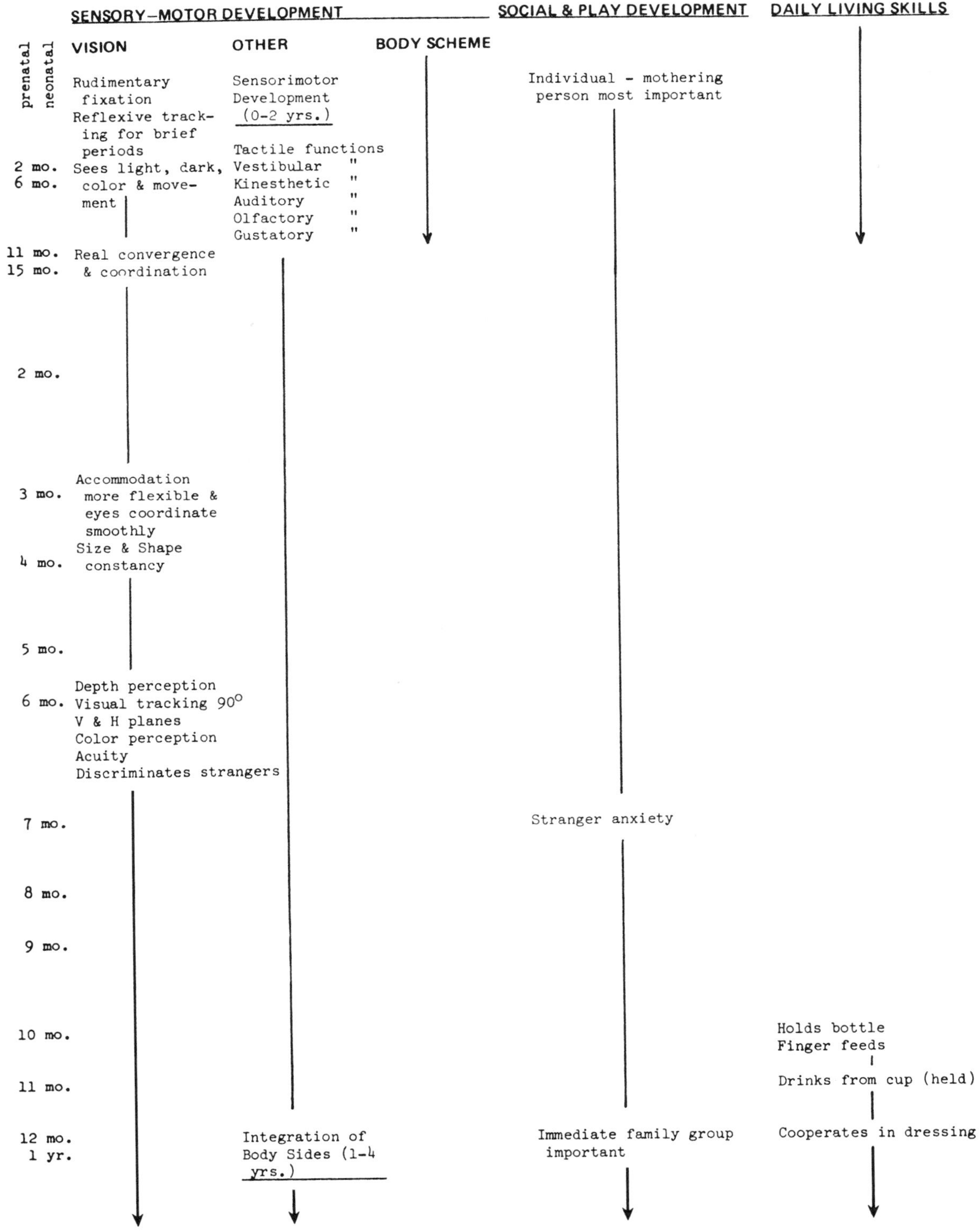

	SENSORY–MOTOR DEVELOPMENT			SOCIAL & PLAY DEVELOPMENT	DAILY LIVING SKILLS
	VISION	OTHER	BODY SCHEME		
prenatal neonatal	Rudimentary fixation Reflexive tracking for brief periods	Sensorimotor Development (0-2 yrs.) Tactile functions	↓	Individual - mothering person most important	↓
2 mo. 6 mo.	Sees light, dark, color & movement	Vestibular " Kinesthetic " Auditory " Olfactory " Gustatory "			
11 mo. 15 mo.	Real convergence & coordination				
2 mo.					
3 mo.	Accommodation more flexible & eyes coordinate smoothly				
4 mo.	Size & Shape constancy				
5 mo.					
6 mo.	Depth perception Visual tracking 90° V & H planes Color perception Acuity Discriminates strangers				
7 mo.				Stranger anxiety	
8 mo.					
9 mo.					
10 mo.					Holds bottle Finger feeds
11 mo.					Drinks from cup (held)
12 mo. 1 yr.	↓	Integration of Body Sides (1-4 yrs.)		Immediate family group important	Cooperates in dressing

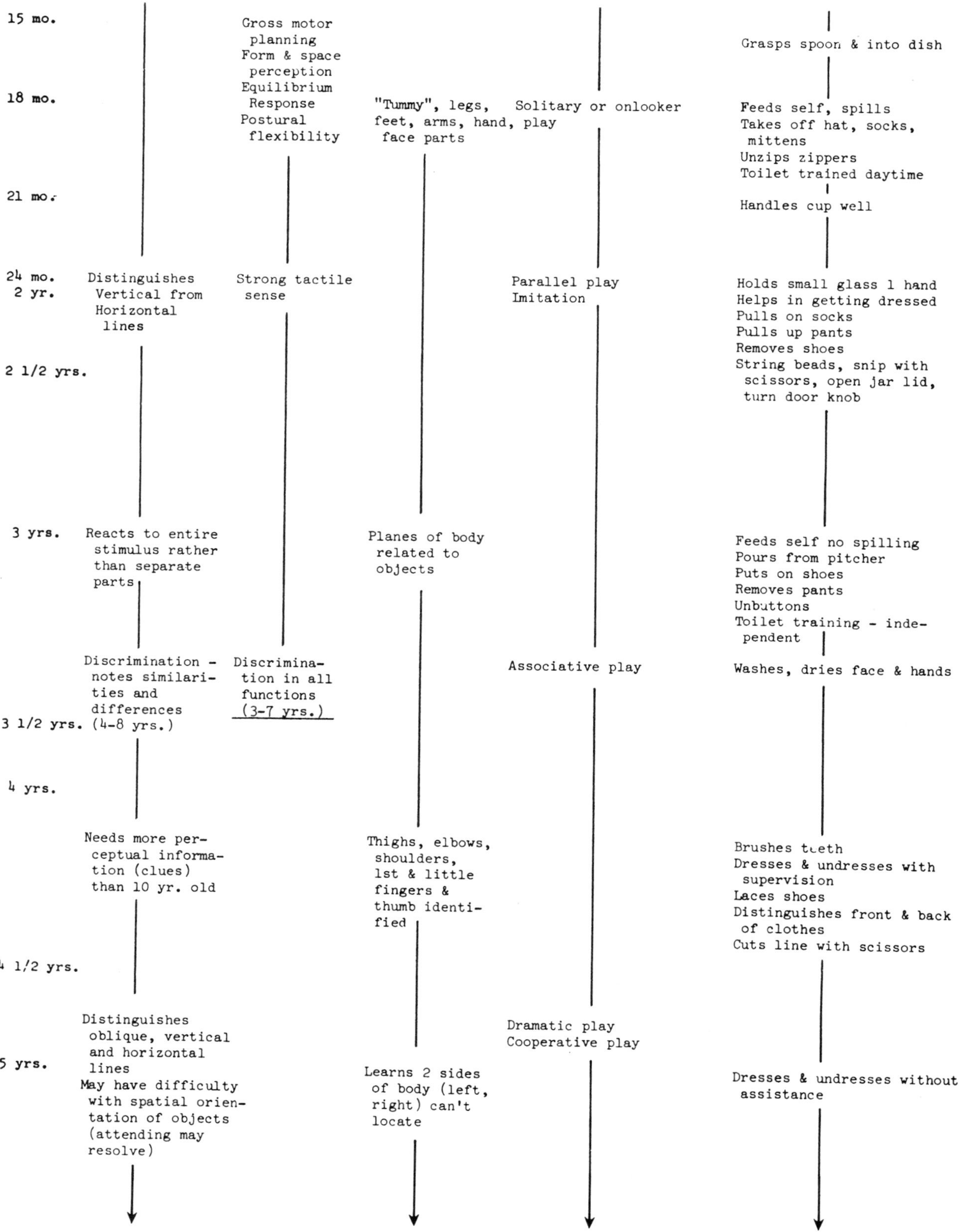

Age					
15 mo.		Gross motor planning Form & space perception Equilibrium Response Postural flexibility			Grasps spoon & into dish
18 mo.			"Tummy", legs, feet, arms, hand, face parts	Solitary or onlooker play	Feeds self, spills Takes off hat, socks, mittens Unzips zippers Toilet trained daytime
21 mo.					Handles cup well
24 mo. 2 yr.	Distinguishes Vertical from Horizontal lines	Strong tactile sense		Parallel play Imitation	Holds small glass 1 hand Helps in getting dressed Pulls on socks Pulls up pants Removes shoes String beads, snip with scissors, open jar lid, turn door knob
2 1/2 yrs.					
3 yrs.	Reacts to entire stimulus rather than separate parts		Planes of body related to objects		Feeds self no spilling Pours from pitcher Puts on shoes Removes pants Unbuttons Toilet training - independent
3 1/2 yrs.	Discrimination - notes similarities and differences (4-8 yrs.)	Discrimination in all functions (3-7 yrs.)		Associative play	Washes, dries face & hands
4 yrs.	Needs more perceptual information (clues) than 10 yr. old		Thighs, elbows, shoulders, 1st & little fingers & thumb identified		Brushes teeth Dresses & undresses with supervision Laces shoes Distinguishes front & back of clothes Cuts line with scissors
4 1/2 yrs.					
5 yrs.	Distinguishes oblique, vertical and horizontal lines May have difficulty with spatial orientation of objects (attending may resolve)		Learns 2 sides of body (left, right) can't locate	Dramatic play Cooperative play	Dresses & undresses without assistance

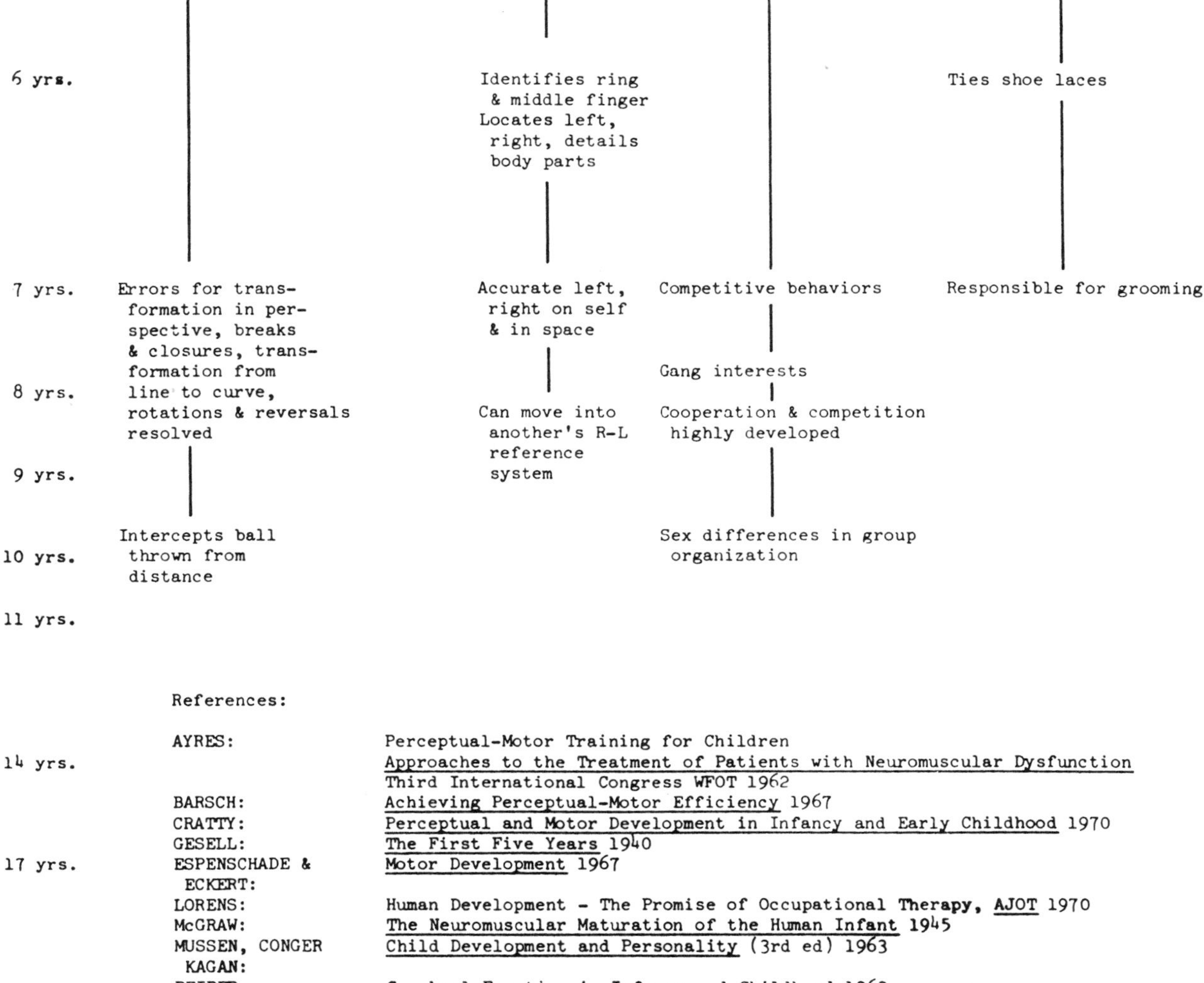

6 yrs.
Identifies ring & middle finger
Locates left, right, details body parts
Ties shoe laces
7 yrs.
Errors for transformation in perspective, breaks & closures, transformation from line to curve, rotations & reversals resolved
Accurate left, right on self & in space
Competitive behaviors
Responsible for grooming
Gang interests
8 yrs.
Can move into another's R-L reference system
Cooperation & competition highly developed
9 yrs.
Intercepts ball thrown from distance
Sex differences in group organization
10 yrs.
11 yrs.

References:

AYRES:	Perceptual-Motor Training for Children
	Approaches to the Treatment of Patients with Neuromuscular Dysfunction Third International Congress WFOT 1962
BARSCH:	Achieving Perceptual-Motor Efficiency 1967
CRATTY:	Perceptual and Motor Development in Infancy and Early Childhood 1970
GESELL:	The First Five Years 1940
ESPENSCHADE & ECKERT:	Motor Development 1967
LORENS:	Human Development - The Promise of Occupational Therapy, AJOT 1970
McGRAW:	The Neuromuscular Maturation of the Human Infant 1945
MUSSEN, CONGER KAGAN:	Child Development and Personality (3rd ed) 1963
PEIPER:	Cerebral Function in Infancy and Childhood 1963

14 yrs.

17 yrs.

Compiled by:

Mary K. Cowan, M.A., O.T.R.

Appendix M. ACRONYMS

In compiling this listing, emphasis has been placed on the inclusion of acronyms frequently used in the profession of occupational therapy. Those identifying specific evaluation instruments have not been included.

AA Alcoholics Anonymous
AAMD American Association of Mental Deficiency
ACLD Association for Children with Learning Disabilities
AD activities director
ADA American Dental Association
ADL activities of daily living
AE above elbow
AJOT *American Journal of Occupational Therapy*
AK above knee
AHA American Hospital Association and American Heart Association
AHCA American Health Care Association
ALS amyotrophic lateral sclerosis
AMA American Medical Association
AMI acute myocardial infarction
ANS autonomic nervous system
ANSI American National Standards Institute
AOA American Orthopedic Association
AOTA American Occupational Therapy Association
AOTAPAC American Occupational Therapy Association Political Action Committee
AP angina pectoris and anteroposterior
APA American Psychiatric Association
APHA American Public Health Association
APTA American Physical Therapy Association
ARC Association of Retarded Citizens
AROM active range of motion
ASA American Society on Aging
ASAHP American Society for Allied Health Professions
ASCOTA American Student Committee of the Occupational Therapy Association
ASHA American Speech-Language-Hearing Association
ASHT American Society of Hand Therapists
AV atrioventricular
BE below elbow
BEH Bureau of Education of the Handicapped
BK below knee
BP blood pressure
BSA body surface area
CA cardiac arrest
CARF Commission on Accreditation of Rehabilitation Facilities
CAT computerized axial tomography
CCU critical care unit
CD chemical dependency
CDC Center for Disease Control
CEC Council of Exceptional Children
CMHC community mental health center
COPD chronic obstructive pulmonary disease
CORF comprehensive outpatient rehabilitation facility
COTA certified occupational therapy assistant
COTA/L certified occupational therapy assistant, licensed
CP cerebral palsy
CPR cardiopulmonary resuscitation
CVA cerebral vascular accident
DB decibel
DIP distal interphalangeal
DLS daily living skills
DJD degenerative joint disease

DOT *Dictionary of Occupational Titles*
DPH Department of Public Health
DRGs diagnostic related groups
DSM III *Diagnostic and Statistical Manual (of Mental Disorders),* 3rd Edition
DTs delirium tremens
EEG electroencephalogram
EKG electrocardiogram
EMG electromyography
EMI educable mentally impaired
EMR educable mentally retarded
ENT ear, nose, and throat
EPI evaluation of personal independence
EST electroshock therapy
FWPR field work performance report
FAOTA Fellow, American Occupational Therapy Association
GTO Golgi tendon organ
HA hepatitis
HHS Health and Human Services (Department of)
HMO health maintenance organization
HSV herpes simplex virus
ICD Institute for the Crippled and Disabled
ICD 8 *International Classification of Diseases,* 8th Edition
ICU intensive care unit
IEP individualized education plan
IP interphalangeal
IQ intelligence quotient
ITP individualized therapy plan
IV intravenously
JCAH Joint Commission on Accreditation of Hospitals
LE lower extremity and lupus erythematosus
LOT licensed occupational therapist
LOTA licensed occupational therapy assistant
LPN licensed practical nurse
LVN licensed vocational nurse
MBD minimal brain dysfunction
MD doctor of medicine and muscular dystrophy
MG myasthenia gravis
MMT manual muscle test
MP metacarpophalangeal
MS multiple sclerosis
NA Narcotics Anonymous
NARC National Association for Retarded Citizens
NARP National Association of Retired Persons
NDT neurodevelopmental treatment
NHO National Hospice Organization
NIH National Institutes of Health
NLN National League of Nurses
NMS nervous, muscular, and skeletal systems
NSPB National Society for the Prevention of Blindness
NVOILA National Voluntary Organization for Independent Living for the Aging
OPD outpatient department
OT occupational therapy
OTA occupational therapy assistant
OTA/L occupational therapy assistant, licensed
OTAS occupational therapy assistant student
OTJR *Occupational Therapy Journal of Research*
OTR occupational therapist, registered
OTR/L occupational therapist, registered, licensed
OTS occupational therapy student
PA physician's assistant
PIP proximal interphalangeal
PM perceptual motor
PNF proprioceptive neuromuscular facilitation
PNS peripheral nervous system
POMR problem oriented medical record
PPS prospective payment system (Medicare)

PRE	progressive resistive exercise
PROM	passive range of motion
PSNS	parasympathetic nervous system
PT	physical therapy
PTA	physical therapy assistant
RD	registered dietician
RDS	respiratory distress syndrome
RN	registered nurse
RO	reality orientation
ROH	roster of honor (AOTA)
ROM	range of motion
RPT	registered physical therapist
RRT	registered respiratory therapist
SBA	stand-by assistance
SEIMC	special education instructional material centers
SNS	sympathetic nervous system
SOAP	subjective, objective, assessment, plan (used in documentation)
SCORE	Service Corps of Retired Executives
SNFs	skilled nursing facilities
TB	tuberculosis
TBSA	total body surface area
TD	terminal device
TIA	transischemic attack
TMI	trainable mentally impaired
TMR	trainable mentally retarded
TNR	tonic neck reflex
UE	upper extremity
UMN	upper motor neuron
USES	United States Employment Service
VC	vital capacity
VD	venereal disease
VMI	visual-motor accuracy
VISTA	Volunteers in Service to America
WAT	work adjustment training
WFOT	World Federation of Occupational Therapy
WHO	World Health Organization

Material for the preceding listing was drawn from chapters of this text as well as from the following sources:

Hopkins H, Smith H (eds) *Willard and Spackman's Occupational Therapy,* 6th Edition. Philadelphia: JB Lippincott Co., 1983

Miller BF, Keane, CB: *Encyclopedia and Dictionary of Medicine, Nursing, and Allied Health,* 3rd Edition. Philadelphia: WB Saunders, 1983

Occupational Therapy Newspaper, Rockville, MD: American Occupational Therapy Association, Vol. 38, 1984

Trombly CA, Scott AD: *Occupational Therapy for Physical Dysfunction.* Baltimore: Williams and Wilkins Co., 1977

Appendix N. Activities Questionnaire

NAME____________________________ SEX_____ AGE_____ BIRTHDATE__________
BIRTHPLACE________________________ RELIGION________ MARITAL STATUS______
WORK BACKGROUND____
FAMILY BACKGROUND____

INSTRUCTIONS: Place an "X" before each of the activities that you are interested in; add comments if you wish.

____ BAKING
____ COOKING
____ CANNING
____ PICNICS
____ RESTAURANT DINING
____ PARTIES

____ RADIO
____ TELEVISION
____ RECORDS
____ MOVIES
____ SINGING
____ DANCING
____ PLAY INSTRUMENT

____ TYPING
____ CREATIVE WRITING
____ READING
____ BOOK REVIEWS
____ MICROCOMPUTER
____ HAM RADIO
____ AVIATION
____ PHOTOGRAPHY
____ FOREIGN LANGUAGE STUDY
____ CURRENT EVENTS
____ GARDENING

____ DRAMATICS

____ BIBLE STUDY
____ CHURCH/SYNAGOGUE SERVICES
____ CHOIR
____ LECTOR
____ USHER
____ MISSIONARY PROJECTS

____ CERAMICS
____ WOODWORKING
____ NEEDLEWORK
____ WEAVING
____ PAINTING/DRAWING
____ CALLIGRAPHY
____ UPHOLSTERY
____ METALWORK
____ OTHER ARTS AND CRAFTS

____ CHECKERS
____ CHESS
____ BACKGAMMON
____ CARDS
____ OTHER GAMES
____ JIG SAW PUZZLES
____ CROSSWORD PUZZLES

____ WALKING
____ SHOPPING
____ FISHING
____ SCENIC TOURS
____ ART GALLERY
____ MUSEUM
____ ZOO
____ CONCERTS

____ PLAYS

____ OTHER ACTIVITIES:

BRIEFLY DESCRIBE THE ACTIVITIES YOU PARTICIPATED IN YESTERDAY:

____

____

INTERVIEWER:_____________________________________ DATE:____________

INDEX